AVOIDING COMMON NURSING ERRORS

AVOIDING COMMON NURSING ERRORS

EDITORS

JEANNIE SCRUGGS GARBER, DNP, RN

Senior Research Scientist
Center for Health Services Research
Carilion Clinic

Assistant Professor, Nursing
Jefferson College of Health Sciences
Roanoke, Virginia

MONTY GROSS, PHD, RN, CNE

Associate Professor, Nursing
Carilion Clinic
Jefferson College of Health Sciences
Roanoke, Virginia

ANTHONY D. SLONIM, MD, DrPH

Senior Staff, Medicine and Pediatrics
Carilion Clinic

Professor, Virginia Tech-Carilion School of Medicine
Roanoke, Virginia

SECTION EDITORS

BETSY HARGREAVES ALLBEE, BSN, CIC
JEANNIE SCRUGGS GARBER, DNP, RN
MONTY GROSS, PHD, RN, CNE
SHEILA LAMBERT, RN, MSN, CCRN
RICKY J. McCRAW, MBA, RN, CMTE
ANTHONY D. SLONIM, MD, DRPH
TERESA A. SLONIM, RN

SERIES EDITOR

LISA MARCUCCI, MD

Assistant Professor of Surgery
Division of Trauma and Critical Care
Department of Surgery
Thomas Jefferson University
Philadelphia, Pennsylvania

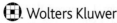 Wolters Kluwer | Lippincott Williams & Wilkins
Health
Philadelphia · Baltimore · New York · London
Buenos Aires · Hong Kong · Sydney · Tokyo

Acquisitions Editor: Brian Brown
Product Manager: Ryan Shaw/Erika Kors
Senior Manufacturing Manager: Benjamin Rivera
Marketing Manager: Angela Panetta
Design Coordinator: Stephen Druding
Production Service: SPI Technologies

530 Walnut Street
Philadelphia, PA 19106 USA
LWW.com

Printed in China

Library of Congress Cataloging-in-Publication Data

Avoiding common nursing errors / editors, Jeannie Scruggs Garber, Monty Gross, Anthony D. Slonim.
   p. ; cm.
   Includes bibliographical references.
   ISBN 978-1-60547-087-0
   1. Nursing errors—Prevention. I. Garber, Jeannie Scruggs. II. Gross, Monty. III. Slonim, Anthony D.
   [DNLM: 1. Nursing Process. 2. Medical Errors—prevention & control. 3. Nursing—methods.
WY 100 A961 2010]
   RT85.6.A96 2010
   610—dc22

                                              2009020195

Care has been taken to confirm the accuracy of the information presented and to describe generally accepted practices. However, the authors, editors, and publisher are not responsible for errors or omissions or for any consequences from application of the information in this book and make no warranty, expressed or implied, with respect to the currency, completeness, or accuracy of the contents of the publication. Application of the information in a particular situation remains the professional responsibility of the practitioner.

The authors, editors, and publisher have exerted every effort to ensure that drug selection and dosage set forth in this text are in accordance with current recommendations and practice at the time of publication. However, in view of ongoing research, changes in government regulations, and the constant flow of information relating to drug therapy and drug reactions, the reader is urged to check the package insert for each drug for any change in indications and dosage and for added warnings and precautions. This is particularly important when the recommended agent is a new or infrequently employed drug.

Some drugs and medical devices presented in the publication have Food and Drug Administration (FDA) clearance for limited use in restricted research settings. It is the responsibility of the health care provider to ascertain the FDA status of each drug or device planned for use in their clinical practice.

To purchase additional copies of this book, call our customer service department at (800) 638-3030 or fax orders to (301) 223-2320. International customers should call (301) 223-2300.

Visit Lippincott Williams & Wilkins on the Internet: at LWW.com. Lippincott Williams & Wilkins customer service representatives are available from 8:30 am to 6 pm, EST.

10 9 8 7 6 5 4 3 2 1

Dedication

This book is dedicated to nurses around the world who work tirelessly to care for their patients' interests and to our nursing colleagues at Carilion Clinic and the Jefferson College of Health Sciences who teach us every day about clinical excellence and the value that nursing adds to patient care.

ACKNOWLEDGMENTS

Authors
We would like to acknowledge and thank each one of the contributors for their hard work in turning this into a product that can help our patients. Your efforts in identifying real problems and converting them into succinct stories from which our colleagues can learn are very much appreciated.

Debby Lee
Thanks for the help you provided to keep our team organized and on track with this project.

Dr. Lisa Marcucci
Thanks again for your continued support, inspiration, and advice on this project.

This book has been developed as a component of the "Avoiding Common Errors" series. The book consists of 500 common problems encountered by bedside nurses and is organized around major nursing content areas like medical and surgical nursing and their subcomponents. Since this book is written by and for practicing nurses, each vignette represents a real or perceived error in caring for patients identified by these clinicians.

As a guiding principle for the inclusion of scenarios, the authors considered problems that occurred in their practice that they believed would not have occurred if someone had told them what to do prior to caring for their patients. The scenarios are not meant to represent all-encompassing explanations, but rather to highlight "what to do," in terms of the key nursing process steps of assessment, planning, implementation, and evaluation, to avoid the error's occurrence. Each scenario is accompanied by Suggested Readings that the reader can access for additional information related to the described problem.

We are hopeful that this book will be helpful as a companion textbook for nursing courses, as a practical guide for bedside care, and as a handy and easy-to-read reference.

JEANNE SCRUGGS GARBER
MONTY GROSS
ANTHONY D. SLONIM

The editors welcome comments and suggestions regarding this book and request that they be sent to: insidesurgery@gmail.com

CONTRIBUTORS

BETSY HARGREAVES ALLBEE, BSN, CIC
Manager, Clinical Effectiveness-Infection Control
Carilion Clinic
New River Valley Medical Center
Christiansburg, Virginia

NANCY F. ALTICE, RN, MSN CCNS, ACNS-BC
Cardiology Clinical Nurse Specialist
Carilion Clinic
Roanoke Memorial Hospital
Roanoke, Virginia

JENNIFER L. BATH, RN, BSN, SANE-A
Forensic Nurse Examiner
Carilion Clinic
Roanoke Memorial Hospital
Roanoke, Virginia

CATHERINE A. CHILDRESS, RN, MSN
Assistant Professor
Carilion Clinic
Jefferson College of Health Sciences
Roanoke, Virginia

ALICE M. CHRISTALDI, RN, BSN, CRRN
Physical Rehabilitation
Carilion Clinic
Roanoke Memorial Hospital
Roanoke, Virginia

MELISSA H. CRIGGER, BSN, MHA, RN
Assistant Professor
Carilion Clinic
Jefferson College of Health Sciences
Roanoke, Virginia

DORIS S. DUFF, BS RN, CEN
Emergency Department Education/P.I. Coordinator
Carilion Clinic
Roanoke Memorial Hospital
Roanoke, Virginia

VANESSA FREVILLE, RN, MSN, CPN
Pediatric Intensive Care Unit
Carilion Clinic Children's Hospital
Roanoke, Virginia

JEANNIE SCRUGGS GARBER, DNP, RN
Senior Research Scientist
Center for Health Services Research
Carilion Clinic
Assistant Professor, Nursing
Jefferson College of Health Sciences
Roanoke, Virginia

ELIZABETH A. GILBERT, RN BA
Unit Director Emergency Services
Carilion Clinic
Roanoke Memorial Hospital
Roanoke, Virginia

MONTY D. GROSS, PHD, RN, CNE
Associate Professor, Nursing
Carilion Clinic
Jefferson College of Health Sciences
Roanoke, Virginia

SAMUEL EMERSON HARVEY
Medical Affairs
Carilion Clinic
Roanoke Memorial Hospital
Roanoke, Virginia

EDWARD HUMERICKHOUSE, MS, MD
Carilion Clinic
Roanoke Memorial Hospital
Roanoke, Virginia

SHEILA LAMBERT, RN, MSN, CCRN
Director, Pediatric Services
Carilion Clinic Children's Hospital
Roanoke, Virginia

LEA E. LINEBERRY, RNIII, BSN, CCRN, CPN
Pediatric Intensive Care
Carilion Clinic Children's Hospital
Roanoke, Virginia

RICKY J. McCRAW, MBA, RN, CMTE
Senior Director, Emergency Department
Carilion Clinic
Roanoke Memorial Hospital
Roanoke, Virginia

BONNIE L. PARKER, RN, CRRN
Rehabilitation
Carilion Clinic
Roanoke Memorial Hospital
Roanoke, Virginia

KATHERINE M. PENTURFF, RN, CAPA
Carilion Assessment, Registration & Education for Surgery
Carilion Clinic
Roanoke Memorial Hospital
Roanoke, Virginia

LYNDA COOK SAWYER, RN, BSN, MBA
Director, Mother/Baby & Wellborn
Carilion Clinic
Roanoke Memorial Hospital
Roanoke Virginia

ANTHONY D. SLONIM, MD, DrPH
Senior Staff, Medicine and Pediatrics
Carilion Clinic
Professor, Virginia Tech-Carilion School of Medicine
Roanoke, Virginia

TERESA A. SLONIM, RN
Consultant, Surgical and Obstetrical Nursing
North Potomac, Maryland

MARY S. WARD, RN, BS, OCN
Oncology Nurse Educator
Carilion Clinic
Roanoke Memorial Hospital
Roanoke, Virginia

JULIE MULLIGAN WATTS, RN, MN
Oncology Clinical Nurse Specialist
Carilion Clinic
Roanoke Memorial Hospital
Roanoke, Virginia

FRANCINE B. YATES, RN, BSN
Thoracic Surgery Care Unit
Carilion Clinic
Roanoke Memorial Hospital
Roanoke, Virginia

CONTENTS

PART II: SPECIFIC NURSING AREAS

SECTION D: BEHAVIORAL AND PSYCHIATRIC NURSING

SECTION E: MEDICAL NURSING

SUBSECTION I: CARDIOLOGY

SUBSECTION II: CRITICAL CARE

1

NURSING RETENTION BEGINS WITH ASSURING APPROPRIATE SUPPORT FOR THE BEDSIDE NURSE

LYNDA COOK SAWYER, RNC, BSN, MBA

WHAT TO DO: ASSESS

Good nurses come to the profession because they care. They have perfected the art of caring during childhood and young adulthood and at some point have had their art form reinforced and been led or directed to a career that can utilize this talent. Then, in nursing school, the student nurse is trained in the science of healthcare. When complete, the lucky recruiting facility receives exceptionally enthusiastic new nurses that are ready to apply their knowledge of healing sciences through the already perfected art of caring.

State governments, professional organizations, regulatory bodies, malpractice juries, and evidence-based medicine have stepped into the void in many states to set a legal minimum for nurse-to-patient ratios in the high-risk areas of hospitals and surgical centers in an attempt to ensure appropriate staffing of licensed nurses at the bedside. In addition, lower nurse-to-patient ratios (nurses with smaller numbers of patient assignments) have superior patient outcomes and separately, the healthcare consumer began to shop around for appropriate care. As a result, more nurses were at the bedside with fewer patients assigned, but without physical assistance for non-nursing activities, which has not helped the overall status of patient care, and nurses continue to leave the profession in record numbers.

Nursing as a discipline needs to take a leadership role in financing the cost of lower cost employees in the workplace to assume the non-nursing activities of daily patient care and protecting and retaining a pool of licensed professional nurses. Assistance with non-nursing tasks will allow nurses to apply their science appropriately and share their art generously with their patients.

SUGGESTED READINGS

Garret C. The effect of nurse staffing patterns on medical errors and nurse burnout. *AORN J.* 2008;87(6):1191–1204.

Marquis B, Huston C. *Leadership Roles and Management Functions in Nursing: Theory and Application.* Philadelphia: Lippincott Williams & Wilkins; 2008.

2

TAKE CARE OF YOURSELF; YOU WILL BE A BETTER NURSE AND YOUR PATIENTS WILL RECEIVE BETTER CARE. PAUSE TO FIND SPACE TO BE STILL EVERY DAY

LYNDA COOK SAWYER, RNC, BSN, MBA

WHAT TO DO: PLAN

Closed eyes and ten controlled, deep, and measured breaths are all that are needed to change that physiologic feeling of panic. When your clinical day rushes over you and your flight response is kicked into high gear, STOP. Find a space—an equipment room or a bathroom—where you can close your eyes and practice your deep breathing. Oxygen to your brain will provide you the clarity you need to go forward with purposeful actions and intentions.

Close your eyes. Relax your shoulders downward. Relax your facial muscles. Inhale through your nose as deeply as you can, extending your abdomen outward. Hold that breath for a moment and then, slowly exhale completely through pursed lips while counting slowly and rhythmically, relaxing your shoulders even more deeply as your breath is expelled. Your body will begin to release its tension and your internal pace will become slow. Do it again. At first, you may not be able to clear your mind of the buzz of activity it is generating, but as you continue with this type of breathing, your concentration will be diverted. The counting and the deliberate actions of relaxing your shoulders will bring a peace that will triumph over the buzz. Open your eyes slowly when you are done with all ten breaths.

This type of moment is yours to take. No one will give it to you—no one can. You must learn to recognize the need, find the place, make the time, and give yourself permission to relax.

Nursing is a fantastic career full of its euphoric moments and tragedies. However, most of the time, your day-to-day activities will occur in the middle areas of your emotional continuum. The pure act of caring for a patient and creating an environment of healing is what we are doing.

But, caring for seven, eight, or nine of them and their families and visitors, your co-workers, and medical staff can leave us drained. And an emotionally drained nurse is headed directly for depression, burnout, and poor patient care.

Make the time to take care of yourself.

You need a life outside of your job, not just a room to eat, sleep, change clothes, and go back to work. You need friends on the job and off. You need to create a life that allows you to receive and give emotionally outside of the workplace. Taking care of yourself is not selfish. In the words of our sister profession, "Put the oxygen mask on yourself, first, then help others."

SUGGESTED READINGS

Benson H, Klipper M. *The Relaxation Response*. New York: Harper-Collins; 2000.

Bhat V. *The Power of Conscious Breathing in Hatha Yoga*. San Jose, CA: Vasantha Yoga Publications; 1998.

TRAVELING NURSES NEED TO PLAN THE CARE THEY WANT TO PROVIDE FOR THEIR PATIENTS FROM THE FOUNDATION UP

JEANNIE SCRUGGS GARBER, DNP, RN

WHAT TO DO: PLAN

Traveling nurses are often used to meet patient care demands at hospitals across the country. These nurses are creating personal and professional experiences tailored to their own interests. They are able to select the location, facility, and contract length and are frequently heard commenting on how wonderful it is to avoid the internal politics of an organization. Travelers also have an amazing opportunity to see many parts of the country and earn higher salaries.

Travelers are hired by travel agencies who then contract with hospitals to employ the nurse. The contracts are generally short term. Sign-on bonuses, salaries, and benefits vary from one company to another. Nurses who are considering traveling as a career, either short- or long-term, must consider the following during contract negotiations:

- Licensure issues in various states
- Length of contract being negotiated
- Hourly rate and shifts offered
- Financial allowances for housing, car, insurance, meals, etc.
- Moving expenses/reimbursement
- Living quarters options
- Agency and hospital policies regarding permanent assignment/employment options
- Liability insurance

Hospitals that use travelers generally contact a nursing agency with their request and then interviews are set up with potential candidates. Many facilities will make job offers based on phone interviews due to the expense of on-site interviews. The agency will finalize all contract negotiations with the nurse before relocation to the hospital occurs. All issues including salary, housing, malpractice insurance, health insurance, and stipends are negotiated with the agency and not the hospital where the nurse will be assigned.

Table 3-1 provides the positives and negatives associated with travel nursing.

The nursing shortage, with predicted shortfalls of 400,000 nurses by 2020, will provide unique opportunities and challenges for nurses. Nurses should consider their personal and professional goals when deciding whether or not to travel as a nurse.

SUGGESTED READINGS

Associated Press. On the road again. *Mod Healthc*. 2001;31(25):56.

TABLE 3.1	TRAVELING NURSES: THE POSITIVES AND NEGATIVES	
TOPIC	POTENTIAL POSITIVE THOUGHT	POTENTIAL NEGATIVE THOUGHT
Experience	Diverse experience from various places, organizations, and cultures within the country	Does not provide consistent exposure to standards, protocols, and opportunities to achieve excellence within an organization
Investment in organizational culture	Able to remain neutral or less emotional during organizational changes and chaos	May be aloof or detached from organizational changes that impact the work environment or patient care
Relationship with colleagues	Minimal opportunity to develop collegial relationships	Relationships do not hinder professional performance or efficiency
Acceptance by permanent employees	Accepted as a rescuer to support the nursing staff	Resented due to pay and ability to maintain distance from internal issues

KNOW YOUR EMOTIONAL IQ

JEANNIE SCRUGGS GARBER, DNP, RN

WHAT TO DO: ASSESS

A question that has been asked many times in the world of business is: Why are some people successful while others are not—even when skills seem equal? Daniel Goleman (as cited by Koonce, 1996) wrote the first book about emotional intelligence and presented an argument that our thinking was as important as, if not more important than, our intellect in determining how successful we are in the workplace. Several definitions of emotional intelligence have emerged over time with the "simplest one suggesting that it is nothing more than 'interpersonal intelligence'" (McQueen, as cited by Robertson, 2008). Another definition by Mayer, Caruso, and Salovey (as cited by Robertson, 2008) is based on reasoning and problem-solving skills with emotion as the framework. Goleman's characteristics of emotional IQ were presented as self-awareness, impulse control, persistence, confidence and self-motivation, empathy, and social deftness (Fisher, 1998). All of these factors are critical for the successful leadership of healthcare professionals and organizations.

Research to substantiate the theory that Goleman presented in 1995 has continued. According to a study conducted by Fisher, traits such as trustworthiness, adaptability, and collaboration were considered key to achieving success. Once one accepts the concept of emotional intelligence as critical to success, the question becomes: What characteristic of emotional intelligence is the most important? Fisher suggests that persuasion is one of the most significant characteristics because it requires listening and understanding others' perspectives while creating a shared vision or goal. Healthcare providers surely use the power of persuasion in dealing with interprofessional and patient–provider relationships.

Over the course of many years, tools to measure emotional intelligence have been developed. Peer reviews are also a possible way to assess emotional intelligence, assuming the right questions are asked. Asking for feedback can be intimidating but it is necessary to achieve an understanding of how one is perceived by others.

Organizations and researchers continue to educate, evaluate, and experience emotional intelligence and determine its importance for advancing healthcare leadership and the delivery of safe patient care. As opportunities to develop these skills arise, leaders can foster the growth of their employees by providing behavioral exercises that allow one to integrate these concepts into the patient care arena and interdisciplinary care.

SUGGESTED READINGS

Fisher A. Success secret: A high emotional IQ. *Fortune.* 1998;138(8). Available at: http://web.ebscohost.com/ehost/detail?vid=4&hid=9&sid=9359cf64-1af2-452d9d0ec23df02fd619%40sessionmgr2&bdata=JnNpdGU9ZWhvc3QtbGl2ZQ%3d%3d#db=heh&AN=1210193. Accessed July 18, 2008.

Koonce R. Emotional IQ, a new secret of success? *Training Devel.* 1996;50(2):19.

Robertson K. Emotional intelligence and healthcare leadership. Master's project. Jefferson College of Health Sciences, 2008.

CULTURAL AWARENESS IN HEALTHCARE

JEANNIE SCRUGGS GARBER, DNP, RN

WHAT TO DO: ASSESS

Health disparities exist. At a personal level, the delivery of differential care to patients based on a demographic characteristic like age, race, gender, religion, or ethnic origin is important for healthcare providers to understand and eliminate. Further, to accomplish this, providers need to be knowledgeable and have awareness that diverse cultural backgrounds have different health practices of which the provider may have limited understanding.

Healthcare professionals are able to experience some of the most intimate times in people's lives such as childbirth, terminal illness, recovery, and death. However, one's ability to provide support to multicultural patients in these situations may be challenging, particularly if the patient's norms and values are different from those of the providers. One of the more common concerns regarding cultural awareness is stereotyping. Unfortunately, providers, as human beings, quickly make assumptions about others based on their past experiences or what they have been taught over time. Healthcare professionals must not allow themselves to categorize patients based on personal demographics and must remain culturally aware and sensitive. Language is so engrained as a part of culture and affects the ability for communication and literacy that providers need an appreciation for what is embedded in language. While many organizations have elaborate translation and interpretation services to meet the communication needs of a diverse language patient population, nurses recognize that these services are often artificial methods for improving communication and often the context of the "conversation" is lost through an interpreter.

These cultural practices and norms are important to understand when providing care. On a daily basis, medical errors originate from problems related to miscommunications among and between providers with the same language and the cultural background— imagine the exponential increase in potential for error when the providers and patients have language or cultural differences.

Many nursing and medical schools are creating courses that focus on cultural competence. Much of the research being conducted is in healthcare education surrounding faculty awareness and student perspectives. Seasoned healthcare professionals also need education and support in obtaining new knowledge about cultural competence so that safe patient care can be provided for anyone—regardless of culture. It is impossible to separate culture from the person, and nursing practice is rooted in caring for the well-being of the whole person; therefore, further exploration of cultural competence is important for practice, education, administration, and research.

SUGGESTED READINGS

Burchum J. Cultural competence: An evolutionary process. *Nurs Forum*. 2002;37(4):5–15.
Flaskerud J. Cultural competence column: Can we achieve it? *Issues Ment Health Nurs*. 2007;28:309–311.

ASSESS YOUR PATIENT'S HEALTH LITERACY

JEANNIE SCRUGGS GARBER, DNP, RN

WHAT TO DO: ASSESS

An American definition of literacy is the ability to read and write English (Osborne, as cited by Chang & Kelly, 2007), and many Americans cannot read or write English. Health literacy is the "degree to which individuals have the capacity to obtain, process, and understand basic health information and services needed to make appropriate healthcare decisions." The *Quick Guide to Health Literacy* also reports that nearly 9 of 10 adults do not possess the skills necessary to manage their health and prevent disease and 14% of adults have health literacy that is below a basic level.

Some of the most obvious tasks that require health literacy include

- Navigation of the healthcare system
- Sharing health history information
- Engaging in caring for oneself
- Understanding likelihood and risk (mathematical processes)
- Knowledge of health topics
- Ability to understand relationships between cause and effect

These definitions and tasks create significant concerns for patients and healthcare providers as patients attempt to complete medical paper work and insurance forms and to provide accurate personal information. Osborne (as cited by Chang & Kelly, 2007) writes that patients may be embarrassed and may not be willing to admit they are unable to follow directions. Nurses are in a position to address literacy concerns for patients and provide them with guidance and support that will result in improved patient and provider understanding.

In 2001, the World Health Organization recognized the need for improved health literacy worldwide. Nurses are in a position to address literacy concerns for patients and provide them with guidance and support that will result in patient knowledge understanding and healthcare provider knowledge understanding. Nurses are obligated to evaluate patient learning needs and provide education at the appropriate level so that information can be understood. The nurse must be aware of literacy and cultural issues to provide adequate information.

It is the responsibility of healthcare professionals to improve health literacy. Professionals must work collaboratively to develop successful strategies to address this overwhelming concern. Healthcare organization leaders are responsible for creating and maintaining cultures of quality and safety, and health literacy is a top priority.

SUGGESTED READINGS

Chang M, Kelly A. Patient education: Addressing cultural diversity and health literacy issues. *Urol Nurs.* 2007;27(5):411–417.

Hochhauser M. What did the Dr. say? Improving health literacy to protect patient safety. The Joint Commission, 2007. Available at: http://www.nifl.gov/pipermail/healthliteracy/2007/000679.html. Accessed July 18, 2008.

Quick Guide to Health Literacy (n.d.). Fact sheet. Available at: http://www.health.gov/communication/literacy/quickguide/factsbasic.htm. Accessed July 18, 2008.

USE SIMULATION TO ASSIST IN EDUCATING AND PRACTICING YOUR CRAFT: PRACTICE MAKES PERFECT... AND MAY PREVENT HARM TO A PATIENT

JEANNIE SCRUGGS GARBER, DNP, RN

WHAT TO DO: PLAN

Simulated clinical learning may be one of the answers to help address patient safety and reduce patient errors. Simulation is not intended to take the place of person-to-person experience but can serve as an adjunct where errors can be made and no one is harmed. Simulation can be used in almost every healthcare scenario from taking a patient's past medical history to executing a complex trauma scenario. Simulation is growing in popularity and may prove to be the next major initiative that directly impacts how healthcare professionals are educated and how competencies are validated. Gaba (2004) suggests that the continued growth of simulation in healthcare will be dependent on the results experienced by those using and conducting educational and outcomes research.

The Institute of Medicine recommends the use of simulators to prevent human error. Simulation is a harm-free mechanism to teach and evaluate complex problem solving, critical thinking, and decision making in clinical situations. Simulation may also be used to teach and assess skills related to teamwork, interprofessional relationships, collaboration, leadership, communication, feedback, delegation, human resource issues, etc. Simulation is being implemented at a rapid pace and can be used with inexperienced and experienced healthcare providers. The opportunities for incorporating simulation in innovative ways are becoming more and more diverse. The *Journal of Simulation* has highlighted several innovative areas for development including

- Resource planning
- Improving patient flow and reducing queues
- Estimating required future expenditures
- Informing and influencing policy
- Assessing the cost-effectiveness of new technologies
- Epidemiologic simulation
- Developing simulation methodology in healthcare
- Developing techniques to improve the healthcare professional's understanding and confidence in simulation
- Healthcare-related simulation educational issues
- Simulation tool use and development for healthcare applications

While the major emphasis in healthcare simulation scenarios deal with "macrosimulation" where providers interface with other providers or a mannequin, other opportunities to evolve "microsimulation" scenarios that are computer- and algorithm-based, dependent upon statistical modeling, and can provide insight into such issues as patient flow, patient care, and outcomes by testing new clinical approaches prior to implementation.

There are numerous practical and research implications for simulation as a method to improve patient safety.

SUGGESTED READINGS

Farrar C, Frendy K, Hamlin A, et al. Creating a culture of patient safety with computerized patient simulators. *Tenn Nurse*. 2007;70, p. 9.

Gaba D. The future vision of simulation in healthcare. *Qual Saf Health Care*. 2004;(Suppl.1): pp. 2–10.

PROVIDE INTERPROFESSIONAL EDUCATIONAL EXPERIENCES FOR YOUR NURSES...YOU MAY BE SURPRISED BY WHAT THEY (AND THE DOCTORS) LEARN

JEANNIE SCRUGGS GARBER, DNP, RN

WHAT TO DO: PLAN

Healthcare professionals must work together to provide quality patient care. Unfortunately, human factors may make teamwork and collaboration difficult to accomplish. Teaching professionals how to work best together has been discussed and evaluated in many different ways. Interprofessional education (IPE) is the term used to describe the process when two or more health disciplines are engaged in learning together. The Centre for the Advancement of Interprofessional Education defines IPE as occasions when two or more health professionals learn with, from, and about each other to improve collaboration and the quality of care. Changing healthcare professional education from a model that is siloed to one that encourages teamwork, collaboration and a spirit of equality is emerging as a model of the future. The IPE model creates much hope for improving the quality and safety of patient care and the quality of the work environment.

Several universities have used this concept to create their nursing, medical, pharmacy, and other allied health programs' curricula. The courses are generally focused on student interaction, communication skills, and an opportunity to understand the perspectives of each profession. Students, in general, have very little knowledge of other healthcare disciplines' curricula or professional roles. Individuals usually form their thoughts and beliefs about the different healthcare professions before entering a program. These thoughts, feelings, and beliefs are developed over time and are reflections of life experiences.

Unfortunately, there is a division between education and practice, and the time has come for us to not only focus on how we educate healthcare professionals before they begin practicing but to continue to educate and influence how we work together after we begin to practice. Interprofessional teams can create dynamic changes in how patient care is delivered.

Achieving the relationships necessary to support the environment for interprofessional and collaborative education is easier said than done. The barriers most often identified regarding implementation of IPE are related to politics, organization, education, and culture. Healthcare organizations are similar to other businesses in that politics—who knows who, who likes who, and who gets listened to—is many times the circumstance that creates the opportunity for progress. Organizational structure can also be a barrier if power and control are key measurements of success for certain roles. Perhaps the most important barrier for IPE is the culture of the organization. A culture that supports IPE is likely open to new ideas and ways of problem solving and encourages interaction and collaboration between individuals across disciplines. If the culture is more traditional or hierarchical, IPE may be more difficult to achieve.

Organizations must create work environments that are engaging, encouraging, and inspiring. We must give healthcare professionals the education, tools, and support to make a difference in patient outcomes and the success of our organizations.

SUGGESTED READINGS

Hixson-Wallace JA, Hash RB, Hodges HF, et al. Interprofessional education: Beginning to cross the bridge. Paper presented at the *Annual Meeting of the American Association of Colleges of Pharmacy*, Sheraton San Diego Hotel & Marina, San Diego, CA, USA, July 2006. Available at: http://www.allacademic.com/meta/p125341_index.html. Accessed June 26, 2008.

Kearney A. Facilitating interprofessional education and practice. *Can Nurse*. 2008;104(3):22–26.

McKenlay E, Pullon S. Interprofessional learning—the solution to collaborative practice in primary care. *NZ Nurse*. 2008;13(10):16–18.

Reeves S, Zwarenstein M, Goldman J, et al. Interprofessional education: Effects on professional practice and health care outcomes. *Cochrane Database Systemat Rev 2008*. Issue 1. Art. No.: CD002213.DOI: 10.1002/14651858.CD002213.pub2.

Steven A, Dickens C, Pearson P. Practice based interprofessional education: Looking into the black box. *J Interprof Care*. 2007;21(3):251–264.

GOAL SETTING FOR PROFESSIONAL NURSING

SHEILA LAMBERT, RN, MSN, CCRN

WHAT TO DO: PLAN

Goal setting for nurses is important to create a climate of professionalism, accountability, and teamwork. Since goal setting can be motivational and empowering for the individual, it is important to work with the individual in this process. This process is the collaborative responsibility of the nurse and the leadership team and will better achieve improved performance and outcomes than a goal that is imposed upon the individual from their leadership.

Two factors should be in place for goal setting and attainment to be effective. First, the individual needs some self-awareness of his/her strengths, growth needs, style, and interests. Second, the individual needs the support and direction from leadership including instruction, providing the appropriate tools, and creating a suitable environment for growth and appropriate risk taking. Goal setting is a method of directing the energies of individuals toward their organizational and professional objectives.

At a minimum, the individuals should set goals for themselves for the upcoming year. This process is done collaboratively with leadership. Goals should be very specific and objectively measurable. For instance, a defined goal of "present a thirty minute lecture on bronchiolitis at the January staff meeting" as opposed to "develop an educational offering on a pediatric illness" assists the individual with an understanding of the goal and the performance expectations. Individual goals should include items such as educational goals such as attempts at certification and degree advancement, and personal goals such as communication strategies and peer relations. Goal setting for an individual should include areas for growth and special interests for the individual. Perhaps they have a strong desire to learn more about a certain process or initiative—this can be supported by leadership through goal development.

Goals for an individual service area are also important for the professional growth of each individual nurse, supporting the mission and vision of that particular area. Leadership should develop educational requirements (team goals) for professional staff, increasing the standard for the team as a whole based upon individual progress. These requirements include attendance at staff meetings, educational offerings, and attempts at certification. In addition, leadership should assist individuals in setting operational goals such as cost containment and staffing accountability. These two processes overlap with each other. Goal development based on an individual and the team's needs will help develop a sense of accountability to one's self professionally and to the team as a whole.

When setting goals as professionals, an action plan on how to best achieve this goal can be included. This plan should include a deadline to accomplish it—3 months, a year, or 2 years. A statement of current and future performance, as evidenced by progress to the goal, should be included. It is important that the individuals believe in the goal as a way to make a difference in their professional growth. The plan should include potential obstacles that may need to be overcome to achieve this goal. Goals should be realistic yet challenging. If goals are unachievable, the individuals will be set up for failure and that is good neither for them nor for the organization. Goal setting must be fair and reasonable to have the commitment from the individual.

Leadership responsibilities for individuals' goal attainment include working with the individuals at mid-year to assess their progress since they will be held accountable for these goals at their end-year review. This process necessitates a formal meeting where the individuals review their goals set forth at their yearly review and their progress on attaining these goals. Should the opportunity for improvement be present, the leader provides mentorship on how to best meet these goals. Action plans should be reviewed to ensure they remain appropriate and realistic. Mutual goal setting between leadership and individual nurses creates an environment of shared respect, trust, and teamwork. The individuals understand that leadership is invested in their success and strives to help them achieve this success.

SUGGESTED READINGS

Latham GP, Locke EA. Goal setting—a motivational technique that works. *Organ Dyn*. 1979;68–80. Available at: http://www.business.umt.edu/Faculty/li/MGMT340/Goal%20Setting.pdf. Accessed August 14, 2008.

Negotiation and conflict resolution are critical to teach your staff

Sheila Lambert, RN, MSN, CCRN

WHAT TO DO: PLAN

Conflict is found in all aspects of society and nursing is not immune. How nurses maintain relationships and resolve conflict in the workplace is an important skill for nursing professionals. However, conflict within the nursing profession has traditionally generated negative feelings with many nurses who use avoidance as their primary coping mechanism. Avoidance methods of conflict resolution are linked to higher occupational stress. Conversely, addressing issues openly is linked to much lower stress. Negotiation and conflict resolution are important skills to support teamwork, staff satisfaction, and retention. As leaders within nursing, we must be adept at this to ensure the team's success.

As nursing leaders, it is our responsibility to mentor staff in conflict resolution and create a culture of transparency and openness. Conflict is normal; it does not denote failure—it means we are human and thus have our own ideas that may not necessarily mesh with others. Negotiation in conflict management consists of finding a resolution, working out the issues that will leave both parties feeling respected and valued. Key elements in conflict resolution and negotiation to be used by staff and nurse leaders would include empathy, anger management, social adaptation, and listening skills.

So how do we do this? When conflicts arise, it is important to address them quickly. If staff members approach you, they want your assistance—they need your help. After determining the issue, ask the individuals what they would like to see as an outcome. Perhaps they just want to talk or possibly they really need resolution; either way it is important enough that they have requested your time. If this issue warrants further discussion, bring the individuals together for discussion. Was there a miscommunication? Was there a process issue? Perhaps the two personalities involved in the conflict just do not work well together and that is okay too. It is important to create a nonpunitive environment to aid in open discussion and growth.

With the healthcare environment today, there is a great emphasis on nurse retention. Creating a better understanding of embedded issues and creating an open but confidential environment to deal with conflict and job difficulty are suggested as ways to reduce turnover. A specific issue such as an unfavorable job assignment or more complex issues such as unmet expectations can cause conflict and job dissatisfaction. It is important to address these issues quickly and effectively.

Great team effectiveness is enhanced through conflict resolution. There must be an emphasis on interpersonal skills, team communication, and self-awareness. Nurse leaders must know their work environments and staff well to create a climate of openness and respect.

SUGGESTED READINGS

Seren S, Ustun B. Conflict resolution skills of nursing students in problem-based compared to conventional curricula. *Nurse Edu Today*. 2008;28(4):393–400.

Tabak N, Orit K. Relationship between how nurses resolve their conflicts with doctors, their stress and job satisfaction. *J Nurs Manag*. 2007;15(3):321–331.

KNOW HOW TO MANAGE A BAD EVENT THAT OCCURS ON YOUR UNIT—CARING FOR STAFF AND REPORTING APPROPRIATELY

SHEILA LAMBERT, RN, MSN, CCRN

WHAT TO DO: PLAN

Bad events occur in hospitals. This is demonstrated everyday at work, in the newspaper, or on the nightly news. How these events are managed is important to the patient, the family, the individuals involved, and the overall healthcare team. Bad events can occur in the most efficient and safety conscious areas. No area is immune. Obviously, healthcare providers do not come to work with the intention of harming their patients. As a result, these events are devastating experiences not only for the patient and family but also for the healthcare providers and team. When these events occur, what do we do, as nursing leaders, to support our staff and ensure that the event will not be repeated?

Significant commitment is required from healthcare organizations and leaders to develop a framework for open disclosure, to ensure its quality, and to support healthcare providers in the process. Organizations also need to address the emotional needs of healthcare professionals in the aftermath of an adverse event. Finally, adequate systems for debriefing and incident analysis need to be in place to learn from adverse events and avoid recurrence.

First, we must address the issue with total transparency and honesty to both the patient and the institution. Research has found that open disclosure remains uncommon although the ethical duty to disclose is widely acknowledged. Barriers to open disclosure include discomfort and a lack of training on how to disclose, a fear of litigation, and a culture of infallibility among healthcare professionals. However, patients clearly expect open disclosure that includes an explanation of what happened, an apology for harm done, an assurance that appropriate action will be taken, and an explanation of what will be done to learn from the event and prevent recurrence.

Most institutions have clear processes in place for reporting. The entire incident should be thoroughly investigated within a short time frame to determine if this was a process issue (the process was not clear, appropriate, or up to date) or a practice issue (failure to follow the appropriate process). This involves the work of a team that includes those individuals directly involved, the nurse leader within the environment, and a team of facilitators specially trained to navigate through this process. Through this work, we can determine our next step. The next step may include a root cause analysis, a peer review, further education, or disciplinary action.

In reviewing these events, it is important to create an environment of opportunity as opposed to one of punishment or remediation. If leadership approaches bad events in a negative way, this greatly increases the risk of staff avoidance in reporting bad events in the future. In an environment where bad events are not reported, this significantly affects patient safety as each bad event offers an opportunity to learn and grow and decreases the chance of the event occurring again.

SUGGESTED READINGS

Manser T, Staender S. Aftermath of an adverse event: Supporting health care professionals to meet patient expectations through open disclosure. *Acta Anaesthesiol Scand.* 2005;49(6):728–734. doi:10.1111/j.1399–6576.2005.00746.x.

Keeping our patients satisfied with their care

Sheila Lambert, RN, MSN, CCRN

WHAT TO DO: IMPLEMENT

As nursing leaders, our approach to keeping our patients satisfied with their care starts with keeping our staff satisfied with their work and environment. This is a lofty but attainable goal. Patient satisfaction has become an established indicator of the quality of healthcare; however, nurses may experience difficulty creating a satisfying environment with their patients when they are not feeling positive about their own role. Job satisfaction is a true indicator of patient satisfaction.

When applicants for potential nursing positions are asked during interviews why they are leaving their current position, how often do we hear, "No one ever tells me I am doing a good job" or "All we hear is the negative"? Many of these applicants come with glowing references from their supervisor. The problem is that the supervisor never told the individual. It is up to the leadership to create a positive climate, to show appreciation for the hard work the nurses do, and to compliment them...often.

In addition to creating a positive work environment, it is essential that the leadership be very clear about its expectations regarding the care of the patients. For instance, if the approach to care is one of family-centeredness, educate the staff on this thoroughly and often. Clear standards and expectations of staff should be communicated at every opportunity. In an environment of transparency, the staff is not left to guess if they are supporting the vision of the institution or if their goals are in alignment with the team.

Another indicator of staff job satisfaction is the quality of nurse–physician relationship and the atmosphere this creates. Daily interactions between nurses and physicians strongly influence the nurses' morale and retention rates. Nurse–physician relationships must be addressed by the leaders since they greatly impact the environment and culture of the workplace. These could be positive or negative relationships; however, it is imperative to understand this dynamic.

Another significant item in patient and staff satisfaction is nurse–patient ratios. Appropriate ratios are specific to individual areas; however, it is important to assess ratios of individual departments to determine appropriateness. A major job dissatisfaction for nurses is being so busy with a patient assignment that it prevents them from providing the care they would like to provide. While it is very useful to have data to support adequate ratios (based upon acuity), it is also essential to query the staff on the appropriateness of their workload.

Studies demonstrate that patients cared for on units that nurses felt had adequate staff, good administrative support for nursing care, and good relations between doctors and nurses were more than twice as likely as other patients to report high satisfaction with their care. Improved nurse work environments in hospitals have the potential to simultaneously increase nurses' job satisfaction and increase patients' satisfaction with their care.

SUGGESTED READINGS

Mahon PY. An analysis of the concept "patient satisfaction" as it relates to contemporary nursing care. *J Adv Nurs*. 1996; 24(6):1241–1248.

Rosenstein AH. Nurse–physician relationships: Impact on nurse satisfaction and retention. *Am J Nurs*. 2002;102(6): 26–34.

Vahey DC, Aiken LH, Sloane DM, et al. Nurse burnout and patient satisfaction. *Med Care*. 2004;42(2):1157–1166.

Know how to avoid workplace violence

Sheila Lambert, RN, MSN, CCRN

WHAT TO DO: PLAN

For 1999, the Bureau of Labor Statistics estimated a total of 2,637 nonfatal assaults on hospital workers, a rate of 8.3 assaults per 10,000 workers. This rate is over four times higher than the rate of nonfatal assaults for all private sector industries, which is 2 per 10,000 workers. OSHA defines workplace violence as violence or the threat of violence against workers. It can occur at or outside the workplace and can range from threats or verbal abuse to physical assaults, even to homicide. In fact, workplace violence is one of the leading causes of job-related deaths.

There are a number of interventions that can be implemented to assist in protecting staff from workplace violence. While not every incident can be prevented, interventions can reduce the incidence dramatically. The best protection employers can offer is to establish a zero-tolerance policy toward workplace violence against or by their employees. A workplace violence prevention program should be established with all employees educated on the policy and developing a clear understanding that all claims of workplace violence will be investigated and resolved promptly. Staff should be encouraged to accurately report all incidents of workplace violence regardless of how incidental they feel the event may have been. It is important to create a culture of transparency; staff should feel comfortable reporting without feeling they will get into trouble. Safety education for employees will allow them to understand what conduct is not acceptable, what to do if they witness or are subjected to workplace violence, and how to protect themselves from future incidents.

One key step in avoiding violence through preparation is to take a thorough look at the workplace to find existing or potential hazards for workplace violence. For instance, has furniture been arranged to prevent entrapment of staff? Is the workplace free of clutter with nothing available to throw at workers or use as weapons? Is there a secondary door for escape in case the main door is blocked?

The type of clients or customers served is a good indicator of the risk of workplace violence. Clearly, those that serve mentally ill clients, substance abusers, and criminals have a much higher risk of onsite assault. But healthcare workers in non–mental–health practices face an almost identical level of risk. High stress situations such as illness or the loss of a loved one can trigger violent behavior. Employers should educate their staff on "Universal Precautions" for violence much as we do for universal precautions such as wearing gloves. A universal precaution for violence infers that violence should be expected but can be avoided or mitigated through preparation.

It is important to give employees the tools they need to avoid workplace violence. Staff education on conflict resolution in the workplace will decrease the risk of hostile employees acting out. They should also be trained in managing anger, dealing with aggressive persons in a nonviolent way, and stress management. In addition, typically, individuals will exhibit signs preceding outbursts of violence, such as an increase in complaints, withdrawn moods, rule breaking, and inappropriate comments to other employees. Staff should be aware of these signs of impending violence, alert supervisors to any concerns about safety or security, and report all incidents immediately in writing.

SUGGESTED READINGS

http://www.wsib.on.ca/wsib/wsibsite.nsf/Public/Workplace Violence. Accessed August 14, 2008.

http://www.trainingtime.com/npps/story.cfm?nppage=154. Accessed August 14, 2008.

SUPPORT YOUR STAFF THROUGH CONTINUED PROFESSIONAL GROWTH OPPORTUNITIES

SHEILA LAMBERT, RN, MSN, CCRN

WHAT TO DO: EVALUATE

Nurse leaders want the most knowledgeable nurses on their staff. For this to occur, staff must remain current in literature and process. Ideally, one would like to think that nurses, as professionals, would seek these opportunities independently and strive for excellence on their own. However, in this day of staffing shortages, overtime expectations, and attempting to achieve work–life balance, nursing leaders must be creative in supporting their staff through their continued professional growth.

Supporting and encouraging professional growth of one's staff requires commitment from both financial and time perspectives. The expectation of participating in growth opportunities must be set and clearly communicated to the staff. Expectations must be measurable, realistic, and achievable. This expectation must be communicated prior to employment since it is important for the potential hires to have communicated with them the growth and educational opportunities that they will be expected to participate in as a nurse working in a particular area. By communicating this preemployment, nurses come on board with a clear understanding of what is expected.

Since participation in educational opportunities is expected, it is important that numerous opportunities be provided to them. For instance, if staff are expected to attend six lectures per year in their area of practice, it is important that such lectures be arranged as opposed to asking staff to seek them out on their own. This requires a commitment from physicians and ancillary staff to provide these opportunities to build the staff. In addition, scheduling multiple offerings on the same day will demonstrate a respect for staff's time. If there is a code review requirement, scheduling this at the same time as a lecture can help to reduce the time the nurse has to come in to work on a day off. Both of these processes illustrate a commitment from the leadership to help the staff achieve these requirements.

It is essential to hold the staff accountable if the requirements are not met and have a predetermined process for demonstrating how this will be reflected in their annual review. This expectation should be clearly communicated to the staff. There should be no surprises to the staff in this practice—transparency is essential. It is important to be consistent in the application of this approach and maintain the integrity of the review; each staff should experience the same outcome if he/she has not met this standard. Conversely, a process should be set for the staff member that exceeds this requirement.

Celebrate individual accomplishments when the staff members achieve certain milestones; let them know that you are aware and proud of them. If a staff member achieves certification, put up signs, buy lunch for the staff member the next time she is working, talk about it at staff meetings, and reinforce the accomplishment in a positive way to demonstrate your pride and support of the individual accomplishment and the success that it brings to the team. This will also further encourage other staff members to achieve these milestones as well.

The message is very clear—we require you to achieve certain educational requirements to further aid in your professional growth; however, we will bring these to you, we will pay you for these, and we will celebrate your successes with you! It is a win-win!

SUGGESTED READINGS

Hallin K, Danielson E. Registered nurses' perceptions of their work and professional development. *J adv Nurs.* 2008;61(1):62–70.

REMEMBER THAT THE NEW INTERN ON THE FLOOR WHO THINKS HE KNOWS EVERYTHING WAS IN DIAPERS (OR AT LEAST MIDDLE SCHOOL) WHEN YOU GRADUATED FROM NURSING SCHOOL

SHEILA LAMBERT, RN, MSN, CCRN

WHAT TO DO: IMPLEMENT

No matter how far we come in nursing, there is an unmistakable chain of command. Perhaps physicians learn this in medical school or maybe they feel a sense of entitlement from being a "real" doctor for a week or two. Or, maybe, they are intimidated by their new level of accountability and mask this with an air of assertiveness and confidence. Another option is that they simply don't know what they don't know. Have a nurse on the floor who is unofficially tasked with keeping them on track. While it is certainly not in our job description or credentials, if they work in a teaching hospital, they are a part of a team that ensures patient safety even in an environment of learning.

As with all physician orders, the nurse must carefully check interns' orders prior to implementing them; however, with the new intern, it is important for the nurse to be even more meticulous with this process. In addition, nurses with experience have the ability to pick up on subtle changes in patient status that less experienced eyes such as those of an intern may overlook.

What can nurses do to assist in the intern's development while assuring a culture of patient safety and mutual respect? Communication is a valuable tool in this process, which will continue to support the team while preventing errors and improving overall patient care. As with all communications between colleagues in healthcare, showing professional courtesy and a professional attitude at all times is very important. Interns report a greater frequency in communication issues with nurses than do more highly qualified physicians.

Keep in mind that the way you say things is many times far more powerful than what you are actually saying.

Know your facts before approaching the intern, make sure that the information you are going to convey is accurate and correct. If this information is not received favorably—for instance, a Tylenol dose is too high and the intern refuses to change the order—what do you do then? Follow the chain of command—go to the second-year resident and follow the chain up to the attending if necessary. It is important to refuse to sign off on an incorrect order and protect the patient at all times. This process is equally important in terms of patient assessment. For instance, your patient's status is declining and the intern is not conceptualizing the gravity of the situation—go to the second-year resident with the information, not only will you protect the patient, the intern may actually learn something that lasts their entire career.

The majority of interns are not arrogant or disrespectful but rather, simply don't know what they don't know. While most interns will be wonderful physicians, we must be hyper-vigilant with their patients, orders, and procedures. We must draw on our years of experience in patient care to assist them in their practice. The lines are definitely blurred in this process—while the physician is responsible with tasking the nurse through orders and progress notes, the nurse may in many instances have more experience than the physician. Nurses must be empowered to initiate these communications at difficult times. This can be done when the culture of the environment is one of mutual respect, transparency, and honesty.

SUGGESTED READINGS

http://intqhc.oxfordjournals.org/cgi/content/abstract/3/1/11.

KNOW WHICH DOCTOR TO CALL

JEANNIE SCRUGGS GARBER, DNP, RN

WHAT TO DO: IMPLEMENT

Nurses in every nursing position have been in the situation where they have asked themselves, Which physician do I call? The roles of nurses and physicians have evolved tremendously in the past decades and role confusion has increased within the professions and interprofessionally. Knowing whom to call for what is quite complex. Nurses who are caring for patients in the hospital need to be aware of the many physician and physician-extender roles such as primary care physician, subspecialist, intensivist, hospitalist, resident, and nurse practitioner or physician assistant. Each hospital should have an established protocol for whom to call and under what circumstances. However, nurses still have to make the decision on which provider they need to reach to obtain the communication required to care for the patient.

Deciding to contact the physician can be a stressful process for many reasons. The nurse may be concerned with the physician's response to the call. Nurses are reporting more and more that physicians are verbally abusive, especially with night calls. Diaz and colleagues report that "physician abuse of nurses is common, with 64% of nurses reporting that they experienced some form of verbal abuse from a physician at least once every 2 to 3 months." A defined protocol and process for physician contact is helpful in minimizing contact of the wrong physician and will provide guidance that supports the nurses' action to call.

Nurses should be aware of the physicians caring for the patient and should work with the primary physician to develop the on-call plan for the patient. In teaching hospitals, the complexity can be even greater, as they often have a detailed process outlined for when the medical student, first-year, second-year, third-year, and chief resident may be contacted and at what point the attending physician is called. This process can be helpful; however, consultants, hospitalists, and physician extenders are now a part of the process and the complexity of whom to call continues. The nurse and other healthcare providers need to be informed of and aware of the on-call protocols so that they can work together to provide the safest environment regarding physician availability. Collaboration is the key to making the right call to the right person at the right time. Nurses should rely on conversations with the patient, if appropriate, and other healthcare providers to guide their decision of whom to call and when. The nurse should also be aware of the protocols available to them in policy, procedure, or from other resources within the organization. In order to promote patient safety, minimize risk to the patient, and facilitate productive communication, the nurse must rely on critical thinking skills and problem solving skills to initiate and carry out calls to the physician regarding patient care.

SUGGESTED READINGS

Diaz AL, McMillin JD. A definition and description of nurse abuse. *West J Nur Res.* 1991;13(1):97–109.
Porto G, Lauve R. Disruptive clinician behavior: A persistent threat to patient safety. *Patient Saf Qual Healthc.* 2006; July/August. Available at: http://www.psqh.com/julaug06/disruptive.html. Accessed June 19, 2008.

FOLLOW THE POLICY AND PROCEDURE

ANTHONY D. SLONIM, MD, DRPH

Policies and procedures (P and P) are necessary evils in today's clinical environment. Most clinicians are easily frustrated with both the number and content of these documents. For many years, the P and P were used as the vehicle to ensure compliance with regulatory standards for a state department of health or the Joint Commission. As a result, they were often wordy and did not facilitate the delivery of care. There are a number of important reasons for the nurse to understand the context of policies and procedures in the delivery of patient care. First, these documents represent the organization's guidance and approach to delivering care. Second, the procedure provides a "how to" guide for infrequent or confusing processes. Finally, the P and P are the approaches that the organization uses to reduce variability in patient care and improve patient safety.

Healthcare professionals and organizations are held to multiple levels of accountability. These are diagrammatically represented in Figure 17-1. There are laws that provide the foundational elements for practice. In the case of the professional, these are discipline-specific and often held within the nurse practice act or the physician practice act of the state governing practice. Similarly, the laws provided by state and local departments of health assist healthcare organizations in providing care that is consistent with legal doctrine and statutes. The next hierarchical element is regulations. A number of regulations that specify important tenets that the professional nurse is responsible for subscribing to may also be found in the nurse practice act. These elements constitute a number of "rules" that need to be followed to ensure appropriate

practice. Similarly, the healthcare organization also has regulations, with performance expectations, provided by the major accrediting body, the Joint Commission. The Joint Commission provides guidance as to the major regulations that the healthcare organizations should follow to achieve and maintain certification. Finally, certification is another mechanism that is usually crafted to demonstrate some level of accomplishment. For professionals, certification is usually offered by professional organizations in a specific discipline. Nurses can be certified in a number of disciplines including critical care, emergency nursing, oncology, and administration. Usually, certification implies familiarity and excellence with a core body of knowledge and practice. Physicians also have certifications referred to as Board Certification. These are again linked to a body of knowledge. Certification examinations in medicine and its subspecialties are governed by the American Board of Medical Specialties. Healthcare organizations also have important certifications of which they can avail themselves. Usually, these represent the demonstration of expertise in specific areas or with specific patient populations.

The healthcare organization has a number of strategies at its disposal to help the employees in delivering care to patients and ensure compliance with applicable laws, regulations, and certifications. Policies and procedures are the most commonly used mechanisms. Policy documents should be easy to understand and should articulate the institution's guiding principle. For example, "this hospital is a nonsmoking facility". The procedure usually contains some of the descriptive elements that allow the policy to be "put into action." For example, there should be guidance for caregivers on what to do if a patient wants to smoke, how to offer consultation for smoking cessation, and locations for visitors to smoke if they desire. There should also be a mechanism to guide nurses on what to do if they cannot comply with the policy, including how to escalate up the chain of command for guidance. By having a standardized and streamlined approach to providing care, organizations hope that there will be similarity in the application of care at the bedside.

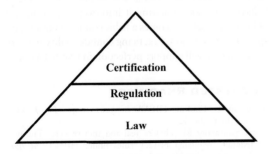

FIGURE 17.1: The levels of accountability governing the healthcare professionals and organizations.

SUGGESTED READINGS

http://www.nursingboard.state.nv.us/nurse%20practice%20act/. Accessed August 18, 2008.

www.Jointcommission.org. Accessed August 18, 2008.

www.abms.org. Accessed August 18, 2008.

PRACTICE STRICT CONFIDENTIALITY TO MAKE IT A HABIT

JULIE MULLIGAN WATTS, RN, MN

WHAT TO DO: PLAN

In 1996, the United States House and Senate enacted the Health Insurance Portability and Accountability Act (HIPAA). The purposes of this law are to improve portability and continuity of health insurance coverage in the group and individual markets, to combat waste, fraud, and abuse in health insurance and healthcare delivery, to promote the use of medical savings accounts, to improve access to long-term care services and coverage, to simplify the administration of health insurance, and so on. Simply stated, the law is meant to prevent barriers to health insurance, such as limiting exclusions for preexisting conditions and offering access to health benefits for those who lose other health coverage. The law helps guarantee that patients will have access to health insurance at new places of employment without having to start with a new insurer at their new place of work. The law also guarantees that health information will not be shared with individuals, businesses, and employers or released to healthcare providers without the approval of the individual.

The U.S. Department of Health and Human Services (DHHS) issued the HIPAA Privacy Rules in 2002 as a way to implement the HIPAA law by outlining standards that address the use and disclosure of individuals' health information called "protected health information." The goal of the Privacy Rule is to simplify the HIPAA law and ensure the strict confidentiality of patient information while allowing the proper access to information to provide quality healthcare.

Across the country, massive education took place at healthcare institutions and businesses so that the employees could comply with the law and companies would avoid the infractions of the HIPAA law and Privacy Rules. When hospitals or individual employees of hospitals or medical offices do not comply with the laws, civil and criminal penalties may be placed against the individual or business. Consistent with that, employees of entities covered by HIPAA can penalize their employees who violate confidentiality within their institutions. In the past few years, there have been reports of hospitals that have fired employees because of infractions of the HIPAA law. In fact, attention has been given to this issue in the national media when infractions of confidentiality occurred, involving celebrity patients such as George Clooney and Britney Spears.

For employees working in hospitals, it is imperative that they practice strict adherence to issues of confidentiality at all times. Sharing confidential information, even with one's boss, administrators, or trusted colleagues, can lead to an environment of careless rules and loss of the employee's self-regulation regarding confidential practices. When employees do not consistently practice behaviors that are required to be in compliance with the HIPAA law, they may find themselves becoming less vigilant over time and fall into a relaxed state of awareness.

There are many opportunities for falling down on confidential practices if one is not vigilant. The routine patient care activities of nurses provide multiple opportunities to lose site of privacy practices. Nurses carrying their daily work-list may drop it in the parking lot. A patient's name may be mentioned in a phone conversation that is overheard by other patients and visitors. Nurses could mention a patient's name to a family member around the dinner table without a thought of confidentiality. Within the hospital, nurses may feel that patient privacy is maintained but charts may be left open in view of the visitors. Clinical conditions or postoperative reports may be shared in public places such as waiting rooms or hallways. Attempts at privacy are made during clinical conferences when names are omitted but, often, the patient's name is clearly visible on scans or slides that are projected on a screen during presentations at clinical conferences or tumor boards.

A difficult situation can arise when the patient discussed at a conference is an employee of the hospital and multiple employees are involved in the care and present for the discussion. A nurse can fall under the assumption that many people are aware of the employee/patient's condition and make a terrible "slip" in confidentiality to other employees who are not involved. As with any other behaviors, consistently practicing a behavior and incorporating it into every situation will help ensure that it becomes a habit that does not require special consideration. Practicing confidentiality in every circumstance will support perfection in that behavior.

SUGGESTED READINGS

Anderson F. Finding HIPAA in your soup. *Am J Nurs.* 2007;107(2):66–72.

Frank-Stromborg M. They're real and they're here: The new federally regulated privacy rules under HIPAA. *Medsurg Nurs.* 2003;12(6):380–385, 414.

U.S. 104th Congress. Public Law 104–191, Health Insurance Portability and Accountability Act of 1996. Available at: www.aspe.hhs.gov/admnsimp/pl104191.htm. Accessed May 5, 2008.

Remember that Cutting Costs for a Particular Patient Does Not Solve the Healthcare Financial Crisis

Anthony D. Slonim, MD, DrPH

WHAT TO DO: PLAN

Healthcare expenditures have continued to rise dramatically over the last several decades. Nurses and other professionals are rightly concerned not only about the costs associated with healthcare but also the value that is derived from healthcare. Despite the expense paid for healthcare in the United States, the outcomes from the delivered services do not compare favorably with other developed countries. As a result, there is considerable discussion about what nurses can do to improve the way that services are delivered.

Many nurses, in their effort to do their part in solving the healthcare financial situation, will raise concerns about expenses. Often, talks on rounds about "this is wasteful," "they're going to die anyway," and "I cannot believe that we're spending all this money, but for what?" enter into the discussions. These statements are not misguided or said with a spirit of meanness; they are statements that come from the experiences of these nurses having watched considerable expense at the end of life. However, this approach for cost containment at the bedside of the individual patients will neither achieve what we need to achieve as a society in terms of healthcare nor provide the appropriate care for the patients.

Nurses do need to be involved in the ongoing debate about resource use in healthcare, and as front-line providers, they are often engaged in delivering services that require expensive resources. While nurses caring for patients need to be concerned about wasting supplies and equipment, they should not be entertaining "rationing" based on individual patients or patient demographics like end of life. The savings accomplished one bedspace at a time will do nothing to impact the more global problem of waste in healthcare and is insufficiently standardized so as to ensure freedom from bias.

Importantly, nurses do have a role in helping to thoughtfully address the bigger issue by encouraging standardized, cost benefit, cost effectiveness analyses on patient populations that may be high consumers of healthcare. When these studies are performed legitimately with attention to the needs of specific populations, important lessons can be learned, resulting in opportunities to reduce waste, at the population level, without disenfranchising an individual patient or family.

Nurses have a role in ensuring that care is delivered efficiently, without waste, and with the best possible outcomes. However, these analyses need to be performed in a standardized way that is free from bias.

SUGGESTED READINGS

Wu AW. Principles of outcome assessment. In: Goldman L, Ausiello D, eds. *Cecil Textbook of Medicine*. 22nd Ed. Philadelphia: Saunders; 2004, pp. 33–38.

ENSURE THAT PATIENTS GET TREATED EQUITABLY

ANTHONY D. SLONIM, MD, DRPH

Equity in healthcare is one of the dimensions of healthcare quality that has been discussed for many years. This dimension implies that patients will not receive differential care based on personal demographics. Providing care that is different based on patient level characteristics is overt discrimination and has no place in healthcare. However, considerable evidence has been accumulated regarding inequities in healthcare based upon age, race, gender, insurance status, and ethnicity. These differences are related to access to healthcare services and providers and result in differences in outcome that affect individual patients and their families. Nurses as patient advocates are involved in these inequities in the delivery of care and need to improve their understanding of how these challenges affect patients and work with their colleagues to eliminate them.

Differences in healthcare exist. They exist because some procedures, medications, and care for one group of patients are not as effective as they are for other groups of patients. In addition, some patients and families exercise their right to self-determination and make choices about their care or participation in research protocols and experimental therapies. None of these represent the inequitable delivery of healthcare services. However, when services that have equal effectiveness are offered differently because of a personal characteristic, then healthcare inequities exist.

It is well recognized that there is variability in practice among nurses. Some nurses perform a task one way while others perform it slightly differently. Both are working within the context of an appropriate standard of care but they perform procedures, deliver medications, and execute tasks somewhat differently. Policies and procedures usually govern this practice.

Similarly, the prescription of healthcare services, medications, and treatments is associated with variability, but it is still within the range of an acceptable standard of care. Nurses have a role in understanding, on behalf of their patients, why one patient may receive one treatment while another patient would receive a different, perhaps less effective, therapy when practices are supposed to be grounded in evidence-based medicine principles. There may be medical reasons or there may not be.

Understanding the application of procedures, tests, and therapies in the area of specialty and then advocating on behalf of the patient for the equitable application of those procedures, tests, and therapies are essential parts of the professional nurse's role in modern healthcare.

SUGGESTED READINGS

Duffy SA, Jackson FC, Schim SM, et al. Racial/ethnic preferences, sex preferences, and perceived discrimination related to end-of-life care. *J Am Geriatr Soc.* 2006;54(1):150–157.

Guthrie BJ. Mental health inequities: Conceptual and methodological implications. *Arch Psychiatr Nurs.* 2007;21(4): 234–235.

Larson E. Racial and ethnic disparities in immunizations: Recommendations for clinicians. *Fam Med.* 2003;35(9): 655–660.

Miller PS. Racial disparities in access to care within the cardiac revascularization population. *J Natl Black Nurses Assoc.* 2007; 18(2):63–74.

Smeltzer SC. Improving the health and wellness of persons with disabilities: A call to action too important for nursing to ignore. *Nurs Outlook.* 2007;55(4):189–195.

Young L, Little M. Women and heart transplantation: An issue of gender equity? *Health Care Women Int.* 2004;25(5): 436–453.

21

Know your patient's PT/INR before giving Coumadin

Alice M. Christaldi, RN, BSN, CRRN

WHAT TO DO: ASSESS

Few drugs that are given to patients today require as much attention to detail as does the oral anticoagulant warfarin (Coumadin). This drug requires frequent lab testing, has a narrow therapeutic window, requires careful attention to diet, and has potentially deadly side effects. Side effects can include bleeding in the patient, petechiae, hematomas, black tarry stools, or brown tinged urine. If the patient experiences shortness of breath, sudden bouts of weakness, tachycardia, and low blood pressure, he or she needs to be assessed for acute bleeding.

Coumadin is considered a Vitamin K antagonist. It inhibits the coagulation factors that are dependent on Vitamin K for activation, which include clotting factors II, VII, IX, and X, and it also inhibits the anticoagulant proteins C and S. This drug is stored in the liver and excreted in urine.

Anticoagulant effects are produced within 24 h, but the peak effect requires at least 72 h. This explains the rationale of starting patients on intravenous heparin at the same time that Coumadin therapy begins. When the patient's international normalized ratio (INR) reaches the therapeutic range after 48–72 h, the heparin can be tapered and discontinued.

There are many reasons to place a patient on Coumadin therapy. The primary diagnoses include atrial fibrillation, valvular heart disease, venous thromboembolism prevention and treatment, and major surgery. To evaluate the effectiveness of the anticoagulant therapy, lab tests are required. Prothrombin time (PT) and international normalized ratio (INR) are monitored. The INR is chosen as the standard measurement of anticoagulant therapy because PT values vary widely. Therapeutic INR target range is generally 2–3. Patients with prosthetic heart valves require a range of 2.5–3.5.

Testing is done daily until the patient stays in the target range for 48–72 h, and then it can be done two to three times a week for several weeks; eventually it can be done monthly. Many factors affect these numbers, including certain drugs such as cimetidine, erythromycin,

fluconazole, miconazole, and proprandolol. These have been shown to raise the INR and increase the risk of bleeding. Factors that lower INR and raise the risk of thrombosis include use of avocados (in large amounts), barbiturates, tube feedings and food containing high levels of Vitamin K (e.g., broccoli, cauliflower, kale, spinach, and liver), nafcillin, and sucralfate. Also, be alert for herbal remedies such as garlic, green tea, ginkgo biloba, ginseng, and St. John's wort that interfere with absorption.

In the hospital setting, any drug that requires dosages based on a daily lab result merits a red flag. Special care must be observed when the drug is "held" for testing or surgery. Too often, it is not resumed on schedule because it gets overlooked in the paperwork. It is very important for the prescribing physician to specify the date on which the drug is to be resumed. Medication administration records (MAR) should include the drug, route, frequency of dosing, time, and dose. If the drug is "held" because of a high INR, then the MAR needs to be clearly marked "No Coumadin Today" and list the date.

When a patient goes for a procedure, such as a surgery, all orders need to be rewritten post-operatively. The blanket "resume all meds" order should not be acceptable. If the Coumadin was held before surgery, it would be very easy to miss it altogether and it would not be resumed.

If the patient develops an elevated INR, treatment must be initiated based on this number. Repeat testing of the INR will be necessary. The dose of Coumadin may be reduced or held for a day or two. If the INR is greater than 5, oral Vitamin K may be given. Should the patient develop active bleeding, intravenous Vitamin K and fresh frozen plasma will be administered. Remember to check the laboratory value prior to administering the drug to prevent overdosing.

SUGGESTED READINGS

Hirsh J, Guyatt G, Albert GW, et al. The seventh ACCP conference on antithrombotic and thrombolytic therapy: Evidence based guidelines. *Chest*. 2004;126:172S–173S.

Porter RS (ed.). Pulmonary embolism. *The Merck Manual Online Medical Libraries*. 18th Ed. Available at: http://www.merck.com/mmpe/sec05/ch050/ch050a.html?qt=warfarin&alt=sh#S05_CH50_T004. Accessed March 29, 2008.

NEVER GIVE ORAL MEDS VIA IV ACCESS; KNOW YOUR ROUTES

ALICE M. CHRISTALDI, RN, BSN, CRRN

WHAT TO DO: PLAN

Do not draw up oral medications into a parenteral syringe; obtain an oral syringe from pharmacy. Oral syringes cannot be connected to an intravenous port; they will not fit. This is to prevent the oral medication from being given intravenously by mistake.

It is imperative to be familiar with common medications that are given on your unit and their routes. Even with the advent of computer-aided medication administration, knowledge is the key to patient safety. A computer does not know why a certain medication is ordered; it takes the critical thinking skills of the nurse to determine if it is indeed the right medication for the right patient. The trained eye of a nurse can note the patient's response to a medication. Be aware of the five rights of medication administration which include the right patient, the right time, the right route, the right dose, and the right drug.

Be aware of the ordered routes of medications. If the patient is NPO and all meds go through a feeding tube, the order should reflect that. If a medication cannot be crushed, check with the pharmacy to see if it is available in a solution form or notify the physician and have it changed to an appropriate formulary. Make sure the Medication Administration Record reflects the proper route. Mistakes could occur if a staff member is not aware of the NPO status and gives the medications by mouth. Keep Medication Administration Records updated, with proper routes clearly listed.

Do not borrow medications from another patient and use it for your patient. That bypasses the pharmacy's double check system. This medication may not be available because the pharmacy is clarifying the order with a physician or possibly another nurse already gave the medication, yet failed to document it properly. Always allow the checks within the pharmacy system to work so that an error does not reach the patient.

There are safeguards built into medication administration systems; do not bypass them. Utilize the technology that is available, but realize that technology paired with savvy nursing knowledge is unbeatable in helping to prevent medication errors.

SUGGESTED READINGS

Cohen H, Robinson ES, Mandrack M. Getting to the root of medication errors: Survey results. *Nursing.* 2003;33(9):36–46.

David U. Medication safety...your call to make a difference. *Alta RN.* 2007;63(8):10–11.

PROPER ADMINISTRATION OF ENOXAPARIN (LOVENOX) INJECTABLE

MELISSA H. CRIGGER, BSN, MHA, RN

WHAT TO DO: IMPLEMENT

Remember that the administration of enoxaparin requires appropriate administration technique and monitoring of appropriate laboratory values. Enoxaparin is used for the treatment of deep vein thrombosis (DVT), pulmonary embolism, myocardial infarction, unstable angina, and prophylaxis for DVT. The most frequent adverse effects for enoxaparin include bleeding, anemia, and thrombocytopenia. Hypersensitivity reactions include fever, urticaria, rash, and chills. Enoxaparin is administered through the subcutaneous route.

With the administration of enoxaparin, the nurse must remember to check for any allergies that the patient might have to the medication. The nurse also should determine where the last injection site was in order to rotate to a new site. Continued injections to the same area can lead to tissue damage. Prior to the administration, the nurse should always review the patient's identification bracelet, provide privacy, and cleanse the appropriate site with alcohol. Syringes prefilled with enoxaparin contain an air bubble. The air bubble is never expelled prior to injection. Remember, to enhance absorption, the injection should be given via the right/left anteriolateral or posteriolateral abdominal wall. The injection should be administered deep into the subcutaneous tissue and the syringe should never be aspirated. The site should not be massaged.

Assessment is of utmost importance for the patient receiving anticoagulant therapy. This includes inspection of the injection site for bruising, redness, warmth, tenderness, and swelling. The nurse should also assess for signs of bleeding, which include bleeding from the gums, heme-positive stools, black tarry stools, reductions in hematocrit, and bleeding from other orifices. Notification of the physician should occur immediately if any of these signs occur.

When caring for the patient receiving enoxaparin, the nurse must remember to review lab reports, including the monitoring of complete blood counts (CBCs). Since thrombocytopenia is a potential adverse effect, the platelet count and hematocrit should be monitored. Should either decrease, the physician should be made aware of these changes. The nurse should also monitor stools for signs of bleeding. Stool specimens for occult blood should be obtained periodically while the patient is receiving enoxaparin. The monitoring of the drug's effectiveness is not measured by the PT/PTT as it is with traditional heparin. Instead, the use of a Factor X assay is the method for monitoring the effectiveness.

Patients receiving Lovenox require adequate teaching. This includes having the patient report any unusual bleeding as well as complaints of dizziness, rash, itching, fever, or swelling. The patient should also be educated about the importance of notifying the physician should any of the symptoms occur. The patient must also be aware of the potential for increased bleeding and should not take aspirin or NSAIDs without consulting his or her physician. For the patient receiving home injections, the nurse must always educate the patient on proper administration technique.

SUGGESTED READINGS

Deglin JH, Vallerand AH. *Davis's Drug Guide for Nurses*. 10th Ed. Philadelphia: FA Davis Company; 2007, pp. 589–593.
Timby BK. Parenteral medications. In: *Fundamental Nursing Skills and Concepts*. 9th Ed. Philadelphia: Lippincott Williams & Wilkins; 2008, pp. 812–813.

Before administering insulin, make sure you know whose blood sugar you are treating

Monty D. Gross, PhD, RN, CNE

WHAT TO DO: ASSESS

The Institute of Medicine's 1999 report suggested that medical errors accounted for 44,000–98,000 deaths each year. An exact number is unknown; nonetheless, medication errors are a significant component of medical errors in U.S. hospitals. Although medication errors can occur at any stage of the process, they most often occur during the prescription and administration phases. These problems are compounded when the nurse relies upon assistance from other providers on the team.

Many medication errors could be prevented with better staff communication or a different procedure. For example, the checking of glucose levels and administration of insulin are common procedures that are complicated in their approach. A patient care assistant (PCA) will often test and report on blood sugar values for patients. The PCA then needs to tell the nurse the patient's name and room number instead of using a phrase with a pronoun like "her blood glucose was 221." It is often better to state, for example, "Mrs. Smith's blood glucose in room 48B is 221." On the other hand, the nurse should request specific identification information instead of assuming the patient the PCA was referring to was the patient in the room a PCA had just exited. The nurse should also check the source of documentation in the patient's bedside chart to verify that the reading was documented. This step would reveal the actual reading for the correct patient. Often, PCAs will jot a quick note on the blood glucoses on a scratch pad or paper towel and document it in the record later.

It may also be possible to avert the error when the nurse enters the room to administer the insulin. The nurse can ask the patient to verify that, in fact, his/her glucose was just read and the reading was the result of the test. This step, however, may not be possible when the patient is unable to communicate.

While nurses in today's busy hospital environments are already multitasking and delegating responsibilities to other members of the healthcare team, clarity in communications, particularly while the nurse is directing others or working off information coming from others, becomes important for assuring patient safety.

SUGGESTED READINGS

Institute of Medicine. Report brief: Preventing medication errors, June 2006. Available at: http://www.iom.edu/CMS/3809/22526/35939/35943.aspx. Accessed June 29, 2008.

Institute of Medicine. *To Err Is Human: Building a Safer Health Care System.* Washington, DC: National Academy Press; 1999.

Meadows M. Strategies to reduce medication errors: How the FDA is working to improve medication safety and what you can do to help. *FDA Cons Mag.* 2003;37(3). Available at: http://www.fda.gov/FDAC/features/2003/303_meds.html. Accessed June 29, 2008.

PATIENTS WITH PENICILLIN ALLERGIES MAY SAFELY RECEIVE ANTIBIOTICS FROM OTHER DRUG CLASSES

ANTHONY D. SLONIM, MD, DrPH

WHAT TO DO: PLAN

Antimicrobial therapy has revolutionized the care of patients suffering from infectious diseases and allowed cures from previously devastating conditions. It is important to remember that drugs come in a variety of "classes." These classes have similar characteristics like the mechanism of action, metabolism, and toxicities. Nurses can remember the characteristics of the class and the idiosyncrasies of specific agents, thereby ensuring that patients get the medications they need without experiencing allergic or toxic effects of the drug.

Penicillins are a group of drugs that belong to a drug class known as β-lactams. The β-lactam antibiotics are so named because their chemical structure consists of a β-lactam ring that provides the opportunity for the medication to work at its site of action. There are four subclasses to this group of β-lactams. They are the penicillins, the cephalosporins, the monobactams, and the carbapenems. Overall, these drugs have similar structures, mechanisms of action, metabolism, and excretion (renal). They also share some important toxicities.

Penicillins consist of a group of drugs with broad antibacterial capabilities and are available in oral and parenteral dosage forms. Depending on the agent selected, these drugs cover many bacterial classes of both the Gram-positive and Gram-negative spectra and also include aerobic and anaerobic activity if the appropriate drug is selected. The most common adverse reaction from penicillins is hypersensitivity reactions that range in severity from rashes with hives to life-threatening anaphylaxis, which occurs rarely. Importantly, patients are often unclear about what reactions, if any, they might have experienced but will often report that they were told in the distant past that they experienced an "allergy" to penicillin. It is important to get clarity from the patient on just what type of reaction occurred since the benefits of these drugs in treating a specific infection may outweigh the risks of a mild adverse reaction that can be treated. When an important adverse reaction from a drug is recognized, alternative agents can often be identified or if an alternative is not identified, the patient can receive the drug after being appropriately desensitized.

It is important for the nurse to remember the cross-reactivity that can occur between the drug and the other members of the class. For example, cephalosporins, which belong to the β-lactam group with penicillins, cross react for adverse reactions approximately 8%–15% of the time. This is important, but again it depends upon what reaction occurred. If the reaction is life-threatening anaphylaxis, it may be best to choose a non-β-lactam alternative to treat the patient's infectious disease. However, if the adverse reaction is a mild rash or unknown, the risk of adverse reaction may be low enough to support the administration of the cephalosporin despite the allergy to the penicillin. Other members of the β-lactam class including monobactams and carbapenems do not share this cross-reactivity with either cephalosporins or penicillins and can be safely administered despite penicillin sensitivity.

SUGGESTED READINGS

Cunha BA. Antimicrobial selection in the penicillin-allergic patient. *Drugs Today (Barc)*. 2001;37(6):377–383.

BE EXTRA VIGILANT WITH CLOSE-SOUNDING DRUG NAMES

MONTY D. GROSS, PhD, RN, CNE

Medication errors are believed to be one of the most common causes of death resulting in less than 7,000 deaths and a significant number of permanently disabled individuals (Meadows, 2003). One source of medication errors is a result of administration of medications with similar sounding names for different drugs. Drug name similarity represents an extra concern at the end of a long hard shift. During this period, nurses are multitasking: responding to call bells, preparing report for the next shift, answering telephone calls from physicians and diagnostic labs, and attending family members seeking a patient's status and other updates. However, medications still need to be administered. When two drugs have similar names and similar routes of administration, it is especially easy to get confused. For example, both dobutamine and dopamine are often kept in the coronary care unit and infused simultaneously. Both the drugs are available in 250 mL bags at the same concentration and are administered by the same multichamber infusion pump at the same site. When the pump begins to beep, that is the time to change the bag with another 250 mL and ensure that you identify the right drug and connect it to the correct IV tubing.

Although medication errors are often viewed as a system wide issue (Crane & Crane, 2006), you need to remember to be extra vigilant when administering medications, especially when names of the medications are similar. At a quick glance at the label, both dobutamine and dopamine can appear the same. When your mind is racing with the other tasks you are also responsible to complete, it is hard to focus on just one task at a time. Medication administration is a task that should be the sole focus of your attention during the time when you go through the rights of medication administration.

First, ensure you have the right medication. Compare the medication label to the medication administration record (MAR) several times. Second, ensure you have the right patient. Check the room number, bed number, and client's identification band. Ask the patient to verbalize his or her name to you. Third, give the medication at the right time. In general, the time frame of medication that should be given is from 30 min before to 30 min after the time stated on the MAR. Fourth, administer the medication via the correct method or route. Fifth, administer the correct dose. Do the math. Have it double-checked for critical drugs such as insulin, potassium chloride, heparin, or other high alert drugs as specified by Joint Commission on the Accreditation of Healthcare Organizations (JCAHO) and hospital policy. Finally, remember to document your actions. This action communicates that the drug was indeed administered and reduces the chance that another nurse could inadvertently give a medication.

Medication errors are too common in hospitals. Focus your attention on medication administration instead of multitasking and remember to use the rights of medication administration.

SUGGESTED READINGS

Crane J, Crane FG. Preventing medication errors in hospitals through a systems approach and technological innovation: A prescription for 2010. *Hosp Top*. 2006;84(4):3–8.

Meadows M. Strategies to reduce medical errors. *FDA Cons*. 2003;37(3):20–27.

Smith S, Duell D, Martin B. *Clinical Nursing Skills: Basic to Advanced Skills*. Upper Saddle River, NJ: Pearson; 2008.

BEWARE OF DRUGS WITH SIMILAR-SOUNDING NAMES OR SIMILAR APPEARING PACKAGING

KATHERINE M. PENTURFF, RN, CAPA

WHAT TO DO: PLAN

A parent with small children would probably never store a bottle of brown-colored poison in the refrigerator next to a bottle of cola. However, medicines with names that sound alike or look alike are frequently stored side by side in medication cabinets, pharmacies, hospitals, and physician offices around the country, and errors when dispensing them can be just as fatal. Healthcare professionals who prescribe, dispense, or administer medications have likely encountered medication errors involving look-alike or sound-alike (LASA) drug names. LASA medication errors occur when drug products that look alike when poorly written in cursive, such as Avandia and Coumadin, or sound alike when spoken, for example, Flomax and Volmax, are confused for one another.

In an attempt to avoid sound-alike names in new drugs, the pharmaceutical industry uses testing protocols that incorporate practitioner testing and computer analysis. To minimize confusion between drug names that look or sound alike, the FDA reviews approximately 400 brand names a year before the drugs are marketed and about one third of these are rejected. Some examples of LASA drugs include Darvon/Diovan, Amaryl/Reminyl, Dilacor/Pilocar, amrinone/amiodarone, and fentanyl/sufentanil. Look-alike errors can also occur when LASA medications use similar bottle colors, label colors, and label designs (Fig. 27-1).

A number of efforts are underway to reduce the incidence of medical errors stemming from similar-looking or similar-sounding names. Joint Commission on the Accreditation of Healthcare Organizations (JCAHO) offers these general safety strategies to avoid mixing up LASA drugs:

- Be familiar with both JCAHO's LASA list and similar lists from other agencies.
- Determine the purpose of each medication before administering it.
- Note the use of boldface, color, or capital letters, which JCAHO calls "tall man" letters, to call attention to the difference between similar drug name (e.g., VinBLAStine and VinCRIStine).

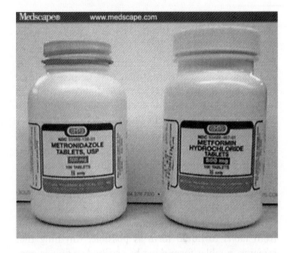

FIGURE 27.1. Look-alike labels for Metronidazole and Metformin.

- List both the generic and the brand names of a drug, whenever possible.
- Store drugs with similar names in different locations.

One of the last defenses against any kind of medication dispensing error is the patient. Patients should be informed regarding the purpose of each of their medications and what they look like, and they should be encouraged to ask questions regarding any medicine that does not look like or is not spelled like what they are accustomed to.

SUGGESTED READINGS

Drug mix-ups threaten patient safety. Available at: www.medscape.com/viewarticle/573465_2. Accessed March 31, 2009.

Metules T, Bauer J. JCAHO's patient safety goals, Part 2: Preventing med errors. Available at: http://rn.modern medicine.com/rnweb/article/articleDetail.jsp?id=394868. Accessed August 24, 2008.

Rados C. Drug name confusion: Preventing medication errors. *FDA Cons Mag.* Jul–Aug 2005;39(4). Available at: www.fda.gov/fdac/featu res/2005/405_confusion.html. Accessed March 31, 2009.

ADMINISTERING MEDICATION THROUGH A FEEDING TUBE

BONNIE L. PARKER, RN, CRRN

WHAT TO DO: IMPLEMENT

Feeding tubes are often seen in the acute care setting and come in many varieties; they may be placed either as nasogastric tubes (NG) or percutaneously placed tubes. There are a variety of sizes ranging from small bore tubes such as the Dobhoff and the red rubber jejunostomy tubes to larger tubes such as the gastrostomy tubes or the large bore NG tubes. They are used for patients who are unable to take nutrition or medication orally and may be in place for a few days, weeks, or years.

The first step in giving medications through any tube is to attempt to get as many medications converted from tablet to liquid form as possible. Anything that remains in tablet form must be crushed as fine as possible and dissolved in warm water. Medications that have lumps or sediment are more likely to clog the tube, especially the fine bore tubes. The greater the number of medications and the more often they are given, the greater the risk of clogging the feeding tube. It is important that the tube be thoroughly flushed with water after each use. When crushing medication, the container used for crushing the meds must be cleaned after each use and the nurse must wash her hands to avoid contamination with other medications. Often medications are not compatible with one another in dissolved form and should be crushed, dissolved, and given separately with a flush between each. It should be kept in mind that enteric coated pills and time-released medications should not be crushed and cannot be given through feeding tubes. Doing so could cause the patient to receive too large a dose of medication too quickly.

The pharmacy should be consulted regarding medications that should be given on an empty stomach and for determining how long any tube feeding that the patient may be receiving should be stopped before and after giving the medication. Some tube feeding formulas may interfere with certain medications.

For medication administration, the patient should be in an upright position and remain upright for at least 30 min after the medications are given. Stop tube feeding if it is infusing and access the feeding tube with a 60 mL syringe; check tube placement and residual. Remove the plunger from the syringe and insert the tip into the feeding tube. Flush the tube with 30 mL of water, pour the dissolved medication into the syringe and allow it to flow slowly into the feeding tube.

If giving more than one medication, flush between each drug with a small amount of warm water. When all of the medication has been instilled, flush the tube with at least 30 mL of warm water. Instilling cold liquids into a feeding tube can cause abdominal cramping and should be avoided. Remember to chart the amount of fluids used on the patient's Intake and Output totals.

If the feeding tube is becoming sluggish or difficult to flush, attempt to instill some warm water or carbonated beverage. Allow them to sit in the tube for 20 min and then flush. This procedure may need to be repeated several times. If the tube is still not patent, an order from the physician for pancreatic enzymes may need to be obtained. The enzymes should be crushed, mixed with 5 mL of warm water, and instilled according to the facility protocol. If the tube still remains clogged, it will need to be replaced.

SUGGESTED READINGS

McConnell E. Administering medication through a gastrostomy tube. *Nursing*. 2002;32(120):22.

Prosser B. Common issues in PEG tubes—what every fellow should know. *Gastrointest Endosc*. 2006;64(6):970–972.

PRECIPITATE IN THE SYRINGE IS A WARNING SIGN NOT TO GIVE THE MEDICATION!

BONNIE L. PARKER, RN, CRRN

WHAT TO DO: IMPLEMENT

Safe medication administration requires a nurse to use her skills, knowledge, and attention. Many medical mistakes involve medication, and hence it is important for a nurse not only to ensure that she is administering the right medication to the right patient but also to be aware that one medication can accidentally be given with another incompatible one. Many medications are incompatible with each other, which affects their efficacy and side effect profiles.

This issue is most serious with medication administered intravenously (IV). Since IV medications create immediate results, the adverse responses also occur more rapidly and dramatically. Great care must be taken that the medications given through the same lumen of an IV be compatible. Every medication administration environment should have an IV drug compatibility chart, a drug book, or computer reference readily available to check drug compatibility. Any outstanding questions of compatibility should be referred to a pharmacist. When administering a medication through the port of an IV line, the nurse should watch for any signs of incompatibility such as precipitate, bubbles, cloudiness, or color change. Occasionally, color change could be a normal and expected result of drug administration. A pharmacist should be contacted if an unexpected color change is detected.

Maintenance IV fluids containing electrolytes are often incompatible with other drugs. To administer medications in these lines, stop the infusion, flush the line before and after the administration, and then restart the infusion. Many hospitals have a list of medications that are not to be mixed with other drugs such as heparin, Dilantin, Lasix, or diazepam. It is also not recommended to mix anything with TPN because of the electrolyte concentration, viscosity, and the increased risk of infection.

Some medications are given frequently enough to be considered routine, such as antiemetics or pain medications. These drugs, such as Phenergan or morphine, are at a high risk for syringe or line incompatibility. For example, Toradol, ordered frequently as a postoperative analgesic, may accidentally be mixed in the same syringe with Phenergan. The result is a thick, white substance that would not be able to be administered through the syringe. These drugs should be given separately with the line flushed between doses.

SUGGESTED READINGS

Rosenthal K. Preventing IV drug incompatibilities. In: *IV Therapy Made Incredibly Easy*. 3rd Ed. Philadelphia: Lippincott Williams & Wilkins; 2006.

Rosenthal K. Avoiding common perils of drug administration. *Nursing*. 2007;37(4):20.

DRUGS WITH A NARROW THERAPEUTIC INDEX ARE AFFECTED BY CHANGES IN DIET, HEALTH CONDITION, OR OTHER MEDICATIONS AND NEED TO BE MONITORED CAREFULLY

KATHERINE M. PENTURFF, RN, CAPA

WHAT TO DO: ASSESS

When a patient is admitted to the hospital, especially in an emergency, there may be a delay from the time he is admitted until his medication history is obtained. Delays may continue until the medication list is reconciled and the patient's usual medications are resumed, provided that they are continued at all while the patient is hospitalized. The hospitalized patient also frequently experiences a major change in dietary intake. These changes in routine can upset the fine balance often needed in maintaining some medications within a therapeutic range. When medications such as warfarin, digoxin, and phenytoin are not maintained within a therapeutic range, not only are they not providing the benefit to the patient as intended but they may also have dangerous or even fatal side effects.

Warfarin (Coumadin) is indicated for the prophylaxis or the treatment of venous thrombosis and thromboembolic complications due to atrial fibrillation or cardiac valve replacement and to reduce the risk of death, recurrent MI, or stroke following a myocardial infarction. The dose is individualized for each patient based on the patient's PT/INR levels and the therapeutic range varies depending on the indication for use. Warfarin has a narrow therapeutic index, and blood levels may be dramatically altered if a patient starts, stops, or changes any medication or if he experiences a sudden change in diet, especially eating or stopping foods rich in vitamin K. Even weight loss can affect the amount of drug needed to maintain therapeutic levels. Inadequate dosing can result in a thrombotic event; toxicity can result in hemorrhage.

Digoxin (Cardoxin, Digitek, Lanoxicaps, and Lanoxin) is one of the cardiac glycosides used in the treatment of mild to moderate heart failure and for the control of ventricular response rate in patients with chronic atrial fibrillation. Recommended dosages of digoxin require titration because of the individual sensitivity of the patient to the drug, the presence of associated conditions, and the use of other medications. The dose of digoxin prescribed is based on clinical grounds; however, measurement of serum digoxin concentrations can be helpful in determining the adequacy of digoxin therapy. Digoxin toxicity can be caused by high levels of digoxin in the body or by a decreased tolerance to the drug. Patients with decreased tolerance may experience digoxin toxicity even though they have digoxin levels within the defined normal limits. Symptoms of toxicity can include visual changes, nausea, vomiting, confusion, loss of appetite, and irregular or slow pulse.

Phenytoin (Dilantin) is an anticonvulsant that is indicated for the control of generalized tonic-clonic and complex partial seizures and the prevention and treatment of seizures occurring during or following neurosurgery. The dosing of phenytoin is very individualized, and the drug may be administered once, twice, or thrice daily. The optimal dosage is often based on the therapeutic blood levels. Phenytoin's metabolism may be affected by many other drugs, such as phenobarbitol, amiodarone, cimetidine, omeprazole, paroxetine, and fluoxetine, and its absorption is reduced by taking it with antacids or enteral feedings. Symptoms of toxicity include slurred speech, lethargy, rapid eye movement, confusion, low blood pressure, and hallucinations, but it is rarely fatal.

SUGGESTED READINGS

Digitalis toxicity. Available at: www.drugs.com/enc/digitalis-toxicity. html. Accessed August 24, 2008.

Lanoxin, RxList—the Internet Drug Index (Professionals), Copyright © 2008 by RxList Inc. Available at: www.rxlist. com/cgi/generic/dig_ids.htm. Accessed August 24, 2008.

Medline Plus. Coumadin. Trusted health information for you. 2007. Available at: www.rxlist.com/cgi/generic/warfarin_ids. htm. Accessed August 24, 2008.

Monson K, Schoenstadt A. Dilantin toxicity. 2007. MedTV. Available at: http://epilepsy.emedtv.com/dilantin/dilantin-toxicity-p2. html. Accessed August 24, 2008.

PATIENT-CONTROLLED ANALGESIC PUMP SETTINGS REQUIRE INDEPENDENT TWO-NURSE VERIFICATION

MARY S. WARD, RN, BS, OCN

WHAT TO DO: IMPLEMENT

Patient-controlled analgesia (PCA) pumps are utilized for delivery of narcotic analgesia that allows for continuous infusion of pain medication and bolus control by the patient for breakthrough pain. While common in postoperative settings and in areas of pain management, these pumps are employed throughout the inpatient hospital setting. Syed et al. (2006) highlighted 17 independent potential human-related errors in PCA administration. These errors range from inappropriate tubing attachment to pharmacy dispensing, but by far, the most common area for error is the programming of the pump by the nurse. The Institute for Safe Medication Practices (ISMP) made multiple recommendations based on cases of fatal or near fatal overdoses of opiates to patients related to programming errors and other problems associated with these pumps.

The first and most important recommendation is that the nurse who programs the pump must be educated on its use. PCA pumps utilized in many settings today are complex computers offering many choices of settings to the nurse. A practitioner who uses the equipment without proper training puts the patient at risk. Errors can occur in choosing the wrong drug, the wrong concentration of drug, the wrong rate for a continuous infusion, the wrong bolus for a PCA infusion, a miscalculated or omitted lockout, or lockout interval. Many pumps offer choices during the set up process; the wrong choice, off by one decimal point, can significantly underdose or overdose the patient. Underdosing the patient leads to inadequate pain relief that may lead to more errors if the misprogrammed pump is used by another nurse for bolus dosing.

ISMP made several recommendations to avoid these potentially fatal errors. Protocols and standard order sets can significantly reduce the amount of confusion and misread orders. Decreasing the number of choices on the pumps for the different drugs, stocking only one concentration of a particular drug, and using the warnings on smart pumps will also decrease potential errors. The proactive measure that all institutions and all individual nurses can perform is an independent double-check system prior to starting any PCA infusion. This check should include the drug, concentration, continuous infusion, and PCA bolus with any lockout intervals. This check should be made against the original physician orders and signed by the nurses who verify them. The actual cartridge in the machine should be viewed by the nurses doing the verification to confirm that the syringe in the pump matches the concentration on the setting. Each time a new caregiver assumes care of the patient, these settings should be reverified and documented. This double-check should also be done any time a change is made to the PCA settings.

Opiate toxicity is potentially lethal and is definitely preventable. Patients on PCAs should be closely monitored and nurses should obtain and maintain competence for the equipment they use to ensure their patient's safety.

SUGGESTED READINGS

Institute for Safe Medication Practices. Misprogram a PCA pump? It's easy! *ISMP Newslett.* July 29, 2004. Available at: http://www.ismp.org/Newsletters/acutecare/articles/20040729_2.asp. Accessed April 3, 2008.

Institute for Safe Medication Practices. More on avoiding opiate toxicity with PCA by proxy. *ISMP Newslett.* May 29, 2002. Available at: http://www.ismp.org/Newsletters/acutecare/articles/20020529.asp. Accessed April 3, 2008.

Syed S, Paul JE, Hueftlein M, et al. Morphine overdose from error propagation on an acute pain service. *Can J Anesth.* 2006;53(6):586–590.

Vicente K, Kada-Bekhaled K, Hillel G, et al. Programming errors contribute to death from patient-controlled analgesia: Case report and estimate of probability. *Can J Anesth.* 2003;50(44):328–332.

Hydromorphone IV concentration is up to seven times that of IV morphine

Mary S. Ward, RN, BS, OCN

WHAT TO DO: PLAN

Nurses caring for patients with acute and chronic pain face many challenges. Pain assessment is now widely considered the fifth vital sign and pain management is considered a patient right by many hospital standards. Morphine has long been considered the standard against which narcotic concentrations are measured. Hydromorphone is a synthetic derivative of morphine and both drugs are used for the control of acute and chronic pain. Morphine and hydromorphone are prescribed for patient-controlled analgesia pumps, intermittent IV push, and for oral administration. However, the strengths of the drugs are quite different.

The Institute for Safe Medication Practices (ISMP) has reported many medication errors related to confusion in morphine/hydromorphone administration. There are several identified factors that lead to this risk. The most obvious is the similarity in their names. Name confusion has led to several documented medication errors. The ISMP has made a formal recommendation that the name be changed. All facilities should make certain that, minimally, hydromorphone be identified with tall man lettering—hydromorPHONE. The name preference should be Dilaudid to reduce confusion altogether. The potency of IV Dilaudid is seven to eight times that of IV morphine and oral Dilaudid is approximately four times more potent than oral morphine. A patient who mistakenly receives 10 mg of IV Dilaudid instead of 10 mg of IV morphine will receive the equivalent of 70–80 mg of IV morphine. For an opioid naïve patient in particular, this dosing may be fatal.

Another reason nurses may mistake Dilaudid for morphine is that they are frequently stocked in the same strengths in the same medication dispensing areas. Even when mechanisms such as barcodes are in place, many hospital systems have override capabilities that allow nurses to administer medications in emergent situations with a physician's order. It is highly recommended that hospitals not stock the same strengths of both drugs in same areas and that if an additional strength of one drug is needed, it be dispensed individually from the pharmacy.

Finally, nurses who lack education regarding equianalgesic dosing are also at a high risk for medication error with these drugs. When a patient requires an opiate switch from morphine to Dilaudid, the nurse is responsible for being aware of at least an approximate amount that the patient would require for adequate pain management without risking overdosing the patient or putting him or her into respiratory depression, cardiac arrest, or even a fatal event. The nurse can consult an equianalgesic chart, such as Table 32-1, to evaluate the morphine dose the patient is getting and determine if the dose of Dilaudid is approximately equivalent. If the nurse is unsure, the pharmacy should be contacted for consultation. Any dose above 4 mg IV push of Dilaudid should be verified with a second practitioner.

TABLE 32.1	OPIOID EQUIANALGESIC DOSES	
ORAL (MG)	DRUG	PARENTERAL (MG)
30	Morphine	10
20	Oxycodone	N/A
7.5	Hydromorphone	1.5
N/A	Fentanyl	0.1 (100 mcg)
200	Codeine	130
20	Hydrocodone	N/A

SUGGESTED READINGS

Armstrong SC, Cozza KL. Pharmacokinetic drug interactions of morphine, codeine, and their derivatives: Theory and clinical reality, Part 1. *Psychosomatics*. 2003;44(2):167–171.

ISMP Medication Safety Alert. An omnipresent risk of Morphine–Hydromorphone mix-ups. July 1, 2004. Available at: http://www.ismp.org/Newsletters/acutecare/articles/20040701.asp. Accessed April 3, 2008.

33

ADMINISTERING MONOCLONAL ANTIBODIES? KNOW THE SIGNS OF HYPERSENSITIVITY

MARY S. WARD, RN, BS, OCN

WHAT TO DO: ASSESS

Monoclonal antibodies are molecules that have been developed in the treatment of cancer and autoimmune disease. Their mechanisms of action vary from inducing direct cell death, or apoptosis, to "tagging" target cells and stimulating the body's own immune system against the offending cells and directing complement-mediated cell destruction. Each antibody is cell-determinant (CD) antigen specific. Monoclonal antibodies have given physicians a new category of weapons in the arsenal to fight many diseases including cancer, rheumatoid arthritis, Crohn disease, and many other autoimmune and neurologic diseases. New applications of existing drugs are ongoing and new drugs in this class are in development. This is a class of drug with many possibilities.

These drugs are not without their own complexities. Unlike many drugs that are used in cancer therapy, monoclonal antibodies do not have the common side effect profiles of many antineoplastic drugs: granulocytopenia, alopecia, nausea, vomiting, and diarrhea. However, monoclonal antibodies do present the practitioner with one challenge: as a group, they have a significant degree of infusion complications. More specifically, according to the National Cancer Institute's terminology criteria, these drugs cause acute infusion reactions. Nurses know that any drug, particularly drugs given intraparenterally, can potentially cause patient reactions. Most of these reactions are commonly referred to as hypersensitivity reactions or allergic reactions and are mediated by IgE antibodies initiated after the patient has had several exposures to a medication. Mild reactions of this type produce rashes, itching, drug fever, and flushing. More severe reactions induce bronchospasms, edema, hypotension, anaphylaxis, and even death. On the contrary, acute infusion reactions are prompted by cytokine release typically tumor necrosis factor-α and interleukins. These reactions can look very similar but onset is prompted by the initial infusion of a medication, usually within the first 30–120 min of the first infusion. Symptoms can range from those that are similar to allergic/hypersensitivity reaction symptoms of pruritus and rash to rigors, chills, headache, abdominal pain and cramping, nausea, vomiting, diarrhea, dizziness, hypotension or hypertension, tachycardia, and diaphoresis.

When a patient experiences any kind of hypersensitivity reaction, the first response of the nurse should be to stop the infusion. Maintain the line for treatment and expect to administer medications such as histamine blockers, diphenydramine, cimetidine, acetaminophen, steroids, and possibly bronchodilators. When the symptoms have subsided, the infusion may be restarted at half the rate depending on the drug and severity of symptoms.

The best treatment for infusion-related reactions, however, is prevention. Nurses who are aware that the drugs they are administering have the infusion reaction potential should also be prepared to administer prophylactic medications, such as acetaminophen, diphenydramine, and possibly a steroid, prior to the infusion. Patients who have a history of allergy to food or medications are at an increased risk for infusion reactions and all patients should be carefully monitored throughout infusions and afterward for delayed cytokine reactions. Vital signs should be taken note of frequently. It is essential that the administering nurse be alert for any sign of infusion reaction; no two patients are alike; signs of infusion reaction vary widely and prompt intervention is vital.

SUGGESTED READINGS

Gobel BH. Chemotherapy-induced hypersensitivity reactions. *Oncol Nurs Forum.* 2005;32(5):1027–1035.
Lenz H-J. Management and preparedness for infusion and hypersensitivity reactions. *The Oncologist.* 2007;12:601–609.
Winkler U, Jensen M, Manzke O, et al. Cytokine-release syndrome in patients with B-cell chronic lymphocytic leukemia and high lymphocyte counts after treatment with an anti-CD20 monoclonal antibody. *Blood.* 1999;94(7):2217–2224.

DON'T FORGET TO CALCULATE DOSE CONCENTRATIONS WHEN CALCULATING RITUXAN TITRATIONS

MARY S. WARD, RN, BS, OCN

WHAT TO DO: IMPLEMENT

Rituxamab, or Rituxan, is a chimeric monoclonal antibody used principally in cancer treatment, but FDA also approved it for rheumatoid arthritis therapy. The typical dose for cancer treatment is $375 \, mg/m^2$ given alone or in combination with chemotherapy for the management of non–Hodgkin B–cell lymphomas. Rituxan targets the over expressed CD20 antigen on those cells. Chimeric antibodies contain a murine component derived from mouse or hamster antibodies that causes the large percentage of acute infusion-related reactions noted with Rituxan administration, especially during the first administration. Thirty to seventy percent of patients receiving Rituxan experience some type of infusion-related symptoms ranging from headache, hypotension, fever, rigors, chill, abdominal pain and cramping, nausea, diarrhea, rash to anaphylaxis. These symptoms may be significantly reduced with prophylactic medication administration of acetaminophen and diphenhydramine.

One of the significant challenges for the nurse administering Rituxan is dose calculation. The administering guidelines require that the first dose be started at $50 \, mg/mL$ for 30 min. If the patient tolerates this well, the infusion is titrated by $50 \, mg/mL$ every 30 minutes to a maximum dose of $400 \, mg/mL$. The patient should be monitored at each titration for symptoms of infusion reaction and vital sign changes. If the patient tolerates the first infusion with no difficulties, the second and subsequent infusions may be started at $100 \, mg/mL$ with titrations of $100 \, mg/mL$ every 30 min to the maximum of $400 \, mg/mL$.

The titrations and monitoring of the patient are a challenge, and this is further complicated by mixing guidelines, which state that Rituxan may be mixed in a concentration of $1–4 \, mg/mL$. Therefore, the first calculation the nurse is required to perform is the calculation of the drug concentration of the infusion bag. For example, for a patient with a BSA of $2.0 \, m^2$, the drug dose is $750 \, mg$. If this is mixed in a $250 \, mL$ bag, the drug concentration is $3 \, mg/mL$. If this is the patient's first infusion, the rate would be $16.6 \, mL/h$. The same drug amount could be mixed in a larger volume of $500 \, mL$, yielding a drug concentration of $1.5 \, mg/mL$ and increasing the infusion rate to $33.3 \, mL/h$.

The same drug amount in these same bags could be started at twice the rates if this is not the patient's first infusion and as long as he has tolerated his first infusion without difficulty. In the first example, a $100 \, mg/mL$ rate would be $33.3 \, mL/h$ and in the second, a $100 \, mL/h$ rate would be $66.6 \, mL/h$.

It should be emphasized that this step of calculating drug concentration should not be overlooked by the administering nurse. Assuming a concentration or standardizing a starting rate may result in too rapid an infusion of drug, which could result in Rituxan toxicities. If, for example, a nurse decides to start Rituxan infusions at 25 or $50 \, mL/h$ and increase in 25 or $50 \, mL/h$ increments, it would not take many dose adjustments at 3 or $4 \, mg/mL$ concentrations to reach or exceed the manufacturer's guidelines. The only time standardizing a rate is acceptable would be if the pharmacy has standardized mixing guidelines with an accompanying titration schedule for the drug and this is understood between pharmacy and nursing.

If a patient exhibits signs of acute infusion reaction, the nurse should discontinue the infusion and anticipate administering medications such as acetaminophen, diphenhydramine, and possibly steroids and bronchodilators. When the symptoms of the reaction subside, the infusion may be restarted at half the rate at which it was stopped.

It should be noted that Rituxan has black box warnings; significantly, pulmonary toxicities, and that too rapid infusions of the drug may put the patient at risk for the development of these toxicities. Careful calculations and monitoring of the patient during infusion are necessary to decrease these risks.

SUGGESTED READINGS

Lenz H-J. Management and preparedness for infusion and hypersensitivity reactions. *The Oncologist*. 2007;12:601–609.

Rituximab. DynaMed. Available at: www.dynaweb.ebscohost.com/Detail.aspx?id=233544&sid=61556d. Accessed April 24, 2008.

Second nurse verification of dose and rate is a simple, cost-effective measure to reduce medication errors with high risk drugs

Mary S. Ward, RN, BS, OCN

WHAT TO DO: PLAN

Medications that top the Institute for Safe Medication Practices' (ISMP) *High-Alert Medications* list are those with narrow safety margins and great risk potential for patient harm and include drugs in classes such as adrenergic agonist/antagonists, antiarrhythmics, antithrombotics, chemotherapy, inatropics, narcotics/opiates, neuromuscular blocking agents, and TPN. Patients in ICUs are at a high risk for medication errors with these classes of drugs; it is suggested that for an ICU patient, 1 in 10 infusions is either prepared or administered in error. The majority of the errors are administration errors. But patients don't have to be in ICU to receive TPN, chemotherapy, anticoagulant therapy, or IV narcotics. The potential for error with these medications exists in all areas of patient care where these drugs are administered. Errors range from misconnected IV tubing to wrong dose, wrong time, omitted dose, physiochemical incompatibilities, and wrong infusion rate.

Research and new technology developments have decreased the likelihood of medication error. Computer-based prescriber order entry (CPOE), bar coding of medications, medication reconciliation processes, and "smart pump" technology have all contributed to reducing medication error and adverse medication events. For the administering nurse, pumps with built-in drug libraries that have soft and hard "Guardrail" dose limits alert the operator when administration limits have been exceeded. Soft limits give an alert that can be bypassed once the message screen is acknowledged. The hard limit cannot be bypassed and the pump must be reprogrammed to operate.

Some drugs may have titration and dosing parameters that fall within the hard limits of the drug libraries but could still potentially be harmful to a patient. Patients who are on an unfractionated heparin drip protocol for deep venous thrombosis, for example, may be on this infusion for several days. This may involve a complex protocol with PTT draws timed at 6 h intervals, weight-based dose adjustments, and bolus heparin injections that are calculated and adjusted according to the PTT results. Small miscalculations or pump maladjustments can accumulate over a period of days and contribute to greater patient harm.

Chemotherapy is also on the ISMP's list of high-alert medications and oncology nurses are acutely aware of the high risk nature of these drugs due to individual dose calculations and pump settings. Some of the drugs are titrated as well, a characteristic shared by other drugs on ISMP's list. Some of the recommendations that The Oncology Nursing Society has made to reduce the risk of chemotherapy medication error may be employed in other settings to reduce the risk of error with High-Alert medications from other classes of drugs.

One recommendation is to have independent second nurse verification for the dose calculation. In the case of heparin administration, having a second nurse verify the weight-based dose is an assurance that the first nurse is correctly calculating the dose, especially true if the weight was obtained in pounds instead of kilograms. Verifying the weight in pounds, which needs to be divided by 2.2 lb/kg instead of multiplying by 2.2 lb/kg, is an important distinction. The second verification should be of the initial bolus dose and the initial rate of the infusion. Once the pump is set, a verification of the pump settings should also be done. This step is critically important and should not be overlooked. Smart pump technology is only as smart as the person programming the pump, and human programming error accounts for the majority of medication errors resulting in incorrect infusion rates or incorrect doses.

It should be emphasized that these verification steps by a second nurse must be done independently from the first nurse. The checks should not be done "over the shoulder" of the first nurse as it can lead to an inherent prejudicial prejudgment of the information. This second nurse verification should also be implemented any time a change is made to the infusion: change in dose or infusion rate. It is not necessary to have a verification when hanging a new bag unless changes are made to the pump settings. All verifications should be noted on the patient's medical record.

Medication errors are a preventable hospital safety issue. They occur in up to 19% of all hospitalized patients. Nurses are busy and most medication errors tend to occur during the busiest times of the day, when nurses are fatigued, or when there is short staffing. However, taking the time to make a quick double-check of the medication infusion dosage and rates that have the highest potential for error can reduce the rates of error and the adverse medication events that result from them.

SUGGESTED READINGS

Fanikos J, Flumara K, Baroletti S, et al. Impact of smart infusion technology on administration of anticoagulants (Unfractionated Heparin, Argatroban, Lepirudin, and Bivalirudin). *Am J Cardiol.* 2007;99(7):1002–1005.

Institute of Safe Medication Practices. *ISMP's List of High-Alert Medications.* 2008. Available at: www.ismp.org. Accessed May 10, 2008.

Kane-Gill S, Webber RJ. Principles and practices of medication safety in the ICU. *Crit Care Clin.* 2006;22(2):273–290.

Keohane CA, Bates DW. Medication safety. *Obstet Gynecol Clin.* 2008;35(1):37–52.

Always use two patient identifiers prior to administering medications

Julie Mulligan Watts, RN, MN

WHAT TO DO: PLAN

As the cost of healthcare goes up and reports of mismanagement, waste, and errors appear in the national media, the public has begun demanding better quality of healthcare. Medical errors are common and are very costly to our society. The Institute of Medicine (IOM) drew attention to medical errors in a series of articles about the state of the U.S. healthcare system. In a far-reaching plan, the IOM proposed strategies to reduce medical errors. This plan affects caregivers, health institutions, governmental agencies, and regulatory bodies.

In order to decrease errors caused by improper identification of patients, the Joint Commission on the Accreditation of Healthcare Organizations (JCAHO) has required healthcare organizations to comply with National Patient Safety Goals (NPSGs). One recommendation includes the use of two methods of identifying patients when performing procedures and administering medications. The JCAHO requires that at least two patient identifiers (neither of which may be the patient's room number) be used whenever administering medications or blood products, taking blood samples, or providing other treatments and procedures. The intent of this recommendation is to ensure that the correct patient receives the medication or procedure.

Some of the most common ways of identifying patients to become compliant with the regulation are through asking the patient's name, asking for identifying information, and checking the patient's identification bracelet. Patient identifiers can include the patient name, birthday, assigned ID number, photograph, or bar coding. The verification of the two identifiers should take place before a procedure is started and before any medication is given. The patient identifiers can vary based on where the patient is treated in a health organization. For example, the inpatient unit may use a bar-coded armband whereas the blood bank may use a separate armband specific to the blood bank.

Approximately, 14% of chemotherapy errors involve patient identification. Outpatient areas and ambulatory treatment areas may pose a challenge because sometimes outpatients do not wear armbands. Patients and family members may come in and out of busy waiting rooms during long treatments. Wait times may be long and patients may become impatient. While waiting for chemotherapy treatments in a crowded outpatient clinic, patients have been known to answer to other patients' names when called for treatment. Some patients want to receive their treatment faster and others think that all the treatments are the same, so they answer to an incorrect name. Nurses need to remember the recommendations of the JCAHO and use the two recommended methods of identifying patients prior to administering medications, especially in a crowded, sometimes confusing, clinical setting. Patients can use their name, social security number, date of birth, or any other information included on their chart as their identification information. The incorporation of these safety principles will ensure that the correct patients receive the correct treatments.

SUGGESTED READINGS

Catalano K, Fickenscher K. Complying with the 2008 national patient safety goals. *AORN J.* 2008;87(3):547–555.

Kohn L, Corrigan J, Donaldson M, eds. *To Err is Human: Building a Safer Health System.* Washington, DC: National Academies Press; 1999.

Schulmeister L. Chemotherapy medication errors: Descriptions, severity, and contributing factors. *Oncol Nurs Forum* 1999;26:1033–1042.

The Joint Commission on the Accreditation of Healthcare Organizations. *Meeting the Joint Commission's 2008 National Patient Safety Goals.* Oakbrook Terrace, IL: Joint Commission Resources Inc; 2007.

KNOW HOW TO TREAT HYPOGLYCEMIA IN YOUR DIABETIC PATIENTS

FRANCINE B. YATES, RRT, RN, BSN

WHAT TO DO: IMPLEMENT

Diabetes is becoming a more common illness in the United States. With greater numbers of people chronically living with diabetes, it is essential that nurses in all inpatient settings become competent in the care of the diabetic patient. An ongoing complication that diabetic patients may experience is low blood glucose levels or hypoglycemia.

Hypoglycemia is defined as a blood glucose level of less than 50 mg/dl and can occur when an individual takes too much insulin or other hypoglycemic medications or after a strenuous workout while not correctly balancing either the medications or the energy output with diet intake. It can occur at anytime of the day or night and symptoms may occur suddenly and without warning. Signs and symptoms of hypoglycemia include sweating, tachycardia, nervousness, hunger, and occasional palpitations. Other signs and symptoms are headache, inability to concentrate, confusion, slurred speech and numbness and tingling in the lips and tongue, emotional changes, and erratic behavior.

A hypoglycemic patient must be treated immediately and an observant nurse will recognize the signs and symptoms quickly and respond appropriately. In some cases, the patients may not be able to speak and, if they do, it may not make sense. Treatment for hypoglycemia is to supplement the patient with a source of sugar; if they can follow commands, fruit juice or regular soda, hard candies, or two teaspoons of sugar or honey may be administered. If the patient is unable to swallow and has a patent IV, then one ampule of D50 is usually sufficient to raise the blood glucose.

It is important, however, to always remember the five rights of medication administration even with juice or soda. That is, if juice or soda is part of the hypoglycemic orders, the nurse should ensure that they are never given through an IV site—this would destroy the vein and surrounding tissue and seriously harm the patient. Also, remember that if hard candy or lifesavers are administered, the patient must be alert enough not to choke on them.

All nurses, new graduates and seasoned nurses, should develop and maintain the competencies and resources to care for and educate their diabetic patients. Nurses who anticipate caring for diabetic patients may consider precepting on a diabetic unit or obtaining continuing education credits in diabetic management to enhance their knowledge of these complex patients.

SUGGESTED READINGS

Greene H, Ruiter HP, Atkins N, et al. Diabetes expertise: A subspecialty on a general medical unit. *Medsurg Nurs.* 2002;11(6):281–288.

Smeltzer SC, Bare BG. Assessment and management of patients with diabetes mellitus. In: *Brunner & Suddarth's Textbook of Medical-Surgical Nursing.* 9th Ed. Baltimore: Lippincott Williams & Wilkins; 1999, pp. 973–1025.

ALL IV ELECTROLYTE REPLACEMENT THERAPY SHOULD BE INFUSED VIA PUMP

FRANCINE B. YATES, RRT, RN, BSN

WHAT TO DO: IMPLEMENT

During a hospital admission, patients often suffer from disruptions in electrolyte balance of key electrolytes such as sodium, potassium, calcium, magnesium, phosphorous, and chloride. Because each electrolyte has essential functions within the body, it is important that these imbalances be corrected to protect the patient's health and safety. Disruptions of electrolyte levels, either too high or too low, can have serious effects on the function of already impaired organs and systems.

It is important to identify the underlying cause of the imbalance so that it too can be corrected. Conditions such as burns, chronic medical conditions, renal failure, trauma, heart failure, poor diet, improper fluid intake, and medications can all be sources of electrolyte imbalance. Once the imbalance and underlying cause or causes are identified, they can be treated appropriately. If the imbalance is mild, a few changes in diet and nutrition may be all that is necessary to move in the right direction. If the disorder is more severe, supplements, either oral or IV, may be given. IV replacement therapy of electrolytes is typically reserved for patients with significant electrolyte imbalance or who are exhibiting signs and symptoms of serious electrolyte imbalances. Patients receiving electrolyte replacement treatment will need to be monitored closely during the infusions.

It is important to note that when electrolytes are replaced intravenously, they must always be infused by an infusion pump and should be administered slowly and not as an IV push bolus. If administered too rapidly, they can cause an imbalance in the opposite direction, leading to a rapid elevation of the serum levels and an excess of the electrolyte. This can be life threatening for the patient; therefore, it is important to closely monitor patients for arrhythmias, neurologic disorders, tetany, EKG changes, or other signs of electrolyte imbalance.

Excessively high levels of electrolytes can be as dangerous as having levels that are too low and treatments to lower electrolyte levels may require longer periods of time or the infusion of other electrolytes. For example, if serum potassium levels are dangerously high, it may be necessary to give calcium IV which antagonizes the action of potassium on the heart.

The nurse who is caring for patients receiving electrolyte replacement therapies should maintain focus on a few essentials. All IV electrolyte replacements should be administered slowly by infusion pump and not as IV push bolus. The second point to remember is that patients need to be monitored closely during replacement therapies and part of that monitoring should include serum levels that will need to be drawn to monitor the electrolyte levels; the results of these should be read and analyzed prior to administering subsequent doses of the replacement therapy. If a physician prescribes oral supplements to be taken, it is important that patients have their serum levels drawn periodically to make certain that they need to continue taking the supplement. Finally, the patient receiving an electrolyte infusion should be monitored for vital signs, respiratory status, EKG changes, arrhythmias, and neurologic status. Electrolyte imbalances can harm a patient, but replacing them inappropriately can do more harm.

SUGGESTED READINGS

Smeltzer SC, Bare BG. Fluid and electrolytes: Balances and disturbances. In: *Brunner & Suddarth's Textbook of Medical-Surgical Nursing*. 9th Ed. Baltimore: Lippincott Williams & Wilkins; 1999, pp. 211–229, 973–1025.

ALWAYS CHECK THE MEDICATION PACKAGE NAME THREE TO FOUR TIMES BEFORE GIVING THE MEDICATION TO YOUR PATIENT

FRANCINE B. YATES, RRT, RN, BSN

WHAT TO DO: PLAN

Nurses wear many different hats when practicing bedside nursing and one of the main hats that means the most to our patients is the "dispenser of medications." Our patients may appreciate our kind and gentle ways; they may relax when we speak warmly and kindly with them; and they may smile at our clever sense of humor and the funny phrases printed on one of our pins chosen carefully just for this response; but they do trust us completely when we bring them their medications. We have all heard stories of patients simply taking the blue pill without questioning because their nurse gave it to them and then suffering a terrible reaction from a medication because it was not the right one. Do not let this happen to your patients.

Check your medication package three times before you give the medication and once more before you toss the packaging into the trash. Large facilities usually have some sort of computerized dispensing machine to aid in the prevention of medication administration errors by assisting up-front—you type in the patient's name and the patient's ordered medications appear; you choose one and the drawer pops open. There are a few hospitals that continue to dispense a patient's medications to his or her own bin.

Regardless of where your facility stores patient medications, train yourself to the following:

Check No. 1: Read the name on the sealed packaging of the medication as you are physically removing it from its storage place. It is not outside of human nature to load a drawer with wrong medications or reach into the drawer or bin right next to the intended one or return a medication to a wrong slot.

Check No. 2: Take the packaged medication to the patient's chart and compare the drug name and dosage with the written order or the Medication Administration Record (MAR). Learn or reteach yourself not to break the packaging while at the Nurses' Station or in the Med Room and drop the medication into a pill cup. Instead, carry the packaged medication to the patient's bedside.

Check No. 3: After checking two identifiers on the patient's ID armband with the patient's MAR that you carried in with you, *read the packaged medication name aloud from the package* to the patient and explain what the medicine is and does—do not just wave the package in the air and speak from memory. This would negate the check step. Read and say to the patient, "Mrs. Jones, this is Inderal. It is a blood pressure medication." This check prevents the possible error in two ways: (1) it provides you with another opportunity to know that the medication you are holding in your hands is the medication you intended to bring to the patient and (2) it gives the knowledgeable patient—if conscious and coherent—valuable information that she could use to let you know she is or is not supposed to have a blood pressure medication. (If the patient is unconscious or incoherent, the statement of the medication name and action still serves as an extra precaution for your own consciousness.) There are many medication errors that could have been prevented if the patient had known to ask or the nurse had initially offered the name and the action of the medication the patient was about to consume. In addition, never argue with a patient who tells you he is not supposed to receive that medication. Apologize and reassure him you will go back and check again. This is a very minor inconvenience to arrest the possibility of incorrectly medicating your patient.

Check No. 4: Read the package one last time before you dispose of it. It is a good habit. Reassure yourself one last time that the medication you intended to give is the one you just watched the patient take. If, after the above checks, you discover that it is the wrong drug or dose, you will know and be able to quickly attain new orders—possibly before a severe reaction occurs.

SUGGESTED READINGS

Roach S, Ford S. *Introductory Clinical Pharmacology*. Philadelphia, PA: Lippincott Williams & Wilkins; 2006.

Taylor C, Lillis C, LeMone P, et al. *Fundamentals of Nursing: The Art and Science of Nursing Care*. Philadelphia, PA: Lippincott Williams & Wilkins; 2006.

LABEL ALL MEDICATIONS AT THE TIME OF USE

JEANNIE SCRUGGS GARBER, DNP, RN

WHAT TO DO: PLAN

The nurse is responsible for monitoring the integrity of the medication delivery system, understanding the therapeutic value of the medication, and evaluating the patient's response to the therapy. Labeling medications is a part of maintaining the integrity of the system.

Regardless of which accrediting organization mandates safe medication practices, including labeling of medications, the patient safety rationale for the practice of labeling is easily conceptualized. The Joint Commission on Accreditation of Healthcare Organizations (JCAHO) national patient safety standard MM.4.30 specifically addresses the proper labeling of medications.

JCAHO STANDARD MM.4.30 (FORMERLY TX.3.5.1)

"Medications are appropriately labeled. Medications must be labeled in a standardized manner according to organizational policy, applicable laws and regulations, and standards of practice to minimize errors. This requirement applies to any medication that is prepared but not administered immediately (i.e., this requirement does not apply to a medication prepared and administered immediately in the emergency department or operating room). At a minimum, labels must include the drug name, strength, and amount (if not apparent from the container); the expiration date when the medication is not used within 24 hours after preparation; the expiration time when expiration occurs within less than 24 hours after preparation; and the date prepared and the diluent for all compounded IV admixtures and parenteral nutrient solutions.

A label does not need to be affixed to containers of IV solutions that are labeled by the manufacturer if nothing is added to the solution.

When preparing individualized medications for multiple patients or when the person preparing the individualized medication is not the person administering the medication (e.g., when pharmacy prepares an IV admixture for administration by nursing staff), the label should also include the patient's name and location. Directions for use and any applicable cautionary statements (e.g., requires refrigeration, for IM use only) should also be added to the label or attached as an accessory label."

This patient safety goal applies to all healthcare facilities where medications are administered. Unlabeled medication containers (vials, syringes, ampules, IV fluids, etc.) must always be discarded.

Medication administration is a process with great risk as medication errors can produce life-threatening consequences. Labeling medications according to these standards helps minimize negative patient outcomes and improve medication administration safety.

SUGGESTED READINGS

Buckner S. Medication administration. In: Potter P, Perry A, eds. *Fundamentals of Nursing*. Canada: Mosby-Elsevier; 2009, pp. 686–770.

Healthcare Publishing News. New JCAHO labeling requirements in effect: What CSMM staffers need to know. 2006. Available at: http://findarticles.com/p/articles/mi_m0BPC/is_/ai_n16070938. Accessed July 31, 2008.

The Joint Commission. Joint commission requirements: Labeling medication for anesthesia. Available at: http://www.jointcommission.org/AccreditationPrograms/Office-BasedSurgery/Standards/FAQs/Medication+Management/Preparing+Dispensing/Label_Med_Anesthesia.htm. Accessed July 31, 2008.

MEDICATION ADMINISTRATION: TECHNOLOGY CHANGES YOUR MEDICATION ADMINISTRATION PROCESS

JEANNIE SCRUGGS GARBER, DNP, RN

WHAT TO DO: PLAN

Medication administration is a complex process within a hospital. Significant advances in technology have occurred in the past 10 years that have had a major impact on the safety of medication administration. The 1999 Institute of Medicine report highlighted that 44,000–98,000 people die annually in US hospitals because of medical errors and that medication errors account for approximately 7,000 of those deaths annually. Although these numbers are alarming, it is not surprising considering the many variations and steps to the medication administration process. Technology is improving the process yet human factors will always have to be considered in the assessment of safe medication administration.

Computerized physician order entry systems have made a major impact on patient safety regarding medication administration. The purpose of implementing these new technologies has been to improve patient outcomes and change clinical delivery systems throughout very complex organizations. As technology has brought new processes and improved patient safety, it has also brought new challenges.

Nurses are the point of care delivery regarding medication administration; therefore, they must practice with knowledge and accountability to prevent error. Nurses must practice the "five rights" of medication administration (right person, right medication, right time, right dose, and right route) without variation. Each step must be carefully carried out making sure that error is minimized.

The nurses must make sure that the correct medication is administered. They must compare the drug with the order and can use any electronic mechanisms available for support. If there is any doubt about an order or medication, it is the nurse's responsibility to double-check the original order. The nurse must also always check the computerized system before giving a drug. In our 'real time' world of immediate order entry, printed worksheets become outdated as soon as they are printed. It is possible that a new medication may have been added, discontinued, or modified from the time the worksheet was printed. Orders may have been electronically entered on the units or even remotely depending on the order entry technology available at the institution.

Healthcare providers, and especially nurses, shoulder the burden for safe medication administration practices. The ultimate goal is to provide the patient with the medication prescribed so that the intended outcome can be achieved with minimal risk to safety and well-being.

SUGGESTED READINGS

Colpaert K, Claus B, Somers A, et al. Impact of computerized physician order entry on medication prescription errors in the intensive care unit: A controlled cross-sectional trial. *MedScape Today*. 2006. Available at: http://www.medscape.com/viewarticle/523538. Accessed July 31, 2008.

Kremsdorf R. Medication safety tools: Evaluation of vendor offerings for computerized physician order entry and medication administration. *The Informatics Rev.* 2003. Available at: http://www.informatics-review.com/thoughts/tools.html. Accessed August 1, 2008.

KNOW HOW TO PLAN FOR THE ADMINISTRATION OF INVESTIGATIONAL MEDICATIONS

ANTHONY D. SLONIM, MD, DRPH

WHAT TO DO: PLAN

Hospitals engaged in clinical trials research often have medications administered to patients using a protocol. Ensuring the delivery of safe and effective care to these patients is critical, yet there are a number of vulnerabilities in the medication administration process as a result of being a participant in the research. Nurses working in these institutions need to do what they can to ensure their patients' safety.

A large component of potential medication problems with investigational drugs are out of the hands of the pharmacy or the nurse. These include differences related to the packaging, including labeling problems, insufficient information related to dose, concentration, and expiration, and problems with the drug name, which is often referred to by a number and not a name. There are problems related to the study itself, which for many reasons requires that the medication not be identifiable and look similar to the placebo. This places the pharmacist and the nurse in an awkward position since they are often familiar with what they are administering. Finally, there are some important points that are under the control of nurses and pharmacists. Being able to store the medication in a safe location where it is clearly identified as a study drug is important. Recognizing patient side effects and reporting them to the quality department, the pharmacy, and the institutional review board are important. It is essential to ensure that the nursing unit has received an approved protocol to govern the use and administration of the drug, including inclusion and exclusion criteria of participants, a signed informed consent, and the contact information of the principal investigator or designated official responsible on a 24 × 7 basis, should problems in patients arise.

Clinical trials are important for advancing medical knowledge and treatment. Patients participating in these trials provide a great service and should be commended. It is our job to ensure that all required information for the administration of a particular agent is available and critical processes are outlined so that patients are protected appropriately. We should also encourage industry representatives and scientists to continually improve these important safeguards.

SUGGESTED READINGS

ISMP Medication Safety Alert. Product-related issues make error potential enormous with investigational drugs. November 1, 2007. Available at: http://www.ismp.org/Newsletters/acutecare/articles/20071101.asp. Accessed August 25, 2008.

KNOW HOW TO REVERSE THE ANTICOAGULANT EFFECTS OF HEPARIN AND WARFARIN

ANTHONY D. SLONIM, MD, DRPH

The administration of a medication in the correct dose and to the correct patient is important and can otherwise lead to serious consequences. While observing the patient for adverse effects of the drug, the nurse should be aware of specific antidotes that in the right circumstances can help to reduce the side effects.

Anticoagulant medications are available to treat a number of clinical conditions. The two major agents used are warfarin and heparin. These two agents work by different mechanisms and their use is monitored clinically by the laboratory. In serious overdoses of warfarin, wherein the patient's PT or INR are elevated and the patient is bleeding, the administration of vitamin K can help reduce these effects. Vitamin K can be administered orally, subcutaneously, and intravenously. While it is true that there is the potential for adverse reactions, such as anaphylaxis related to intravenous administration of vitamin K, their occurrence is rare. What is more important is a consideration of what will happen when the anticoagulant effect is reversed. Patients may become prothrombotic and begin to clot, which may be more problematic than the bleeding that was being experienced. Fresh frozen plasma (FFP) can also be administered to assist with warfarin overdose; while this is nonspecific antidote, the provision of clotting factors will help to improve the bleeding from warfarin.

Heparin is another example of an anticoagulant. Heparin is used commonly to treat thrombotic disorders and to prevent the development of deep venous thrombosis due to immobility in the hospital setting. Heparin has a specific antidote known as protamine that allows heparin activity to be reduced. Protamine combines with heparin forming a complex that is free from anticoagulant activity. One milligram of heparin is administered for every 100 units of heparin remaining in the body. It is administered slowly by an intravenous route. Protamine itself has anticoagulant activity when given in excess and should be used only in the doses recommended. Protamine can also be used to reverse the effects of low molecular weight heparin, but the dosage adjustment is less precise. Approximately 1 mg of protamine reverses 1 mg of low molecular weight heparin.

Knowing the appropriate antidote is particularly helpful when a patient is experiencing an adverse reaction related to an anticoagulant.

SUGGESTED READINGS

Hambleton J. Drugs used in disorders of coagulation. In: Katzung BG, ed. *Basic and Clinical Pharmacology*. 9th Ed. New York: McGraw Hill Company; 2004, pp. 543–560.

USE DRUGS FOR THEIR INTENDED PURPOSES

ANTHONY D. SLONIM, MD, DrPH

Medications are an important part of the nurse's armamentarium to help cure disease and add comfort. Yet, there is a tendency to become "sloppy" with language and be imprecise in what is intended. The downside is that a patient may get the wrong drug for a given indication because the wrong term was used. It is important for the nurse to know what drug is being used and discuss its effect profile both with the family and with other providers.

One of the biggest challenges in the intensive care unit (ICU) setting is the use of sedatives, analgesics, and neuromuscular blockers. Sedatives are used to produce somnolence and amnesia during a procedure or ICU course. Sedatives usually do not have analgesic properties. Analgesics, on the other hand, are intended to relieve pain. Analgesics also have sedative properties that can benefit the patient. Neuromuscular blockers are another drug class used in the ICU. These drugs inhibit skeletal muscle responses and prevent the patient from moving. They have neither sedative nor analgesic properties. It is important that when neuromuscular blocking agents are administered, appropriate sedation and analgesia are also provided.

For many providers, the term sedation is used broadly to cover these three specific classes of drugs. Unfortunately, this imprecise language provides difficulty for the novice nurse or family who may not understand the differences in these medications. Drugs should be used for their intended purposes. If the patient needs pain medication, analgesics should be administered, not sedatives or neuromuscular blocking agents. If the patient needs to have ventilation facilitated because of patient–ventilator dyssynchrony, any of the agents may be appropriate and may be used in a tiered approach starting with sedation and progressing to neuromuscular blockers.

Always use drugs for their intended purpose and avoid the use of casual language when speaking to the family or other providers since it may lead to misunderstandings and medication errors.

SUGGESTED READINGS

Sedation, analgesia, and neuromuscular blockade of the critically ill adult: Revised clinical practice guidelines for 2002. Available at: http://www.medscape.com/viewarticle/424699. Accessed August 25, 2008.
Society of Critical Care Medicine and American Society of Health-System Pharmacists. Clinical practice guidelines for the sustained use of sedatives and analgesics in the critically ill adult. *Am J Health-Syst Pharm.* 2002;59:150–178.

KNOW WHAT TO WATCH FOR IN YOUR ELDERLY PATIENT RECEIVING MULTIPLE MEDICATIONS

ANTHONY D. SLONIM, MD, DrPH

ANTHONY D. SLONIM, MD, DrPH

WHAT TO DO: ASSESS, PLAN, AND EVALUATE

Aging slows down a number of physiologic processes. This has important implications for the use of drugs in the population of elderly patients. The nurse needs to understand the role physiology plays in the healthcare of these patients and be alert to adverse effects of medications.

The elderly, even with normally functioning organs, experience a number of pharmacokinetic changes that alter the ways in which drugs act and side effects that become apparent. While absorption is not dramatically affected by age alone, distribution, metabolism, and elimination are. The distribution of a drug is affected by its binding to plasma proteins. The elderly have lower concentrations of albumin and reduced fat stores which affect the loading and maintenance doses of some medications. Drug metabolism is also affected by aging. The elderly have problems with the liver's ability to metabolize medications. Similarly, since the kidneys are the major organs involved in elimination and age-related reductions in elimination, regardless of increases in creatinine, they reduce the ability of the elderly to eliminate medications.

When all these pharmacokinetic changes in the elderly are considered, the nurse is faced with several important medication issues that need to be reconciled. First, the loading dose, dosage, and interval of medications may need to be adapted for the elderly. Second, because metabolism and excretion are slowed, toxic levels or adverse side effects from the buildup of medications, their metabolites, or the synergistic effects of multiple drugs need to be considered. Finally, the nurse needs to work as a patient advocate advancing a care plan that is functional, affordable, and does not create complications once the patient leaves the hospital. In addition, it is notable that the elderly often have poor nutrition and eat irregularly. This may also affect the medications they take and the ability of the medications to have their intended effects.

The elderly need to have a medication profile that has the fewest medications needed to ensure their intended effects. These medications need to be clearly explained and written down so that the patient can follow the regimen. The drugs need to be affordable, since the regimen the patient is discharged on will change if they are unable to acquire the drugs. The medications need to integrate appropriately with the patient's diet. Finally, the patient needs to be aware of the side effects that arise from toxicity problems due to inadequate metabolism or elimination.

SUGGESTED READINGS

Katzung BG. Special aspects of geriatric pharmacology. In: Katzung BG, ed. *Basic and Clinical Pharmacology*. 9th Ed. New York: McGraw Hill Company; 2004, pp. 1007–1014.

ENSURE THAT OVER-THE-COUNTER (OTC) MEDICATIONS ARE ASSESSED ON ADMISSION

ANTHONY D. SLONIM, MD, DRPH

WHAT TO DO: ASSESS

Patients will often use self-prescribed, over-the-counter (OTC) medications to alleviate common symptoms and complaints. A number of medications are now available over the counter, which provides patients relief from a number of common concerns without the need to consult a physician. These include cold remedies, topical agents for sore muscles, acne, and wounds, analgesic agents for pain including aspirin, acetaminophen, and naproxen, and a number of agents for gastrointestinal symptoms including indigestion, diarrhea, and constipation. Importantly, the patient may not realize the interactions, effects, and problems that may arise from their use. Hence, the nurse needs to understand what medications, including OTCs, the patient is using so that the health-care team is appropriately informed about their use.

A major problem has recently been identified in OTC cold remedies administered to children less than 2 years of age. Not only do these products not improve the symptoms in a standardized way, but the side effects of these medications may lead to harm and potentially even death. Parents need to be alert to only prescribe symptomatic relief to their young children on the advice of their child's healthcare provider.

The OTC industry is marked by a number of products that can be provided topically to relieve pain or the symptoms of acne. Many patients think that because a product is not ingested there is no absorption into the systemic circulation. The same holds true for prescription eye drops, which are often taken by the elderly, but not remembered as a part of the medication list. These drugs can interact particularly with cardiac medications and cause harm to patients.

Another category of products that needs to have thoughtful use is aspirin. Aspirin is used frequently for its anti-platelet effects and the benefits in preventing adverse cardiac events. No one would argue with the benefits of aspirin. However, when the patient is admitted to the hospital, the adverse platelet effects continue. Hence, patients receiving invasive or operative procedures may bleed more than expected because of the failure of platelets to form appropriate hemostatic plugs.

Finally, the use of gastrointestinal (GI) products, particularly those that alter GI motility, may create adverse effects if the patient has a condition like *C. difficile* colitis or antibacterial associated diarrhea. The patient wants to control the symptom of diarrhea, but the underlying condition needs to be treated. Agents that improve constipation may adversely affect the absorption of some prescribed medications.

OTC medications are particularly helpful for common conditions affecting broad masses of the population. The nurse should remember that these drugs may interact with prescription drugs or cause unwanted side effects just as much as prescribed medications. One way to prevent this is to ensure that these OTC medications are included in the medication list at admission and discharge.

SUGGESTED READINGS

FDA Center for Drug Evaluation and Research. Public health advisory: Nonprescription cough and cold medicine use in children. Available at: http://www.fda.gov/cder/drug/advisory/cough_cold_2008.htm. Accessed August 25, 2008.

FDA Consumer Health Information. Use caution with over-the-counter creams, ointments. Available at: http://www.fda.gov/consumer/updates/otc_creams040108.html. Accessed August 25, 2008.

REASSESS THE MEDICATION LIST AFTER AN INVASIVE OR OPERATIVE PROCEDURE

ANTHONY D. SLONIM, MD, DRPH

WHAT TO DO: ASSESS AND EVALUATE

The care of the postprocedure or postoperative patient requires that the nurse have special skills and talents. While the major emphasis in this postprocedure period of time is on getting the patient settled in, assessing for pain, checking the wound or dressing, and ensuring that the vital signs are stable, the next step needs to include an assessment of the plan of care, not only related to the operative procedure but also to how that plan fits within the context of the patient's medical problems and medications.

A major part of this assessment includes an analysis of the preprocedure medications and the postprocedure orders. Hopefully, there has been a thoughtful approach applied to what needs to be continued, modified, or discontinued from the preprocedure medications and the nurse is in a unique position to assist with this by identifying omissions or commissions in the care. The nurse should never accept a "continue all preoperative orders" as the postprocedure medical plan of care. This places the nurse outside of the scope of practice and poses undue burden for what should be a medical function.

Some commonly forgotten medications after a procedure include antimicrobial agents, including a stop date. If the patients received their procedure while hospitalized for an infectious disease, like pneumonia, the physician should make a thoughtful approach about an antimicrobial agent that adequately covers both of these conditions and should ensure that the pneumonia treatment continues for an appropriate duration after the empiric coverage for the procedure is discontinued. Prophylactic agents for deep venous thrombosis, stress ulcer prophylaxis, and stool softeners for patients on narcotics are often forgotten on the postoperative medication orders and provide an important opportunity for follow-up. Finally, pain medications may also be forgotten and will need to be addressed in the short-term before a patient's pain gets out of hand. Similarly, antiemetics and other symptom relief medications may not have been on the preprocedure medication list and should hence be included.

Another omission in care arises from the failure to recognize why the patient is taking a particular drug that has multiple indications. For example, with large numbers of patients taking anticoagulants for many reasons, there needs to be a consideration of their continuation postprocedure. This, in part, depends upon the reason for their initiation but also needs to be done with an understanding of what occurred in the operating room. The patient taking warfarin preprocedure for prophylaxis for a mechanical heart valve may be transitioned to heparin during the perioperative period. It is necessary to remember that the patient will need to be transitioned back to warfarin or another long-term anticoagulant strategy when the postprocedure concerns have abated. Failure to remember the original indication may lead to errors in discontinuation of a drug when it is essential to the patient's condition.

Commissions in care can also occur from failure to reconcile preprocedure and postprocedure medications. Preoperative medications, like β-blockers, that are continued on the postprocedure orders with a patient in shock on dopamine are good examples. There are a number of good reasons to provide patients with β-blockers preprocedure, but if the course in the procedure or the patient's condition establishes a relative contraindication, then the orders need to be reevaluated.

SUGGESTED READINGS

Joint Commission International Center for Patient Safety. Where should reconciliation occur? Medication Reconciliation. Available at: http://www.wsha.org/files/64/medication rec-all.ppt#266,20. Accessed August 25, 2008.

REMEMBER THAT A LOADING DOSE OF A DRUG IS SOMETIMES NEEDED TO ACHIEVE APPROPRIATE THERAPEUTIC LEVELS

ANTHONY D. SLONIM, MD, DrPH

WHAT TO DO: IMPLEMENT

The loading dose of a drug is the amount of drug that needs to be administered to quickly achieve an adequate serum level and desired therapeutic effect. The loading dose is most frequently used for those medications that have long half-lives. The nurse needs an understanding of this pharmacodynamic principle but more importantly needs to recognize the drugs that need to be provided with a loading dose to achieve appropriate patient care.

There are several medication classes in which a loading dose becomes important. These are areas where the clinical situation requires quick control through the actions of the medication. While this is not an exhaustive list, these do represent common examples to illustrate the importance of a loading dose in clinical care. Further questions can be answered by a hospital pharmacist.

The first group of drugs is commonly in the critical care unit or emergency department of the hospital. Arrhythmias occur frequently in the setting of the emergency department, the cardiac care unit, and the intensive care unit. Regardless of where they occur, several antiarrhythmic agents require loading doses to achieve appropriate serum levels and get control of the arrhythmia. Digoxin is a medication that has been used for quite a long time. It has been used as an inotropic agent and as an antiarrhythmic agent. A rapid loading dose can be achieved for digoxin in just a few hours and help to stabilize rapid cardiac rhythms. Lidocaine is also an antiarrhythmic agent that can be used to acutely stabilize ventricular arrhythmias in a number of settings. Esmolol is used to control blood pressure or treat rapid cardiac rhythms.

Milrinone is a drug that is used as an inotropic agent. It can be used without a bolus in some circumstances, but the use of a bolus is important when inotropic support is needed acutely.

Anticonvulsants are another group of agents that can be used to quickly stabilize the patient with status epilepticus. The use of both phenytoin and Phenobarbital helps to stabilize the acutely ill seizure patient by achieving rapid serum levels with a bolus of medication.

Finally, antibacterial agents, like gentamycin, can be used to achieve appropriate serum levels quickly and begin to act. For these drugs, the drug continues to work by an intracellular mechanism after the serum levels have decreased; hence, it is important to ensure that appropriate dosing is accomplished.

Nurses need to understand appropriate principles of drug therapy to ensure that their patients receive the care they need when they need it.

SUGGESTED READINGS

Holford NHG. Pharmacokinetics and pharmacodynamics: Rational dosing and the time course of drug action. In: Katzung BG, ed. *Basic and Clinical Pharmacology*. 9th Ed. New York: McGraw Hill Company; 2004.

KNOW THAT ADENOSINE NEEDS TO BE PUSHED QUICKLY AT THE CLOSEST IV PORT TO THE PATIENT AND THE NURSE SHOULD BE PREPARED FOR ASYSTOLE

ANTHONY D. SLONIM, MD, DRPH

WHAT TO DO: PLAN AND IMPLEMENT

Adenosine is a nucleoside analog that is used in the treatment of supraventricular tachycardia (SVT). It has a rapid onset and short duration of action, making it particularly useful for the patient who is acutely ill with SVT. However, there are a couple of very important nursing implications that need to be taken care of if the patient is to receive appropriate care.

First, patients with SVT who receive adenosine often have a brief period of asystole while the rhythm abates. This is usually self-limited, and the patient usually returns to the SVT or to sinus rhythm if the medication was successful in terminating the arrhythmia. For a small group of patients, however, the asystole may be prolonged, which makes the healthcare team very nervous. A smaller group of patients may actually require resuscitation from their asystolic event. Therefore, it becomes important for the nurse to ensure that the code cart is at the bedside and ready to be used if needed.

Second, adenosine causes a very intense feeling of warmth and light-headedness in patients. The patient needs to be warned prior to the administration of medication that these events will occur. Not only may these symptoms be intense, but they can also make the patient fearful. Fortunately, these events too are often short-lived and do not recur. The nurse should warn the patient that they may occur.

Finally, because of its short half-life, adenosine needs to be pushed rapidly through the intravenous line at the closest port to the patient. This is often accomplished with two syringes, one containing the medication and the other containing the flush solution. It is important for the nurse to label the syringes so that they remember which syringe is the medication and which is the flush, and this ensures that they are administered in the appropriate order.

Adenosine is an important medication for the treatment of SVT and nurses should remember the important caveats that accompany its use.

SUGGESTED READINGS

Jacobson C. Narrow QRS complex tachycardias. *AACN Adv Crit Care*. 2007;18(3):264–274.

McIntosh-Yellin NL, Drew BJ, Scheinman MM. Safety and efficacy of central intravenous bolus administration of adenosine for termination of supraventricular tachycardia. *J Am Coll Cardiol*. 1993;22(3):741–745.

KNOW THE REVERSAL AGENTS FOR NARCOTICS AND BENZODIAZEPINES

ANTHONY D. SLONIM, MD, DRPH

Narcotics and benzodiazepines are two drug classes that are very valuable to patients. Narcotics help in the treatment of moderate to severe pain and benzodiazepines assist with sedation, anxiolysis, and amnesia for procedural sedation. There is a synergy between both the effects and complications of these medication classes particularly with respect to respiratory depression, which usually manifests itself as hypoventilation and hypercarbia. While the respiratory rate is monitored during the administration of these medications, one of the major problems is that most patients are monitored with pulse oximetry, and oxygen saturation does not begin to decrease until late in the course of hypoventilation.

Importantly, the nurse has several options when the patient begins to experience medication-related hypoventilation after assurance that the airway is maintained, breathing is adequate, and circulation is appropriate. The first option is to reduce the dose of one or the other agent depending upon what symptom needs to be controlled. The second is to increase the interval between the medications. Finally, the nurse can administer a reversal agent. Naloxone is the agent that is used to reverse narcotic-induced respiratory depression. Naloxone is also a narcotic and works by competitively inhibiting the narcotic at the receptor. Naloxone has a short half-life and if the duration of action for the narcotic is longer than that of naloxone; repeated doses may need to be given. It is also important that naloxone be administered in a small dose and incrementally increased to the desired effect. For patients who are chronically addicted to narcotics, the administration of naloxone may induce a state of withdrawal and need to be given with caution to these patients.

For benzodiazepine-induced respiratory depression, the administration of flumazenil can be helpful to counteract this complication. Flumazenil can also be administered sequentially to ensure that the adverse effect is counteracted without over-reducing the therapeutic effects of the medications.

Nurses have an important role in the administration of narcotics and benzodiazepines. The nurse needs to know what opportunities are available to counteract respiratory depression induced by these agents.

SUGGESTED READINGS

Schumacher MA, Basbaum AI, Way WL. Opioid analgesics and antagonists. In: Katzung BG, ed. *Basic and Clinical Pharmacology*. 9th Ed. New York: McGraw Hill; 2004, pp. 497–516.

Trevor AJ, Way WL. Sedative hypnotic drugs. In: Katzung BG, ed. *Basic and Clinical Pharmacology*. 9th Ed. New York: McGraw Hill; 2004, pp. 351–366.

BE AWARE OF PATIENTS TAKING SSRIS WITH PAIN MEDICATIONS AND MIGRAINE PREPARATIONS

MELISSA H. CRIGGER, BSN, MHA, RN

WHAT TO DO: ASSESSMENT

Remember that the patient receiving selective serotonin reuptake inhibitors (SSRIs) for depression must be cautious with using migraine and pain medications. SSRIs are used as a first line of treatment for depression. SSRIs block the reuptake of serotonin and in turn increase the level of serotonin. Examples of SSRIs include fluoxetine, sertraline, paroxetine, citalopram, and escitalopram. As with other types of antidepressants, the nurse caring for the patient receiving SSRIs should be aware of the potential interactions that can occur with other medications, including pain medications and migraine preparations.

Migraine preparations such as triptans (e.g., Imitrex and Zomig) act as selective agonists of the 5-HT receptor, which causes vasoconstriction of the large intracranial arteries. When a patient is receiving triptans as well as SSRIs, there is a potential for drug interactions, which include symptoms of weakness, hyperreflexia, and incoordination. The nurse caring for the patient who is prescribed triptans and SSRIs should always educate the patient on possible drug interactions that occur. The patient should also be educated to notify the physician should these symptoms occur. If the patient is admitted to the acute care facility, the nurse should be aware of potential symptoms of drug interactions and notify the physician immediately if weakness, hyperreflexia, or incoordination is observed.

Pain medications such as opioids (e.g., morphine) are also a concern for the patient taking SSRIs. Morphine binds to opiate receptors in the central nervous system, thus producing central nervous system depression. One concern for the patient taking SSRIs in conjunction with opioid analgesics is that central nervous system depression can increase. The nurse must make sure that the patient is aware of this possible drug reaction as well as the signs and symptoms of central nervous system depression, which include sedation, confusion, and respiratory depression. As stated earlier, the nurse who is caring for the patient in the acute setting should be aware of and report these symptoms to the physician immediately. The nurse must make sure that he/she assesses vital signs, including respiratory rate. The assessment should also include obtaining orientation to all four spheres (person, place, time, and situation) as well as alertness of the patient. As there is a potential for increased central nervous system depression, the nurse must also educate the patient to notify different providers of any changes that occur related to medications.

Ambulation can also be a concern for the patient receiving opioid analgesics with SSRIs. The patient may require assistance with ambulation and should be instructed to contact the nurse when wanting to ambulate. Upon discharge, the patient should also be educated on avoiding alcohol in combination with these two types of drugs. Alcohol, which is also a central nervous system depressant, can further potentiate the effects of both medications.

SUGGESTED READINGS

Deglin JH, Vallerand AH. *Davis's Drug Guide for Nurses*. 10th Ed. Philadelphia, PA: F. A. Davis Company; 2007.

Varcarolis EM, Carson V, Shoemaker N. Mood disorders: Depression. In: *Foundations of Psychiatric Mental Health Nursing*. 5th Ed. St. Louis, MO: Saunders-Elsevier; 2006, pp. 343–345.

Watch for "Picking Errors" When Using Technologies to Administer Medication

Anthony D. Slonim, MD, DrPH

The administration of medications is getting more complex with the addition of a variety of technologies at different parts of the medication process. There are computers at the point of order entry, computers in the pharmacy to assist with order processing, computer dispensing cabinets for drug distribution, and medication administration verification systems and pumps to assist with medication administration. One of the more common errors in medication delivery related to administration is picking errors.

A picking error occurs when a healthcare professional selects the incorrect drug from a list or cabinet. This is particularly problematic because drugs spelled similarly, with similar sounding names, or with different concentrations are often placed adjacent to one another on the pick list or in adjacent drawers in the medication cabinet.

At the point of prescribing, a letter of the alphabet is often entered to begin the pick list. The computer then brings up the list of medications that begin with that letter to allow the ordering process to be easier. However, the prescriber is then presented with the list and can select from the list rather than identifying a specific drug. When the provider is fatigued, rushed, or inattentive, the wrong drug is selected and verified.

Unfortunately, once this occurs at the point of order entry, there is no downstream method for fixing this problem.

In the pharmacy, the pharmacists will see the order and then begin the processing process. Here, the medication needs to be prepared from the numerous bins in the pharmacy. It is important to keep similar drugs or drugs with different concentrations physically separated from each other. For example, place the 1,000 units per mL and 10,000 units per mL of heparin vials on physically different shelves to avoid confusion.

Nurses face a similar problem from dispensing cabinets when they begin the pick list with a letter and may select the incorrect drug from the list. This is compounded since the drawer opens automatically. If the incorrect drug has been placed in the drawer or the nurse does not validate that the correct drug has been selected, an administration error can occur.

Nurses are receiving additional help from the numerous technologies available to assist in medication delivery. Unfortunately, these new processes also create new challenges that need to be kept in mind by all providers involved in providing medications to patients.

SUGGESTED READINGS

Beso A, Franklin BD, Barber N. The frequency and potential causes of dispensing errors in a hospital pharmacy. *Pharm World Sci.* 2005;27(3):182–190.

KNOW THE CONTINUUM OF THE SYMPATHETIC AGONISTS

ANTHONY D. SLONIM, MD, DrPH

WHAT TO DO: PLAN

The sympathetic nervous system is particularly important for organ function throughout the body. It assists with functions as disparate as assuring adequate heart rate during excitement to breaking down fats for energy. It is a central component of the "fight or flight" response. Importantly, there are a number of drugs available to modulate the sympathetic nervous system and the nurse needs to understand the continuum of these drugs since the activation of different receptors will lead to different effects. This discussion is quite simplified, but is essential to understand the role these drugs have in clinical practice in the intensive care unit for maintaining heart rate and blood pressure (Fig. 53-1).

There are a number of pharmacologic agents that activate sympathetic receptors. The two receptors that are important here are the alpha (α) and beta (β) receptors. Alpha receptors are classified into two groups: α_1 and α_2. The α_1 receptors are responsible for increasing peripheral vascular resistance, elevating blood pressure, and vasoconstriction. The α_2 receptors inhibit norepinephrine release. Similarly, the β receptors are classified into β_1 and β_2. The β_1 receptors are responsible for increasing myocardial heart rate and contractility and the release of renin to ensure that intravascular volume is maintained. The β_2 receptors vasodilate, bronchodilate, relax uterine smooth muscle, and increase the release of glucagon and muscle and liver glycogenolysis.

SUGGESTED READINGS

Howland RD, Mycek MJ. Adrenergic agonists. In: *Lippincott's Illustrated Reviews: Pharmacology*. 3rd Ed. Philadelphia: Lippincott Williams & Wilkins; 2006.

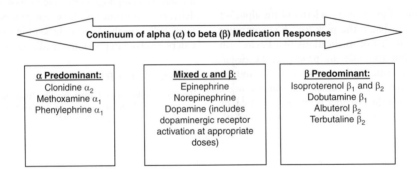

FIGURE 53.1. Understanding the adrenergic receptors and the medications that stimulate them provide the nurse with the opportunity to select the correct drug for the correct indication.

KNOW HOW TO MIX AND ADMINISTER DRUGS APPROPRIATELY

ANTHONY D. SLONIM, MD, DrPH

WHAT TO DO: PLAN

Drug incompatibility is a problem that occurs when two drugs or compounds are either mixed or administered together or with a diluent, which react chemically inactivating their effects and causing potential harm. There are well recognized lists of compatibility charts available in the pharmacy and in a number of reference texts. However, the problem often arises when the nurse needs to administer medications in an emergency and has insufficient intravenous access as may occur in the ICU.

Phenytoin is a drug that has specific requirements for mixing. It cannot be mixed in dextrose-containing solutions because it will form a precipitate. This has been, in large part, eliminated with the use of phosphenytoin. However, the nurse also needs to recognize that it is not the mixing alone, but also the administration that can cause a problem. Total parenteral nutrition (TPN) contains high concentrations of dextrose. The administration of phenytoin through a TPN line can lead to the same precipitate as if the drug was mixed in dextrose.

Another common example is electrolyte-containing solutions. The co-administration of bicarbonate with calcium salts can cause a precipitate to form. The nurse who is administering medications, particularly in emergent situations like a code event or when a patient is critically ill and there is a lot of commotion at the bedspace, needs to be sure which IV line he or she is using for the infusion of drugs to ensure that incompatible electrolyte solutions are not inadvertently mixed.

Natrecor, a relatively new drug, binds to a variety of medications including heparin, insulin, bumetanide, enalaprilat, hydralazine, and furosemide. The lines should be flushed in between the administration of these medications. Further, heparin-bonded catheters, used in many ICUs, may also contain enough heparin to interact with Natrecor and reduce the effective dose.

While the mixing of drugs usually falls to the pharmacy, in some places, the nurse will be responsible for the mixing and administration. In these cases, the nurse should refer to compatibility charts to ensure that the medications are compatible.

SUGGESTED READINGS

Natrecor. RxList: The Internet drug index. Available at: http://www.rxlist.com/cgi/generic/natrecor_ids.htm. Accessed September 1, 2008.

Always look for the patch...

Anthony D. Slonim, MD, DrPH

WHAT TO DO: ASSESS

Many medications are now administered in transdermal formulations. These include fentanyl, nitroglycerin ointment, clonidine, scopolamine, nicotine, and a variety of hormones. Many of these are administered while the patient is hospitalized, but patients often come into the hospital taking these medications from home and the nurse may be unaware of their presence. The nurse needs to look for transdermal patches during their initial assessment and ensure that when they administer a new dose of the drug they find the old patch and remove it from the patient's skin to prevent overdose.

There are several other important reminders for patients (and nurses) when handling these medications in this formulation. The medication should be placed on clean, dry, and hairless skin. Remember that you should not place the patch on abraded or irritated skin because it will speed up the absorption of the drug. When you remove the old patch, you should avoid getting the medication on your hands; if you do, wash your hands immediately and thoroughly. Discuss the medication and how it works with the patient. Patients often do not believe that medication can be administered this way. The absorption of the drug can also be increased by rubbing the patch or applying heat or a warming blanket, which should be avoided.

If your patient experiences a side effect related to the drug, look for the patch and remove it. This is particularly important for patients who become hypotensive and have multiple nitroglycerin patches in place or become somnolent due to excessive narcotic administration from fentanyl patches.

Transdermal medications provide outstanding benefits to patients when used appropriately. The nurse needs to be familiar with their use and educate their patients on how to use them and what to watch out for.

SUGGESTED READINGS

McConnell EA. Using transdermal medication patches. *BNet Business Network*. 1997. Available at: http://findarticles.com/p/articles/mi_qa3689/is_199707/ai_n8767414/print?tag=artBody; col1. Accessed September 1, 2008.

Roth JV. Warming blankets should not be placed over transdermal medications. *Anesth Analg*. 2002;94:1043. Available at: http://www.anesthesia-analgesia.org/cgi/content/full/94/4/1043. Accessed September 1, 2008.

KNOW HOW TO MANAGE A PATIENT'S HOME INFUSION PUMP

ANTHONY D. SLONIM, MD, DrPH

WHAT TO DO: PLAN

With increasing frequency, technologies formerly relegated to hospital use are being used in the home environment. Most important among these devices is medication infusion pumps. It is important for the inpatient nurse to note that these pumps may contain a variety of medications ranging from insulin to pulmonary vasodilators to chemotherapeutic agents to patient controlled analgesia. The nurse needs to not only understand what the medications do and whether or not they can be discontinued during the inpatient stay, but also realize that these pumps are very different in terms of their programming, and the nurse may need additional consultation from elsewhere in the hospital to ensure the patient's safety.

When patients present to the hospital and have a medication infusing, it is important to ensure that the device is working properly. Many hospitals require that the device be checked by the biomedical department to ensure that it is working appropriately and does not allow free flow. The nurse should assess what medication is in the device, at what dose it is being administered, and how it is being monitored. Next, the nurse needs to ensure that the device is connected appropriately to the patient. The patient, if conscious, or the family can often provide feedback regarding this point. Finally, the nurse needs to know from the physician what the plan is in continuing or discontinuing the device for the hospitalization. This is important. The nurse needs to have an order for administering medications by the home device. The order needs to be appropriately specific to allow the nurse to assess that the correct drug and dose are being administered. Often, the care of these pumps and their medications may be under the direction of a different physician with specialty experience. For example, home infusions of pulmonary vasodilators may be under the supervision of a cardiologist or insulin infusions may be under the direction of an endocrinologist. Nonetheless, the nurse needs specific direction on what the admitting physician wants to do with the device and medication even if it means obtaining consultation from the subspecialist.

The care of patients with home infusion devices has allowed the patient to be cared for in a more comfortable environment. However, the nurse responsible for admitting a patient with a home device to the hospital needs to understand how that device will be used during the hospitalization and needs to ensure that all required information is available to appropriately and safely administer the medications.

SUGGESTED READINGS

Joint Commission Resources. *Front Line of Defense: The Role of Nurses in Preventing Sentinel Events*. Chicago, IL: Joint Commission Resources; 2001, pp. 34–36.

ANALYZE THE MEDICATION ADMINISTRATION PROCESS

ANTHONY D. SLONIM, MD, DrPH

WHAT TO DO: PLAN

The administration of medications has become more complicated over time as the way medications are delivered to patients during hospitalization has changed. Unfortunately, most of the time, the incremental changes are added without appreciating how they will affect other parts of the delivery system. For example, when narcotic problems occur, a double check or new form is put in place so that the error will not occur again; however, no one takes a look at the whole process to determine if this redundancy will add extra work to the nurses or even be successful in averting another error.

A Failure Mode Effects Analysis (FMEA) is a useful tool that can be used on an individual nursing unit to proactively examine at-risk processes such as medication administration to determine if there are opportunities to streamline the process and improve its effectiveness. The FMEA can be performed with the providers who know the process best and can be facilitated by a member of the quality department or pharmacy safety team.

In an FMEA, the process from medication ordering through administration to the patient is "mapped out." This allows providers to see opportunities to reduce risk or add safety checks. What is valuable about mapping out the system is that an added safety check can be visualized with its impact on the broader process. Importantly, this is done proactively before an error occurs. The FMEA should include all efforts by the nursing staff to validate that medications are being administered safely, including the midnight chart check and its effectiveness, the assurance of the five rights for medication safety, and the use of double identifier for administering medications to a patient. If the unit has data available about their medication errors, the FMEA can provide additional information on the major risk points and identify the priorities for intervention.

The FMEA is one tool available to nursing units to analyze important processes and can be used to interrogate the medication delivery process to assure its safety.

SUGGESTED READINGS

Adachi W, Lodolce AE. Use of failure mode and effects analysis in improving the safety of i.v. drug administration. *Am J Health Syst Pharm.* 2005;62(9):917–920.

Failure mode and effects analysis. A hands-on guide for healthcare facilities. *Health Dev.* 2004;33(7):233–243.

Nickerson T, Jenkins M, Greenall J. Using ISMP Canada's framework for failure mode and effects analysis: A tale of two FMEAs. *Healthc Qual.* 2008;11(3 Spec No.):40–46.

Riehle MA, Bergeron D, Hyrkäs K. Improving process while changing practice: FMEA and medication administration. *Nurs Manage.* 2008;39(2):28–33;quiz 34.

Wetterneck TB, Skibinski KA, Roberts TL, et al. Using failure mode and effects analysis to plan implementation of smart i.v. pump technology. *Am J Health Syst Pharm.* 2006;63(16):1528–1538.

USE PROTOCOLS FOR THE ADMINISTRATION OF HIGH-RISK INFREQUENTLY USED MEDICATIONS

ANTHONY D. SLONIM, MD, DrPH

Variability is the enemy of safe healthcare, particularly when medications are used infrequently and in high-risk situations. To combat the variability in the delivery of these medications, protocols should be established that provide guidance in delivering these medications the same way each time for separate indications, particularly when there is a time imperative for getting the medication infused. The best example of this problem is the use of thrombolytic agents for acute myocardial infarction and ischemic stroke.

The use of thrombolytic agents has revolutionized the care of acute ischemic stroke and myocardial infarction. The problem is that this medication is administered acutely in both these situations. The timing interval, bolus dosing, and total dosing regimens are similar enough to be dangerous for providers who handle patients with both these diagnoses and rely upon memory. As a result, the availability of a standardized protocol for each indication helps allow providers a ready reference to improve the care for patients, particularly when these medications may be prepared without the availability of a pharmacist.

The standardized protocol does not need to be fancy. In fact, it is more important that it be simple and used frequently. A simple flow diagram that is laminated and kept in the medication bin where the drug is kept provides a hand tool for administering this medication safely. Since the medication is administered based on strict criteria for both these diagnoses, the criteria can also be included to ensure that appropriate patient selection occurs.

High-risk, low-volume events in healthcare can create big safety problems for patients. A protocol, guideline, or algorithm can be a simple and effective way to ensure that thrombolytic agents are administered to patients who need them in the right dose and schedule.

SUGGESTED READINGS

Cannon CP. Thrombolysis medication errors: Benefits of bolus thrombolytic agents. *Am J Cardiol.* 2000;85(8A):17C–22C.

Richards CF, Cannon CP. Reducing medication errors: Potential benefits of bolus thrombolytic agents. *Acad Emerg Med.* 2000;7(11):1285–1289.

Shapiro J, Bessette M, Levine SR, et al. HandiStroke: A handheld tool for the emergent evaluation of acute stroke patients. *Acad Emerg Med.* 2003;10(12):1325–1328.

Ensure That Medications Are Administered Safely to Vulnerable Pediatric Patients

Anthony D. Slonim, MD, DrPH

WHAT TO DO: IMPLEMENT

Pediatric patients represent a population at particular risk for medication errors for a number of reasons: the dosing of medications is weight dependent, they are unable to identify themselves to providers, they cannot recognize errors by the color of the liquid or pill, and their immature physiologic systems may be incapable of rebounding from a serious overdose. Hence, ensuring that medications for hospitalized children are administered keeping a number of safety checks in mind is important.

Approximately 2.5% of medication errors in children result in harm. As a result, the Joint Commission has identified a number of important medication safety checks for administering medications to hospitalized children particularly when those children are cared for in adult hospitals. The major categories of recommendations include standardization of medication delivery processes, engaging pharmacy oversight in the delivery of medications, and the use of appropriate technology to ensure safety.

Specific actions that can assist in assuring that medications are delivered safely include assuring that children are weighed consistently in kilograms prior to the administration of medications. Medication dosages should be calculated in both the total dose and dose per kilogram to ensure that the appropriate limits are not reached. Oral syringes should be used to administer oral medications and unit doses are preferred to multidose formulations. Specialty expertise should be available for pediatric patients from a pharmacy perspective and continuing education should be available to advance the pharmacists skills. In the pharmacy, separate areas for the preparation of pediatric medications should be available to ensure that focused attention is applied to these formulations.

Pediatric patients are vulnerable to medication errors for a number of reasons. However, with appropriate attention, these patients can receive their medication safely.

SUGGESTED READINGS

The Joint Commission. Preventing pediatric medication errors. 2008;39. Available at: http://www.jointcommission.org/SentinelEvents/SentinelEventAlert/sea_39.htm. Accessed September 1, 2008.

KNOW HOW TO HELP YOUR PATIENTS WITH THEIR ADDICTION TO SMOKING

ANTHONY D. SLONIM, MD, DRPH

WHAT TO DO: IMPLEMENT

Nicotine is a drug that is a major ingredient in tobacco and has strong addictive potential. Nicotine is readily absorbed through exposure to the oral and gastrointestinal mucosa, lungs, and skin. The effects of nicotine include euphoria, relaxation, and arousal. Within a few days, tolerance begins and dose escalation is required to achieve the same effect. Most importantly, the addictive potential is manifested by its withdrawal syndrome and this is where nurses can be most helpful to their patients.

Cigarette smoking is a risk factor for a number of diseases including coronary artery disease, hypertension, cerebrovascular disease, chronic lung disease, and cancers of the oral mucosa, gastrointestinal, pulmonary, breast, and reproductive organs. Its use contributes to preventable healthcare. Nurses in the outpatient arena have a role in counseling patients who smoke about the risks to their health. The greatest impact of these interventions comes from nurses who are nonsmokers and who not only encourage their smoking patients to quit, but also offer help in accomplishing the task.

For patients admitted acutely to the hospital, smoking is not allowed, particularly because of its interference with therapy with acute medical conditions. However, the dependence on nicotine will lead to a withdrawal syndrome characterized by irritability, anxiety, restlessness, and difficulty concentrating. Patients will also begin to eat more. Nurses can be helpful in identifying these symptoms as they occur, and also intervening on the patient's behalf to obtain appropriate medications to treat the symptoms of withdrawal. Nicotine is available in both transdermal and chewing gum forms to allow the patient to wean from the physical dependence without the associated symptoms. In addition, buproprion is an antidepressant that acts specifically to reduce nicotine cravings.

The nurse is uniquely positioned to assist the patient with cravings from nicotine. Importantly, in addition to pharmacologic support, behavior modification techniques including relaxation and guided imagery may be helpful as well.

SUGGESTED READINGS

Grilli CM. Plant the seeds of success for smoking cessation. *Nursing*. 2008;38(Med Surg Insider):8–10.

Howland RD, Mycek MJ. Central nervous system stimulants. In: *Pharmacology*. 3rd Ed. Philadelphia, PA: Lippincott Williams & Wilkins; 2006.

Ingersoll KS, Cohen J. Combination treatment for nicotine dependence: State of the science. *Subst Use Misuse*. 2005;40(13–14):1923–1943, 2043–2048.

Rose JE. Nicotine addiction and treatment. *Ann Rev Med*. 1996;47:493–507.

KNOW THAT HEPARIN'S SIDE EFFECTS ON PLATELETS OCCUR FROM TWO DIFFERENT MECHANISMS

ANTHONY D. SLONIM, MD, DrPH

Heparin is a commonly used anticoagulant to treat thrombotic events. It acts through binding to Antithrombin III and inactivates the body's intrinsic coagulation factors. One of the major side effects of heparin is thrombocytopenia, which occurs by two different mechanisms. The first type is due to a nonimmunologic reduction in the platelet number. This type usually occurs relatively quickly after the administration of heparin and does not pose a significant danger. The second type requires activation of the platelets by an immunoglobulin reaction that causes the platelets to clump and can lead to thrombosis. This type is rare and occurs within 1–2 weeks of initiating heparin therapy.

Thrombocytopenia is a common condition that results from a number of factors, one of which is heparin use. Thrombocytopenia resulting from heparin usually follows one of the above-mentioned two patterns. It is usually sufficient to stop the heparin and see if the platelet count rises unless the patient requires on-going anticoagulation. There are rare circumstances when it may be necessary to obtain a hypercoagulable workup or send a heparin-induced thrombocytopenia antibody. However, these instances are rare.

The treatment for these conditions is to discontinue heparin therapy including the heparin present bonded to central venous catheters, in intravenous flushes, and as solutions to maintain the patency of arterial and central venous catheters. Patients who require anticoagulation but who have an adverse effect to the actions of heparin can receive one of the direct thrombin inhibitors. Drugs in this class include lepirudin and danaparoid which can be used to treat patients with heparin-induced thrombocytopenia.

SUGGESTED READINGS

Boggio LN, Oza VM. Argatroban use in heparin-induced thrombocytopenia. *Expert Opin Pharmacother*. 2008;9(11): 1963–1967.

Howland RD, Mycek MJ. Drugs affecting the blood. In: *Pharmacology*. 3rd Ed. Philadelphia: Lippincott Williams & Wilkins; 2006.

Warkentin TE, Greinacher A, Koster A, et al. Treatment and prevention of heparin-induced thrombocytopenia: American College of Chest Physicians Evidence-Based Clinical Practice Guidelines. 8th Ed. *Chest*. 2008;133(6 Suppl):340S–380S.

BE CAREFUL IN TREATING THE SYMPTOMS WITHOUT TREATING THE DISEASE

ANTHONY D. SLONIM, MD, DRPH

WHAT TO DO: IMPLEMENT

Nurses are often faced with patient complaints about symptoms and need to be a mediator to both raise potential problems that may be a concern and offer treatment options to improve their care. However, while advocating on behalf of the patient, the nurse needs to recognize those times when symptom control is either insufficient or inappropriate. The following examples provide some specific guidance.

Nausea is one of the most unpleasant symptoms experienced by patients. It may occur related to the primary disease or as a side effect of a medication. Unfortunately, some of the side effects of the typical classes of antiemetics are sedating. Hence, the patient experiencing nausea in the post-ictal phase of status epilepticus or after a concussion, whose mental status and neuro checks need to be monitored frequently to detect a deterioration, may become inadvertently somnolent from the medication and the ability to complete the neurologic examination becomes limited.

A similar situation arises when a patient with a serious head trauma is mechanically ventilated in the intensive care unit for a traumatic brain injury. Sedation is often used to facilitate the ventilation, but it can often obscure the findings of the neurologic examination and prevent the team from recognizing important warning signs.

Diarrhea is another problem. No one likes to endure this symptom. However, stopping the diarrhea by using a medication makes sense only if you know that the etiology of the diarrhea is not caused by bacterial gastroenteritis or *C. difficile* colitis, which have complications of their own. Similarly, the administration of antacids is fine if the patient is experiencing indigestion, but if the pain is a unique manifestation of angina, the drug may be incorrect.

Finally, the use of acetaminophen for fever is helpful to alleviate the symptoms if the underlying cause of the fever is known and the pattern recognized. Unfortunately, the symptomatic treatment of fever without a known cause may only alleviate the symptom and the patient may be septic and require a diagnostic study and antibacterials to treat the underlying sepsis.

Medications provide a wide armamentarium to combat physical symptoms that are unpleasant. Every intervention has a risk and a benefit associated with it and before the nurses advocate for a particular benefit, they should have also weighed the risks.

SUGGESTED READINGS

Howland RD, Mycek MJ. Anti-inflammatory drugs and autocoids. In: *Pharmacology*. 3rd Ed. Philadelphia: Lippincott Williams & Wilkins; 2006.

Howland RD, Mycek MJ. Gastrointestinal and antiemetic drugs. In: *Pharmacology*. 3rd Ed. Philadelphia: Lippincott Williams & Wilkins; 2006.

ASPIRIN: KNOW WHEN TO USE AND WHEN NOT TO...

ANTHONY D. SLONIM, MD, DrPH

Aspirin has a number of beneficial effects and is an economic choice for therapy. Aspirin works on cyclooxygenase, a precursor to prostaglandins, which are a major inflammatory substance of the body. Aspirin then gets deacetylated to salicylate, which is how it manifests its major effects.

Aspirin has three major actions. It is an antinflammatory, antipyretic, and analgesic agent. As an antiinflammatory agent, aspirin inhibits prostaglandins and is particularly beneficial in those diseases in which prostaglandin-mediated inflammation is apparent, including rheumatoid arthritis. Aspirin reduces fever from a number of causes by causing peripheral vasodilation and sweating. Again, the action for this is centered on the inhibition of prostaglandins. Finally, through the same mechanism, aspirin also reduces mild to moderate pain, particularly if inflammation is involved.

While there are a number of benefits attached to the use of aspirin, there are also a number of side effects, most of which are mediated by the same inhibition of prostaglandins. Patients may experience gastrointestinal distress and epigastric discomfort after aspirin ingestion. Because of its effects on the kidneys, aspirin can induce interstitial nephritis and sodium and water retention. Platelet aggregation is irreversibly reduced with the administration of aspirin. This can work to the benefit of the patients with acute coronary syndromes, but can also work against them when they have been taking aspirin consistently and require an invasive procedure that puts them at risk for hemorrhage. Finally, the administration of aspirin to children is contraindicated in all but the fewest circumstances. Reyes syndrome, a deadly disease characterized by hepatitis and cerebral edema is initiated by aspirin administration.

Aspirin is beneficial in a number of circumstances including pain relief, fever relief, and inflammation reduction. It is also beneficial in thrombotic situations like acute coronary syndromes. Because of its mechanism of action, its effects, both good and bad, manifest themselves in all areas where prostaglandins mediate disease.

SUGGESTED READINGS

Howland RD, Mycek MJ. Anti-inflammatory drugs and autocoids. In: *Pharmacology*. 3rd Ed. Philadelphia: Lippincott Williams & Wilkins; 2006.

KNOW HOW TO COUNSEL WOMEN ABOUT THEIR OSTEOPOROSIS

ANTHONY D. SLONIM, MD, DrPH

WHAT TO DO: IMPLEMENT

Postmenopausal women experience a loss of bone mass over time, which makes them susceptible to fractures. There are a number of strategies that women can follow to reduce this loss, including eating a balanced diet that is rich in calcium and vitamin D, performing weight-bearing exercises, and leading a healthy lifestyle. For women in whom this is not enough to improve their skeletal health, a number of medications may be helpful.

The bisphosphonates are a group of drugs that are useful in osteoporosis. The bisphosphonates work by inhibiting osteoclastic bone resorption. As a result, for the duration of the drug's use, the patient experiences a slowing of bone loss and consequently may have fewer fractures. These drugs are administered orally except for pamidronate. These medications are usually well tolerated and have few side effects. Selective estrogen receptor modulators, for example, raloxifene, also act to prevent osteoporosis and improve bone density. This drug does not increase the risk of cancer like other estrogen agents. Finally, calcitonin is a drug that is administered intranasally to reduce bone resorption. It is tolerated well in most women.

Osteoporosis is an important problem for post-menopausal women since it is associated with fractures that can compromise a woman's independence and quality of life. The administration of medications, in addition to living a healthy lifestyle may improve a woman's risk for fractures. Fortunately now, there are medications that are effective, well tolerated, and with minimal side effects.

SUGGESTED READINGS

Howland RD, Mycek MJ. Erectile dysfunction, osteoporosis and obesity. In: *Pharmacology*. 3rd Ed. Philadelphia: Lippincott Williams & Wilkins; 2006.

KNOW THE COMMON DRUGS OF ABUSE AND THEIR EFFECTS

ANTHONY D. SLONIM, MD, DrPH

WHAT TO DO: ASSESS

Drug abuse involves the use of an illegal or a legal drug for nonmedical indications. The reasons why people use drugs are as varied as the drugs they abuse. Nurses caring for patients need to assess drug use since these drugs often induce physiologic dependence and abstinence will then incite a withdrawal syndrome that will be physiologically and psychologically distressful for the patient. Several drug categories are commonly abused including sedative hypnotics, opioids, stimulants, hallucinogens, and marijuana.

Sedative agents include drugs like benzodiazepines and barbiturates. These drugs are often prescribed for the relief of anxiety because they induce a state of relaxation, which increases their potential for abuse. These patients may present somnolent, unarousable, or with inadequate respiration. After ensuring that the As, Bs, and Cs are intact, these patients can often sleep through their "high." Flumazenil is a specific antidote that can be used to counteract the respiratory depression of benzodiazepines. Withdrawal from these addictive agents may present as seizures or excitable syndromes; therefore, a gradual tapering of these drugs for the addicted patient is in order. These drugs have a synergistic effect with alcohol and should never be co-ingested.

Opioid analgesics are clinically useful agents to combat pain. Some members of this class including heroin are used for the euphoric state they produce. These drugs can be taken orally, ingested, or smoked. Patients will present as somnolent, unarousable, and with respiratory depression. After establishing the As, Bs, and Cs, of resuscitation, the patient can sleep through their "high." Naloxone is a narcotic antagonist that helps overcome the effects of an opiate overdose. Unfortunately, the half-life of naloxone is usually shorter than the ingested drug. Hence, it may need redosing. However, it may not be good for the chronically addicted patient since it can precipitate an acute withdrawal syndrome. The withdrawal syndrome for opioids includes a well characterized "abstinence" syndrome with lacrimation, yawning, sweating, and tremors. This evolves into muscle cramps, abdominal pain, and anxiety that are uncomfortable for the patient.

Stimulants are a group of drugs that leads to euphoria and confidence. Drugs listed here include amphetamines and cocaine. These drugs are widely abused and overdoses can lead to seizures, arrhythmias, accelerated hypertension, and stroke. The patient presents in a hyperexcitable frame of mind and needs time to calm down in a safe and quiet environment. Withdrawal of these drugs often leads to depression and symptoms associated with a depressed mood.

Hallucinogens include phencyclidine (PCP), lysergic acid diethylamide (LSD), and marijuana. These drugs are used for the ability to create a vivid, dreamlike state that is associated with euphoria. Overdoses can be treated in a calm environment that protects the patients. Benzodiazepines may be useful.

Patients who use drugs for recreation will often present to care for the drug use or for other conditions. The nurse needs to be familiar with these common symptoms and most importantly assess the chronic use and physical dependence to prevent the withdrawal syndrome.

SUGGESTED READINGS

Trevor AJ, Katzung BG, Masters SB. Drugs of abuse. In: *Katzung and Trevor's Pharmacology Examination and Board Review.* 7th Ed. New York: Lange; 2005.

KNOW THE INS AND OUTS OF INTRAVENOUS CONTRAST FOR CT SCANS

ANTHONY D. SLONIM, MD, DrPH

Computerized tomography (CT) has revolutionized diagnostic and therapeutic capabilities in all body regions allowing improved visualization of anatomic structures and pinpoint precision for drainage procedures. The use of CT, depending upon the organ being imaged, can be enhanced by the use of radiocontrast media. The nurse is often in the position of monitoring the patient's preprocedure and postprocedure and should be familiar with the different types of agents.

Contrast material can be classified as ionic and nonionic. Ionic contrast is safe, but has a higher risk of side effects. Hence, nonionic contrast is used for patients at risk of complications from the introduction of the dye. The major complication is contrast nephropathy, which is diagnosed with a 1 mg/dl increase in the serum creatinine within 48 h of the administration of the contrast study. Risk factors for contrast nephropathy include age, diabetes, renal insufficiency, and dehydration. The possibility of performing the CT without contrast should be considered when the serum creatinine rises above 1.5 mg/dl. If it must be performed with contrast, adequate hydration and the use of N-acetyl cysteine or theophylline may be beneficial in preventing contrast-induced kidney disease.

Aside from contrast nephropathy, the use of contrast is associated with a few other side effects including the feeling of warmth during injection and a metallic taste. Anaphylaxis is rare and occurs in less than 1% of patients. Patients at risk for anaphylaxis may have had prior reactions to contrast, have a history of allergies or asthma, or have allergies to shellfish. If contrast needs to be used, nonionic agents should be used and appropriate prophylaxis including the premedication with steroids 12 h and again 2 h prior to the procedure should be provided. H_2 antagonists and antihistamines can also be used for prophylaxis 2 h prior to the procedure.

Nurses play an important role in the preprocedure and postprocedure management of the patients undergoing CT scans. They need to know the complications of the procedure and the fact that several things can be done to prevent the complications if they are known in advance.

SUGGESTED READINGS

Dillon WP. Neuroimaging in neurologic disorders. In: Kasper DL, Braunwald E, et al., eds. *Harrison's Principles of Internal Medicine*. 16th Ed. New York: McGaw Hill; 2005, pp. 2350–2355.

Kelly AM, Dwamena B, Cronin P, et al. Meta-analysis: Effectiveness of drugs for preventing contrast-induced nephropathy. *Ann Intern Med*. 2008;148(4):284–94. Erratum in: *Ann Intern Med*. 2008;149(3):219.

DON'T ALLOW YOURSELF TO BE "OVER ALERTED" AND BECOME COMPLACENT

ANTHONY D. SLONIM, MD, DrPH

The introduction of technology into the medication administration process has dramatically improved medication safety for patients. However, there continues to be less than optimal success because providers continue to override the technological systems that were put in place to help their patients.

There are alerts and alarms at a number of contact points in the medication delivery process. In an integrated provider order entry system, the prescriber will receive dosage alerts; the pharmacist will receive dosage, interaction, and allergy alerts; and the nurse will be alerted prior to administration. Many of these alarms and alerts are redundant, which is a good news in an integrated system. Hopefully, someone is paying attention to the warning message, right? However, providers often become complacent to these alerts because of their frequency. As a result, the alerts lose their impact.

Nurses in particular receive alerts from a number of different sources. For example, there are alerts at the medicationp-dispensing cabinets where the nurse acquires the drug. There are also alerts, usually in a different system, at the point of administration with barcode technology. For intravenous medications, there are programming opportunities with guardrails that offer yet another series of alerts and alarms for nurses to respond to. Nurses quickly become adept at distinguishing an important alert from one that is unimportant. However, this complacence may result in a medication error.

The Institute for Safe Medication Practices has highlighted a number of opportunities to reduce over-alerting in electronic systems. First, the sensitivity of the alarm system should be turned down so that high risk alerts come through. Second, the institution should prioritize a few alerts that are very important for implementation. Third, those alerts that are bypassed should be identified and the system should be updated. Finally, the alert should be printed on the label.

Technology has made important improvements in medication safety. Nurses need to know how to work within these systems and how to have others help improve the system for the benefit of patients.

SUGGESTED READINGS

ISMP Medication Safety Alert. 2007;12(3):1–3. Available at: http://www.ismp.org/newsletters/acutecare/archives/NL_20070208.pdf. Accessed September 1, 2008.

KNOW WHERE TO GET DRUG INFORMATION WHEN YOU NEED IT

ANTHONY D. SLONIM, MD, DrPH

Nurses are busy. They have a heavy patient load, are stuck with new equipment and technologies that slow them down, have sicker patients than ever before, and have fewer people to help with problems. Despite all these challenges, there is still never a good explanation for administering a drug that you are not familiar with or whose side effects you are not aware of. Come on, you know this; your nursing instructor told you this during your early months of nursing school. It is the reason why they made you create all those drug cards (as if you just couldn't buy them at the bookstore). The reason is that as a professional you have an obligation to know what the foreign chemical you are about to give the patient in front of you is supposed to do. So, now that you know you should know, how do you get the information?

In fact, there are a number of very good references for the nurse to identify the indications, contraindications, interactions, and side effect profiles of drugs. First, most nursing units have drug handbooks that place this information at your fingertips. Second, one of the big advantages of computerized drug information is that the appropriate ranges and alerts are programmed into the system. Remember, though the programming was done by humans, mistakes may be present there, so do not rely on the computer if you are unfamiliar with the drug or do not understand what the drug is used for. Third, the pharmacy usually has a number of specialty drug references, as will your unit if you are in a specialty area like the intensive care unit or dialysis unit. Fourth, there is always the opportunity to learn from colleagues on the unit or pharmacists in the pharmacy. Specialty pharmacists are becoming a more and more important component of the healthcare team and have extensive knowledge about the medications in their areas. Finally, a number of important online references are readily available and free to professionals. Searching the internet for some of these so that you can use them efficiently in your practice is helpful.

As a nurse, you should never feel that you do not have ready access to a reference to help you identify what medications you are giving your patients, whether they are indicated and what you need to watch for. Know what is available to help you do your job for your patient.

SUGGESTED READINGS

Nursing Drug Handbook 2009. 29th Ed. Lippincott Williams & Wilkins, Philadelphia, PA; 2009.

BE CAREFUL WHEN GIVING PATIENTS DRUG SAMPLES

ANTHONY D. SLONIM, MD, DRPH

WHAT TO DO: IMPLEMENT

Drug samples exist in many hospital clinics and physician offices. They are brought by pharmaceutical representatives so that they can be given to patients for a trial of therapy, for short-term courses of therapy, or as a method for helping an indigent patient. The problem is that these drug samples provided by an office practice require attention to detail since nurses have now moved from their usual role in the process of administering medications to one of processing and dispensing medications, which is usually relegated to the expertise of the pharmacist.

You are probably saying, "What is the big deal? It is just a matter of slapping a sticker on the box and handing it to the patient." In fact, for liquid medications that need to be reconstituted, following the directions for reconstitution is important. The storage and quality control checks that are in place in the pharmacy need to be in place for the sample closet. Who is keeping the log and the lot numbers? Who is managing a recall when it occurs? Who has the list of patients given each drug?

There is considerably more responsibility in the management of a sample closet than handing out a few boxes of drugs and wishing the patient well. Nurses need to remember their scope of practice, which in most states does not provide for processing or distribution of medication.

SUGGESTED READINGS

Buppert C. Who can legally dispense drug samples? Available at: http://www.medscape.com/viewarticle/519748. Accessed September 1, 2008.

Paparella S. Sample medications can be dangerous. *J Em Nurs.* 2006;32(2):172–174.

KNOW THE RISKS OF NOT EDUCATING YOUR PATIENTS ON THEIR MEDICATIONS PRIOR TO DISCHARGE

ANTHONY D. SLONIM, MD, DRPH

The discharge order has been written for Mrs Smith; your patient in 842 is asking to go to the bathroom; and radiology is calling for Mr Jones to perform the stat head CT. You wonder how you are going to pull off Mrs Smith's discharge, reconcile her medications, and accomplish your other tasks.

Nurses everywhere face these challenges on a daily basis. The Institute for Safe Medication Practices performed a survey to help identify some of the barriers to adequately educating patients on their medications. Not surprisingly, time constraints were a common reason why medication education was not performed. What is surprising is that many nurses were unaware that preprinted information was available to help them educate their patients. Either it was not in a place that was accessible or was simply unavailable. Finally, very little was known about how to help patients avoid medication errors.

Since the survey was performed, the Joint Commission has added medication reconciliation to the list of discharge requirements. This is a good thing. When you think about the effort that goes into helping a patient recuperate during a hospitalization, consider how poorly healthcare providers perform at ensuring that patients know what to do to prevent a relapse or readmission. Then, you recognize the need for these standards. Having the standards by themselves will not ensure that it gets done.

Nurses need to work with their hospitals to ensure that they have the tools they need to adequately educate patients about their after-hospital care to prevent post-discharge medication errors or confusion in the medication regimen. This attention to medication safety is in everyone's interest.

SUGGESTED READINGS

ISMP Medication Safety Alert. 2003. Helping to remove the barriers to patient education. Available at: http://www.ismp.org/Newsletters/acutecare/articles/20031002.asp. Accessed September 1, 2008.

71

REMEMBER TO PERFORM A DISCHARGE ASSESSMENT AND VITAL SIGNS

MONTY D. GROSS, PHD, RN, CNE

WHAT TO DO: ASSESS

Prior to discharging a patient, it is a good practice to perform an assessment and check vital signs. A thorough assessment is normally performed at the beginning of every shift. However, multiple issues could develop between the time the assessment was conducted and when the patient leaves the hospital at the time of discharge. For example, a suture could open or a dressing could loosen, exposing a wound to the environment. The dressing might need to be changed due to drainage. A fever could develop or blood pressure rise. Therefore, it is wise to perform a quick assessment just prior to sending the patient out the door.

The patient's vital signs should be assessed and documented immediately prior to the patient leaving the unit for home or an alternate destination such as a rehabilitation facility or nursing home. Checking vital signs at the time of discharge will provide an opportunity for the nurse to verify that they are within the patient's normal range. If they are not, the physician can be contacted, the discharge postponed or cancelled, and steps taken to ensure the patient is stable.

Some hospitals have policies requiring that vital signs be checked and documented within 30–60 min of discharge. Others rationalize that a problem-focused assessment is more valuable than vital signs at discharge. Examples of problem-focused assessments include wound assessment for the patient with a sutured laceration and temperature checks for the patient with fever or pneumonia. The rationale is that checking vital signs takes time, could delay discharge, may miss an important clinical issue, and may be relatively insensitive for identifying the patient's problems. It is also important to ensure that if aberrant vital signs are identified, the nurse escalates the information appropriately to the physician.

Taking time to perform an assessment including vital signs can provide important information. Simple oversights such as forgetting to remove a peripheral intravenous catheter, not reassessing an elevated blood pressure or temperature, or not double checking a wound dressing can be identified and appropriate interventions initiated. This last check prior to sending a patient out the front door is worth the time it takes. Remember to conduct an assessment and check vital signs at least 1 h prior to discharging a patient.

SUGGESTED READINGS

Patient hemorrhages, dies just outside of the hospital: Jury blames discharge nurse. *Legal Eagle Eye Newslett Nurs Prof.* 2008;16(5).
Zimmerman P. Cutting edge discussion of management, policy, and program issues in emergency care. *J Emerg Nurs.* 2006;32(4):333–338.

Handoffs of care: Providing seamless care

Monty D. Gross, PhD, RN, CNE

WHAT TO DO: IMPLEMENT

The number of transfers of patient care that occur during a patient's stay in a hospital is staggering. Transfers, also known as handoffs, from one care provider to another are points of vulnerability where information can be omitted or not clearly communicated, which leaves the patient susceptible to injury or omission of care. Care handoffs occur when the responsibility for patient care changes as the result of a change in the patient's location or provider.

The Joint Commission on Health's 2009 National Patient Safety Goal is to improve communication among and between caregivers. The organization is to implement a standardized approach to handoff communications, including an opportunity to ask and respond to questions. The primary objective of a handoff is to provide accurate information about a patient's care, treatment and services, current condition, and any recent or anticipated changes. The information communicated during a handoff must be accurate to meet patient safety goals.

There are a variety of formats for an effective handoff of care. The Institute for Healthcare Improvement provided the SBAR Handoff Report Tool. The tool is used for handoffs of care to provide seamless transfer of care. The acronym SBAR stands for *S*ituation, *B*ackground, *A*ssessment, and *R*ecommendation.

Another format used at the University of Virginia is the IDEAL handoff of care. IDEAL stands for *I*dentify the patient, *D*iagnosis, current condition, and recent *E*vents or changes in condition, *A*nticipated changes in condition or treatment, what to watch for in the next level of care or contingency plans, and *L*eave time to ask questions or clarify questions.

Either of these handoff tools provides a snapshot of important information that will allow for immediate seamless care. It does not provide unnecessary information or every detail of care. Too much information can hide important information the caregiver needs. Remember to use a handoff of care tool to improve communication among caregivers.

SUGGESTED READINGS

Dracup K, Morris P. Passing the torch: The challenge of handoffs. *Am J Crit Care*. 2008;17(2):95–97.

Institute for Healthcare Improvement. SBAR Handoff Tool. Available at: http://www.ihi.org/IHI/Topics/PatientSafety/SafetyGeneral/Tools/SBARHandoffReportTool.htm. Accessed June 29, 2008.

National Patient Safety Goals. Joint Commission on the Accreditation of Healthcare Organizations. 2006 Comprehensive Accreditation Manual for Hospitals: The Official Handbook (CAMH). Joint Commission Resources, Inc. 2005. Available at: http://www.jointcommission.org/PatientSafety/NationalPatientSafetyGoals. Accessed June 29, 2008.

University of Virginia. Handoff of care: Frequently asked questions. Available at: http://www.healthsystem.virginia.edu/internet/e-learning/handoff_faq.pdf. Accessed June 29, 2008.

Help to establish a "patient first" mindset: "They ARE my patients"

Jeannie Scruggs Garber, DNP, RN

Nurses who work in a hospital setting would have certainly heard the words, "they are not my patients" from another nurse. You might have heard it when the call bell rang and the nurse answering it was too busy to go to the patient's room; it could be either that the nurse taking care of the patient had a reputation that influenced whether or not others would help with his or her patients, or that the individual was uncomfortable with the patient's situation. Regardless of the reason, the underlying situation is that the nurse has not put the patient's needs first. Quality patient care suffers when healthcare providers' attitudes prevent a patient-first mindset.

When the patient's needs are not at the center of decisions (e.g., who answers the call light?), care may be delayed, errors may be made, or patient safety may be at risk. A student nurse's description of what happens when the patient's needs are not at the center of decision making is helpful for the students regardless of their level of experience or tenure in nursing.

"There were the nurses my friend Julie had to deal with, who, when her patient was having a seizure and she screamed 'Help!' from the doorway, actually looked at her and said, 'That's not my patient.' WHAT?! Yes, people are actually like this. And I don't think they started like this— I think that over time they developed this attitude towards patients. Maybe these nurses will never go home at night and cry over a patient, but I would rather cry every night than lose my ability to care about other human beings."

We must do better in our profession to prevent situations like the one described by this student nurse. Patients rely on nurses to help them in times when they are fearful and cannot help themselves.

Patient–nurse interactions are sometimes posted on the Internet and allow providers to view the experience through the lens of the patient. One particular case of a patient regarding an emergency room experience describes a patient asking to use the bedpan. The nurse, within hearing distance of the patient, argues with another nurse about whose patient she is and proceeds to discuss how assignments were made unfairly. She then walks away to go on a break and the patient does not get the bedpan.

Delvin states that "Patients and their families were fed up with hearing nurses say 'sorry that is not my patient,'" and so this served as a catalyst to develop a service course for nurses to help to improve patient satisfaction. A hospital in Southern California adopted behavioral standards of communication that read: "It is unacceptable to make the statements, 'I don't know' or 'That's not my patient.' The appropriate response is, 'I'm sorry, I don't know, but I will find a person who can answer that for you.'" Nurses make an impact on patients' lives in many ways. The way nurses speak to patients and respond to their requests may be the most important skill needed to provide safe care. The poem below, written by djtphn1, captures the essence of the importance for the statement, "they ARE my patients":

Today, I will open my eyes…
Today, I will only see the truth…
Today, I will take responsibility for my own actions…
Today, I will not blame…
Today, I will only see what I could have done differently
And that my patient is your patient
And yours, mine…
And that your patient could be my mother, father, sister or brother…
Today, I will know that each person I lay my hands on
Has a family, a history, a journey, that I pray
Does not end with me.....
But if it does
Today I will find comfort in knowing that I did
Everything possible to ensure that my patient was cared for
The way I would care for one of my own,
And today I will know that I am a good nurse
Just because of that…
Today, I will care about each person I have the privilege
To cross paths with and I will know that the
Magic of nursing
Happens in the wee hours of the morning
When there is no one else around,
Where secrets are shared over bedpans
And trust is implicit
Just because I am a nurse…
Today, I will believe in nursing
Once again!

Suggested Readings

Confessions of a student nurse. 2008. Available at: http://lilk8tob.spaces.live.com/Blog/cns!D17A28AACD396F0B!1691.entry. Accessed June 20, 2008.

Delvin K. NHS nurses told to smile more, gossip less. Telegraph. co.uk. 2008. Available at: http://www.telegraph.co.uk/news/uknews/1578419/NHS-nurses-told-to-smile-more-and-gossip-less.html. Accessed June 20, 2008.

djtphn1 (n.d.). A nurses prayer. A Nurses Prayer: Today I Will. Available at: http://hubpages.com/hub/A-Nurses-Prayer-Today-I-Will. Accessed June 19, 2008.

Kushell E, Bowers N, Gillespie T. The rise and fall of one unit's patient satisfaction scores. *J Healthc Qual*. 2007. Available at: http://www.nahq.org/journal/ce/article.html?article_id=287. Accessed June 20, 2008.

Nurse wretched. Sunny side up: Dispatches from paradise. 2006. Available at: http://dgm.typepad.com/sunny_side/2006/04/nurse_wretched.html. Accessed June 20, 2008.

INTERDISCIPLINARY COMMUNICATION, INCLUDING A CASE MANAGER, CAN BENEFIT YOUR PATIENT AT THE END OF LIFE

MELISSA H. CRIGGER, BSN, MHA, RN

WHAT TO DO: IMPLEMENT

Remember that communication is essential in most healthcare experiences, but it becomes particularly important when performing discharge planning for the terminally ill. Communication is necessary for establishing a caring relationship. In the acute care setting, communication can be both verbal (words or written language) and nonverbal and is influenced by several factors including:

- Perceptions
- Values
- Emotions
- Sociocultural background
- Knowledge
- Roles and relationships
- Environment
- Space and territoriality

When caring for the terminally ill patient, communication of discharge plans is very important. The patient's prognosis, treatment, and end-of-life preferences should be addressed by the physician. One concern, however, is that the physician may lack experience working with a multidisciplinary care team or may have insufficient knowledge of the hospice process or its availability. Many medical schools lack curricula in end-of-life care. According to Roscoe and Schonwetter, "physicians must work to educate their patients about end-of-life care options and must initiate discussions of treatment preferences, ideally long before a serious diagnosis is made or shortened prognosis is given." However, physicians may not be prepared to perform this necessary work.

Communication of the plan is critical. For the case manager who is in charge of discharge planning, it is important to ensure that communication between the physician and the patient regarding hospice care occurs prior to his or her carrying out the discharge plan. The patient should be aware of the case management consult for palliative care prior to the case management meeting. The case manager should evaluate the patient's current knowledge prior to discussing the actual plan and should also share with the ordering physician what has already been discussed and determine any areas where additional information will need to be provided (e.g., insurance coverage for hospice services). The case manager should remember to always provide detailed descriptions of the hospice benefit and clarify any patient misconceptions.

Another area of communication that needs to be ensured by the case manager is that discharge planning occurs with the inclusion of the family. For the patient who will be cared for by hospice in the home, the family must be educated on the covered services. One misconception of family members is that hospice provides 24×7 care when, in fact, the family will assist in providing basic care. According to Harrison and colleagues, when discharge planning for hospice services included case management, collaboration between providers and family members improved and length of stay and unnecessary utilization of inpatient services was reduced.

When providing discharge planning, the case manager must be aware that the patient can display different emotions based on current stage of grief. The patient can be anxious or depressed regarding the current prognosis. For the anxious patient, the case manager must remember to provide clear and concise communication. The case manager must make sure that discharge planning discussions occ ur in an environment with minimal noise and a closed door for privacy. For the depressed patient, the case manager must remember to provide information in a clear and concise manner. The case manager should be honest and demonstrate empathy for the patient. Using good communication skills goes a long way to promote a caring relationship with the patient.

SUGGESTED READINGS

Elkin MK, et al. *Nursing Interventions & Clinical Skills*. 4th Ed. St. Louis, MO: Mosby Elsevier; 2007, pp. 20–37.

Harrison JP, Ford D, Wilson K. The impact of hospice programs on U.S. hospitals. *Nurs Econ*. 2005;23(2):55, 78–84, 90.

Roscoe LA, Schonwetter RS. Improving access to hospice and palliative care for patients near the end of life: Present status and future direction. *J Pall Care*. 2008;22(1):46–52.

DO NOT ASSUME THAT A PATIENT GOING TO A NURSING HOME DOES NOT NEED EDUCATION AND SELF-MANAGEMENT SKILLS

NANCY F. ALTICE RN, MSN CCNS, CNS-BC

WHAT TO DO: IMPLEMENT

Much of the patient education provided at discharge is intended to help patients manage their care needs at home. When a patient is being discharged to a long-term care environment such as a skilled nursing facility, questions arise about the necessity of completing discharge education. Typically, there are special forms that are used to communicate pertinent information to the receiving facility, and the assumption is sometimes made that the patient is not capable of self-management in the long-term care environment. Recently, many hospitals have been faced with demonstrating the quality of care that they provide by submitting quality data that can be accessed by the public. The Joint Commission included specific patient education requirements in the Core Measures quality initiative, specific to heart failure. The requirement to provide specific education to heart failure patients only applies if the patient is being discharged to home. This is obviously an issue that requires an individualized approach. The simple rule, "do what is best for the patient" applies here.

Many patients who must reside in long-term care environments have had a decline in their memory and cognitive function. Teaching complex information to these patients would obviously have little benefit, if any. However, family education is still very important. Families need to be able to monitor the condition of their loved ones and be able to participate in their care as much as possible. If the patient requires a special diet, the family should be made aware so that they do not bring foods that could cause harm or discomfort to the patient. They should be aware of any major side effects of the medications the patient is currently taking so that observations can be appropriately reported to the nursing home staff.

Many patients who are discharged to a long-term care environment do remain in control of their own decision making for most aspects of their care but are physically too frail to return to a home environment with less than 24 h supervision. These patients should receive education about their condition, signs and symptoms to report, activity, diet, and medications. Although they will not have complete control over their diet, they can make informed choices that will eliminate foods that might be troublesome for their condition. Many long-term care facilities do not offer an extensive range of special diets; so patients may be offered broader choices than they received in the acute hospital environment, but with dietary education, they can choose wisely. Although a licensed person will administer medications in most long-term care environments, an informed patient will be able to monitor his or her response to treatment better.

Remember that for many patients, the skilled nursing facility is just a stepping stone to eventual return to home. Providing education about self-management of chronic conditions will help patients succeed and hopefully prevent unexpected readmissions to the hospital.

SUGGESTED READINGS

Joint Commission (2007). Performance measurement initiatives. Available at: http://www.jointcommission.org/Performance Measurement/ PerformanceMeasurement/default.htm. Accessed April 10, 2007.

Willette EW, Surrells D, Davis LL, et al. Nurses knowledge of heart failure self management. *Prog Cardiovasc Nurs.* 2007; 22(4):190–195.

CAN THE PATIENT REALLY AFFORD THOSE MEDS?

NANCY F. ALTICE RN, MSN CCNS, CNS-BC

WHAT TO DO: PLAN

Medication noncompliance is a costly problem. Not only does it cause increased morbidity and mortality for individual patients but it also increases healthcare costs when these patients return for additional medical care. There are a number of reasons that patients do not follow through with obtaining all of their prescriptions. Cost of medications is one of the major factors.

Often, patients have no idea what a medication will cost until they are at the pharmacy picking up their medications. If the price is too high, they may have no choice at the moment but to leave those prescriptions at the pharmacy. If specific medications are commonly prescribed for a particular population, it is helpful to alert patients to the average cost at the time the prescription is written. Explain the importance of continuing the medications. Do not assume that patients with insurance or Medicare can afford their medications. Most plans have co-payments which add up to a sizable amount when the patient is on multiple medications. Although there are various assistance programs available, the eligibility requirements vary. Helping patients navigate their options is an important aspect of providing comprehensive care. It is hard to maintain awareness of all the options available. Some of the resources to assist with this may be case managers, social workers, pharmacists, and physician office staff.

Although finances are a sensitive subject for patients and providers, it is important to address the issue before patients go to the pharmacy and make an unwise decision to discontinue their medications.

SUGGESTED READINGS

Dutcher R. When the patient won't take the medicine. *Pharmacy Times*. 2007. Available at: http://www.pharmacytimes.com/issues/articles/2007–02_4420.asp.

Jackevicius CA, Li P, Tu JV. Prevalence, predictors, and outcomes of primary nonadherence after acute myocardial infarction. *Circulation*. 2008;117(8):1028–1036.

THE COMPLAINING OR CONTROLLING FAMILY MAY REALLY JUST BE FEARFUL

NANCY F. ALTICE RN, MSN CCNS, CNS-BC

WHAT TO DO: ASSESS

Families of patients need support when faced with illness and changes in quality of life for their loved ones and potentially for themselves. Often, serious illness and particularly complications of the illness or treatments add to the stress that is felt by all involved. Each person handles these stresses in a unique way. For a few families, the coping behaviors are perceived as negative. They may make negative comments about the care that their loved one is receiving. They may play the role of a staff member for each other and may ask the actual staff member not to be involved in their loved one's care. Some families keep written notes about many details of the patient's care. Some families may react by being absent at crucial times when decisions need to be made. These behaviors usually increase stress for the staff and can impact quality of care for the patient. Occasionally, staff will request not to be assigned to the patient due to their discomfort in handling the family.

Open communication is often the key to resolving family conflicts. Most families desire to talk with the physician at least daily. In many cases, there are multiple physicians taking care of the patient, and this often leads to overlapping and sometimes seemingly conflicting information being given. Whenever possible, it is helpful to have a consistent person such as a primary staff nurse, clinical nurse specialist, case manager, unit manager, or patient advocate who is able to serve as an "interpreter" for the family. This person's role is to assess the families understanding and clear up any points of confusion or at least help them understand that some information such as the ultimate outcome is beyond their grasp when prognosis is uncertain. Acknowledging the difficulty of not knowing is appropriate and reassures the family that their needs are understood.

Scheduling a family conference that can be attended by multiple care providers including physicians and family members is often well worth the effort to resolve family concerns and to inform the healthcare team of concerns or patient history, wishes, etc. that may not be known to everyone. Families are not outsiders in the patient's life and should not be excluded from important information about the patient's care, progress, and prognosis.

Families who keep written notes are not always attempting to intimidate staff with the threat of legal action. They are often writing down information that is unclear to them so that they can share it word for word with other family members or can look up information on the Internet when they have access. Some families have expressed that they want to be able to tell the patients what has happened to them during the time that they have been sedated or unconscious. Offering to contribute information for their writings is one way of breaking down the tense atmosphere that often exists when families are stressed.

Remember to anticipate what information the family may want to know. Volunteer information without the family having to ask. Be sure to keep the family informed of any significant change in condition, either good or bad, to assure them that they will be kept informed. Often, families are afraid to leave the hospital for their own personal care or rest because they are afraid they will not be there when needed. Recognize that negative remarks or behaviors may just be a sign of their fear.

SUGGESTED READINGS

AACN Protocols for Practice: Creating Healing Environments. 2nd Ed. 2007. Available at: http://www.aacn.org.

Davidson JE, Powers K, Hedayat KM, et al. Clinical practice guidelines for support of the family in the patient-centered intensive care unit: American College of Critical Care Medicine Task Force 2004–2005. *Crit Care Med*. 2007;35(2):605–622.

Baker MK, Miers A, Sulla S, et al. Families: From difficult to exceptional-one team's journey. *J Nurs Care Qual*. 2007;22(3): 272–278.

Objectively Validate the Information Your Patients Provide

Anthony D. Slonim, MD, DrPH

WHAT TO DO: EVALUATE

Patients experience demoralizing and uncomfortable circumstances during care in which they lose control of their environment. For some, the underlying condition or the embarrassment of sharing information with the healthcare provider prevents the healthcare team from knowing important information that could ultimately improve their condition or prevent harm. It is important for clinicians to listen to their patients and to "hear" what they are saying. On occasion, it becomes necessary to validate the situation through further assessments, team meetings, laboratory, or radiographic testing. Several important situations highlight this point, which needs to be remembered to prevent harm. These include elderly falls, pregnancies, child abuse, alcohol, and tobacco use.

The elderly patient often experiences functional decline with increasing age. Activities that were previously well tolerated and performed independently become more difficult. Hospitalization, and importantly bed rest, worsens both the physical and mental condition of the elderly. As a result, an appreciation of their condition needs to be consistently validated. The aged patient may require assistance in getting out of bed, going to the rest room, and walking, which were performed independently a day or two before. In addition, unfamiliar environments complicate their surroundings and create additional obstacles and barriers to independence. A provider can never assure that, despite what seems to be full understanding, the elderly patient actually will follow the entire directions provided. Putting a call bell in place, instructing when to call for assistance, and waiting for feedback may be insufficient despite the patient's understanding of the directions. Direct observation and repetitive assessments of the patient's status are important to prevent devastating falls and other injuries during hospitalization. When falls or injuries occur, the denial of pain or discomfort may also be insufficient to rule out a serious injury since patients often act out of a desire to please their provider. Therefore, confirmatory examinations and follow-up testing, based on the clinical situation, are indicated.

Pregnancy is an important life event but can also be unexpected for the woman. A series of routine questions for the woman during her child bearing years, including the timing of the last menstrual period and the occurrence of sexual intercourse without contraception, is a routine component of the initial assessment for the patient. More importantly, despite the patients' best intentions, they may not remember the answers to these questions, particularly when they are stressed because of an immediate health concern. In these circumstances, it becomes important to validate the pregnancy with an objective test to ensure that the woman and potentially her fetus are not harmed by medical interventions or diagnostic testing.

Child abuse is an important societal ill and parents have a defined role in providing protection to their children. When young children present with injuries that are suspicious for abuse, it is important that the clinician listen and attend to the concerns of the parents with a nonjudgmental approach, but be appropriately concerned for the safety of the child. It also becomes important to recognize that parents may be legitimately concerned about an injury and may not know how it occurred. Children may be cared for in other settings including day care and with babysitting, so the parent may not be the cause of the injury and may be bringing the child to medical attention with legitimate concerns. There are important clues as to when the parent may not be meeting their parental obligations and be injuring the child. These include discrepancies in the story between the two parents, an injury that is out of proportion to the story, or an injury that does not match with the developmental age of the child. All of these should represent "red flags" to the provider, and appropriate reporting should take place to protect the child if the provider has suspicions that cannot be allayed through further assessments.

Alcohol and tobacco use are important habits with adverse health effects. It is not uncommon for patients to underestimate the amount of alcohol and tobacco used on a consistent basis. When acute concerns about alcohol use are raised, laboratory testing can be used to detect the level of alcohol in the blood and validate if the symptoms may be associated with this use.

While clinicians often want to believe what their patients tell them, there are often circumstances when the validation of what the patient says either through repeated assessments or through corroboration with formal testing is important and is in the patient's interest to prevent harm.

SUGGESTED READINGS

Corsinovi L, Bo M, Ricauda Aimonino N, et al. Predictors of falls and hospitalization outcomes in elderly patients admitted to an acute geriatric unit. *Arch Gerontol Geriatr*. Jul 30, 2008 [Epub ahead of print] PMID: 18674824 [PubMed—as supplied by publisher].

Carroll NV, Delafuente JC, Cox FM, et al. Fall-related hospitalization and facility costs among residents of institutions providing long-term care. *Gerontologist*. 2008;48(2):213–222.

Gushurst CA. Child abuse: Behavioral aspects and other associated problems. *Pediatr Clin North Am*. 2003;50(4):919–938.

Mathews B, Walsh K, Fraser JA. Mandatory reporting by nurses of child abuse and neglect. *J Law Med*. 2006;13(4):505–517.

Porteous J. Oh, by the way, the patient is pregnant! *Can Oper Room Nurs J*. 2008;26(2):35, 37–39, 41–22.

KNOW WHEN TO PUT ON YOUR ISOLATION GOWN

BONNIE L. PARKER RN, CRRN

WHAT TO DO: IMPLEMENT

In a healthcare setting, isolation precautions are employed to reduce the spread of microorganisms to patients, staff, visitors, and families. Isolation can only be effective if all those involved in the patient's care follow established isolation precaution guidelines. Contact precautions are the most frequently used precautions and are implemented to reduce the transmission of diseases that can be spread by close contact or direct contact with infectious pathogens. Among these diseases are methicillin-resistant *Staphylococcus aureus* (MRSA), vancomycin-resistant enterococci (VRE), shingles, and chicken pox.

Personal protective equipment (PPE) is designed to protect mucous membranes, airways, skin, and clothing from contact with infectious organisms. All PPE is intended to be applied before entering an isolation room and removed before leaving the room. When a patient is on contact isolation precautions, an isolation gown and gloves should be applied before entering the room whenever close contact or soiling is anticipated. It is presumptuous of nurses to assume that they will not touch the patient or anything in the room when entering to administer a medication or to check on a patient. Many patients will wait until the nurse is present to ask for help. That quick medication administration may rapidly become a bedpan assist, change of position in bed, or another unplanned task. With several patients in isolation, donning PPE for every trip into a room may appear inefficient, but saving a minute now may prevent the transmission of disease and expense later. Many of these pathogens have a long life once dried on hard surfaces. For example, MRSA can live 7 days on a dry surface; so uniforms can become contaminated when the nurse brushes against the side rail, or over bed table. The nurse can then carry the organism down the hall to another patient, to the nurses' station, to her coworkers, to her car, and to her family.

Properly applying PPE begins with the handwashing. Next, the isolation gown is applied fully covering the body from neck to knees and arms to wrist. After the gown, if the patient is on droplet or airborne precautions, apply a mask, fitting it snuggly to the face and below the chin. If splashing of contaminated fluids such as blood, mucus, or urine is anticipated, goggles should be applied. Finally, gloves would be donned, covering the cuffs of the gown. Gloves should be changed whenever torn or heavily soiled.

PPE removal begins with the gloves by turning them outside in so that the outsides are not touched. The mask is removed next by touching only the strings which they tie in the back or the earloops. Finally, the gown is removed by pulling the neck tape loose and pulling the arm out so that the gown is turned inside out and only the insides are exposed. Hands should be washed before leaving the room. Following facility guidelines for infection control and isolation precautions can reduce the spread of infectious organisms and protect not only patients but also staff and others in the community.

SUGGESTED READINGS

Siegel JD, Rhinehart E, Jackson M, et al. *Guideline for Isolation Precautions: Preventing Transmission of Infectious Agents in Healthcare Settings*. 2007, pp. 49–129. Available at: http://www.cdc.gov/ncidod/dhqp/pdf/guidelines/Isolation2007.pdf. Accessed August 19, 2008.

KNOW HOW TO CARE FOR A URINARY CATHETER

BONNIE L. PARKER RN, CRRN

Urinary catheters are some of the oldest documented medical equipment used in the 1st century to treat urinary retention. Urinary catheters are commonly used during hospitalization, in as many as 12.6% of hospitalized patients. Catheters are used to protect skin, to relieve pain caused by frequent bedpan use, to treat urinary retention, and in intensive care units (ICU) as an accurate monitor of output to assess fluid status and renal function. Catheters are also the leading cause of urinary tract infections (UTIs). In addition, as of October 1, 2008, Medicare payment guidelines will no longer cover hospital acquired UTIs. Therefore, it is imperative that urinary catheters be removed when no longer needed and not be used whenever they can be avoided. The rate of infection with urinary catheter use is directly related to the length of time that a catheter is left in the place. When catheters are medically necessary, it is important to provide the best care possible to prevent complications that can arise from their use. Bacteria can enter the urinary tract in one of these three ways: upon catheter insertion, tracking up the catheter tube into the urethra, or by growing in the space between the urethra and the catheter tubing. As many as 30% of catheterized patients will grow bacteria in their urine, 6% of those may progress to a UTI, and as many as 4% may develop bacteremia, which could potentially result in death.

When a urinary catheter is inserted, it is very important to follow strict aseptic techniques. The sterile gloves included in most pre-packaged kits may not fit hands that are very large or very small; this may require obtaining a separate pair of sterile gloves before starting the procedure. During insertion for a female patient, if the urinary meatus is missed and the catheter is accidentally inserted into the vagina, a new sterile catheter needs to be used for the next attempt.

After the catheter is inserted, it is important to maintain routine hygiene to keep the perineal region and the catheter itself clean by cleaning with warm water and soap at least once per 8 h shift and more often if the patient is incontinent of stool. The bag should be hung on the bedside making sure that it is below the level of the bladder at all times. Not only is infection a concern, but the catheter may also be pulled accidentally by a confused patient or by staff when transferring the patient. Pulling a catheter out while the balloon is still inflated can cause damage to the urethra and is very painful. After the catheter is inserted and the balloon inflated, the tubing should be secured to the patient's leg with either a tape or a catheter holder, keeping the tubing below the level of the bladder. Securing the catheter will prevent it from being pulled out if it is caught on bed rails or a wheelchair.

To obtain a urine sample from a catheter, clamp the tubing for 20 to 30 min; clean the port with alcohol and allow it to dry. With a sterile syringe, access the port and draw out 20 mL of urine. Empty the urine from the syringe into a sterile specimen container, label it, place it in biohazard bag, and send it to the lab. Remember to unclamp the tubing; forgetting to unclamp the tubing will cause bladder distention, backflow of urine into the kidneys, and discomfort for the patient.

SUGGESTED READINGS

Ellis H. The Foley catheter. *J Perioper Pract*. 2006;16(4).

Fallis W. Indwelling Foley catheters is the current design a source of erroneous measurement of urine output? *CritCare Nurse*. 2005;25(2):44–51.

Godfrey H, Fraczyk L. Preventing and managing catheter-associated urinary tract infections. *Br J Commun Nurs*. 2005;10(5):205–206, 208–212.

Seymour C. Audit of catheter-associated UTI using silver alloy-coated Foley catheters. *Br J Nurs*. 2006;15(11).

REMEMBER TIMELY PAIN MANAGEMENT

BONNIE L. PARKER, RN, CRRN

WHAT TO DO: ASSESS, PLAN, AND EVALUATE

One overriding concern that many patients face with medical treatment is pain. Recent court cases have resulted in decisions against medical personnel for inadequate pain control. Pain can be defined as an unpleasant feeling or a state of discomfort and can range from mild to severe. Pain is also subjective, that is, pain is simply what a patient says it is. People have a wide range of reactions to pain; some hide it, not wanting to accept its existence, and others distress over what appears to be a minor injury. What is an insignificant nuisance to one patient is a crippling event to another. Nurses must accept patients' impression of their pain and treat it effectively. All patients have the right to receive adequate pain relief. Some nurses may choose to administer pain medication according to their own impression of the patient's pain, that is, if the patient appears to be relaxed and comfortable, the nurse may not administer the medication as quickly as when a patient appears uncomfortable. This should be avoided; every patient has the right to adequate and prompt pain relief and a patient's level of pain cannot be assessed by appearance alone.

Pain is now considered by many as the fifth vital sign and patients should be assessed at least once every shift for the presence and degree of pain. Not assessing pain sufficiently has been found to be a major factor in unrelieved pain. One successful method of pain assessment is the Numeric Pain Scale that allows the patient to rate his pain from 0 to 10, with 0 being no pain and 10 being the most severe pain. Another scale that is useful with non-English-speaking patients and nonverbal patients is the Faces Pain Rating Scale. It uses six faces with varying expressions from smiling to tearful to rate pain. Patients who are unresponsive or unable to answer questions can be assessed by physical assessment signs such as monitoring vital signs, observing facial expressions, protection of a body area, massaging, and agitation and moaning.

Acute pain occurs suddenly; it is usually related to injury or inflammation; and it is usually of short duration. It is typically treated with a combination of pain relievers and treatment of the underlying cause. Chronic pain may be constant or intermittent, may or may not be related to an illness or injury, and lasts more than 6 months. People who have experienced chronic pain for an extended period of time may display no outward signs of discomfort when in pain. Treatment of chronic pain may utilize several treatment modalities, including narcotic and non-narcotic pain relievers, physical therapy, heat or cold packs, or transcutaneous electrical nerve stimulation (TENS) units. Repositioning a patient or providing support for an affected limb may also offer some relief. Patients expect nurses to be strong advocates for them and to be proactive in seeking treatment plans that relieve their suffering.

SUGGESTED READINGS

Cadden K. Pain management. *Nurs Manage*. 2007;38(8):31–35.
D'Arcy Y. Pain management standards, the law, and you. *Nursing*. 2005;35(4):17.
D'Arcy Y. Pain management by the numbers: Using rating scales effectively. *Nursing*. 2007;37(11):14–15.
Fishman S. Fifth vital sign. American Pain Foundation. Available at: http://www.painfoundation.org. Accessed April 6, 2008.
McCaffery M, Pasero C, Ferrell B. Pain control: Nurses'decisions about opioid dose. *Am J Nurs*. 2007;107(120):35–39.

ENSURE APPROPRIATE POSITION OF THE DOBHOFF TUBE PRIOR TO FEEDING

BONNIE L. PARKER, RN, CRRN

WHAT TO DO: ASSESS AND EVALUATE

A Dobhoff tube is a small bore, weighted nasogastric (NG) tube inserted in patients who need an enteral route for nutrition and medication. It is inserted like a standard NG tube but verification before use must be made with an abdominal X-ray. Dobhoffs are frequently used to provide short-term nutrition to patients whose oral ingestion is insufficient. The Dobhoff causes little irritation to the soft tissues of the sinuses or throat. Placement should be checked when the tube is first placed, prior to giving any feeding, prior to giving medication, after episodes of coughing or vomiting, after suctioning, if the length of the tube exiting the nose differs from that of the insertion time, or if the patient has sudden respiratory difficulty.

The biggest disadvantage with a Dobhoff tube is that a check for gastric residual for placement cannot be done as with larger tubes. This makes verification of placement and assessment of the feeding process more difficult since it is not feasible to do a chest X-ray before each access of the tube. Dobhoffs should be marked at the insertion point at which they enter the nostril once placement has been verified by X-ray. This serves as a guide to the nurse to indicate if the tube has been pulled out or has migrated further into the gastrointestinal tract. The Dobhoff has a weighted end and can be carried further down the gastrointestinal tract by peristaltic movement.

The small caliber of the Dobhoff tube makes it more prone to becoming dislodged without the patient exhibiting significant symptoms. Therefore, it is important to thoroughly assess the patient. An episode of vomiting can dislodge the tube while it may still be securely taped in place and appear to be in proper position. If a patient with a Dobhoff tube experiences an episode of forceful vomiting, check to ensure the tube is still taped securely and the insertion mark is in the correct location at the nares. Assess the patient for any shortness of breath, signs, and symptoms of airway compromise and/or other significant physical changes. If any of these signs or symptoms is present, an abdominal X-ray may need to be performed to verify correct placement. Contact the physician and inform him of the episode, any symptoms the patient may be experiencing, and the patient's complaints. To avoid complications for the patient, it is important to stop using the tube until proper placement has been confirmed.

SUGGESTED READINGS

Best C. Nasogastric tube insertion in adults who require enteral feeding. *Nurs Stand*. 2007;21(40):39–43.

Kawati R, Rubertsson S. Malpositioning of fine bore feeding tube: A serious complication. *Acta Anaesthesiol Scand*. 2005;49:58–61.

KNOW THE PROPER CARE OF A PERIPHERAL IV SITE

BONNIE L. PARKER, RN, CRRN

WHAT TO DO: EVALUATE

Just about every patient admitted to the hospital will have an intravenous catheter (IV) inserted. The most commonly used IV is placed into a peripheral vein, usually in the hand or arm and very rarely in a leg or foot. These catheters are used for fluid replacement therapy, medication administration, and blood transfusions and should be changed according to hospital policy.

Complications of peripheral IVs include infiltration of fluid into the tissue surrounding the IV site, which may be caused by dislodgement of the catheter. Signs of infiltration include a beeping infusion pump, a site that is cool, swollen, and hard, or complaints of pain or burning at the site. If these signs or symptoms occur, stop the IV fluids, elevate the extremity, and apply warm compresses to facilitate reabsorption. Document the findings and restart the IV in a new location. To avoid infiltration, secure the IV to the skin with an occlusive dressing and tape the tubing to prevent the IV catheter from being pulled as the patient moves. The site should be assessed at least every two hours.

Another complication of peripheral IV sites is inflammation of the vein which may be caused by injury during insertion, tension on the catheter from being moved or pulled on, irritation due to long-term therapy or irritating medications, large bore IVs, or infection. Treatment and prevention of inflammation include securing the IV site properly and tubing to the skin. To prevent infection, sterile technique must be used when inserting an IV, and every time the line is accessed, the port must be thoroughly cleaned with alcohol utilizing a scrubbing action.

Extravasation of tissue-destroying fluid is also a complication of IV therapy. Extravasation of IV fluids occurs when medications that are damaging leak into the surrounding tissue. The consequences can be severe up to and including amputation. Among the most harmful medications are vancomycin, imipenem, nafcillin, chemotherapeutic agents, phenergan, and phenytoin. When giving any of these drugs, the medication must be infused per hospital policy and the site checked frequently. If an extravasation occurs, the infusion must be stopped immediately and protocols to treat the extravasation must be followed. These guidelines may be drug-specific and the procedures that must be followed may be dictated by individual facilities' specific guidelines. The best prevention for all IV site complications will always include sterile technique, good ongoing assessment skills, and patient education.

SUGGESTED READINGS

Hudson K. IV therapy. *Dyn Nurs Edu.* October 21, 2004. Updated December 2006;5–7. Available at: http://dynamicnursing education.com/class.php?class_id+29&pid=15.

Cook L. Choosing the right intravenous catheter. *Home Healthc Nurse.* 2007;25(8):526.

DISTRACTIONS CAN LEAD TO MEDICATION ERRORS

BONNIE L. PARKER, RN, CRRN

WHAT TO DO: PLAN

"Quiet! Hospital Zone." It is a sign that is frequently posted on streets near hospitals, but as nurses advance in their career, they find that hospitals are anything but quiet. People are talking and calling out to each other; medication carts and stretchers rattle and bang as they ramble down the hall; phones and call bells ring; and overhead announcements blare. What effect does all this noise and confusion have on the nurse? A nurse is a busy person, with patient assessments to perform, notes to write, medications to give, and treatments to administer.

Administering medications is one of the most detailed duties a nurse must perform and one that has the highest potential of resulting in a mistake. Noise and interruptions that cause distractions can cause mistakes. Having a large patient load and changes in routine can add to the feeling of pressure, and the need to hurry can cause a reduction in concentration when rushing to complete a medication pass. According to Pape (2006), a nurse is interrupted as often as six times per hour during a shift and many of these interruptions occur during medication administration. Administering medication requires a nurse's undivided attention; it is important that she be able to focus on the task at hand.

As the population ages and the patients admitted to the hospital have increasing needs that require more care, distractions become more frequent, demanding a nurse to be ever more vigilant. It is a frequent occurrence to have a medication prepared to hand to a patient and be interrupted or called away. When the nurse returns, she may mistakenly hand it to the wrong patient because of the distraction. In nursing school, every student nurse is taught to double-check the labels of all medications, compare patient armbands, check and recheck, not just one time, but several times. If a nurse's attention is diverted in the middle of medication administration, she must go back and recheck to ensure that she has the correct medications and doses for the correct patient. It has been estimated that as much as 47% of medication mistakes have been caused by distractions.

One suggestion for reducing distractions would be to reduce the level of noise in the environment. For example, turning down or completely turning off background music, setting telephones and bells to a softer ring, setting pagers, beepers, and cell phones to vibrate, and turning off computer speakers unless needed. Reducing the level of ambient clutter can also reduce distractions that could lead to a mistake. Therefore, medication carts, medication stations, and nurses' stations should be cleared of unnecessary clutter.

It is after medications have been opened and placed in a cup to give to the patient that most mistakes occur due to distraction. With the exception of a patient emergency, it is imperative to stay with the patient throughout the medication pass to verify that you are handing the correct medication to the correct patient and to ensure that he takes the medication given to him.

SUGGESTED READINGS

Jackson M, Wesley R. A systematic approach to preventing medication errors. The U.S. Pharmacist Continuing Education Program. Available at: http://www.uspharmacist.com. Accessed May 3, 2008.

Pape T. Workaround error. *Nursing*. February 2006. Available at: http://www.webmm.ahrq.gov.

Smetzer J. Medication management. *Nurs Manage*. 2001; 32(12):44–48.

KNOW HOW TO IDENTIFY PATIENTS

KATHERINE M. PENTURFF, RN, CAPA

WHAT TO DO: IMPLEMENT

Throughout healthcare settings, failure to correctly identify patients results in medication errors, transfusion errors, testing errors, wrong person procedures, and the discharge of infants to the wrong families. Because patient misidentification is the cause of multiple errors within the healthcare system, the Joint Commission listed improving patient identification accuracy as the first of its National Patient Safety Goals introduced in 2003, and it continues to be an accreditation requirement.

One of the most widely used methods of patient identification utilized is the patient armband. Armbands typically include the patient's name and other identifying information and are attached to the patient in a "permanent" fashion that requires destruction of the band by its removal, preventing reuse by another patient. While this is a very simple, accurate, and cost-effective method of patient identification, it cannot be used exclusively to identify patients. A study conducted at the Veterans Affairs Medical Center in West Los Angeles, California, compared wristband identification errors for 712 hospitals. Phlebotomists checked patient wristbands over two million times finding over 67,000 errors. Missing armbands constituted a significant portion of the errors. The Joint Commission now recommends the use of two identifiers for patient identification, such as the name, date of birth, social security number, or phone number. Neither identifier should be the patient's room number. When identifying patients on admission to a facility, patients should be asked to state and not confirm their own information in full. "Can you tell me your full name?" should be asked, instead of "Are you Mary Smith?" Many patients may not hear well or are reluctant to admit that they do not hear well; so they choose to be "nodders"—smiling and nodding agreeably, regardless of whether they heard or understood what was spoken. In addition, patients, especially non-English-speaking patients, may give more than one name or date of birth. Identification of non-English-speaking patients may need to be made through an interpreter. If none is available, a language bank or language line should be accessed by phone if necessary. Patients should be educated on the importance of correct patient identification in a positive manner, respecting the patient's right to privacy. It should also be stressed that patients should use their legal name at all times while undergoing treatment. Some patients prefer nicknames or the use of a former name, especially if a name change is a recent occurrence. If their insurance carrier has not yet been notified, patients may express a concern that healthcare bills will not be covered by insurance if the name on their insurance card does not correspond to the name on the bills.

If a patient is unable to identify himself or herself, guidelines should be in place for consistent initial identification on admission and the use of ID armbands that remain on the patient throughout the stay. The recent increase in the use of electronic scanning has greatly decreased the number of misidentification, but it is only as accurate as the armband was when it was placed on the patient, and only as long as it remains on the patient.

SUGGESTED READINGS

The Joint Commission International Center for Patient Safety. Patient safety solution 2: Patient identification. Available at: www.jcipatientsafety.org/25087/.

Schraag J. Patient identification. *EndoNurse*. Available at: www.endonurse.com/articles/patient_safety/596_641feat4.html. Accessed April 1, 2006.

IDENTIFYING PATIENTS WITH LATEX ALLERGY

KATHERINE M. PENTURFF, RN, CAPA

WHAT TO DO: ASSESS

Although patients are usually quick to alert their surgeon to their drug allergies, they often do not realize the importance of alerting them to a latex allergy. Patients coming into the hospital for any reason, including surgery, should be asked directly if they have had problems in the past relating to rubber or latex. True latex allergy is present in 1%–5% of the general population, with an increased prevalence in atopic individuals. Latex allergies are increased in populations with chronic occupational exposure to latex, such as healthcare workers, rubber industry workers, and EMS providers. The highest prevalence of latex, allergy in a single group, up to 68%, is found in patients with spina bifida or congenital urogenital abnormalities.

Latex exposure is associated with one of three syndromes: irritant dermatitis, delayed (Type IV) hypersensitivity reaction, or immediate Type I hypersensitivity. Irritant dermatitis is a result of mechanical disruption of the skin due to the rubbing of latex gloves. It is not an allergic reaction but is responsible for the majority of latex-induced skin rashes and is often mistaken for Type IV hypersensitivity. Type IV hypersensitivity reaction causes a distinctive contact dermatitis with symptoms typically developing within 24–48 h of topical exposure to latex in a sensitized person. The dermatitis may predispose patients to further sensitizations or infections. The most serious and least common syndrome is immediate Type I hypersensitivity. It is mediated by an immunoglobulin E (IgE) response specific for latex proteins. It can occur following skin, mucous membrane, or visceral/peritoneal contact. It can also follow inhalation of latex-laden particles or bloodstream exposure to soluble latex proteins

following intravascular access procedures. Symptoms generally begin within minutes of exposure and may include localized or generalized urticaria, rhinitis, conjunctivitis, bronchospasm, laryngospasm, hypotension, and full-blown anaphylaxis. Type I allergy has been implicated clearly in intraoperative and intraprocedure anaphylaxis and can be fatal without immediate treatment.

Patients with hypersensitivity and their families should be educated to identify and avoid latex in home, work, and medical/dental settings. A "red flag" when interviewing a patient for possible latex sensitivity indicates allergies to such foods as banana, avocado, and chestnuts. Patients with known or suspected latex allergy who seek care must be kept within a latex-safe environment to prevent serious complications including all patients with spina bifida. Patients with type I hypersensitivity should carry subcutaneous epinephrine kits at all times and should obtain and wear a MedicAlert-type bracelet identifying their allergy.

The U.S. Food and Drug Administration has cleared the marketing of the first device made from a new form of natural rubber latex, guayule latex. It has some of the same desirable properties of traditional latex, such as flexibility and strength. Available data on the new guayule latex show that even people who are highly allergic to traditional latex do not react on first exposure to guayule latex proteins.

SUGGESTED READINGS

Behrman AJ, Howarth M. Latex allergy. Available at: www.emedicine.com/emerg/topic814.htm. Last Updated: November 28, 2007.

U.S. Food and Drug Administration. FDA clears glove made from new type of latex. Available at: www.fda.gov/bbs/topics/NEWS/2008/NEW01822.html. Accessed August 19, 2008.

KNOW HOW TO REACH THE ATTENDING PHYSICIAN

ANTHONY D. SLONIM, MD, DrPH

WHAT TO DO: IMPLEMENT

Complex pediatric care is often provided in pediatric hospitals that do outstanding work delivering clinical care, advocating for the most vulnerable of our patients, performing cutting edge research for children, and teaching the next generation of pediatric providers. While education is a core function of many children's hospitals, the staff must remember that the attending physician remains in charge of the case and should be notified particularly when difficulties arise in the delivery of care with a trainee.

Medical trainees at all levels including medical students, pediatric residents, and subspecialty fellows continue to work under an apprenticeship model of delivering care. While residents and fellows are employed, they are learning their craft from senior clinicians who are providing them with guidance. However, it must be remembered that the care they are delivering is real and since they are learning, they may not know when they do not know something, are confused, or do not know how to ask for assistance.

The experienced pediatric nurse is an important participant in the delivery of excellent care for children and needs to be able to identify when care provided by trainees is less than optimal and escalate it appropriately to the child's attending physician. The advocacy role of the nurse is very important in this area since families may become concerned with a child's care or confused by mix messages that trainees bring and will often raise these concerns with the nurse who has an obligation to notify the attending physician.

While there are important elements to clinical documentation, documenting that a trainee has been notified is only half of the nurse's job when a child's needs are not being met. If nurses remain dissatisfied with the responses of the trainee, they should feel comfortable escalating until their concerns are addressed. This is not only a professional responsibility, but a child's life may depend upon it.

SUGGESTED READINGS

Kennedy TJ, Lingard L, Baker GR, et al. Clinical oversight: conceptualizing the relationship between supervision and safety. *J Gen Intern Med*. 2007;22(8):1080–1085.

Singh H, Thomas EJ, Petersen LA, et al. Medical errors involving trainees: A study of closed malpractice claims from 5 insurers. *Arch Intern Med*. 2007;167(19):2030–2036.

Verbal Orders Should Never Be Routine—Always Read Back and Wait for Confirmation

Katherine M. Penturff, RN, CAPA

WHAT TO DO: PLAN

When healthcare workers are employed in a specific, specialized area for a prolonged period of time, there may be a tendency to fall into a predictable routine. This can be exhibited when responding to certain expected complications such as respiratory depression, hypotension, and pain management in the postanesthesia care unit or PACU. In this setting, these complications are routinely treated by a standing order set that gives options to be chosen by the ordering physician. Many physicians tend to order the same medications routinely for the same type of complication, leading to a sense of predictability. It becomes very comfortable for the nurse to assume what Dr Gynecologist is going to say when he is called about Mrs Hysterectomy's post-op nausea, and that familiarity can lead to verbal medication order errors.

The National Coordinating Council for Medication Error Reporting and Prevention (2008) defines medication error as any preventable event that may cause or lead to inappropriate medication use or patient harm while the medication is in the control of the health care professional, patient, or consumer. Such events can stem from professional practice, healthcare products, procedures, and systems. Errors may involve prescribing, order communication, product labeling, packaging, nomenclature, compounding, dispensing, distribution, administration, education, monitoring, or use. Giving and receiving verbal orders is a common practice in hospitals but there has been little systematic study of them. Although the potential for harm arising from the miscommunication and misunderstanding of verbal orders has been recognized, there is very little research examining their complexity. Verbal orders carry the risk of introducing an error from many sources and, therefore, should be minimally used. They can be misunderstood, misinterpreted, or miswritten. In 2003,

Joint Commission on the Accreditation of Health-care Organizations (JCAHO) began examining each organization's process for taking verbal orders as part of its recommendation to improve the effectiveness of communication among caregivers. The National Coordinating Council for Medication Error Reporting and Prevention has established a protocol for clarifying verbal orders, which includes such guidelines as

- Name of the patient
- Age and weight of the patient, when appropriate
- Drug name
- Dosage form (e.g., tablets, capsules, inhalants)
- Exact strength or concentration
- Dose, frequency, and route
- Quantity and/or duration
- Purpose or indication (unless disclosure is considered inappropriate by the prescriber)
- Specific instructions for use
- Name of the prescriber, and telephone number when appropriate
- Name of the individual transmitting the order, if different from the prescriber

Leaders of healthcare organizations should promote a culture in which it is not only acceptable but also strongly encouraged for staff to question prescribers when there are any questions or disagreements about verbal orders.

SUGGESTED READINGS

Center for the Advancement of Patient Safety (CAPS). U.S. Pharmacopeia. Available at: http://www.usp.org/pdf/EN/patientSafety/capsLink2002–10–01.pdf. Accessed August 19, 2008.

National Coordinating Council for Medication Error Reporting and Prevention. Recommendations to reduce medication errors associated with verbal medication orders and prescriptions. Available at: http://www.nccmerp.org/council/council2001–02–20.html. Accessed August 19, 2008.

WHEN YOU ARE IN THE PATIENT'S AND LOVED ONES' PRESENCE, YOU ARE NOT INVISIBLE OR SLY. REMEMBER, THEY ARE HYPERSENSITIVE TO YOUR EXPRESSIONS, YOUR TONE, AND YOUR ACTIVITIES. THEY HOLD WHAT YOU "DON'T DO" IN THE SAME REGARD AS "WHAT YOU DO"

LYNDA COOK SAWYER, RNC, BSN, MBA

WHAT TO DO: PLAN AND IMPLEMENT

Human beings are admitted to hospitals and treatment facilities for healthcare-related reasons. Some suffer from chronic illnesses and their visit may not be the first; some are admitted for an emergency or acute illness or a traumatic event, and some, as for hospital childbirth, are admitted for a happy reason. Regardless of the reason, they realize they are in a hospital and not in their own home.

Our homes are where we all feel relatively in control. The home may be spotless or a cluttered mess; our refrigerator, cupboards, glassware, silverware, and sink all await our whims of hunger and thirst; even our bathroom contains the soaps and lotions we care to use and the toilet paper we most prefer. Our beds are comfortably lumpy, double, queen- or king-sized, and our sheets smell like our sheets, and even the pillows on our bed are familiar in shape and smell and are recognizable to our head and neck. The phone's ring is known to us; the television control and channels are of our choice; the sounds of the house setting, doors opening and closing, stairs creaking, and the footsteps of our loved ones as they navigate the structure are all known to our souls and ingrained into our daily waking and sleeping patterns. It is home.

A hospital room, on the other hand, is nothing like home. No matter how many times people have been admitted to one, it is not like home. It is likely that they cannot eat when, where, and what they like; the bathroom is foreign and the toilet paper is never right. The toiletries, if brought from home, do not perform in the same soothing manners. The lighting is all wrong.

The hospital bed, while interestingly functional, becomes a brick after only a few hours. The sheets are rough and way too white. The blankets are thin, uncomfortable, and never seem to stay on the bed. The pillows are smaller bricks covered in vinyl, slipped into a rough and too white pillow case, and positioned under the head for maximum neck discomfort, obviously. The phone ring is too loud and making a call to the outside world is initially impossible and the television has every available channel except the one that is showing their favorite show. The sounds of carts, alarms, overhead pages, other rooms' phones, toilets flushing, strangers talking, and foreign doors opening and banging shut again add little to their peace of mind and ability to heal. The windows do not open and they often cannot reach or find the light cord. The temperature control is mysteriously hidden and if found, seems to control very little of the actual temperature. They are not at home.

This is the hourly ordeal of your patients and their families. Disney likens your physical entrance into the room as "stepping onto the stage." With every accoutrement of the room being foreign to the inhabitants, you become the variable entity. With consciousness (and many semiconscious states), the bed- or chair-bound patient becomes acutely aware of the human presence. Visiting family and friends will go silent and become vigilant observers as you enter the room and go about your business.

What you do and say and how you do it and say it will be taken in by all who observe and hear you. Indeed, even your voice and chosen words via the Nurse Call System when answering a call light will be attributed to your "performance." You need to project calmness, kindness, caring, and compassion. Smile. Introduce yourself first to your patient, then to the visitors. Shake hands, when able. Touch your patient. When establishing rapport for the first time with any particular patient, sit down. Tell your patient, and by virtue of being in the room, the visitors, what you are there to do, how long you will be there, and how to reach you if you are needed before you come back.

Observe. Is this patient safe? Is your patient in pain? If allowed, does he have fresh ice and water? Is the patient ergonomically positioned in the bed? Are the flimsy sheets and blankets arranged neatly on the bed? Are the call bell, light cord, and telephone within reach? Does the trash need to be removed off of the overbed table, side table, countertops, and window ledges? Are the trashcans overflowing? Is the linen basket full? Are there towels on the bathroom floor or old meal trays on the sink counter? Are there flowers or plants to be admired? Do they need to be watered? Take care of these issues. Someone may have told you that these issues are not your job. They were wrong.

Know that every time you enter a patient's room (step on stage), all eyes and ears are on you. What you do or do not do are the deciding factors for the patient and his or her visitors as to whether or not you care. And, you cannot possibly be an effective nurse if it has been determined that you "do not care." Take the time to care: listen more than you speak; see more than you hear; do more than just your job.

SUGGESTED READINGS

Kinni T. *Be Our Guest: Perfecting the Art of Customer Service*. Los Angeles, CA: Disney Editions; 2003.

Lee F. *If Disney Ran Your Hospital: 9 ½Things You Would Do Differently*. Bozeman, MT: Second River Healthcare; 2004.

HEALTHCARE PROVIDERS MUST ADDRESS END-OF-LIFE ISSUES HONESTLY TO GIVE PATIENTS OPTIMAL CARE

MARY S. WARD, RN, BS, OCN

WHAT TO DO: IMPLEMENT

Patients approaching the end of life require unique qualities in their caregivers, nurses, and physicians. It is well documented that many physicians, even oncologists, are untrained and reticent about discussing the end of life and palliative care options for their patients. The dying process presents many ethical, moral, spiritual, and physical challenges to the healthcare team. Nurses are often the initiators of discussion with patients and caregivers and should act as advocates for them with physicians as appropriate. Patients have many genuine fears about the dying process: fear of needless pain and suffering and loss of control. The SUPPORT trial of over 9,000 end-of-life patients indicated that many of these fears are justified. Of those who remained conscious of the end of life, over 50% had moderate to severe pain at least half the time in the last 3 days of life, 46% of DNR orders were written in the last 2 days of life, and only 47% of physicians were actually aware of their patient's DNR status.

All patients deserve the opportunity to have some input into their end of life. The percentage of patients whose DNR orders are written at the last minute indicates that these issues are often not dealt with until the patient is very near death. For the majority of these patients, the process is much longer and it is the nurses' and physicians' responsibilities to allow the patient to acquire the information about his status to be able to assume some control over his life. The patient should be able to decide whether he would prefer quality of life, with more control, over life prolonging treatment with more side effects. Often, treatment options are not presented in this light and in the framework of the patient's overall prognosis.

The most important reason for allowing the patient full disclosure of his condition is to allow him and his loved ones to complete his life's tasks. He may have some goals he would like to complete before he dies. There may also be some relationships that need closure

or some visits to be made. Perhaps he needs to complete a will.

To address these issues, the nurse should first evaluate the patient's level of understanding about his prognosis and what the physician has already told him. The nurse should also evaluate the patient's emotional state and the support system in place and his readiness to engage in any discussion of this nature. The discussion should focus on the patient's goals; he should be asked what his goals are and treatment should be directed toward achieving them as much as is reasonable. The nurse must actively listen to the patient and be in tune with emotional cues. The information that the nurse gathers should then be communicated to the physician so that he can be prepared to carry the discussion further with the patient and family members.

It should be stressed that at no time should any caregiver convey to the patient a sense of abandonment. Often in end-of-life care, the patient is transferred from the home to the hospital and then to a nursing home or to a hospice setting for palliative care. In each of these transitions, it is imperative that all caregivers convey to the patient that the care is being transferred and done on a continuum.

The end of life can be a meaningful time for both patients and families. When healthcare providers avoid discussions until the patient is actively dying, they have deprived all of those involved of rich times together in completing a person's life. It is part of a nurse's responsibility to be willing to step in and initiate discussion of these issues when appropriate.

SUGGESTED READINGS

Balaban RB. A physician's guide to talking about end-of-life care. *J Geriatric Intern Med*. 2000;15:195–200.

Ngo-Metzger Q, August KJ, Srinivasan M. End-of-life care: Guidelines for patient-centered communication. *Am Fam Phys*. 2008;77(2). Available at: www.aafp.org/afp. Accessed April 8, 2008.

Quill TE. Initiating end-of-life discussions with seriously ill patients: Addressing the "Elephant in the Room." *J Am Med Assoc*. 2000;284(19):2502–2507.

THE PROPER REMOVAL OF URINARY CATHETERS IS NECESSARY TO AVOID HARM TO THE PATIENT

MARY S. WARD, RN, BS, OCN

WHAT TO DO: IMPLEMENT

Urinary catheterization is a common nursing procedure undertaken by properly trained staff for a number of indications. Among these are relief of urinary retention, preoperative and perioperative bladder decompression, surgical repair of the urethra and surrounding structures, instilling medication into the bladder, accurate measurement of output, and sterile urine collection. Staff members are properly trained in catheter placement under sterile conditions, and all assistive staff members should be carefully trained in proper catheter maintenance and care to reduce injury to the patient.

Even though urinary catheters are quite common in the medical setting, they are not without their own risks. The most common risk associated with catheters is, of course, catheter related urinary tract infection. However, there are documented cases of complications arising from misplacement of the catheter upon insertion as well as complications that arise from mechanical injury due to the catheter dwelling or removal. The catheter may be inserted too far into the bladder and actually be placed in one of the ureters. This may cause ureteral trauma and pain. Other complications can be urethral trauma, retention of the balloon in the urethra, bladder perforation, and rectovesicular fistula formation.

While much of the injury to the patient may come from the catheter insertion or malfunction, occasionally, a poorly thought-through shortcut by a practitioner may be the cause of harm to the patient. Most catheters are made of a rubber or plastic tube that has a side port into which the nurse instills up to about 10 mL of sterile water into a balloon that inflates a few centimeters from the end of the catheter tip. The purpose of the balloon is to keep the catheter in the bladder and hold the tip in place, allowing the drainage of urine. The proper way to remove the catheter is to use an empty 10 mL syringe and withdraw the water from the balloon and gently allow the catheter tip to slide out.

However, every good nurse always carries several things in her pockets, one of which is a good pair of scissors. If a syringe is not quickly available and a staff member tries to use scissors to cut the end of the catheter to release the water from the balloon, significant injury to the patient could result. The catheter end has a tendency to be quickly pulled into the bladder once the water has been released from the balloon. Once this happens, a urologist will need to be consulted to remove the remainder of the catheter tip from the bladder. This puts the patient at risk of injury from the procedure as well as great risk for infection.

SUGGESTED READINGS

Kim MK, Park K. Unusual complication of urethral catheterization: A case report. *J Kor Med Sci*. 2008;23: 161–162.

Lewis SM, Heitkemper MM, Dirksen S. *Medical-Surgical Nursing*. St. Louis: Mosby; 2007, pp. 1288–1289.

IMPROVE NURSE–PHYSICIAN COMMUNICATION TO IMPROVE PATIENT OUTCOMES

MARY S. WARD, RN, BS, OCN

WHAT TO DO: PLAN

Nurses are educated to be advocates for their patients and every contemporary nursing curriculum contains some component of communication skills. These communication skills seem to do little for a nurse who needs to call an on-call physician at 3 AM or come face to face with a harsh and demanding physician on a critical care unit. Nurses tend to withdraw or find themselves in an abject role in their relationships to other members of the healthcare profession, particularly physicians. Current trends and evidence, however, indicate that this attitude is detrimental for all involved: nurses, physicians, other healthcare team members, and, most importantly, the patient. Nurses, especially in an inpatient or long-term care setting, are often with the patient for extended periods of time and more in touch with ancillary members of the healthcare team, such as dieticians, case managers, social workers, etc. In addition, nurses are often in closer communication with family members than many other members of the healthcare team and often have a better overall assessment of the patient and family needs. Often, however, nurses are reluctant to share their observations, insights, assessment findings, or recommendations with physicians and other key decision makers for the patient.

There are several factors that contribute to this lack of communication. Much of it is focused on culture and the structure of the healthcare system. There may be a question as to who is responsible for making decisions for the patient. At times, there may be confusion as to which physician to refer particular problems to, especially if the patient has multiple physician consults. Often, a doctor is called with an issue who refers this to another doctor because it does not fall under his area. When a nurse receives a response like this, she is often more reluctant to make the second phone call to resolve an issue. Other factors that contribute to this reluctance include a culture of implied hierarchy between nurses and physicians, sex differences, and cultural backgrounds. In addition, physicians and nurses have been trained to communicate differently. Physicians are trained to communicate in brief bullet-point statements, whereas nurses are trained to communicate in descriptive detail.

The essential factor to remember is that the patient needs to remain the focus. When communication breaks down, his care is compromised. Breakdown in communication among healthcare members has contributed to a decrease in patient safety, a slowing of services to the patient, and wasted resources, and it can also lead to a loss of important information needed to treat the patient. All clinicians involved in caring for the patient need to have the treatment of the patient as their first goal.

With this primary goal in mind, nurses need to practice open, honest communication with physician colleagues. When approaching physicians, nurses who are organized in their communication and thoughtful in their approach will have more success in being the patient advocate they desire to be. Institutions and individuals, nurses and physicians alike, who approach patient-centered care from the standpoint of a teamwork approach, will meet with far more success than the old-fashioned "silo" approach so often practiced. But nurses need to be willing to step forward with their assessments and make recommendations to their physician colleagues for the sake of their patient's improved outcomes.

There are benefits to improving communication for nurses and physicians as well. Nurses who are involved in their patients' care utilizing a team approach find increased satisfaction, improved personal health, greater longevity, improved personal productivity, and find that they can anticipate their patients' needs rather than always react to them.

SUGGESTED READINGS

Friedman DM, Berger DL. Improving team structure and communication: A key to hospital efficiency. *Arch Surg.* 2004;139:1194–1198. Available at: http://archsurg.ama-assn.org/. Accessed April 15, 2008.

Haig K, Sutton S, Whittington J. A shared mental model for improving communication between clinicians. *Joint Comm J Qual Patient Saf.* 2006;32(3):167–175.

Sachs BP. A 38 year old woman with fetal loss. *J Am Med Assoc.* 2005;294(7):833–840. Available at: www.jama.com. Accessed April 25, 2008.

Shortell SM, Singer SJ. Improving patient safety by taking systems seriously. *J Am Med Assoc.* 2008;299(4):445–447.

TO PREVENT PATIENT INJURY, USE EQUIPMENT FOR THE PURPOSE FOR WHICH IT WAS INTENDED

JULIE MULLIGAN WATTS, RN, MN

WHAT TO DO: IMPLEMENT

Since 2000, patient safety has received much attention by the national media, regulatory bodies, industry, and consumers. The Joint Commission on Accreditation of Healthcare Organizations has made patient safety one of its highest priorities by issuing a number of national patient safety goals and regulations. These regulations are related to infection prevention, reduction of medical errors, improved communication, and a reduction in surgical errors.

In oncology nursing practice, errors are often thought of in terms of errors in cancer treatments, adverse reactions to cancer treatment, vesicant extravasations, and blood product transfusion reactions. Oncology nurses are not exempt from errors that occur in general medical–surgical areas, such as errors with infusion pumps, IV therapy, restraints, high-risk medications, and equipment. Most oncology patients need vascular access at some point in the course of their disease. For patients undergoing chemotherapy, especially over an extended period, vascular access is important. Often, the nurse is involved in selection, maintenance, use, and management of the device. Oncology nurses are also responsible for educating patients and families about home care of devices. Types of venous access devices used in the oncology patient population include peripheral IV access, peripherally inserted central catheters (PICC), tunneled central venous catheters (e.g. Hickman), and implantable vascular access devices (ports). Since the 1980s, the use of peripherally inserted catheters and needles for short-term use has decreased. The reason is that other devices are available that are easily inserted and maintained and well accepted by patients.

Today, peripherally inserted IV access for oncology patients under treatment is only used on a short-term basis; usually for 4 to 7 days. These angiocaths or scalp-vein needles are low-cost devices that are easily

inserted with minimal complications. These devices can be difficult to insert in the very young, the elderly, and those with sclerotic or fragile veins. Peripheral vessels can become irritated from infusions of electrolytes and blood products and chemotherapy. At times, peripheral IV access may be impossible due to the inability to find an acceptable and stable location for needle insertion. When this happens, nurses may turn to practices such as warming of the hand or arm, lowering the extremity to increase venous flow, or both these methods, although there is little literature to support these practices.

If nurses resort to the warming techniques to aid in cannula insertion, it is important that proper equipment be used to warm the hand or arm. Use of towels or cloths that have been warmed in hot water or in places that are not designed for this use, such as a microwave oven, can result in burns and injuries to the patient. Any piece of equipment, if used improperly, can cause injury to a patient. Keeping safety in mind will help reduce risks associated with medical devices. Always be sure that medical devices are never used for something other than their designed purpose. Likewise, be sure that nonmedical devices are not used for patient care. The use of a blanket warmer or heating pad by staff trained in the use of those devices would be the best selection for warming a patient's arm to find an accessible vein for peripheral IV access.

SUGGESTED READINGS

Camp-Sorrell D, ed. *Access Device Guidelines: Recommendations for Nursing Practice and Education.* 2nd Ed. Pittsburgh, PA: Oncology Nursing Society; 2004.

Infusion Nursing Society 2006. Infusion nursing: Standards of practice. *J Infusion Nurs.* 2007;29:1S.

Lenhardt R, Seybold T, Kinberger O, et al. Local warming and insertion of peripheral venous cannulas: Single blinded prospective randomized controlled trial and single blinded randomized crossover trial. *Br Med J.* 2002;325(7371):1038.

Sosin J. Legally speaking: Careful with that equipment! *RN.* 2002;65(2):59–62.

NURSE PRECEPTORS—TEACHING THE NEXT GENERATION OF NURSES

FRANCINE B. YATES, RRT, RN, BSN

WHAT TO DO: IMPLEMENT

When nursing education shifted from learning by apprenticeship to learning by education in the academic arena, there emerged complaints that graduating nurses lacked the abilities to assume patient care immediately after graduation. Most new graduates, regardless of education, could not handle patient workloads or distribute medications competently and lacked organizational skills. Nursing schools only lay the foundation for a career in nursing. The minimal amount of clinical experience that is received is only a taste of what is required of a nurse after graduating. Student nurses are allowed to observe but not to touch. Little can be learned from observation alone.

Intelligent preceptors and instructors are in high demand throughout the medical system. Unfortunately, working as a preceptor brings on many challenges and the criteria for selection may be minimal. The selection of preceptors may be based on who is available and has the time for the task. But more stringent criteria should be established since a good preceptor should be an experienced nurse with multiple clinical skills and expertise as well as good leadership and communication skills.

A new nurse greatly benefits from having an excellent preceptor, one who takes into account her learning style and exposes her to the daily routine of the unit. A good preceptor applies theory to clinical practice and explains the rationale of a procedure while performing it, allowing the recently graduated nurse to understand it better, which will ultimately benefit her patients.

An effective preceptor can help the new nurse transition into a field of clinical competency while minimizing the effects of the transition from nursing student to professional nurse. This allows for less stress, disillusionment, and frustration. The novice nurse needs to develop confidence that she can manage the events of the day and the daily needs of her patients.

A novice nurse will flourish in the orientation period if provided with the right preceptor. The preceptor who is chosen must possess the clinical skills and the educational preparation and knowledge base necessary to effectively train the new nurse. Interpersonal skills are also essential. A preceptor who is cold or has a negative attitude toward the employer will not be beneficial in the overall goal of retention of new nurses.

It is imperative that preceptors are trained, effective teachers. With the nursing shortage growing every year, retention of new nurses is essential. If new nurses are dissatisfied with the length of the orientation period or an unprepared or inefficient preceptor, they may seek employment in a less stressful, less intimidating position within the medical field.

Precepting new nurses is stressful and challenging, yet new nurses must develop competency for patient care. Preceptor courses and training seminars may be beneficial to aid preceptors in developing the necessary skills to effectively teach novice nurses the skills and knowledge that they need to be successful in the nursing arena. This will allow for the retention of the new nurse as well as the experienced preceptor.

SUGGESTED READINGS

Daigle J. *Preceptors in Nursing Education—Facilitating Student Learning*. Kansas State Nurses Association; April 2001. Available at: http://findarticles.com/p/articles/mi_qa3940/is_200104/ai_n8938452/printHow.

Floyd JP. How nurse preceptors influence new graduates. *Crit Care Nurse*. 2003;23(1S):26, 52, 95.

Myrick F. Preceptorship—Is it the answer to the problem in clinical teaching? *J Nurs Edu*. 1988;27(3):136–138.

Machines alarm; patients do not. Nothing is more important than the necessity for routine assessments

Francine B. Yates, RRT, RN, BSN

WHAT TO DO: ASSESS

Increasingly in nursing, especially in the ICU setting, technology plays a large role in patient care. The greater the degree of patient compromise is, the more the technology is required to monitor the patient, practice ongoing assessments, and make sound decisions to treat the patient's fluctuating condition. Monitors are used to measure vital signs such as blood pressure and heart rate; ventilators are used to assist a patient with breathing; and balloon pumps are used to enhance the cardiac output. The more the technology is implemented, the more the training is required for healthcare and nursing staff.

The use of technology and equipment in healthcare requires more attention, time, and energy of the nurses operating them and caring for the patients that require their assistance. Nursing staff members have had to learn to operate, maintain, and troubleshoot many problems that arise to safely and efficiently use the technology. Newer technology has been developed to ensure patient safety, decrease work for the nurse, and monitor patients more accurately. The design is intended to increase patient safety so that the nurse is able to make sound decisions to respond to changes in patient condition quickly and accurately. However, this may not occur always.

Reliance on various technologies and multiple alarms may divert the attention of the nurse from the patient. When an alarm sounds, it attracts the attention of the nurse, as it was designed to, causing the nurse to focus on the equipment and perhaps diverting his or her attention from the patient. The level of care may be compromised due to the emphasis placed on technology and equipment.

The more the equipment and technology are used, the greater the tendency of a nurse to rely on them. Everything appears to be controllable, measurable, and somewhat predictable. However, one must remember that the human body is rarely predictable. This idea can create a false sense of security in the equipment and lead to a reduction in assessment skills. The data provided by the equipment must be validated by observation and not taken at face value. A good example of this occurs when the monitor begins to alarm that the patient is in V-tach causing the nurse to run into the room only to find that the patient is sitting up in bed wondering what the commotion is all about. This is not an uncommon occurrence.

Safe competent nursing practice is the result of knowledge and understanding of the equipment and technology that are used in different practice settings. At some point, a nurse may find a piece of equipment malfunctioning while being used by a patient. The care and outcome of that patient will depend on the critical thinking and extensive assessment skills developed by the nurse. Experience and education of nurses regarding the use of technology, alarms, and the potential for the machine to malfunction will allow for greater competence in operating the equipment and increase the nurse's ability to care for her patients.

SUGGESTED READINGS

Haghenbeck K. Critical care nurses' experiences when technology malfunctions. *J NY State Nurses Assoc.* 2005;Spring/Summer:13–19.

Kiekkas P, Karga M, Poulopoulou M, et al. Use of technological equipment in critical care units: Nurses' perceptions in Greece. *J Clin Nurs.* 2006;15(2):178–187.

Aseptic technique and common sense can help prevent IV site complications

Francine B. Yates, RRT, RN, BSN

The majority of patients admitted to the hospital, regardless of whether they are in an intensive care unit or on a surgical floor, will require some type of intravenous access (IV). The education of and training in peripheral IV insertion should be a crucial part of nursing preparation and competency validation. The nurse should also be knowledgeable regarding the indications for the IV therapy and complications that can follow IV insertion.

To minimize complications, aseptic technique as a minimum standard should be practiced when inserting an IV, though some facilities indicate the use of sterile technique for insertion. The nurse should always keep in mind that thorough and improper handwashing is the first barrier to preventing infection; the first step in any IV insertion procedure is proper handwashing.

The nurse should likewise be conscientious about always using clean or sterile supplies. The site should be scrubbed thoroughly with the appropriate antiseptic solution, such as alcohol, chlorhexidine, or betadine solution. The IV catheter that is inserted must be sterile; therefore, the cap should not be removed until just prior to insertion to prevent contamination of the catheter. After the IV is safely and appropriately inserted, the site should be covered with a sterile adhesive dressing such as Tegaderm. Some facilities may provide a kit that contains all that is necessary to start the IV except the catheter itself. If tape is used to secure the line, it is especially important to ensure that the tape is clean, and not from a roll that has been picked up out of the patient's bed, off their bedside table, or even off of the floor. To maintain strict technique, if the tape happens to roll to the floor, the nurse should never use it for IV sites and should always obtain a new roll of tape. Using tape or dressings that are not clean can greatly increase the risk of infection, both local and systemic. Systemic infections, though less frequent, are more serious and can be life threatening.

Nurses today must not only know how to insert IVs safely but also monitor the site for complications such as infection, infiltration, extravasation, phlebitis, and clotting. IV sites should be flushed routinely and observed closely. Without regular flushes, the catheter may occlude. Infection can occur if aseptic technique is not followed during insertion, dressing change protocols are not followed, and if the site is used for an extended period of time. Nurses must be familiar with and follow individual institution-specific policies and procedures regarding IV catheter placement and management. Knowing the correct insertion and maintenance techniques for a peripheral IV is the first step to minimize the risk of infection and other complications.

SUGGESTED READINGS

Schmid MW. Risks and complications of peripherally and centrally inserted intravenous catheters. *Crit Care Nurs Clin N Am.* 2000;12(2):165–174.

Weigand DJ, Carlson KK. Peripheral intravenous catheter insertion. *AACN Procedure Manual for Critical Care.* 5th Ed. Philadelphia, PA: Saunders; 2005, pp. 667–689.

97

Avoid Incomplete Documentation of the Patient's Hospitalization

Lea E. Lineberry, RNIII, BSN, CCRN, CPN

What to Do: Evaluate

Incomplete documentation can be defined as documentation that is unfinished or fragmented. Documentation is the written presentation of evidence. In nursing, assessment documentation is the legal statement that what is written was performed. The failure of the nurse to complete appropriate assessment documentation is substandard. It represents carelessness and can be used as evidence of negligence or malpractice. With the number of malpractice lawsuits increasing, meticulous documentation is essential. Paperwork is usually the nurse's least favorite task on the daily agenda. Spending time with the patient and providing bedside care is what nurses prefer doing. However, it cannot be emphasized enough that the documentation of the care provided is the evidence that it occurred. The elimination of even simple tasks or events from the chart that occur during a patient's hospital stay can be detrimental to any case should it be called into court. This leaves the nurse open to skepticism and vulnerable to liability.

The nurse must take time to document completely and efficiently. On admission, the nurse must thoroughly document the patient's history. A common error by the nurse is failure to document important history. Medical institutions open themselves and their employees to possible litigation if the admission database is incomplete and proper information is missing. Strides to correct this type of problem have been made as institutions develop quality management programs to audit nursing documentation. Documentation can be considered incomplete if the handwriting is unclear. The medical record provides clinical communication and care planning among clinicians serving the patient as well as a basis for evaluation of the adequacy and appropriateness of care. Nurses often have time constraints, whether due to poor staffing, complicated care issues, or simply wanting to leave work on time, and may tend to write hastily, use poor grammar, or use incorrect spelling when documenting. Extreme care must be made to avoid these pitfalls.

Incomplete documentation is considered unfinished and conveys that the assessment has not been completed by the nurse appropriately. Illegible medical records are open to scrutiny and can be used as evidence in a malpractice suit against the nurse. Clear, legible handwriting and thorough documentation may not keep the nurse out of court but may provide protection for her license and career.

Suggested Readings

Glondys B. Practice brief: Ensuring legibility of patient records. *JAHIMA*. 2003;74(5):64A–64D. Available at: FORE Library: HIM Body of Knowledge. Accessed June 30, 2008.

Leacock-Ballish P, Spader C. Preventing documentation errors. *Nurs Spectrum*. 2005. Available at: http://www.nurse.com. Accessed June 2, 2008.

ENSURE CORRECTIONS IN DOCUMENTATION ERRORS

LEA E. LINEBERRY, RNIII, BSN, CCRN, CPN

WHAT TO DO: IMPLEMENT

Practice-related issues such as errors in documentation are more common in today's nursing society than ever before. The incidence of malpractice lawsuits no longer involve just the institution but may involve the nurse personally as well. The failure of the nurse to correct errors in documentation is problematic and can be used against her in law. Proper documentation can provide strong support for the nurse and demonstrate practice patterns if ever required during testimony.

One way to avoid documentation errors is to be familiar with the policies and procedures that address charting mistakes. The term mistaken entry should be used instead of error when correcting documentation. The simplest and most practical way of error documentation is to draw a straight line through the mistake and initial the mistaken entry. Following hospital policy and adhering to its guidelines for documenting errors should be observed by all practitioners to avoid legal pitfalls.

Some documentation errors often fall into the category of simple mathematics. The intake and output measurements should always be double checked for addition or subtraction mistakes. Inaccurate fluid calculations could mean delayed treatment or a possible fluid overload if additional fluid is given to correct an erroneous low output. The use of a calculator eliminates some of these errors; however, a documentation mistake in the placing of the numerical values would still cause miscalculation. Other numerical mistakes can be made by misplacing values into the wrong column or proper area. If the mean arterial pressure value was placed into the central venous pressure column, erroneous treatment by the physician could occur as he interprets the mistaken value as correct.

Some practical guidelines to be followed to avoid documentation errors include never using correction fluid to cover a mistaken entry or other methods to hide an error. These methods could be argued in court that the nurse was trying to "cover up" something. Always use a single line drawn through the mistaken entry and place the date, time, and initials above the line for clarification of the error. Altering words or entries after being documented in the chart is considered fraud and places the nurse open to litigation. Documentation errors can be corrected if done by following hospital policy and procedure appropriately.

SUGGESTED READINGS

Lynch VA. *Forensic Nursing*. St. Louis, MO: Elsevier; 2003.
Smith L. Handling documentation errors. bNet: Business Network. 2003. Available at: http://findarticles.com/p/articles/mi_qa3689/is_200310/ai_n9317905. Accessed July 2, 2008.

AVOID PLAGIARISM IN YOUR DOCUMENTATION

LEA E. LINEBERRY, RNIII, BSN, CCRN, CPN

Nurses often find that detailed shift documentation can be tedious. As a result, documentation shortcuts are often utilized. One of the quickest means of documentation that leads to "nursing documentation plagiarism" is copying the previous shift nurse's assessment notes. Plagiarism is defined as "taking another person's writing or ideas and use them as their own" (*Webster's New World Dictionary*, 2002). In higher education, this is a form of academic dishonesty. In the field of nursing, it is a form of assessment dishonesty.

Over the years, various charting methods have been developed. Some of these include narrative charting, focus notes, problem oriented charting, and flow sheet systems charting. All forms of nursing documentation that assess the patient's progress become part of the patient's medical record. The nurse's notes become a legal document of the patient's care and emphasize the skills used in implementing such care. In the realm of nursing malpractice, nursing documentation is the heart of analysis. Erroneous charting could be repeated if a charting shortcut is made by copying documented assessment notes from the prior shift. Good documentation can be used in a nurse's defense if ever involved in a malpractice lawsuit and can protect one's license.

Documentation of the nursing process is the responsibility of the nurse and must be done with honesty and accuracy. Nurses who are in a hurry often get caught in the easy ways to simply copy what was documented by the prior shift nurse, especially in flow sheet charting. By simply following suit in the quick check-off manner on many flow sheet charting systems, nurses "assume" that the person documenting before them has documented correctly. An example is the documentation that the patient has briskly reactive pupils when the patient actually had a prosthetic eye that was not documented. Another example would be the documentation that the patient moved all extremities equally when actually the patient is hemiplegic from a prior stroke.

Assessment honesty is the standard by which all nurses must document. As academic honesty is a part of all collegiate institutions, plagiarism can bring harsh consequences. The same is true for assessment dishonesty, the nursing form of documentation plagiarism. Termination from a job or losing a nursing license is never a part of a nurse's career but could happen if some form of erroneous charting ends up in a malpractice suit.

SUGGESTED READINGS

Iyer PW, Aiken T, eds. *Nursing Malpractice*. 2nd Ed. Lawyers & Judges Online Publishing Inc; 2001.
Laird C, ed. *Webster's New World Dictionary*. Hoboken, NJ: John Wiley & Sons Inc; 2002.

TRUST YOUR INSTINCTS—YOU KNOW YOUR PATIENT

ALICE M. CHRISTALDI, RN, BSN, CRRN

WHAT TO DO: IMPLEMENT

Patients are far more complicated than a diagnosis would portray. Nurses today have updated technologies at their disposal such as computerized charting, lab results obtained instantly at the bedside with handheld devices requiring just a drop of blood, and wireless medication barcode scanning, which increases the safety and accuracy of medication administration. When in need of help, nothing can matter more to the patient than a nurse who is advocate, articulate, and proactive with patients as well as one who listens to her instincts. These instincts may take years to develop, and it is often learned through trial and error. A solid education is paramount, which requires not only book learning but also time spent at the bedside.

Nurses are in the unique position of being an advocate for the patient. This requires a collaborative spirit among nurses and physicians. Trust and respect are developed over time, and a team spirit can be fostered which can only benefit the patient. It is vital to be articulate in verbalizing and documenting. Avoid editorializing and keep personal opinions out of it. Be as objective as possible. Don't wait for a better time. When you see something that needs to be addressed, do not wait for the next shift to handle it. It is important to know when to call the physician or when to merely leave a note on the chart for the physician to address in the morning. Be brief, and get to the point. Any nurse who has called a physician at 1 AM already knows this.

Be aware of the standards of care and your institution's policies and procedures. Do not deviate from these policies but be proactive in maintaining their relevance. In our fast paced nursing units, sometimes, listening can be a lost art, but it is vital to listen to our patients. Many give very readable nonverbal cues if only we take the time to look for them. It is not just the medication to be passed or the treatment to be completed, but the patient as a whole to be cared for. Take the time to develop a working rapport with the patient, utilize your instincts, and become articulate in advocating for him.

SUGGESTED READINGS

Austin S. Ladies and gentleman, I present the nursing documentation. *Nursing*. 2006;36(1):56–64.

Hennerman EA. Unreported errors in the intensive care unit: A case study of the way we work. *Crit Care Nurse*. 2007;27(5):27–34; quiz 35.

Mace S. Trust your instincts. Available at: http://include.nurse.com/apps/pbcs.dll/article?AID=20066122101. Accessed May 11, 2008.

USE RESTRAINTS APPROPRIATELY

ALICE M. CHRISTALDI, RN, BSN, CRRN

WHAT TO DO: EVALUATE

Restraint use has been dramatically reduced in hospitals and all but vanishing in nursing homes. It has been mandated by the Joint Commission on Accreditation of Healthcare Organizations (JCAHO) that the use of restraints by healthcare providers be kept to a minimum.

There are many restraint types that have been used in the hospital setting, and they include wrist restraints, vests, locked belts around the waist, and hand mitts. Bed rails are also considered a restraint. If the patient cannot remove the device himself, then this is considered a restraint. Medications that restrict or control a patient's behavior can also be classified as a restraint.

Fall prevention is one of the top reasons for the use of a restraint, as is the protection of therapeutic devices such as endotracheal tubes, intravenous and central lines, and an indwelling urinary catheter. Fifty percent of the elderly (>80 years) who have fallen are being cared for at home. A total of 20% to 30% of these falls cause a reduction in mobility and independence for the elderly and 3% to 5% cause fractures.

If a patient requires restraint to ensure his safety, it is important to visually observe the patient a minimum of every 2h. Fluids and nutrition need to be monitored and provided every 2h, as well as toileting the patient. Meticulous skin care will need to be done and the patient turned frequently to prevent skin breakdown.

Always ensure that if a restraint is necessary, the least restrictive device should be used. Use only approved restraint devices, not a folded sheet or pillowcase wrapped around a wrist. Do not tie the restraint to a movable part of the wheelchair or bed. Check at least every 2h for circulation to the extremity and to ensure that there are no breakdowns in skin integrity under the restraint. If the restraint is ripped, do not attempt to repair it, obtain a new one. Safety pins are not appropriate and could cause injury.

There are now several devices available to alert the staff when a patient is attempting to get out of his bed or chair. Bed alarms can be set to ring when a patient raises his legs off the bed. A device that records a voice telling the patient not to get up can be purchased. A pressure-sensitive pad that activates the recorded voice when the patient attempts to stand can be placed on the chair. It has been found very effective in reminding a patient to call for help before transferring.

If a patient is wandering the halls, check to see if he is hungry, thirsty, or needs to use the restroom. Often these basic body needs will trigger the patient to begin walking about. Constant reorientation may be necessary. Make sure the patient can easily find his glasses, cane, or hearing aid. Check for underlying medical conditions that might be triggering agitation or an increase in wandering. Things such as an infection, especially a urinary tract infection, lack of control of blood sugars, or possibly an, underlying neurologic disorder may be adding to the patient's confusion. Careful assessment of pain is important. The patient may not be able to express his discomfort, so nonverbal cues may be evident. Remember to reassess pain after an intervention to determine if the pain level has improved or further interventions are necessary.

Attempt to reduce stimuli in the patient environment. Hospitals are notoriously noisy places. There are bright lights 24h a day, phones constantly ringing, and televisions blaring. There are no quiet times, even during the night. If possible, arrange care of these patients so that they may indeed get some much-needed rest. Allow for uninterrupted periods of sleep.

Make sure that documentation is appropriate. If you use a flow sheet, make sure it reflects your hospital's policy and is compliant with current standards. Record in real time; do not complete charting either at the beginning or at the end of your shift. Be thorough and accurate in assessment documentation.

Involvement of the family could be an important intervention. They will have valuable clues to the behavior issues that the patient may have. They may also be willing to sit with the patient during difficult times. They should also be made aware every time a restraint is being used. Often they will think that the restraint is used to punish the patient, so good education of the family is necessary.

Fall prevention teams are springing up in hospitals. Ways are being devised to keep the patient safe without the need to physically restrain him. It will require a multidisciplinary approach to work, with involvement from nursing staff, physicians, therapists (including occupational and recreational), and pharmacists. The safety of patients is very important. Sometimes restraints will be the only alternative, but when they are used, they need to be used properly and evaluated frequently.

SUGGESTED READINGS

Caruso LB, Stillman RA. Geriatric medicine. In: *Harrison's Internal Medicine*. Fauci AS et al., eds. Available at: www.accessssmedicine.com/content.aspx?aID=2860353&searchStr=decubitus+ulcer. Accessed March 28, 2008.

Sweeney-Calciano J, Solimene AJ, Forrester DA. Finding a way to avoid restraints. *Nursing*. 2003;33(5):32HN1–4.

REDDENED BONY PROMINENCES SHOULD NOT BE RUBBED

ALICE M. CHRISTALDI, RN, BSN, CRRN

WHAT TO DO: IMPLEMENT

A call is on for better tracking and assessing of pressure ulcers. Admissions to acute care necessitate a thorough evaluation of the skin and extensive documentation of any abnormalities that are found. Medicare reimbursement has changed and hospitals are now being held accountable for the development of hospital-acquired pressure ulcers.

Approximately 10%–18% of hospital patients in general acute care areas develop a pressure ulcer. Eighty percent of these ulcers occur over bony prominences such as heels, sacrum, lateral malleolis, ischia, and greater trochanters. Pressure ulcers can develop even over a short time when there is intense pressure over a bony prominence. Prolonged moisture may reduce skin resilience. Friction that happens when the skin is dragged over bed linen and shear that happens when the skin located over a bone slides over a hard surface act together to increase damage to the skin. The use of a pressure ulcer risk assessment tool such as the Braden Scale may help to identify at-risk patients. Those found to be at high risk for pressure ulcer development may be identified sooner and greater effort can be taken to maintain skin integrity.

Contributing factors to these ulcers include poor nutrition, diabetes, hypotensive episodes causing decreased perfusion, and elderly patients with multiple disease entities. Having a history of an ulcer puts a patient at risk for development of a new ulcer. Incontinence of bowel or bladder is a major contributor to ulcer development.

How we provide care to our patients, especially the elderly, needs to be examined. A daily full bath may not be in the best interest of the patient. Many soaps cause drying and may alter the pH of the skin, which decrease the skin's ability to retain moisture. Water used on the body should be warm, not hot. Creams should be applied to the skin after a bath when the skin is still moist. Contrary to what many nurses were taught, bony prominences should not be rubbed, especially when reddened. This has been shown to increase tissue damage.

Turn the patient every 2 h, and use a flow sheet to document the care and communicate with coworkers. Be mindful of friction and shear when turning patients or getting them out of bed. Use of a bed pad under the patient may help in this regard. Use heel protectors if they are available, and float heels off the bed by placing the feet on a pillow and float the heels off the end. This will relieve any pressure buildup. Do not raise the head of the bed more than 30° if possible; this will aid in preventing the patient from slipping down in bed and possibly causing a shear injury. Use pressure relief mattresses or specialty beds for immobilized patients. Use alternating air mattresses that are now readily available in most hospitals. Keeping pressure off the skin is important and these mattresses allow better pressure redistribution.

Do not overlook the impact of good nutrition as an important adjunct to treatment. Patients will especially need an increase in protein and calories. A dietician should be consulted. Nutritional supplements might be tried, which will also add to adequate hydration. If the patient is incontinent, clean the patient as soon as possible after an incontinent spell. Use of a moisture barrier may be very helpful. Urine and feces hasten the development of a skin breakdown if left on the skin for any length of time.

SUGGESTED READINGS

Baranoski S. Pressure ulcers: A renewed awareness. *Nursing.* 2006;36(8):37–41.

Caruso LB, Stillman RA. Geriatric medicine. In: *Harrison's Internal Medicine.* Fauci AS et al., eds. Available at: http://www.accessmedicine.com/content.aspx?aID=2860353&searchStr=decubitus+ulcer#2860353. Accessed May 3, 2008.

Hess CT. Fundamental strategies for skin care. *Ostomy Wound Manage.* 1997;43(8):32–41.

Use care when charting; Do not confuse < for >; it could make a big difference to the patient

Alice M. Christaldi, RN, BSN, CRRN

Many hospitals today are utilizing fewer and fewer abbreviations and symbols in their approved list for documentation because they have been misread, resulting in medication errors and patient injuries. With the advent of computer and medication systems going paperless, it may be the time to eliminate them altogether. In 2003, the Joint Commission's National Patient Safety Goals stated that all healthcare institutions needed to develop a list of unacceptable abbreviations and symbols that all prescribers had to follow.

Medication errors are the eighth leading cause of death in the United States, with an estimated annual cost of between $17–29 billion . A patient's hospital stay may be increased by almost 5 days because of these errors. The majority of all medication errors occurs during physician ordering.

There are many computerized systems available to help prevent medication errors due to prescribing. Software is available with programmed default values for drug dosages, routes, and frequencies. Prompts are available that warn of potential drug interactions or contraindications. There will no longer be a need for constant calls to prescribers to clarify orders that are illegible.

Regardless of the systems used, pharmacy needs to be an active partner in the medication delivery system. All medication orders need to be reviewed by a pharmacist. There are ways to override even the most basic systems, and care must be taken that they are used only in emergent situations.

There are "high alert" drugs that require closer monitoring of dose, route, time, and correct patient, which can cause serious injury or even death if not given correctly. These include coumadin, heparin, and potassium chloride. These medications should not be stored together and require a double-check during preparation and administration, especially when safety measures are bypassed in an emergency.

Be an advocate for the patient, know why they are receiving a specific medication, and if in doubt, question the order. Know the routine medications that are given on your unit and their doses and routes. If an order does not make sense, do not give it until it becomes clarified to your satisfaction.

Many times, blood pressure medications come with parameters: "hold for blood pressure <90 systolic" or "give 1 mg for any systolic blood pressure >190." We also see orders to hold a medication with any "heart rate <50." It is time to see an end to such orders. A single stroke of a key will have the medication given for the wrong reason or not given at all. And just when you think you got the symbol right, a physician will change the way he usually orders a medication, and you will be holding a medication for any heartrate >50. This is too confusing.

Whoever devised the abbreviations for eye drops certainly made for a confusing time for generations of medical personnel. The "OU, OS, OD" should be immediately eliminated. For years, I would go down a hall chanting O Darn Right eye, OU beautiful eyeS, and the OS I could never remember, so I would only know it by eliminating the other two. It is time for our patients to receive better care.

It is time now to put these outdated symbols and abbreviations away. Errors have resulted from misinterpretation. Patient safety must be our primary concern. Utilize the technology that is currently available to enhance your practice and make it the safest you can possibly attain. Double check those orders that have symbols or abbreviations and make sure you understand the physician's comment before giving any medications.

SUGGESTED READINGS

Banning M. Medication errors: Professional issues and concerns. *Nurs Older People*. 2006;18(3):27–32.

Leape LL, Bates D, Cullen DJ, et al. Systems analysis of adverse drug events. *J Am Med Assoc*. 1995;274(1):35–43.

Mayo AM, Duncan D. Nurse perceptions of medication errors: What we need to know for patient safety. *J Nurs Care Qual*. 2004;19(3):209–217.

ENSURE THAT YOUR PATIENT'S IV HAS BEEN REMOVED PRIOR TO DISCHARGE

BONNIE L. PARKER, RN, CRRN

WHAT TO DO: EVALUATE

Nurses are taught that discharge planning begins at admission and all healthcare settings, outpatient as well as inpatient, have discharge criteria that patients and nurses have to meet: stable vital signs, good pain control, no signs of bleeding, the ability to eat or drink, obtaining a physician's order, completing discharge instructions and patient education, escorting the patient to the door, and documenting the discharge. Your job is done! Or is it?

Many complications occur after a patient leaves the hospital. As many as 19% of discharged patients have had a complication after discharge related to care while in the hospital; 6% of those injuries were preventable. Nurses are human and they work in a fast-paced, high-stress environment. Sometimes little things can be missed in the rush, but it can be those little things that cause difficulties for the patient later.

The Joint Commission has made communication, especially handoff reports between care givers, an important National Patient Safety Goal. A patient can be cared for on as many as five units in a typical hospital stay and, as they move unit to unit, vital information may be omitted. An important step in nursing care is change-of-shift report when nurses can communicate from one shift to the next about each patient: who they are, what is going on with them, their status, and what they need. Many hospitals have developed guidelines for these handoff reports that have different formats. One of the newer standards is the **SBAR** communication format. **SBAR** stands for: **S**—Situation, **B**—Background, **A**—Assessment, and **R**—Recommendation.

SBAR can be used as a template for giving report to a physician when a patient is having a problem or to the next nurse at shift change. Many hospitals that use computer charting also have a guideline for giving report that automatically lists pertinent information. It is important for caregivers to use the communication guideline their facility has chosen to provide a complete picture of the patient and his needs.

As nurses work in a fast-paced manner to complete their assignments, ordinary things may be overlooked. Diligently teaching the patient, arranging follow-up care, and ensuring that the patient is safely delivered to his or her waiting vehicle, the busy nurse may have overlooked the little saline lock hiding under the patient's sleeve. Started on another unit and never used by the current one, it is just one of those small things neglected in report and unexplored until the patient calls back later that day or next week seeking information about the object in his arm.

It is important that nurses assess every patient, even those getting ready to go out the door. Ask him if he has an IV access, look at both arms and hands, check for a PICC or central line, if one is present, inquire about its necessity for discharge, and verify with the discharging physician that he wants the catheter to remain. Of course, if it is to remain after discharge, discharge planning should encompass consideration of this line as well.

SUGGESTED READINGS

Barclay L. Adverse events common after hospital discharge. *Ann Int Med*. 2003;138:161–167.

Kingdom B, Newman K. Determining patient discharge criteria in an outpatient surgery setting. *AORN J*. 2006;83(4): 898–904.

Pittman MA, Morgolin FS. Community health: Crossing the quality chasm: Steps you can take. *Trustee*. 2001;54(7):30–32.

WASH YOUR HANDS BEFORE AND AFTER YOU TOUCH THE PATIENT

JEANNIE SCRUGGS GARBER, DNP, RN

WHAT TO DO: IMPLEMENT

The story of how infection and handwashing were first linked is quite interesting! In the 1800s, several physicians observed a connection between handwashing and infection in women delivering babies. As they promoted handwashing to their colleagues, their ideas were dismissed and criticized. The idea of handwashing was somewhat foreign at the time, especially since indoor plumbing was not yet available. Despite these physicians' warnings and clinical studies supporting their idea, handwashing did not become a universally accepted practice until the late 1800s and early 1900s. When the practice did become accepted, some physicians argued that the practice would negatively impact their business since patients would not need their services.

It is hard to imagine that such a perspective could exist on a practice that is now commonly understood as one to prevent and control infection. However, are practitioners today really that different from those who lived over 100 years ago? Healthcare providers learn and accept that handwashing helps prevent and control infections, yet many still do not follow handwashing policies and procedures. The Centers for Disease Control and Prevention publishes the statement that "handwashing is the single most important means of preventing the spread of infection." The prevention of nosocomial infections depends on healthcare providers practicing proper handwashing. The Centers for

Disease Control and Prevention defines handwashing as the act of washing hands with soap and water and rinsing with water for at least 15 s. The practice of proper handwashing protects both the patient and the provider by preventing and controlling infection.

Ongoing studies continue to reveal that despite training and understanding, handwashing is still not practiced as needed. Hospitals have invested endless resources in initiatives to improve the rate of handwashing and to impact infection rates. This basic procedure is simply not practiced by all healthcare providers. We now have plumbing, hot water, and soap available, yet handwashing compliance continues to be a major concern in hospitals. Hand hygiene must be practiced by all providers before and after interacting with patients and families, regardless of title and role. Adopting this procedure as a habit requires practice and influence by others. Institutions must provide the proper equipment, supplies, and training to support the development and maintenance of proper handwashing technique. Handwashing is a standard precaution that must be practiced to promote a safe patient-care environment.

SUGGESTED READINGS

Case C. (n.d.) Handwashing. Available at: http://www.accessexceleence.org/AE/AEC/CC/hand_backgroun.php. Accessed July 28, 2008.

West K. Infection prevention and control. In: Potter P, Perry A, eds. *Fundamentals of Nursing*. Canada: Mosby-Elsevier; 2009, pp. 655–658.

ASPIRATE FROM CENTRAL LINES AND PICC LINES BEFORE USING

JEANNIE SCRUGGS GARBER, DNP, RN

WHAT TO DO: IMPLEMENT

In order to improve patient safety and minimize risk of complications, healthcare providers must be familiar with the procedure to determine the patency of central lines and peripherally inserted central catheters (PICC) before attempting to administer medications or fluids. If the provider is unfamiliar with the equipment and technique, the patient could be harmed.

The most likely reason why a patient will have a central line is long-term fluid and medication administration, long-term laboratory access, poor venous access, or when an emergent venous access is required. When accessing a central line, it is important to aspirate blood to verify the placement and patency of the line. It is also important to cleanse the access point and maintain closure of all access points except when using the port for aspiration, flushing, or infusing.

PICC lines do not require heparinization, although some institutions continue to include this practice in their procedure. Before accessing a PICC line, aspiration is necessary to minimize the possibility of a medication bolus. The aspiration is accomplished using a syringe and applying slow, consistent pressure to withdraw blood. Any clots or medications used to close off the site will be aspirated. It is also important to flush the line after using. After the aspiration is completed, the catheter should be flushed with normal saline to decrease the possibility of blood clots at the tip of the catheter.

If aspiration of a blood return is not achieved, check the site for positioning and tubing kinks. It may also be helpful to have the patients cough and turn or reposition their head and shoulders. This movement may allow the catheter to move away from the vascular wall and allow aspiration. If after attempting to achieve aspiration there continues to be no blood return, the catheter site should not be used for infusion.

Another consideration when accessing a central line or PICC line is infection control practices. The access site should have a cap and be covered at all times. The port must also be cleansed appropriately prior to attempting to aspirate or administer fluids. These practices will minimize the risk of infection. Catheter placement or movement is also of concern. Some catheters are secured by suture but that does not guarantee proper placement. The provider must be cautious when moving the patient to maintain catheter placement.

SUGGESTED READINGS

Bunce M. Troubleshooting central lines. *RN Web*. 2003. Available at: http://rn.modernmedicine.com/rnweb/article/articleDetail.jsp?id=107207. Accessed July 31, 2008.

Redding J. Demystifying the central line. *Emerg Med Serv*. 2006; 35(9):120–125, 145. Available at: http://www.emsresponder.com/print/Emergency–Medical-Services/Demystifying-the-Central-Line/1$4046. Accessed July 31, 2008.

KNOW HOW TO CARE FOR PERIPHERALLY INSERTED CENTRAL CATHETERS TO PREVENT INFECTION

JEANNIE SCRUGGS GARBER, DNP, RN

A peripherally inserted central catheter (PICC) provides intravenous access that can be used for long-term infusions such as chemotherapy, antibiotics, or nutrition. A PICC is inserted into a peripheral vein by a specially trained healthcare provider, that is, usually a registered nurse, a physician, or a radiology professional.

The most common complications for patients with these lines are:

- Phlebitis
- Hemorrhage
- Thrombosis
- Infection

Signs and symptoms of infection include insertion site redness, inflammation, or drainage. As the line is inserted and dressing changes are done, it is important to apply a clean, dry 2×2 gauze at the insertion site, and not to leave the bloody gauze in place. Bleeding should be stopped prior to covering the site as bloody gauze is a possible breeding source for bacteria that can lead to infection. Other potential concerns are the development of blood clots in the catheter, air inside the line, or an actual break in the catheter. It is important not to use scissors near the catheter and to always aspirate and use caution with insertions to minimize the risks of blood clots and air emboli.

SUGGESTED READINGS

Cancerbackup (n.d.). PICC lines. Available at: http://www.cancerbackup.org.uk/Treatments/Chemotherapy/Line sports?PICCline#6932. Accessed July 30, 2008.

Molchaney C. Inserting and maintaining peripherally inserted central catheters. *Med Surg Nursing*. 1997. Available at: http://findarticles.com/p/articles/mi_m0FSS/is_n6_v6/ai_n18607581/pg_3?tag=artBody;col1. Accessed July 31, 2008.

Runzer N. Central venous catheters, care and maintenance of peripherally inserted central catheters (PICC). 2004. Available at: http://www.bccancer.bc.ca/HPI/Nursing/References?NursingBCCA/C-086.htm. Accessed July 31, 2008.

CLEANING PERIPHERALLY INSERTED CENTRAL CATHETERS

JEANNIE SCRUGGS GARBER, DNP, RN

WHAT TO DO: IMPLEMENT

Caring for a peripherally inserted central catheter (PICC) requires appropriate technique and attention to process to prevent complications such as infection or dislodgement. PICC line dressings are changed according to institutional policy at least weekly, when not being used routinely, and more often, if used frequently.

The insertion site must be assessed within the first 24 to 48 h of insertion to determine if any bleeding or drainage has occurred. The dressing needs to be clean and dry in order to minimize the risk for infection. The dressing should be changed at any time if it is moist, bloody, or loose, and it is very important to note the length of the catheter from insertion site to the end to make sure the catheter is still in its original place.

The common PICC dressing procedure includes the following steps:

- Explain procedure to the patient and others present and wash hands
- Prepare patient's arm for dressing change
- Remove old dressing from the bottom of the dressing upward

- Assess catheter site for redness, swelling, or drainage
- Wash hands and prepare dressing
- Use STERILE gloves (powder free)
- If blood or drainage is present, clean the catheter exit site with the required agent by cleaning the catheter and the skin using concentric circles away from the puncture site
- Allow cleaning agent to dry before applying steri-strips

Proper technique is critical to patient safety. Healthcare providers caring for patients with PICC lines must be trained and educated in the procedure and rationale for actions. The purpose of a dressing is to control bleeding, prevent infection, absorb blood and wound drainage, and protect the wound from further injury. Cleaning the insertion site and maintaining a clean, dry dressing will minimize infection rates for patients with PICC lines and maintain catheter patency for an extended period of time.

SUGGESTED READINGS

ASWCS Chemotherapy Handbook. PICC line protocols. 2005. Available at: http://www.aswcs.nhs.uk/pharmacy/Chemo Handbook/NetworkPolicies/ProtA45.pdf. Accessed July 31, 2008.

KEEP NEWSWORTHY PATIENT INFORMATION CONFIDENTIAL

JEANNIE SCRUGGS GARBER, DNP, RN

WHAT TO DO: IMPLEMENT

Sharing newsworthy patient information with the media must meet the same confidentiality standards as patient information that is not newsworthy. It is the nurse's ethical and legal responsibility to maintain patient confidentiality regardless of how dramatic or intriguing a situation may appear.

In an attempt to regulate how patient information is shared, The Health Insurance Portability and Accountability Act (HIPAA) was established in 2001 and it became effective in 2003. This Act was developed to increase the control patients have regarding how their personal health information is shared. Only specific patient information may be shared and that information must be limited and on a need-to-know basis. Clinicians are privileged to personal and sensitive health information and should always maintain confidentiality within the work group, organization, and the public.

Most healthcare organizations have privacy and confidentiality policies and procedures that outline the process of how patient information is shared with the media. Some organizations allow the patient to determine if and what type of information is to be shared with the media. If the patient "opts in" to allow patient information to be shared, the patient conditions are reported as "undetermined, good, fair, serious, critical, treated and released, and treated and transferred." According to the HIPAA Consumer Bill of Rights and Responsibilities, "consumers have the right to communicate with healthcare providers in confidence and to have the confidentiality of their individually identifiable healthcare information protected." The healthcare provider is in a unique position to ensure that the patient's wishes are realized and not compromised for the sake of a good story.

SUGGESTED READINGS

HIPAA Consumer Bill of Rights and Responsibilities. Available at: http://www.opm.gov/insure/health/cbrr.htm#chpt1. Accessed August 14, 2008.
Wake Forest University Medical Center, Patient Information (n.d.). Available at: http://www.1.wfubmc.edu/news/patient information.htm. Accessed June 11, 2008.

MICROWAVES CAN BE DANGEROUS

ALICE M. CHRISTALDI, RN, BSN, CRRN

WHAT TO DO: IMPLEMENT

The use of microwave ovens has spread from the home kitchen to most hospital departments. I doubt there is a lounge or cafeteria that does not offer its use to staff. Caution must be used, however, in heating anything other than food or liquids for drinking. For the most part, heating supplies that will be used on the patient should be discouraged. Examples of using the microwave to heat wet towels to use for bathing patients, bags of intravenous solutions, antibiotics, and peritoneal dialysis fluid are commonplace. None of these can be recommended. Certainly, microwaves will heat, but the problem is, this is not a controlled heat.

Today's microwaves have high output that can quickly overheat a liquid. Even cheaper, less powerful models can produce a liquid that is too hot for clinical use. Years ago, microwaves had a maximum output power of 600 to 650 W. Many models today exceed 1,000 W. Temperatures may vary between different makes of microwaves, making it hard to standardize the time for heating.

Microwave ovens heat water directly. The energy passes through a container and is absorbed directly by the water. Water will begin to boil at 100°C. Superheating occurs when the liquid is heated to a temperature above this normal boiling point. This leads to instability and the production of steam vapors.

It has been documented that burns in children, attributed to the use of microwaves, were the result of spilling food on their bodies. Burns to the trunk or the face were the most common types of burn, with oral burns running at 0.7%. Food at the very surface of the heated dish may indeed be cooler than what is located deeper inside the dish. An uneven distribution of heat may very well cause the food to explode, eggs being a prime example. It is not recommended that baby bottles be heated in the microwave. The water in the formula heats more rapidly and quickly turns to steam in the closed container.

Hypothermia is a major concern when dealing with trauma cases, diabetic ketoacidosis, major gastrointestinal bleeding, and any condition requiring large volume of fluid replacement. For many years, intravenous fluids used in resuscitation were commonly heated in the microwave oven. There are set algorithms that state how long to heat fluids; however, they do not take into account the power variation on individual microwaves. The fluid may be overheated.

Never heat an intravenous antibiotic in a microwave. It has been shown that heating this medication will reduce its usefulness to fight susceptible bacteria. Be aware of placing closed containers in any microwave oven. Steam will build up inside the container and when opened, there is a real possibility of it being released on the body. Burns to the eyes have occurred this way.

Likewise, heating packed red blood cells in a microwave should never be done. An unknown amount of hemolysis will occur. This will not only destroy the cells intended to improve oxygen delivery but also lead to high levels of potassium and potential cardiac arrest during transfusion. Commercial heaters are readily available and should be utilized when heating any fluids that will be used on patients. This includes intravenous solutions and peritoneal dialysis fluids. They ensure uniform heating of the liquid, without any chance of overheating. Microwave ovens continue to heat as long as the oven is turned on, and superheating may lead to a dangerous release of steam or temperatures that will easily scald.

Place only microwave approved materials in the microwave to avoid fires and burns. Metals in materials such as spoons, forks, and aluminum foil help to concentrate the electric field and may produce sparks. These sparks could start a fire.

Fabrics, such as towels, are also not to be used in microwaves. Example of this is the fire produced by a blanket that had been warmed in a microwave oven and placed on a patient in a hyperbaric chamber. It should be noted that while a container that has been heated may appear cool, what is inside may still be very hot. The uneven heating patterns with the superheating encased in the folds of the blanket were the culprits. Burns can occur when an individual grabs hold of the container not realizing how hot it is.

Microwave ovens have a place on the nursing unit, but they must be utilized wisely. If your unit has the need for a warmer, then commercial warmers appropriate to heat fluids should be purchased, saving the microwave oven to heat water for your cup of tea.

SUGGESTED READINGS

Delaney A. Reliability of modern microwave ovens to safely heat intravenous fluids for resuscitation. *Emerg Med.* 2001;13:181–185.

Medical Device Safety Report. Fire from blanket warmed in microwave oven. Available at: http://www.mdsr.ecri.org/summary/detail.aspx? doc_id=8152. Accessed April 29, 2008.

Millin V. Effect of electro magnetic field leakage from a microwave oven on the efficacy of an antibiotic. *Acupunct Electrother Res.* 2001;26(3):203–205.

Powell EC, Tanz RR. Comparison of childhood burns associated with use of microwave ovens and conventional stoves. *Pediatrics.* 1993;91(2):344–349.

KNOW WHERE YOUR TELEMETRY PATIENT IS AT ALL TIMES

ALICE M. CHRISTALDI, RN, BSN, CRRN

WHAT TO DO: PLAN

A patient may need cardiac monitoring for many reasons. This is no longer performed only in intensive care units, but it occurs on the medical–surgical floors as well. Physicians may order telemetry to determine if an arrhythmia is the cause of syncope, for chest pain or electrolyte imbalances, or to monitor when a change in medications is necessary. Individual units may use monitor technicians right in the unit, or they can be monitored remotely on another wing or floor. Communication is done by telephone. Standards by the American Heart Association have been published in response to a more routine monitoring available for the average medical-surgical patient experiencing a dysrhythmia.

A telemetry pack is applied to the patient's chest by way of leads attached to electrodes. A poor signal can be caused by electrodes that have dried out, dead or weak batteries, or lead wires that may be frayed or entirely broken off. If there are certain dead areas on a unit where the signal is unable to be transmitted, then the patient must be instructed to avoid this area.

The monitor technician will notify the nurse when arrhythmias develop or a problem develops with the signal. If the monitor is showing asystole, it may mean the leads have fallen off, the patient is out of range, or indeed, the patient has no heart rate. The nurse must assess the patient to determine the cause.

If a weak signal continues, the reason must be investigated thoroughly. Possibly, the patient is diaphoretic, very thin with rib bones protruding, or obese. Rearranging the electrodes might aid in getting a stronger signal. A hairy chest is best managed by clipping and shaving the hair under the electrodes to gain a better connection.

Make sure that when a patient is moved to another room or off the unit for a procedure, the monitor tech is notified. Also, the monitor tech needs to be sure that the patient's name and room number are not switched at the central monitor and that he or she is aware in which bed a specific patient is assigned. The monitor technician will call with a possible arrhythmia, but it is up to the nurse to determine if this is indeed the real issue with the specified patient.

Keeping track of your patients is not always easy. Many times, they may leave the unit for testing or surgery or leave the building entirely. Ensure that your unit has a system to track the coming and going of patients which includes informing you when they have moved on.

The best leads for monitoring dysrthythmias are V1 followed by V6. V1 leads are used to distinguish ventricular from supraventricular rhythms. Also, P waves are more prominent in V1. Lead II or Lead III is preferred to monitor atrial fibrillation and atrial flutter. It is the monitor technician's responsibility to provide rhythm strips of any events that might occur during the shift. Also, rhythm strips are routinely run and charted. From these strips, a new diagnosis might be made or the physician may order a change in medications.

No longer is cardiac monitoring the realm of intensive care units. All nurses need a basic understanding of how their hospital's telemetry system functions and of cardiac arrhythmias. It is a collaborative effort of the patient, monitor technician, and nurse to provide a 24-h readable rhythm that is available through telemetry. It is the responsibility of the nurse to quickly and accurately assess the situation when an alarm has been raised and to ensure that a patient stays in range so that monitoring is not interrupted. Check the patient first before treating any arrhythmia to rule out artifact. And, never turn off alarms because they are ringing too much.

SUGGESTED READINGS

American Association of Critical Care Nurses. AACN Practice Alert: Dysrthymia monitoring. Available at: http://www.aacn.org/AACN/practiceAlert.nsf/Files/DYS/$file/Dysrhythmia%20Monitoring%208–2004.pdf. Accessed April 18, 2008.

Drew BJ, Funk M. AHA scientific statement: Practice standards for electrocardiographic monitoring in hospital settings. *J Cardiovas Nurs.* 2005;20(2):76–106.

Scalzo T. Managing a patient on remote telemetry. *Nursing.* 1992;22(3):57–59.

THE IMPORTANCE OF EDUCATING PATIENTS AND FAMILY MEMBERS TO PREVENT A FALL AFTER SEDATING MEDICATION

MARY S. WARD, RN, BS, OCN

WHAT TO DO: IMPLEMENT

When an individual is hospitalized, the disorientation from displacement itself is arguably enough justification to place most patients on falls precautions. But many patients can function in a hospital setting independently, getting to the bathroom or bedside commode without calling for assistance or utilizing minimal assistance from family or visitors. However, this scenario can change dramatically if the patient receives any type of sedating, hypnotic, or narcotic medication.

A patient who may be steady or a simple one-person assist may become a high risk falls patient due to weakness, confusion, increased sedation, dizziness, disorientation, and other side effects of the medication. Medications of this nature may be administered for a procedure, such as EGD, MRI, or CT scan. Narcotics administered for pain, especially for patients who are opioid naïve, as well as other medications that are routinely ordered in hospital settings, such as anxiolytics or sedatives for sleep or histamine blockers for certain treatments such as blood transfusions, place patients at risk. Many times, healthcare workers are aware that these medications have been administered to the patient but that communication may not always be given to the family members or others who care for the patient in the hospital which could lead to disastrous results. If the family or visitors are used to seeing their loved one ambulating without assistance and are unaware that he or she has had sedation for an MRI, colonoscopy, or other procedure and allow the patient up without required assistance, the patient is at significant risk for falling. Likewise, if the patient has received a narcotic or sedative for sleep or antihistamine or other sedating medication for a treatment, family and friends may be unaware of the patient's condition.

Nurses, physicians, and other members of the healthcare team must constantly balance the patient's need for independence and strengthening along with maintaining a safe patient environment. Incorporating the family and concerned visitors into the plan of care is a healthy part of holistically caring for the patient. According to the Centers for Disease Control, the average cost of a fall injury in 1998 was $19,440. This is just the total amount in terms of dollars; it does not take into account the amount of time, quality of life, and emotional costs for patient and family related to a fall. The CDC estimates that 20% to 30% of falls are moderate to severe and many of those are fatal. When a patient's activity status has changed, nurses and other healthcare givers must make educating, not only the patient, but all those who care for the patient in a hospital setting a priority. A well- intentioned visitor or family member may allow a patient who has been sedated to get out of bed with minimal or no assistance because that is what the patient's normal pattern has been. This may result in consequences no one is prepared to face.

Good communication among healthcare givers as to the patient's condition is another key element to keeping the patient safe. Being aware of what types of medications a patient has received for a procedure or treatment is important, as well as being aware of individual characteristics of each patient, such as renal clearance. Elderly patients may have more significant adverse effects such as delirium, confusion, and oversedation to sedating and hypnotic medications. Keeping the patient safe requires communication at all levels.

SUGGESTED READINGS

Agnostini JV, Concato J, Inouye S. Improving sedative-hypnotic prescribing in older hospitalized patients: Provider-perceived benefits and barriers of a computer-based reminder. *J Gen Intern Med*. 2008;23(S1):32–36.

Centers for Disease Control and Prevention. Costs of falls among older adults. Available at: http://www.cdc.gov./mcip/fact. Accessed April 3, 2008.

EDUCATE FAMILIES ABOUT COMMON DANGERS IN THE CONFUSED AND MEDICALLY UNSTABLE PATIENT

JULIE MULLIGAN WATTS, RN, MN

WHAT TO DO: IMPLEMENT

Families are frequent visitors to patients, and some patients are hospitalized for extended time periods. The patient and family may be overwhelmed by a new diagnosis or therapy. Common fears about treatments, procedures, surgeries or chemotherapy, and the side effects of medication can increase the anxiety of both patient and family beyond their normal coping strategies. Families feel that everything is out of their control. Actions that may have been helpful and supportive in earlier times may not be helpful for the current hospitalization. Seeing a loved one in a vulnerable condition can increase fear and the feeling of helplessness.

Often, family members become allies with the nursing staff by assisting in care and encouraging the patient to eat, assisting with and encouraging physical activity, and offering emotional support. This can give family members a sense of accomplishment and add meaning to an otherwise difficult situation. Common fears such as loss of the relationship, fear of pain and suffering, and loss of control can be diminished by nurses offering education to the family about the disease and treatment, providing support to the family, encouraging a sense of control, and developing a good rapport with the family.

Nurses also need to teach the family approaches that support safety during hospitalization. The proper use of the bed, how to safely steer intravenous poles around furniture, how to support the patient when assisting with ambulation, and how to avoid falls and other trauma are important parts of education for the family of a hospitalized patient. Families should be taught measures to minimize infection and bleeding risks. Handwashing, diet limitations, use of personal protective equipment when required, and avoiding exposure to infected bodily fluids are topics to include in family teaching.

Families of patients who are medically unstable or experiencing confusion or delirium should be taught additional measures to ensure the safety of the patient. Families should be educated on the rationale for restraints if required and the avoidance of items that can cause injury such as razors, scissors, knives, matches, and lighters. When infirm or confused patients have access to these types of items, injuries and fires can occur.

SUGGESTED READINGS

Ahrens M. Smoking and fire. *Am J Pub Health*. 2004;94(7):1076.

Carroll-Johnson R, Gorman L, Bush N. *Psychosocial Nursing Care Along The Cancer Continuum*. 2nd Ed. Pittsburgh, PA: Oncology Nursing Society; 2006.

Kobs A. Managing the environment of care. *Nurs Manage*. 1998;29(4):10–11, 13.

ENSURE THAT INVASIVE PROCEDURES GET APPROPRIATE SITE VERIFICATION OUTSIDE OF THE OR

ANTHONY D. SLONIM, MD, DrPH

WHAT TO DO: IMPLEMENT

The performance of an incorrect procedure or the performance of a procedure on the incorrect site or person is one of the preventable occurrences in healthcare organizations. Many organizations including the Joint Commission, the American College of Surgeons, and consumer groups are educating and advocating on methods of assuring that the safety of patients undergoing invasive procedures is ensured. For several years now, the Joint Commission has had a regulatory requirement in place entitled the Universal Protocol that aims to prevent the wrong site and wrong procedure errors. While many operative personnel and surgeons are aware of the requirements for the Universal Protocol, procedures performed outside of the operating room are equally susceptible and require the same, if not higher, subscription to these standards of care.

The Universal Protocol consists of three major steps. The first step is the operative or procedure verification process. This is performed to ensure that both the patient and the team are consistent with the expectations of surgery. Second, site marking by the patient allows the opportunity to identify not only laterality but also the specific body part to receive the procedure. For example, if the right middle finger requires surgery, assurance that the right index finger is not operated on is critical. Finally, a "time out" is called prior to beginning the procedure to ensure that the final verification of the patient, procedure, and site is affirmed. The time out is a team sport and requires all members of the team to participate and affirm the plan. Nurses are critical to the performance of the Universal Protocol and must recognize their professional obligation to ensure that it is performed, both inside and outside of the operating room for invasive procedures.

Outside of the operating room, the pressure on the professional nurse increases even more. Providers in settings like the medical ward or intensive care unit may be unfamiliar with these safety mechanisms or know what they need to do to provide safe care. The nurse in these situations needs to ensure that the procedure is done in a safe manner including following the steps in the Universal Protocol. A provider's unwillingness to engage in these procedures should be taken to the notice of a charge nurse or shift administrator for resolution.

SUGGESTED READINGS

The Joint Commission Universal Protocol. National patient safety goals. Accreditation Program: Hospital; 2008. Available at: http://www.jointcommission.org/NR/rdonlyres/AEA17A06-BB67–4C4E–B0FC-DD195FE6BF2A/0/UP_HAP_20080616.pdf. Accessed August 18, 2008.

Universal protocol for preventing wrong site, wrong procedure, wrong person surgery. 2003. Available at: http://www.jointcommission.org/NR/rdonlyres/E3C600EB-043B-4E86-B04E-CA4A89AD5433/0/universal_protocol.pdf. Accessed August 18, 2008.

MOVE FROM A BLAME-FREE TO AN ACCOUNTABLE PATIENT SAFETY CULTURE

ANTHONY D. SLONIM, MD, DrPH

Considerable knowledge about how to protect patients from harm during the healthcare experience has been gained over the last decade. More importantly, the relevance of the clinical environment in which providers work and patients receive care has received focus. In this effort, healthcare has changed its attention from providers as the sole cause of medical errors to misdirected systems and processes.

Underlying the approach that faulty systems, not providers, are to blame is a need to understand how these systems are put together and perform. The "structure" of healthcare includes not only the bricks and mortar of the hospital and clinic but also the providers and equipment that combine to deliver the care. Processes in healthcare are the series of steps that occur between healthcare providers and their patients and result in the outcome of the experience. Alterations and impediments in either the structure or the process can lead to altered outcomes in the traditional Donabedian approach.

Healthcare organizations have not only attempted to analyze these structures and processes to improve care but also investigated and now recognized the importance of the environment or milieu in determining healthcare outcomes. A number of patient safety culture surveys have been developed so that leaders can understand the culture of their organizations and the likelihood that adverse events will be openly reported and managed in a nonthreatening environment where learning can take place. However, over time, this has moved to the other end of the continuum where

healthcare has moved from a blame-free environment to one that is able to recognize that employees do have accountability in delivering healthcare.

The "Just Culture" movement is an effort to temper the patient safety climate from one that is focused on being blame free to one that holds healthcare providers accountable for reckless and negligent acts. In a just culture, providers have a duty to produce an outcome, follow a procedural rule, and avoid unjustified risk or harm. The importance of establishing these duties is that they provide guidance for providers and their supervisors on the level of accountable action that needs to be assured and the action that becomes necessary if the duty is ignored. In this paradigm, reckless behavior is subject to punishment since it violates a duty on the behalf of the provider to perform.

Providers and organizations need to work together to ensure patient safety. The importance of the established culture in specifying the behavioral norms is critical to this work. A just culture maintains its focus on systems of care and allows providers to be accountable for their actions.

SUGGESTED READINGS

Leape LL. A systems analysis approach to medical error. *J Eval Clin Pract*. 1997;3(3):213–222.

Leape LL, Bates DW, Cullen DJ, et al. Systems analysis of adverse drug events. ADE Prevention Study Group. *J Am Med Assoc*. 1995;274(1):35–43.

Marx D. Patient safety and the "Just Culture." The Just Culture Community. 2007. Available at: http://www.health.state.ny.us/professionals/patients/patient_safety/conference/2007/docs/patient_safety_and_the_just_culture.pdf. Accessed August 18, 2008.

DO NOT ASSUME THAT AN ENDSTAGE PATIENT DOES NOT WANT AGGRESSIVE THERAPY

NANCY F. ALTICE, RN, MSN, CCNS, CNS-BC

WHAT TO DO: PLAN AND IMPLEMENT

Nurses and other medical professionals often express opinions about end of life decisions, especially when patients are elderly, chronically and severely ill, or when quality of life is estimated to be poor. Many people base opinion about quality of life on their own experience and wishes.

A memorable patient had been ill for several years with end stage heart failure and COPD. He had been admitted to the hospital on numerous occasions and was followed by a home health agency. To improve his quality of life and hopefully reduce his numerous trips to the hospital, he was started on IV inotropes that were continued at home for more than 1 year. He had fewer hospital admissions on this regimen but during one of the times that he was in the hospital, he developed sustained ventricular tachycardia while standing at the sink, brushing his teeth. He quickly lost consciousness and in the process, he fell to the floor and broke his ankle. He was successfully defibrillated, brought to consciousness quickly, and subsequently transferred to the CCU. Several of his nurses and physicians remarked that he should have been a DNR and they regretted resuscitating this patient who, in their opinion, had a very low quality of life.

The patient was approached and the cardiac arrest event was explained to him. When asked if he would want to be put through another resuscitation attempt, he thought for a moment and then replied, "Some days I really don't feel well but some days I am able to ride to the grocery store with my wife and I sit on the bench while she does the shopping. Other days, I may be able to go get a haircut. Yes, I think I would want to be treated if something like this happened again."

Patients' views on acceptable quality of life may change over time. No one can predict what patients may want based on their own beliefs. Patients who are capable of understanding their prognosis and the various treatment options should be given the opportunity to discuss their wishes.

SUGGESTED READINGS

Cherniack E. Increasing use of DNR orders in the elderly worldwide: Whose choice is it? *J Med Ethics*. 2002;28:303–307.
Palmer R. A review of nurses' attitudes towards DNAR decisions. NursingTimes.net. 2007. Available at: http://www.nursingtimes.net/ntclinical/a_review_of_nurses_attitudes_towards_dnar_decisions.html.

DO NOT ASSUME AN ADVANCED DIRECTIVE ALWAYS MEANS THE PATIENT WANTS TO BE A DNR IN ALL CIRCUMSTANCES

NANCY F. ALTICE, RN, MSN, CCNS, CNS-BC

WHAT TO DO: IMPLEMENT

Advanced directives are one way a person may document his or her wishes for various types of medical care in the event that he or she becomes unable to express these wishes in the future. Both, care that is desired and care that is not desired, can be included in the document. Likewise, these wishes can be discussed with a medical power of attorney or health care proxy who would speak on behalf of the patient if the patient became unable to discuss his or her wishes in the future.

The majority of written advance directives are written to express a desire to forego futile treatment in the case of terminal illness. However, some advance directives are written to provide additional instructions. A document may specify that the person wants aggressive treatment for a certain time frame prior to omitting specific care modalities such as mechanical ventilation or nutritional therapies. A specific request may be made to have terminal illness confirmed by a second opinion.

Advance directives rarely stand alone in making such important decisions, but sometimes provide the only "voice" for the patient during a critical illness. Healthcare professionals sometimes make the assumption that the presence of an advance directive on the chart means that the patient does not want aggressive treatment. Often, the document states that aggressive treatment is not desired during terminal illness but the definition of terminal illness is frequently subject to interpretation. Many patients would want aggressive therapies if the potential to recover at least partially were present. Whenever an advance directive is in place, it is essential that the person also discusses his or her wishes verbally with key people such as family members and the primary physician.

Always review the content of a patient's advance directive. Remember that advance directives are not intended to be DNR orders and must always be interpreted according to the present clinical situation. If the patient is able to communicate his/her wishes, then obtain current direction from the patient rather than assuming that the advance directive should be followed.

SUGGESTED READINGS

Advance directives and do not resuscitate orders. Available at: http://familydoctor.org/online/famdocen/home/pat-advocacy/endoflife/003.html. Accessed March 31, 2008.

American Bar Association. Healthcare advance directives. Available at: http://www.abanet.org/publiced/practical/directive_recognition.html. Accessed March 31, 2008.

THE HOSPITAL IS NO PLACE TO BE WHEN YOU'RE SICK: HELP TO GET YOUR PATIENTS MOVING ON THE PATH TO DISCHARGE

ANTHONY D. SLONIM, MD, DRPH

WHAT TO DO: IMPLEMENT

The nurse plays an important role as a pivotal member of the multidisciplinary healthcare team. As healthcare has become more complex, providers tend to adhere to the roles that they've been given. Unfortunately, the nurse is often left to pick up what's left. While there are specific roles in many hospitals aimed at patient discharge and care management, the nurse is in a unique position to be able to contribute to this work while at the same time looking out for the patient's best interests.

A number of "guidelines" have been published with specific criteria for when patients need to be admitted to hospitals. When these criteria are not met, there is a presumption that care could be provided in other settings. These guidelines are often written with the intent of ensuring that: 1) there was an indication for the admission, 2) only hospital-dependant services are provided in the hospital setting, and 3) there is justification for payment. While these specific guidelines and criteria for hospital admission take up entire books, the nurse can provide an important service by simply asking the question, Does my patient need to be here?

Whether you primarily practice in the emergency department, the ICU, obstetrics, pediatrics, or on a medical or surgical floor, the question is the same. Hospitals often assist with the placement of patients and transitions of care by creating admission and discharge criteria for specific floors or units. This ensures that patients placed on that unit are cared for by appropriately competent and experienced staff. By asking the question, Does my patient need to be here? the nurse can help to ensure that the patient gets the necessary services. For example, if the patient remains in the ICU, but does not require ICU-specific care—such as a ventilator, a vasoactive or high-risk infusion, or frequent monitoring—the nurse may be able to facilitate transfer of that patient to a more comfortable and family-friendly setting by asking the question. For patients on a medical floor who are eating regular diets, not requiring oxygen, and able to perform activities of daily living, asking the question may facilitate discharge planning and the appropriate establishment of home care therapies and support.

Sometimes, no matter how diligent the nurse and the case management staff, the answer to the question, Does my patient need to be here? is no, but nonetheless the patient remains. These are frustrating examples for many members of the team and may be placing the patient at risk for hospital-acquired complications. The nurse, through key relationships with other members of the healthcare team, is in a unique position to help influence these answers.

SUGGESTED READINGS

http://www.caregiving.org/pubs/brochures/familydischarge planning.pdf. Accessed on April 15, 2009.

http://www.nhchc.org/discharge/Documents/IVB_Exemplary Practices.doc. Accessed on April 15, 2009.

119

KNOW HOW TO CARE FOR THE OVER SEDATED PATIENT ON A PCA

BONNIE L. PARKER, RN, CRRN

WHAT TO DO: PLAN

Patient-controlled analgesia or PCA is often used with postsurgical patients to deliver timely, adequate pain relief. When used properly, PCAs can safely relieve patients of pain and make the nurses work more efficiently by not having to administer repetitive doses of analgesia. Use of the PCA, however, requires that the nurse must be competently trained in its use and must appropriately monitor the patient. Over sedation can be an issue for the patient on a PCA. PCAs allow patients to administer their own medication as needed for pain relief. There is some discussion regarding family-controlled or nurse-controlled analgesia, which may be appropriate under certain circumstances. However, some believe that by limiting the activation of the PCA to the patient alone, the potential for overdoses would be minimized because an over-sedated patient would be unable to push the button for additional medication.

The patient should be closely monitored during the first 24 h of PCA activation until the effects of the medication on the patient can be thoroughly assessed. He should also be monitored closely at night when oxygen saturations may fall due to shallow respirations while sleeping. Capnography, or end-tidal CO_2 monitoring, is recommended to monitor patients for rising levels of carbon dioxide as an early warning of respiratory depression. When used with oxygen saturation, end-tidal CO_2 monitoring gives a more accurate assessment of the patient's overall respiratory condition.

The patient's level of consciousness may progress from being alert and awake to drowsy but arousable to being very drowsy and difficult to arouse. With ongoing medication, the patient's condition may progress further to responding to light stimuli but falling asleep during conversation and then having minimal or no response to physical stimulation. It is possible that a patient who is oversedated may respond to vigorous stimuli but the nurse should avoid thinking that the patient is fine. In order to prevent further complications such as respiratory depression, patients who are difficult to arouse require an immediate response from the nurse.

If the patient has difficulty staying awake or does not respond to stimuli, a more thorough assessment should be performed. Vital signs and oxygen saturation levels should be obtained and the doctor should be notified. An order should be acquired to have the dose lowered or the interval between PCA doses increased. However, the medication should not be just stopped or the control removed from the patient's reach or an antidote administered. To do so may cause him or her to suffer as a result of uncontrolled pain. If the patient is unresponsive, a thorough assessment should be made and the naloxone, an opioid antagonist, may be considered.

PCAs, when used correctly, can be a safe and effective method of pain control but ongoing monitoring and assessments of the patient are necessary to prevent complications. Those who have not taken narcotics in the past are small or obese, are taking other medication that may increase the effects of the PCA medication, or have a history of respiratory difficulties may require more frequent monitoring and adjustment to their PCA dose or rate of delivery.

SUGGESTED READINGS

Cohen MR. Patient controlled analgesia: Pushing for safe pain relief. *Nursing.* 2003;33(11):10. Available at: http://findarticles.com. Accessed May 6, 2008.
D'Arcy Y. Keep your patient safe during PCA. *Nursing.* 2008;38(1):50–55; quiz 56.
Noah V. PCA by proxy: Minimizing the risks. *Nursing.* 2003; 33(12):17.

DEATH COMES IN A VARIETY OF FORMS AND IT IS IMPORTANT FOR THE NURSE TO UNDERSTAND THE DIFFERENCES

ANTHONY D. SLONIM, MD, DRPH

WHAT TO DO: PLAN

There is no more important time for the nurse to support the patient and family than the time of death of the patient. It therefore becomes important for the nurse to understand the three major ways in which people can die and the fundamental nursing differences with each type of death.

First, patients can die suddenly from a cardiopulmonary arrest. These anxiety provoking circumstances are in some ways the easiest to deal with from a medical perspective. A patient is found unresponsive; a code team is summoned; and the appropriate algorithms are followed. Unfortunately, in hospitals, cardiac arrest is associated with significant mortality. From an emotional perspective, these are often challenging because often the patient's death is unexpected, and the family questions why and what happened. For providers, supporting the family through this while simultaneously having their care scrutinized even when nothing wrong was done can be difficult.

Second, patients can also die when they have reached a point when advanced medical interventions are no longer desired and the focus of care changes from being aggressive to providing comfort. At some point in this journey, either the patient or the surrogate decision maker may decide not only to limit further interventions but also to actively withdraw some interventions. For the patient and family, this may be a relief, particularly if the disease has been long and difficult for the patient. In this case, death is often seen as a relief from suffering. Alternatively, withdrawal of care may occur in the acute setting, after trauma, for example, and be more difficult for the family to understand.

Finally, patients may die through a pronouncement of brain death. This type of death is the most difficult for families and providers to understand since the patient's heart, a traditional sign of life, is still beating. The criteria for brain death have been well established for decades. What is important is that brain death, while it may include the withdrawal of life, supporting equipment, does not represent a choice for the family. The role of the providers here is to support the family through their understanding of the diagnosis. This is difficult because many nurses do not understand the differences with brain death and how it differs from the two other types of death.

The nurse needs to have an understanding of the different "types" of death to effectively support the grieving family.

SUGGESTED READINGS

Manno EM, Wijdicks EF. The declaration of death and the withdrawal of care in the neurologic patient. *Neurol Clin.* 2006;24(1):159–169.
Truog RD. Brain death—too flawed to endure, too ingrained to abandon. *J Law Med Ethics.* 2007;35(2):273–281.

121

KNOW HOW TO MANAGE THE COMBATIVE CLIENT AND PROVIDE SAFE CARE

MELISSA H. CRIGGER, BSN, MHA, RN

WHAT TO DO: PLAN

Nurses must promote safety for any patient in the inpatient psychiatric unit. However, for the patient diagnosed with schizophrenia, safety is a top priority. Schizophrenia is the disease process that causes the patient to experience abnormal or bizarre patterns of thinking. The schizophrenic patient can have either positive or negative symptoms. Positive symptoms include delusions, hallucinations, flight of ideas, and loose associations. Negative symptoms include anhedonia, flat affect, and feelings of apathy. The patient will also be poorly dressed and not care about personal hygiene.

There are different types of schizophrenia. The paranoid schizophrenic is characterized as a patient with persecutory or grandiose delusions. The patient may also have hallucinations and can exhibit hostile and aggressive behavior. When caring for the patient with paranoid schizophrenia, the nurse must remember to assess the patient's current condition. This assessment includes general appearance, speech, mood and affect, thought process, and presence of delusions and hallucinations, as well as assessment of judgment and insight.

At times, paranoid schizophrenics will lack the necessary judgment to meet their needs for safety and personal care. Patients may not realize that they need to bathe or they have not eaten or slept. Schizophrenics who experience persecutory delusions (e.g., the nurse is trying to poison me) will choose not to eat for fear that someone is trying to kill them. Delusional patients may also fear that the nurse and/or other patients are out "to get them." Remember, whenever the nurse approaches the patient, it must be in a nonthreatening manner. This includes providing adequate space, knocking when entering the room, and avoiding touch during periods of agitation.

Paranoid schizophrenic patients may become agitated due to auditory hallucinations or delusions that others are going to harm them. This agitation can place both the patient and others in danger. The nurse must remember to observe throughout the shift for signs of increased agitation. This can include an increase of fast-pressured speech, increased volume of speech, increased hostile behavior, which includes hitting and yelling, and increased movements. The nurse should try to avoid confrontation or arguing with the delusional patient. The nurse should attempt to move the patient to a quieter environment. The reduction of external stimulation may assist in reducing the stimuli causing the delusional behavior. The nurse must also present reality to the patient using a "matter-of-fact" approach. For the patient who asks the nurse if she can hear the voices, the nurse needs to state that she does not hear the voices but wants to know what the patient is hearing. Although the nurse does not hear the voice, she still needs to assess the auditory hallucination.

The nurse must also remember that the delusional patient may act in a bizarre manner such as touching others, undressing in front of others, and performing sexual acts such as masturbating in front of others. The nurse should try to redirect the patient away from these situations. This could include taking the patient back to his or her room. The nurse must remember that limit setting and controlling the environment provides the patient with an opportunity to learn new appropriate behaviors. If the patient is touching others or making inappropriate remarks, the nurse should encourage the patient to participate in other activities such as walking. The nurse should try to avoid the use of restraints unless behavior truly warrants potential harm to self or others.

SUGGESTED READINGS

Morrison-Valfre M. The therapeutic environment. In: *Foundations of Mental Health Care*. 3rd Ed. St. Louis, MO: Elsevier-Mosby; 2005, p. 116.

Videbeck SL. Schizophrenia. In: *Psychiatric Mental Health Nursing*. 3rd Ed. Philadelphia, PA: Lippincott Williams & Wilkins; 2006, pp. 275–302.

PREPROCEDURE AND POSTPROCEDURE CARE FOR THE PATIENT RECEIVING ECT

MELISSA H. CRIGGER, BSN, MHA, RN

Preprocedure and postprocedure care for the patient receiving electroconvulsant therapy (ECT) includes educating the patient, monitoring the patient's condition, and symptom management. Major depressive episodes occur when depression symptoms last longer than 2 weeks. These symptoms include depressed mood, anhedonia, changes in sleep patterns, weight changes of greater than 5% that are unintentional, feeling of hopelessness, or suicidal ideation. Antidepressants are usually the first line of treatment for depressive episodes; however, in those patients who do not respond to medications, ECT may be used as an alternate treatment to treat depression.

ECT involves introducing an electric current to the brain, which leads to the creation of a tonic–clonic seizure. The procedure lasts only a few minutes, with the electrical current being delivered in a couple of seconds. Most patients who receive ECT will receive a total of 6 to 15 treatments that are administered over the course of a few weeks. A typical schedule would include treatments on alternate days of the week (e.g., Mondays, Wednesdays, and Fridays). For the patient receiving 12 treatments, the cycle would be complete in 4 weeks. Remember to educate the patient on the importance of following the cycle regimen and the importance of not missing any scheduled procedures.

ECT can be administered as an outpatient or inpatient procedure. Prior to the procedure, the patient should be educated on not taking anything by mouth for 8 h before the procedure. The patient must also avoid and remove fingernail polish/makeup prior to the procedure. The patient is then placed in a hospital gown. The nurse should always check the baseline vital signs prior to the procedure and start an intravenous line for the medication administration. The nurse should alleviate any fears regarding the procedure and should try to avoid using terminology such as "shock treatment." The proper technical terminology is ECT. In the past, patients did not receive sedatives for ECT. Patients were strapped down and allowed to convulse actively. For the patients who have received ECT in the past, it is necessary to assess their current knowledge level and correct any misconceptions.

Just prior to the procedure, the patient will receive an anesthetic and muscle relaxing agent. The two electrodes are then placed on the patient's head in a unilateral (on the same side) or bilateral (on both sides) position. The electric current is delivered and the seizure activity is monitored on an electroencephalogram (EEG).

In postprocedure, the patient receives oxygen and vital sign monitoring. The patient will likely be disoriented or complain of headache. Headaches will be treated based on the symptoms experienced. Another common occurrence in patients receiving ECT is the complaint of feeling tired. Remember to discuss these symptoms with the patient prior to and after the procedure. Short-term amnesia can also occur in the postprocedure ECT patient. Remember to educate the patient on this symptom and to notify the patient that it is only a short-term effect. The patient may also be assessed using a Mini-Mental Status Exam. Once the patient's gag reflex returns, the MD will order the patient to eat.

SUGGESTED READINGS

Morrison-Valfre M. Depression and other mood disorders. In: *Foundations of Mental Health Care.* 3rd Ed. St. Louis, MO: Elsevier-Mosby; 2005, pp. 214–218.

Videbeck SL. Mood disorders. In: *Mental Health Nursing.* 3rd Ed. Philadelphia, PA: Lippincott Williams & Wilkins; 2006, pp. 312–317.

123

KNOW HOW TO CARE FOR THE PATIENT WITH A BORDERLINE PERSONALITY DISORDER

MELISSA H. CRIGGER, BSN, MHA, RN

WHAT TO DO: IMPLEMENT

Nursing care for the patient with a borderline personality disorder includes promoting patient safety, providing satisfactory boundaries in patient–nurse relationships, helping the patient control emotions, and administering pharmacologic agents.

Personality disorders are diagnosed when a person exhibits personality traits that are different from the cultural norm. These personality traits are often maladaptive and interfere with the patient's normal functions. Borderline personality disorder is diagnosed when the patient has increased impulsivity, unstable personal relationships, and unstable thoughts about self-image. It is three times more likely to occur in females and is one of the most common personality disorders seen in inpatient psychiatric facilities.

When caring for the patient with borderline personality disorder, the nurse must remember to assess general appearance, mood and affect, thought processes, judgment, insight as well as self-concept. For the patient with borderline personality disorder, self-image views may change dramatically. At times, the patient may appear needy, and then become angered for no apparent reason (labile emotions). Suicidal ideations and gestures such as self-mutilation are also common in the borderline patient. The patient who shares thoughts of wanting to harm himself/herself should be approached in a nonjudgmental manner. Always remember to have the patient contract for safety. The contract is an agreement made by the patients that they will not harm themselves.

Borderline personality patients also have difficulty maintaining appropriate boundaries with others, including staff. The nurse must remember to establish clear boundaries with the patient. This includes maintaining a regular schedule and routine to follow and notifying the patient that the goal of the nurse–patient relationship is to help the patient develop more appropriate relationships. This may require limit setting in some cases. The nurse should try to avoid being the only staff member that the patient can talk to. This could lead to the transference of feelings to the nurse, which is not productive to meet the patient's goal of developing appropriate relationships.

The borderline personality patient is often impulsive and has difficulty controlling his or her emotions. Inattention from the staff or not having a need met can immediately lead to hostile behavior or the possibility of self-mutilative behavior. The nurse should remember that the borderline personality patient has difficulty controlling behavior. The nurse may need to provide activities such as walking, watching television, playing cards, and listening to music as a distraction technique. This provides the patient with something to do while waiting to have a need met.

Pharmacologic management of personality disorders requires the use of medications to manage individual symptoms experienced by the patient. The patient with borderline personality disorder may exhibit anxiety. Treatment for anxiety includes the administration of SSRIs, MAOIs, benzodiazepines, and, in severe forms of anxiety, low-dose antipsychotics. For those with impulsivity, mood stabilizers such as Lithium and anticonvulsants, such as Tegretol and Depakote, are potential pharmacologic choices. The nurse must remember to observe side effects of medications and to educate the patient on these potential effects. The nurse must also remember to monitor serum blood levels for lithium, Tegretol, and Depakote prior to the administration of these medications due to the potential for toxicity.

SUGGESTED READINGS

Morrison-Valfre M. Personality disorders. In: *Foundations of Mental Health Care*. 3rd Ed. St. Louis, MO: Elsevier-Mosby; 2005, p. 320.

Videbeck SL. Personality disorders. In: *Psychiatric Mental Health Nursing*. 3rd Ed. Philadelphia, PA: Lippincott Williams & Wilkins; 2006, pp. 346–364.

124

KNOW HOW TO CARE FOR THE BIPOLAR PATIENT

MELISSA H. CRIGGER, BSN, MHA, RN

WHAT TO DO: IMPLEMENT

Nursing care for the bipolar patient with mania includes administering psychopharmacology, providing for safety, meeting psychologic needs, and promoting appropriate behaviors. Bipolar disorder is a mood disorder that involves sudden and drastic shifts in emotion. The patient with bipolar disorder can cycle between periods of depression and normal behavior (bipolar depressed) or between periods of mania and normal behavior (bipolar manic). Bipolar disorder occurs equally between males and females, with the average first manic episode occurring in the early 20s. Symptoms of mania consist of angering quickly, pressured speech, flight of ideas, delusion of grandeur or persecutory delusions, bizarre dressing, as well as little intake of food or sleep, but the patient remains hyperactive.

When caring for the bipolar patient, treatment consists of psychopharmacologic agents such as lithium or anticonvulsant agents that are used as mood stabilizers. Lithium's onset of action ranges from 5 to 14 days and requires close observation of serum blood levels. Lithium levels greater than 1.5 mEq/L are indicative of lithium toxicity. Symptoms of lithium toxicity are the same as side effects and include nausea, diarrhea, thirst, sleepiness, lightheadedness, and drowsiness. For most patients, side effects of lithium usually disappear or decrease by the sixth week of therapy. If symptoms continue, the nurse should be aware of the potential for lithium toxicity. Prior to administration, the nurse should review the patient's last lithium level.

Anticonvulsants (Tegretol, Depakote, Neurontin, Lamictal, Topamax, and Trileptal) are also used as mood stabilizers in the bipolar patient. Side effects include dizziness, ataxia, nausea, and vomiting. With the administration of certain anticonvulsants (Tegretol and Depakote), drug serum levels are required to be monitored for toxicity. Again, prior to administration, the nurse should be aware of serum drug levels.

The bipolar patient with mania often has little insight into his or her current behavior. One of the top priorities of the nurse is to provide safety for the patient in the manic phase. The nurse must assess the patient for suicidal ideations and plans to hurt others. Often, the manic patient will take others' belongings and engage others in an aggressive nature. The nurse needs to know the whereabouts of the manic patient and may have to set limits to control inappropriate behavior. The nurse needs to provide the manic patients with an explanation of what is expected of them and what behaviors will not be tolerated. These explanations must be concise, with short simple statements. All staff must follow and consistently set limits to promote appropriate behaviors.

The manic patient receives very little rest and nutrition. Reducing external stimuli (placing the patient in an area without noise or television) can assist the patient with relaxation. Bedtime routines may also assist the patient. Many manic patients are "too busy" to eat. The nurse can provide the manic patient with finger foods that are high in caloric value to ensure adequate nutrition. Food items such as sandwiches and protein bars provide more adequate nutrition.

The patient with mania requires additional attention to provide for safety as well as to meet psychologic needs. Drug levels must be monitored. Communication among caregivers is important to provide consistent instructions to the patient to reduce confusion.

SUGGESTED READINGS

Morrison-Valfre M. Depression and other mood disorders. In: *Foundations of Mental Health Care*. 3rd Ed. St. Louis, MO: Elsevier-Mosby; 2005, pp. 214–216.
Videbeck SL. Mood disorders. In: *Psychiatric Mental Health Nursing*. 3rd Ed. Philadelphia, PA: Lippincott Williams & Wilkins; 2006, pp. 326–333.

Patients who are suspected of becoming detoxified during their hospital stay should be started on CIWA protocol for improved outcomes

Francine B. Yates, RRT, RN, BSN

WHAT TO DO: IMPLEMENT

Ethanol is the most commonly abused compound in the United States with an estimated 17.6 million Americans having some form of alcohol abuse disorder. Alcohol abusers are admitted to the hospital with illnesses such as nutritional and gastrointestinal disorders, diabetes, mental illness, and injuries.

Many nurses, during their career, may have the opportunity to encounter a patient experiencing alcohol abuse withdrawal symptoms. The Clinical Institute for Withdrawal Assessment (CIWA) is a protocol developed by the Mayo Clinic to treat withdrawal symptoms experienced by these patients during their hospitalization. Utilizing CIWA can effectively and safely manage the symptoms of alcohol withdrawal. The use of benzodiazepines within the protocol has reduced the complications of withdrawal even when delirium occurs. The main concern with the protocol is that patients must be properly screened to ensure that it is being initiated on the appropriate patients. This protocol should not be used with patients who can communicate appropriately but have no recent history of alcohol abuse. Conversely, it should not be started on patients that consumed alcohol heavily until the time of admission to the hospital and cannot communicate effectively.

It is essential that all aspects of a patient's history are examined before incorporating CIWA. It is commonly assumed that most alcoholics minimize the amount of alcohol that is consumed per day. It is important not only to look at medical histories but also to speak with family members or significant others regarding the patient's alcohol consumption.

Nurses should be aware that patients may also be admitted with conditions that mimic alcohol withdrawal symptoms such as cardiac disorders, dementia, anxiety disorders, postoperative confusion, or drug withdrawal. It is important for physicians and nurses not to initiate the CIWA protocol on these patients as there could be severe adverse effects or reactions to the benzodiazepines that are given through the protocol.

Although the CIWA protocol can be a useful tool for alcohol withdrawal syndrome, if it is not utilized on the appropriate patient population, the outcomes may be serious or even life-threatening.

SUGGESTED READINGS

Berge KH, Morse RM. Protocol-driven treatment of alcohol withdrawal in a general hospital: When theory meets practice. *Mayo Clini Proc*. 2008;83(3):270–271.

Grant BF, Stinson FS, Dawson DA, et al. Prevalence and co-occurrence of substance use disorders and independent mood and anxiety disorders. *Arch Gen Psychiatry*. 2004; 61(8):807–816.

Hecksel KA, Bostwick JM, Jaeger TM, et al. Inappropriate use of symptom-triggered therapy for alcohol withdrawal in the general hospital. *Mayo Clin Proc*. 2008;83(8):274–279.

PATIENTS WITH PSYCHIATRIC PROBLEMS CAN GET ADMITTED TO ANY UNIT IN THE HOSPITAL: A LITTLE TRAINING CAN GO A LONG WAY

FRANCINE B. YATES, RRT, RN, BSN

WHAT TO DO: PLAN

When a patient with a history of psychiatric condition is admitted through the emergency department for a medical condition like chest pain, the nurses on the medical floors need to know how to manage him. Unless a nurse has specialized in psychiatric nursing at some point in her career, the most exposure she has likely received will have been some brief coursework and clinical rotations in nursing school. Nurses with this type of preparation on medical–surgical and intensive care units may not feel qualified to care for some of these patients. Caring for patients with a psychiatric history can create a lot of stress for the nursing staff who may not feel adequately prepared to undertake this work.

Safety is a top priority for the nurse, the ancillary staff, and the patient. The nurse should attempt to get as clear an assessment of the patient's medical and psychiatric history as possible to understand and address the patient's specific needs. Speak with the patient's physician and inquire about depression, anxiety, paranoia, violent tendencies, suicidal ideation, or any other disorder that may affect the patient's care and staff interaction with the patient. Having a 1:1 sitter assigned to the patient may help the nurse. Maintaining routines, such as giving medications regularly and on time, may help the patient maintain a better sense of emotional balance. It may also help keep the room quiet and limit the amount of contact the patient has with multiple staff members.

The nurse needs to maintain self-control at all times. If the patient refuses his medications, the nurse should remain calm and readdress the issue once the patient has a chance to calm down. If the patient requires some tests to be performed, explain to him or her that they are necessary to rule out any complications that may arise from the symptoms that he or she had complained about earlier. If the patient consistently refuses care on the medical unit, such as refusing medications, IVs, tests, and procedures, then the physician may need to reconsider the admission criteria for the unit. At this point, it may be more appropriate to transfer the patient back to the psychiatric facility. If the patient becomes aggressive or seeks to leave, the attempt to stop him could potentially escalate. The nurse should keep in mind that she can call the physician and security for assistance. To keep situations from escalating, make sure that patients remain on their regular psychiatric medications throughout their hospital admission.

Keep in mind that safety is the first priority for staff and the patient. Patients should receive medications on time to keep their behavior from becoming violent. The nurse or the staff should never try to handle a violent situation on his or her own. Call the physician and security should the need arise. When the patient is cleared off the medical complaint, set up the transfer or discharge as appropriate.

SUGGESTED READINGS

Hermanns MS, Russell-Broaddus CA. "But I'm not a psyche nurse"! *RN*. 2006;69(12):28–31; quiz 32.
Smeltzer SC, Bare BG. Emergency nursing. In: *Brunner and Suddarth's Textbook of Medical-Surgical Nursing*. 9th Ed. 1999, pp. 1929–1930.

PEDIATRIC NURSES SHOULD BE TRAINED TO RECOGNIZE POSTPARTUM DEPRESSION

LYNDA COOK SAWYER, RNC, BSN, MBA

WHAT TO DO: PLAN

Today, in America, 6% to 13% of postpartum women display the signs and symptoms of an affective disorder of depression that could be diagnosed and if found to be major, should be treated. In looking at major depression alone, six of these women could be diagnosed in the first 3 months of postpartum.

Major depression is clinically diagnosed based on a list of clearly defined observances: depressed mood, tearfulness, inability to experience pleasure in normally pleasurable acts—such as eating, exercise, and social or sexual interaction—insomnia, fatigue, appetite disturbance, suicidal thoughts, no desire to provide self with the activities of daily living, routine hygiene, and regular meals, kempt manner, and recurrent thoughts of death. Anxiety is prominent.

The prevalence of major depression among postpartum women is not appreciably different than the typical adult female population, but the inability to care for themselves and their baby makes major depression in the first postpartum year a double strike that could have serious physiologic consequences for the infant. In addition, Cox et al. (1993) found that, in the first 5 weeks postpartum, the odds of a new episode of major depression are three times that of a comparison group of females.

Minor depression is differentiated from major depression in that symptoms are usually transient and short-lived. Signs and symptoms include irritability, hostility, social withdrawal, conflicts with loved ones, and irregular sleep patterns. In postpartum, all the above can be explained by irregular sleep patterns. When sleep does occur, it is usually insufficient to provide the new mother with her usual controls to limit or prevent irritability. These symptoms are usually associated with "the Blues" postdelivery peak 3 to 5 days after birth with spontaneous bursts over the following 2 weeks. Minor depressive symptoms associated with the postpartum woman, however, can reappear many times during the first postpartum year. A strong differentiator between major and minor postpartum depression will be the mother's ability to care for herself and her infant.

The most serious affective disorder is that of postpartum psychosis. Thankfully, postpartum psychosis is extremely rare, occurring in 1.4 to 4.0 cases per 1,000 mothers. Symptoms appear suddenly, usually 2 to 14 days after birth and include delusions, hallucinations, extreme agitation, insomnia, mania, and suicidal or homicidal thoughts. New mothers most at risk for developing psychosis postnatally have personal histories of schizophrenia or bipolar disease or a family history of schizophrenia, bipolar disease, or psychosis.

In the grand scheme of routine medical visits in the first year postpartum, mothers see their pediatric providers a recommended eight times and their obstetric providers only once or twice. Remember then, it would be beneficial for all pediatric nursing personnel to be trained in the clinical signs and symptoms of major and minor postpartum depressive disorders and have the tools available to refer these women to appropriate resources for care.

SUGGESTED READINGS

Bloch M, Daly RC, Rubinow DR. Endocrine factors in the etiology of postpartum depression. *Compr Psychiatry.* 2003;44(3):234–246.

Cooper PJ, Campbell EA, Day A, et al. Non-psychotic psychiatric disorder after childbirth. A prospective study of prevalence, incidence, course and nature. *Br J Psychiatry.* 1988;152: 799–806.

Cox JL, Murray D, Chapman G. A controlled study of the onset, duration and prevalence of postnatal depression. *Br J Psychiatry.* 1993;163:27–31.

Perinatal depression, prevalence, screening accuracy, and screening outcomes summary. Available at: http://www.ahrq.gov/clinic/epcsums/peridepsum.htm. Accessed April 3, 2008.

KNOW HOW TO MANAGE THE CONFUSED PATIENT WITHOUT RESTRAINTS

BONNIE L. PARKER, RN, CRRN

WHAT TO DO: PLAN

Restraining patients is an option for caregivers that should be used only if certain, limited criteria are met. Developing restraint-free environments is the goal of many healthcare settings. Restraints should be used only to protect the patient from harm and as an option when all other approaches have been exhausted. The use of restraints often escalates the behavior and actually may worsen the clinical situation.

Confused patients present a significant challenge to nurses in many healthcare settings. The elderly population is especially at risk for confusion due to the increased incidence of chronic ailments and reduced ability to metabolize and excrete medications. Many patients, but especially the elderly, can become confused when ill, with certain medications or after surgery. This may be a temporary situation or one that has more permanent effects.

Alternatives to restraints should always be attempted first. The initial task for the nurse is a good assessment. Assess the patient for other symptoms and evaluate the admitting diagnosis. Speak to the family to determine if the patient has a history of confusion or this is a new onset of symptoms and ask if there have been any recent changes in the patient's life. The assessment should include a review of the patient's medications including a review of the home medications. Scheduled pain medications may need to be reduced in dosage or their schedule modified. Many medications, such as sedatives and muscle relaxants, can cause severe confusion if stopped abruptly. Evaluate the patient's fluid and electrolytes for any potential causes of confusion.

Rather than putting the patient in restraints, inquire if a friend or family member can stay with the patient.

Many times, having a familiar face that the patients know and trust is enough to calm them down, and the family can be educated to call for assistance if the patient attempts to get out of bed. Another precaution that can be taken is the use of a bed or chair alarm. The sound of the alarm may be enough to remind the patient not to get up and will alert the staff about potential safety concerns. Frequent rounding, keeping a low light on in the patient's room, and ensuring that the call bell is within easy reach are all measures nursing staff should take to reduce the risk of injury from falls for a confused patient. Nurses should also reinforce the use of the call bell and answer calls as quickly as possible.

One of the most common reasons a patient falls is when he is trying to get to the bathroom. As their frame of reference has changed, confused patients may not understand that they cannot safely stand without assistance. One way to help reduce falls is to take the patient to the bathroom on a schedule and offer toileting to a restrained patient at least every 2 h. Once the patient has been assisted to the bathroom, the question arises as to whether the nurse should leave or remain with the patient. Since a confused patient is not likely to remember to use the call bell, the nurse should remain immediately available to the patient, especially if the patient's confusion and unpredictable behavior were assessed to be the cause for concern in the first place. Since chair alarms and restraints do not work on the toilet or bedside commode, staying with the patient while he is using the bathroom may be the safest thing to do.

SUGGESTED READINGS

Burke A. Nursing assistant education. Available at: http://www.nursingassistanteducation.com. Accessed May 3, 2008.

Hall GR, Wakefield B. Acute confusion in the elderly. *Nursing.* 1996;26(7):32–37; quiz 38.

REMEMBER THAT YOUR DEPRESSED PATIENTS MAY HAVE A MEDICAL REASON FOR THEIR DEPRESSION

ANTHONY D. SLONIM, MD, DrPH

WHAT TO DO: ASSESS

Major depression is an important healthcare concern and affects approximately 15% of the population at some point in their lives. In addition, there are estimates that approximately 6% to 8% of patients in the outpatient setting meet established criteria for depression. There are a number of causes for depression. While some of these causes may be related to genetic or biologic predispositions, there are also important medical causes for depression that require assessment.

Depression is a common side effect of major classes of medications. Commonly prescribed medications including antihypertensives, antibacterial agents, steroids, anticonvulsants, and analgesics may cause or contribute to a depressed mood.

While medications are an important contributor to depression, there is often a bit of a "chicken and egg" phenomenon when trying to understand depression in patients with medical illness. Is the medication causing the depression or is the medical condition causing the depression? Often, it is difficult to know. Common medical conditions often lead to depression in our patients. These conditions include new diagnoses of cancer, recent myocardial infarctions, transplants, and critical illness or severe trauma. Nurses are in a unique position to ensure that patients with these conditions are appropriately screened and prophylactically treated for their depressive symptoms.

In addition to the association of depression with medical illness, depression can sometimes be the primary symptom that requires that organic disease be ruled out. For example, diabetes, hypothyroidism, Lyme disease, and fibromyalgia can be the underlying cause for major depressive symptoms that often improve with treatment of the disease.

The nurse needs to be aware of common depressive symptoms, including prolonged changes in mood, alterations in appetite, sleep, and sexual function, changes in weight, and variations between agitation and somnolence. Partnering with our physician colleagues allows an investigation for an underlying cause and treatment of the symptoms so that patients can begin to experience an improved mood.

SUGGESTED READINGS

http://www.emedicinehealth.com/depression/article_em.htm. Accessed on April 15, 2009.

Reus VI. Mental Disorders: Depression in Association with Medical Illness. In: Kasper DL, Braunwald E, Fauci AS, et al. *Harrison's Principles of Internal Medicine*. 16th Ed. New York: McGraw Hill; 2005, pp. 2552–2553.

HEALTHCARE PROVIDERS MUST DEVELOP AN APPRECIATION FOR THE PATIENTS' FEAR AND ANXIETY GENERATED BY TESTS, PROCEDURES, AND DIAGNOSES

FRANCINE B. YATES, RRT, RN, BSN

WHAT TO DO: PLAN

When a patient is admitted to the hospital or sees his physician for an examination or undergoes testing, he is likely to experience some degree of anxiety or fear. Fear of the unknown, news about one's own health, or any impairment of normal bodily function can create anxiety. Healthcare providers often forget the level of fear and anxiety that patients acquire during a hospital stay. It is often helpful to allow the patient adequate time and multiple opportunities to express fear or anxiety. It is also beneficial to let the patient know what to expect before, during, and after a procedure or test. However, this can be overlooked as healthcare providers hurry to finish rounds, administer a medication, document a procedure, and neglect to provide a human touch to discussions with their patients.

Providers may have forgotten or have not ever experienced the trials and tribulations that patients are put through during their stay in the hospital. Unfortunately, providers seldom approach these issues in a focused manner since they lack the communication skills to effectively reduce the level of fear and anxiety of their patients.

In today's society, scheduled appointment times are shorter; the patient is allowed 10 min as compared to 20 min in the past. Patient assignments have increased in all facets of healthcare. The patient interview is shorter and more abrupt. Patients feel as if providers neither listen to what they say nor answer their questions appropriately. They feel as if they are treated with arrogance, and their fears and concerns are dismissed. Patients tend to be less anxious and cope better with whatever news they receive when the physician appears to be more involved and communicative.

A few extra minutes spent with the patient will enhance the provider–patient relationship. The patients will hopefully have the answers they need (why, where, how, and the outcome), and the provider will not have a patient that thinks he made a mistake or one that wants to change physician's midstream.

SUGGESTED READINGS

Ellis-Christensen T. What is bedside manner? Available at: http://www.wisegeek.com/what-is-bedside-manner.htm.
Halpern J. Empathy and patient–physician conflicts. *J Gen Intern Med.* 2007;22(5):696–700.

ALCOHOL ABUSE AND ISOLATION ARE A DEADLY COMBINATION IN GERIATRIC PATIENTS. CONSIDER A CALL TO PROTECTIVE SERVICES: IT COULD SAVE A LIFE

JULIE MULLIGAN WATTS, RN, MN

WHAT TO DO: IMPLEMENT

In the United States, almost 8% of the population above 12 years was classified in 2005–2006 with dependence on or abuse of alcohol in the previous year. A recent study shows that 10% of primary care patients above 60 years had evidence of alcohol dependence. Alcoholism accounts for 1% of all hospitalizations of the elderly, but it often goes unrecognized. Patients with symptoms of alcohol abuse have a higher rate of hospital admissions and are more likely to die than nonalcoholic patients by 4.3%. In spite of this, older alcoholics do not visit the emergency department or outpatient clinics more frequently, and they do not have longer lengths of stay in the hospital. With this in mind, where might you find the older alcoholics in need of assistance? These individuals are found in almost all clinical settings. One study found that in regularly scheduled visits to their primary care physician, more than 10% of elderly patients reported at least two symptoms of alcoholism. As the US population ages, it is expected that adults above 55 years will comprise 25% of the population, and the problems of alcohol abuse will also continue to grow.

Identifying these older patients who abuse alcohol can be difficult. They may be less forthcoming about their use of alcohol because of social stigma and fear of negative responses by caregivers. Severe physical, social, and psychologic effects can result from alcohol abuse in elderly populations, and yet because of age, isolation, and shame, the abuse may be difficult to identify. The elderly may be less mobile and less social and may drink alone. Because of this, their drinking is not obvious to multiple individuals, and they are less likely to be in social situations where drinking interferes with healthy functioning. If they are retired, not driving, and distant from family, the abuse may go unnoticed. Also, physical conditions that are common in the elderly are also related to alcohol abuse. The causes of conditions such as weight loss, inability to sleep, hypertension, dementia, and gastrointestinal problems may not be attributed to alcohol because these are common conditions of aging.

Chronic medical conditions are frequently worsened by alcohol. Also, the use of alcohol, along with multiple medications for chronic conditions, can increase physical risks. Alcohol interferes with more than 50% of the 100 most frequently prescribed medications. Falls, trauma, poor nutrition, and gastrointestinal problems all are problems associated with alcohol abuse in the elderly. Most common physical problems that occur with alcohol abuse are liver diseases, lung diseases (because of association with smoking), ulcers, falls, and mental impairment. Abuse of alcohol often contributes to social isolation, which has a negative impact on interpersonal relationships. The feelings of loss of friends, family members, and career can be worsened when abusing alcohol. The ability to cope with the common losses of aging can be diminished. Alcohol has a profound effect on the nervous system, and many experts believe that 5% to 10% of dementia is related to alcohol. Psychologic effects from alcohol abuse are confusion, decreased coordination, mood and anxiety disorders, and depression. Frequently, individuals use alcohol to self-medicate psychologic problems, which contributes to the pre-existing problems.

In most states, nurses are considered mandated reporters for suspected abuse, neglect, or exploitation of elders or incapacitated adults. Elders who live alone, who are socially isolated, and who abuse alcohol can fall under the definition of a neglected elder. If a nurse identifies physical signs such as fractures, malnourishment, burns, bruises, and cuts, combined with lack of supervision, inappropriate clothing, unsanitary or unsafe housing, or an untreated medical condition, a call to social services or adult protective services may be required. Elderly persons in poor condition may be suspicious, reclusive, and defensive about their living situation, especially when abusing alcohol, but self-neglect needs to be reported because it can save a life.

SUGGESTED READINGS

American Geriatric Society. Foundation for health in aging substance abuse. Available at: http://www.healthinaging.org/agingintheknow/chapter_print_ch_trial.asp?ch=36. Accessed May 11, 2008.

Boyle A, Davis H. Early screening and assessment of alcohol and substance abuse in the elderly: Clinical implications. *J Addict Nurs.* 2006;17:95–103.

U.S. Department of Health and Human Services, Agency for Healthcare Research and Quality. Healthcare for the elderly. Available at: http://www.ahrq.gov/research/apr96/dept6.htm. Accessed May 11, 2008.

U.S. Department of Health and Human Services, Substance Abuse and Mental Health Services Administration. Alcohol dependence or abuse. Available at: http://www.drugabusestatistics.samhsa.gov/2k6state/Ch5.htm#5.1. Accessed May 11, 2008.

Virginia Department of Social Services. Abuse hurts at any age: Mandated reporters can save lives. Available at: http://www.dss.state.va.us/familyB032-02-0121-eng.pdf. Accessed May 11, 2008.

KNOW HOW TO IDENTIFY AND MANAGE THE PATIENT WITH VIOLENT BEHAVIOR TENDENCIES

ANTHONY D. SLONIM, MD, DRPH

WHAT TO DO: ASSESS

Nurses need to know how to effectively assess patients who may be real or perceived threats to staff or to others in the environment because of their violent behavior. While many patients are appreciative of nursing care, others may not be able to appropriately manage their aggression and may strike out physically, leading to potential harm. There are, however, criteria that are associated with the risk of a tendency toward violent behavior. The nurse, by using these criteria, may use appropriate goal setting and de-escalation techniques once these clients are identified.

The major risk domains for violent behavior include demographic characteristics, medical and psychiatric history and diagnoses, social–environmental risks, and cognitive–behavioral risks. By using a standardized approach across each of these domains, nurses can derive a "profile" of risk regarding their client's potential for violent behavior and intervene before the behavior escalates.

From a demographic perspective, these patients tend to be young, unemployed men with limited education. They have a history of violence, often stemming from early childhood, including infractions of the law, and many have been victims of violence themselves. Their medical and psychiatric histories are informative. Some may have experienced traumatic brain injuries, have used illicit drugs, and have antisocial or impulsive character traits. These patients may have access to a weapon and be willing to use it. They are often financially as well as socially dependent upon others and move often. From a behavioral perspective, they have low self-esteem, poor impulse control, and make statements about their intent to harm others.

These characteristics contribute to an important range of risk factors from which nurses can recognize at-risk clients before violent behavior begins. Some precautions to protect nurses include keeping an eye on the client at all times, not allowing themselves to be backed into a room with the exit blocked by the client, having an escape path identified and remaining out of direct reach of the client, remaining open and nonconfrontational but recognizing when they need assistance, and not staying alone with the client.

By using these simple techniques, nurses can identify and manage patients with violent tendencies while protecting themselves and their colleagues from harm.

SUGGESTED READINGS

Littrell KH, Littrell SH. Current understanding of violence and aggression: Assessment and treatment. *J Psychosoc Nurs Ment Health Serv.* 1998;36(12):18–24.

Lowe T, Wellman N, Taylor R. Limit setting and decision making in the management of aggression. *J Adv Nurs.* 2003;41: 154–162.

Rickelman BL. The client who displays angry, aggressive or violent behavior. In: Mohr WK, ed. *Psychiatric Mental Health Nursing.* 6th Ed. Philadelphia: Lippincott Williams & Wilkins; 2006.

KNOW HOW TO HELP THE CLIENT IN CRISIS

ANTHONY D. SLONIM, MD, DRPH

WHAT TO DO: IMPLEMENT

A crisis is due to a mismatch between a threat and the resources available to deal with it. When a client experiences a problem that challenges his usual and customary coping mechanisms, a crisis ensues. The nurse needs to recognize the factors that make it difficult for patients to cope and be able to offer strategies to assist.

Crises occur all the time, but their outcome is determined by a number of factors including the clients, prior experience and ability to manage through crises, the time since the last crisis, their resilience, and their membership in a vulnerable population. In general, females, minorities, and those of lower socioeconomic status tend to have a lesser ability to cope with a crisis. Not all crises are bad. Similar to stress, there can be "good" crises and "bad crises." A good crisis may develop when you give birth to your first child; a wonderful event, but a crisis nonetheless. Similarly, the death of a spouse would be an example of a negative crisis.

The nurse playing the role of crisis intervention counselor can provide a number of useful strategies that the clients themselves may not be able to identify while distressed in the center of the crisis. These include the ability to objectively help with analysis of the event. The nurse can also offer ideas for problem solving and actions for accomplishing them. The nurse may simply be a "sounding board" with whom the clients can discuss their concerns openly and objectively by way of working through the crisis. In this way, the client is not looking for the nurse to provide an answer but simply to listen. Finally, the nurse can help identify methods by which the client can cope with the current crisis and plan for potential future crises.

For patients in crisis, the nurse is an important part of the crisis intervention team and requires the ability to assess and intervene.

SUGGESTED READINGS

Connolly PM. Crisis intervention. In: Mohr WK, ed. *Psychiatric Mental Health Nursing*. 6th Ed. Philadelphia: Lippincott Williams & Wilkins; 2006, pp. 395–410.

KNOW HOW TO ASSESS ALCOHOLISM IN YOUR MEDICAL PATIENTS

ANTHONY D. SLONIM, MD, DrPH

Using drugs or alcohol in a repeated manner is substance abuse. Approximately 10% of the US adult population is estimated to have a problem with substance abuse. These patients may live completely normal lives, have normal relationships, hold full time employment, and perceive that they do not have a problem with alcohol or drug use. Nonetheless, it is important for the nurse, particularly when these patients are admitted for medical reasons, to formally assess their use of alcohol if upon initial screening, a problem has been identified.

The CAGE assessment tool has been a useful and validated tool for the identification of client with a substance use problem for several decades and consists of only four questions. For the nurse, this useful tool allows for patients at risk to receive appropriate detoxification and the prevention of withdrawal. The four questions are as follows:

- Have you ever felt that you should **C**ut down on your drinking?
- Have people **A**nnoyed you by criticizing your drinking?
- Have you ever felt bad or **G**uilty about your drinking?
- Have you ever had a drink or **E**ye opener first thing in the morning?

A positive response to any of these questions indicates that the patient is in need of additional assessment.

SUGGESTED READINGS

Cornwell CJ, Lickteig MK. The client who abuses drugs or alcohol. In: Mohr WK, ed. *Psychiatric Mental Health Nursing*. 6th Ed. Philadelphia: Lippincott Williams & Wilkins; 2006, pp. 687–722.

Ewing JA. Detecting alcoholism: The CAGE questionnaire. *J Am Med Assoc.* 1984;252:1902–1907.

KNOW HOW TO CARE FOR THE ELDERLY PATIENT WITH DEMENTIA

ANTHONY D. SLONIM, MD, DRPH

WHAT TO DO: ASSESS

Dementia is an acquired condition that affects cognition and memory and is serious enough to affect the patient's ability to function socially because of its impact on language, behavior, and thought. The classification of dementia consists of several types including Alzheimer dementia, vascular dementia, and dementia with Lewy bodies. There are several other diseases like Parkinson disease and Huntington disease that may have dementia as a constituent of the syndrome.

Alzheimer dementia is the most common form of dementia, affecting nearly 4 million people in the United States. It usually begins after the age of 65 when patients begin to experience memory loss and have problems finding words. The condition is degenerative, and the patients experience progressive loss of function including their ability to perform their activities of daily living. They can become combative, have difficulty relating to others, and lose continence of bowel and bladder at later stages of the disease.

Vascular dementia occurs from small vessel disease in the brain where hypoperfusion and infarcts manifest themselves. This type of dementia usually occurs at an earlier age in patients with vascular risk factors like hypertension, diabetes, hyperlipidemia, and cardiovascular disease.

Lewy body dementia is named so because of the presence of Lewy bodies in the brains of the affected patients. These patients experience hallucinations, memory loss, language problems, and debilitating motor symptoms.

Patients with dementia have a number of pharmacologic agents available for treatment, some with more modest success than others. Nonetheless, for patients with dementia of the Alzheimer or Lewy body types, cholinesterase inhibitors are the mainstay of therapy. For patients with vascular dementia, the treatment of the underlying cardiovascular function is important to prevent repeated infarcts.

In addition to pharmacologic agents, the nurse has an obligation to keep the patient safe by ensuring that his or her whereabouts is known at all times. As time progresses, the patient may need assistance with activities of daily living, including eating, washing, and drinking. Behavioral strategies may help with some of the agitated behaviors. Most importantly, the nurse must work with the family to support them through the care of this difficult disease.

SUGGESTED READINGS

Cummings JL, Mendez MF. Alzheimers disease and other disorders of cognition. In: Goldman L, Ausiello D, eds. *Cecil Textbook of Medicine*. 22nd Ed. Philadelphia: Saunders; 2004, pp. 2248–2256.

Thomson Heisterman AA. The client with a cognitive disorder. In: Mohr WK, ed. *Psychiatric Mental Health Nursing*. 6th Ed. Philadelphia: Lippincott Williams & Wilkins; 2006, pp. 723–768.

KNOW THAT VITAL SIGNS NEED TO BE INTERPRETED INDIVIDUALLY AND AS TRENDS TO APPROPRIATELY UNDERSTAND THE PATIENT'S CONDITION

NANCY F. ALTICE RN, MSN, CCNS, CNS-BC

WHAT TO DO: ASSESS

Vital signs are an important aspect of every patient's assessment. Obtaining vital signs is usually one of the first skills taught to students in any of the healthcare professions. Along with the technical aspects of obtaining vital signs, normal ranges are taught for each parameter. While individual vital sign readings can provide important information at the extremes, interpretations based solely on single readings can be misleading. Vital sign trends provide much more meaningful information and may provide clues to subtle changes in the patient's condition.

A heart rate between 60 and 100 is considered normal. But there are situations where a specific heart rate may be inappropriate for the clinical situation, even though technically "normal." A patient with a high fever and a pulse rate of 65 should be further assessed to determine if cardiac abnormalities exist that are preventing a normal rise in heart rate. Typically, when the metabolic rate is increased, as occurs with fever, the heart rate will also be increased. Likewise, when a patient who normally has a heart rate of 65 develops a sustained heart rate of 90 while lying in bed, further assessment should be performed. A heart rate of 90 in this clinical situation could indicate that the heart rate is increasing to compensate for a reduction in cardiac contractility or the patient has increased sympathetic nervous system activity, perhaps from pain, anxiety, or a vasodilating drug, and the increased heart rate is the only way the patient can maintain his or her cardiac output.

Blood pressure can also fluctuate under different circumstances and should be considered thoughtfully with regard to the clinical situation. A blood pressure of 120/80 is a sign of trouble when the patient's baseline blood pressure is 170/90. A lowered blood pressure resulting from therapeutic response to an antihypertensive medication would be a welcome situation, but in the absence of such therapy, other causes of these sudden changes should be considered. Perhaps this patient is dehydrated or bleeding. Although a blood pressure of 120/80 has long been considered a "perfect" reading, it could just as easily represent a problem in a person who typically has much higher readings.

Vital signs provide important cues when assessed thoughtfully in view of the patient's clinical situation. Because vital sign measurement is a skill that is often delegated to unlicensed personnel, the readings may not be considered as part of the overall assessment until other abnormalities or patient complaints draw attention to these basic parameters. By the time other abnormalities draw attention to changes in vital signs, valuable time may have been lost, and the patient's condition may have deteriorated rapidly.

Do not forget to look at the basics and do remember to take into consideration the patient's baseline assessment. Look beyond the top of the daily flow sheet. Yesterday's parameters may have been quite different.

SUGGESTED READINGS

Garcia TB, Miller GT. *Arrhythmia Recognition: The Art of Interpretation*. Boston: Jones and Bartlett Publishers; 2004, pp. 436–437.

Glotzer J. Nursing assessment in the inpatient setting. In: Moser DK, Riegel B, eds. *Cardiac Nursing: A Companion to Braunwald's Heart Disease*. St. Louis: Elsevier-Saunders; 2008.

REMEMBER TO TAKE BLOOD PRESSURES CORRECTLY... THEY AFFECT THE PRESCRIBED CARE

JEANNIE SCRUGGS GARBER, DNP, RN

WHAT TO DO: ASSESS

Do you remember how you were taught how to take a blood pressure? Do you know the physiology behind what you are measuring when you take a blood pressure? Is your equipment working correctly? Are you using the correct technique? Are you using the right size cuff? Are the readings accurate? All these questions should be considered by the clinician when measuring blood pressure. This assessment procedure has become so routine that it is easy to minimize the importance of skill and knowledge regarding blood pressure monitoring.

When answering the above questions, Anderson and Maloney encourage clinicians to evaluate the equipment, the patient, and the nurse as blood pressure readings are acquired. The sphygmomanometer should be inspected to make sure that the bulb is free from holes, that the bladder inflates, and that the cuff can be secured tightly to the arm. A major consideration regarding the cuff is to ensure that the correct size cuff is being used. A cuff that is too small may produce falsely high readings. The stethoscope must also be inspected to ensure it is working properly.

Other reminders to the clinician are that blood pressure fluctuates and does not remain constant at any given time; so it is expected to obtain variable readings each time the blood pressure is taken. It is also important to know that body positioning, fluid intake, body temperature, stress, age, weight, smoking, alcohol consumption, and ethnicity also impact blood pressure readings. Considering the many extrinsic, uncontrollable factors that impact blood pressure, it is critical that the skill of the provider and the functioning of the equipment have as little variation as possible.

Procedural reminders that support accuracy of blood pressure monitoring are listed below:

- Know patients' history and why blood pressure (BP) monitoring is necessary
- Select best site to obtain BP (avoid IV site arms, breast surgery side arms, and casted areas)
- Discuss the procedure with the patient
- Palpate the pulse at BP cuff site
- Follow routine process for inflating cuff to higher than past readings
- Deflate cuff SLOWLY! Listen for first sound, and then last sound
- Discuss the finding with the patient and/or the primary care provider

These simple reminders can be essential components that make a blood pressure reading as accurate as possible. Intervention and treatments such as medication selection and dosage, fluid management, and activity level are frequently determined based on blood pressure measurements. Inaccurate readings could lead to errors in treatment and patient safety could be compromised.

SUGGESTED READINGS

Anderson D, Maloney J (n.d.). Taking the blood pressure accurately: Its no off-the-cuff matter. Available at: http://www.steeles.com/catalog/takingBP.html. Accessed June 16, 2008.

UNDERSTAND THE PATIENT'S CONDITION PRIOR TO HOLDING MEDICATIONS BASED ON BP ALONE

NANCY F. ALTICE RN, MSN, CCNS, CNS-BC

WHAT TO DO: EVALUATE

Heart failure is one of the most frequent conditions resulting in hospitalization of patients aged 65 and above, but it also affects people of all ages. Symptoms of heart failure are often improved with medications. There was a time when symptomatic improvement was really all that the medical profession had to offer for this condition. Now, several classes of medications including angiotensin converting enzyme inhibitors (ACEIs), angiotensin receptor blockers (ARBs), aldosterone antagonists, and beta blockers have shown to improve mortality and decrease morbidity in this population of patients. All these drugs can have a profound effect on blood pressure, but their benefits in heart failure go beyond simply lowering blood pressure. In fact, many of the patients who benefit from these drugs have never had high blood pressure.

Heart failure is a condition that encompasses complex interactions of the sympathetic nervous system and the renin–angiotensin–aldosterone system, in addition to mechanical dysfunction of the heart. These complex interactions can lead to worsening symptoms as well as increased mortality. The medications that are most effective in decreasing mortality have to be carefully titrated due to the effects they can have on blood pressure, heart rate, cardiac output, and renal function. Typically, these medications are started at very small doses and gradually increased as the patient's tolerance allows. This often requires frequent adjustments of each medication and consideration of other factors such as diuretic dosage and response and electrolyte balance.

It is helpful to have established parameters regarding when to withhold a medication when the patient is undergoing initiation and titration of these medications.

Some nurses may assume that any of these medications should be held whenever the systolic blood pressure is less than 90 to 100 mm Hg. Considering that the benefits of these medications are not based simply on blood pressure response, there should be a more comprehensive assessment of the patient's status before withholding any of these medications. Ideally, the prescribing physician or other licensed independent provider should be notified. The American College of Cardiology/American Heart Association 2005 Guideline on the Diagnosis and Management of Chronic Heart Failure in the Adult recommends not withholding these medications as long as the systolic blood pressure is at least 80 mm Hg unless the patient has symptoms from hypotension, such as dizziness, visual changes, syncope, or worsening renal function.

When faced with a hypotensive patient who is due for his or her next dose of an ACEI, do not automatically withhold the medication. First, assess symptoms related to hypotension. Second, consider the patient's fluid balance. Could the patient possibly be dehydrated based on observation of the daily weights, intake and output, and lab results? If so, the physician may choose to gently rehydrate the patient rather than withholding medications. Certainly, there are times when holding the medication at least for a few hours will be the best treatment, but this decision should not be based on a single blood pressure reading alone.

SUGGESTED READINGS

Hunt SA, Abraham WT, Chin MH, et al. ACC/AHA 2005 guideline update for the diagnosis and management of chronic heart failure in the adult. *Circulation*. 2005;112:1825–1852.

Springhouse. *Nursing Pharmacology Made Incredibly Easy*. Philadelphia: Lippincott Williams Wilkins; 2005.

WHEN IN DOUBT, GET A 12-LEAD EKG... LEAD II IS NOT ALWAYS THE BEST LEAD FOR INTERPRETATION

NANCY F. ALTICE RN, MSN, CCNS, CNS-BC

WHAT TO DO: EVALUATE

Basic education for dysrhythmia monitoring often encourages students to focus on looking at Lead II because it is usually the best lead for identifying p waves if they are present. Identification of the p wave is essential in determining whether the EKG rhythm originates from the sinus node or from another location in the heart. Lead II is also a good lead for looking at ischemic changes in the inferior wall of the left ventricle. However, Lead II is sometimes not the best lead for measuring the QRS width. Anyone who has experience with measuring the various components of the EKG waves knows that any two people may draw different conclusions when trying to determine where the QRS begins and especially where it ends as it transitions into the ST segment. Even if the QRS measures 0.12 or greater in this lead, it sometimes does not appear wide during casual viewing on the monitor screen and may not draw the attention of the person watching multiple monitors at once. The V leads are sometimes better for this, but there will be individual variations for each patient. Determining the QRS width is important in determining whether conduction through the ventricles is normal. Bundle branch blocks and ventricular dysrhythmias can widen the QRS complex. In lead V-1, the specific configurations of right versus left bundle branch block can be recognized and distinguished from other more variable configurations of the wide QRS complex seen in ventricular tachycardia.

Another important aspect of monitoring for select patients receiving antiarrythmic drugs is measurement of the QT duration. This is measured from the beginning of the QRS to the end of the T wave. It can also be very difficult to determine the end of the T wave in some leads. Failure to recognize a prolonged QT can leave the patient at increased risk of developing Torsades de Pointes, which can be a lethal form of ventricular tachycardia. Especially for QT monitoring, it is essential that the same lead be used for each measurement of the QT interval.

The best way to determine which lead to use is to first look at a 12-lead EKG. Determine which lead shows the most distinct ending of the T wave for that individual patient. This is also a good rule of thumb when choosing leads to monitor for each individual patient. Although Lead II remains an excellent lead for identifying p waves, it is not the only lead in which p waves are clearly seen. If the patient is having any degree of heart block or any ventricular conduction abnormalities including ventricular dysrhythmias, a V lead may provide more comprehensive information.

Because EKG monitoring is a very complex topic, it is essential that decisions about the practice of EKG monitoring be based on sound evidence. In 2004, the American Heart Association Science and Coordinating Committee approved a scientific statement that included detailed recommendations.

SUGGESTED READINGS

Drew BJ, Califf RM, Funk M, et al. Practice standards for electrocardiographic monitoring in hospital settings: An American Heart Association scientific statement from the Councils on Cardiovascular Nursing, Clinical Cardiology, and Cardiovascular Disease in the Young: Endorsed by the International Society of Computerized Electrocardiography and the American Association of Critical Care Nurses. *Circulation*. 2004;110:2721–2746.

Don't just say "all clear"... Look!

Nancy F. Altice RN, MSN, CCNS, CNS-BC

WHAT TO DO: IMPLEMENT

Early defibrillation is a key component of successful resuscitation of patients with pulseless ventricular arrhythmias. Safety of the resuscitation team is stressed in advanced cardiac life support education. It has long been accepted that no one should be in direct contact with a patient during defibrillation due to the possibility of receiving a high voltage shock. For this reason, the person administering defibrillation is responsible for shouting "all clear" to alert everyone. However, during resuscitation, various team members may be intent on executing various procedures simultaneously, such as starting and IV, intubating, administering drugs, or drawing blood for stat tests. The person administering defibrillation is responsible to ensure that no one else is touching the patient. Saying "all clear" may not always be enough to get everyone's attention. Always remember to look at the whole scene as well.

The success rate of resuscitation efforts for hospitalized patients remains low. Research continues to determine better methods to improve success. Currently, there is an emphasis on uninterrupted cardiopulmonary resuscitation to increase survival. A recent study has tested the hypothesis that risk to rescuers in contact with the patient during defibrillation is low. There may eventually be a change in practice based on new research, indicating that CPR should not be interrupted for defibrillation. Until new guidelines are established, remember to maintain a safe environment when performing defibrillation.

SUGGESTED READINGS

2005 American Heart Association Guidelines for Cardiopulmonary Resuscitation and Emergency Cardiovascular Care, Part 5: Electrical Therapies. *Circulation*. 2005;112:IV-35–IV-46. Available at: http://circ.ahajournals.org/cgi/content/full112/24_suppl/IV-35.

Lloyd MS, Heeke B, Walter PF, et al. Hands-on defibrillation: An analysis of electrical current flow through rescuers in direct contact with patients during biphasic external defibrillation. *Circulation*. 2008;117(19):2510–2514.

RECHECK THE FEMORAL PUNCTURE SITE POSTCARDIAC CATHETERIZATION AFTER VIGOROUS COUGHING, GAGGING, OR VOMITING EVEN IF IT IS NOT TIME FOR VITAL SIGNS

NANCY F. ALTICE RN, MSN, CCNS, CNS-BC

WHAT TO DO: EVALUATE

The femoral artery is used for vascular access in a variety of coronary diagnostic and interventional procedures as well as other types of arteriography. Most procedures are uncomplicated but occasionally excessive bleeding may occur at the puncture site in the artery leading to formation of a hematoma or a spontaneous hemorrhage. Numerous factors are implicated in these complications, including anticoagulation, vascular access technique, and postprocedure care. Maneuvers that increase the intra-abdominal pressure, such as coughing, laughing, sneezing, or using the urinal or bedpan can increase pressure at the arterial puncture site. Patients are instructed to hold firm pressure over their dressing site when performing any of these maneuvers. But not all patients are able to follow these instructions for various reasons including sedation, severity of illness, baseline cognitive function, etc.

Patients are routinely monitored very closely following procedures involving femoral artery puncture. Typically, vital signs and peripheral pulses as well as the puncture site are assessed frequently for the first few hours. This is the time of highest risk for bleeding complications. However, even after hemostasis has been obtained, vigorous coughing, vomiting, laughing, etc. could dislodge the hemostatic clot, especially in patients who are receiving anticoagulation.

Remember to reinforce groin instructions with patients following these procedures and recheck the femoral area anytime the patient experiences any of the maneuvers associated with risk. A large amount of blood can accumulate in the groin, leading to hemodynamic compromise if undetected bleeding occurs.

SUGGESTED READINGS

Hamner JB, Dubois EJ, Rice TP. Predictors of complications associated with closure devices after transfemoral percutaneous coronary procedures. *Crit Care Nurse*. 2005;25(3):30–37.

Nikolsky E, Mehran R, Halkin A. Vascular complications associated with arteriotomy closure devices in patients undergoing percutaneous coronary procedures: A meta-analysis. *J Am Coll Cardiol*. 2004;44:1200–1209.

DO NOT ASSUME IT CANNOT BE VT JUST BECAUSE THE PATIENT IS STILL STANDING!

NANCY F. ALTICE, RN, MSN, CCNS, CNS-BC

WHAT TO DO: EVALUATE

Determining the origin of wide complex tachycardia can be based on a variety of clues. Hemodynamic stability is not one of them! Studies have shown that the most common cause of wide complex tachycardia in conscious adults is ventricular tachycardia. The American College of Cardiology (ACC) recommends that when the origin of wide complex tachycardia is unknown, it should be presumed to be ventricular (ACC Guideline, Section IV). A variety of factors other than the origin of the dysrhythmia determines the hemodynamic stability. According to Section IV of the ACC Guideline, "the stability or tolerance of VT is related to the rate of tachycardia, presence of retrograde conduction, ventricular function, and the integrity of peripheral compensatory mechanisms. A presentation with stable, relatively well-tolerated VT does not suggest the absence of heart disease and can be observed in patients with very poor LV function. Even patients with poor ventricular function may not be aware of palpitations during VT. Presentation with stable VT does not in itself indicate a benign prognosis in patients with significant heart disease."

When a patient develops wide complex tachycardia, the cause may be uncertain. While obtaining a 12-lead EKG and additional rhythm strips to aid in determining the origin of the tachycardia, the nurse should also assess the patient frequently for potential deterioration. Hemodynamic instability and heart failure symptoms could develop at any time. Ventricular tachycardia that is not accompanied by hemodynamic compromise can possibly be treated with antiarrhythmic medication. A defibrillator should be readily available in case of sudden clinical deterioration.

SUGGESTED READINGS

ACC/AHA/ESC 2006 Guidelines for Management of Patients with Ventricular Arrhythmias and the Prevention of Sudden Cardiac Death. Ventricular arrhythmias and sudden cardiac death. *J Am Coll Cardiol.* 2006;48:1064–1108. Retrieved from: http://content.onlinejacc.org/cgi/content/full/48/5/e247.

2005 American Heart Association Guidelines for Cardiopulmonary Resuscitation and Emergency Cardiovascular Care, Part 5: Electrical Therapies. *Circulation.* 2005;112:IV-35–IV-46. Available at: http://circ.ahajournals.org/cgi/content/full112/24_suppl/IV-35.

Steinman RT, Herrera C, Schuger CD, et al. Wide QRS tachycardia in the conscious adult: Ventricular tachycardia is the most frequent cause. *J Am Med Assoc.* 1989;261(7):1013–1016.

DO NOT ASSUME THAT A PATIENT IS ON A LOW SODIUM DIET JUST BECAUSE HE OR SHE SAYS, "OH, WE DON'T EAT ANY SODIUM"

NANCY F. ALTICE, RN, MSN, CCNS, CNS-BC

WHAT TO DO: ASSESS

Most patients who are prescribed a low sodium diet have been instructed to "throw the salt shaker away!" For some patients, this was the end of their dietary instruction. Many believe that the salt shaker is the primary source of sodium. But for many people who avoid the salt shaker but continue to eat convenient, processed foods, the daily sodium intake can still greatly exceed the recommended 2 to 3 g sodium diet. When assessing dietary knowledge, it is helpful to ask the patient and family about the typical meals that they prepare and eat. A patient who claims to eat no salt but readily tells you that he typically eats a spam sandwich and canned soup for lunch obviously needs some education. Many patients and families will report that they add salt only during cooking but never at the table, as if there is a difference.

The dietary history is an important part of the admission assessment when the patient is hospitalized. For some patients, the lack of understanding about their dietary restrictions may lead to increasing dosages of medications, readmissions for fluid overload, or a concern of a refractory medical condition. Providing the patients with clarity around the dietary prescription is an important part of therapy that goes a long way in improving their health and the efficacy of the other components of the therapeutic regimen.

SUGGESTED READINGS

Bentley B, De Jong MJ, Moser DK, et al. Factors related to nonadherence to low sodium diet recommendations in heart failure patients. *Eur J Cardiovasc Nurs.* 2005;4(4):331–336.
Heart Failure Society of America. Introduction—following a low sodium diet with heart failure. Available at: http://www.aboutHF.org/module2/default.htm.

PATIENT MONITORS: NURSES... BEST FRIENDS OR ENEMIES?

JENNIFER BATH, RN, BSN, FNE, SANE-A

WHAT TO DO: ASSESS

The invention of cardiac monitors has helped make the nurse's job easier. Cardiac monitors have many advantages. They monitor the patient's heart rate, rhythm, and blood pressure; they alarm to preset limits when the heart rate or blood pressure is too low or high or if the cardiac rhythm is lethal. Unfortunately, these devices are only as useful as the people who use them, and it is easy to fall into the trap of treating the monitor instead of the patient.

Monitor artifacts that occur from the patient swinging the remote telemetry box or unhooking one of the leads can resemble ventricular fibrillation or asystole. The patient often sits up in bed completely unaware of the havoc he or she has caused, which is why it is important for the nurse to assess the patient in the setting of these disturbances and not rely on the monitor itself. While the staff may sometimes overlook the patient and focus on the monitor and what it is showing, there are also times when the patient will have normal vital signs and a normal sinus rhythm, but be highly symptomatic and extremely ill. Therefore, while the information the monitor provides is normal, we cannot forget that the patient is symptomatic.

Monitor alarms are another important benefit for nurses when they work, but they can also be a patient's worst nightmare. Monitor alarms allow nurses to be informed that a problem has arisen with their patient. However, the absence of alarm signals is not always a good thing. Alarms are often silenced because they continuously alarm, or are set with unrealistic parameters, or are turned off altogether. There is also the possibility that the patient was not admitted to the monitor, therefore, his or her rhythm is not being "seen" on the central monitors and the alarms do not sound.

While monitors can help the nurse to keep a closer eye on patients, they may also create a false sense of security if the nurse becomes over-reliant on their use. The monitor needs to be checked frequently, but so does the patient. Patients will provide information on the trajectory of the disease and whether they are feeling better or worse while the monitor cannot. The monitor can only pick up when a change has occurred. Staff that work on units with monitors need classroom training and hands-on experience with the equipment. They need to be able to recognize subtle changes in the rhythm that the monitors cannot. As technologic advances help us do our job better and more efficiently, we need to remember that nothing replaces the knowledge, experience, and intuition of a seasoned nurse.

SUGGESTED READINGS

Drew BJ, Califf RM, Funk M, et al. Practice standards for electrocardiographic monitoring in hospital settings. *Circulation.* 2004;110(17):2721–2746.

Xiao Y, Mackenzie CF, Seagull J, et al. Managing the monitors: An analysis of alarm silencing activities during an anesthetic procedure. In: *Proc IEA 2000/HFES 2000 Cong.* Available at: http://hfrp.umm.edu/alarms/xiao_seagull_mackenzie_jaberi_hfes2000.pdf.

DO NOT JUMP TO CONCLUSIONS WITH CHEST PAIN BEFORE PERFORMING A THOROUGH ASSESSMENT

ALICE M. CHRISTALDI, RN, BSN, CRRN

WHAT TO DO: ASSESS

A thorough assessment is the first step to ensuring appropriate interventions. Some nurses become dependent on a single source of information, such as a monitor, for their assessment. For the most part when you see a rhythm, especially something that looks like ventricular tachycardia, you want to act quickly. How many times does a rhythm look deadly, when it is indeed merely an artifact? Use of a monitor is merely an adjunct to good clinical observation and assessment skills. Knowing what to do when a patient complains of chest pain depends a lot more on observation, a comprehensive assessment, and narrowing down the problem from a list of alternatives.

We have attempted to educate people on the signs and symptoms of myocardial infarction, and of course, chest pain is the number one symptom. When the patient decides to come into the emergency department with complaints of chest pain, he will immediately be listened to, taken right back for treatment, and placed on the monitor. Vital signs and a detailed history are helpful at this point. Information is important to obtain. Questions such as the following should be asked:

- Where does it hurt?
- When did it start?
- What was the person doing when it first started?
- Does the pain increase on palpation?
- Characteristics of the pain: is it sharp, a feeling of pressure on the chest, or is it a dull ache?
- Does the person have associated symptoms like nausea? Has he vomited?
- Does it radiate to the shoulders, arms, neck, or jaw?
- What have they done to try and relieve the pain... taken an antacid, repositioned the body, or applied heat?
- Do actions like taking a deep breath or coughing make it worse?

Further testing will be necessary. Labs will be drawn on; serum cardiac markers (creatinine kinase MB and troponin), electrolytes, coagulation studies and complete blood counts, 12-lead EKG, and possibly chest x-rays will be ordered. Oxygen should be administered to the patient and an intravenous line should be started.

Many times, the source of the chest discomfort is noncardiac in nature. One third of all patients brought into emergency department with chest pain symptoms are found to have costochondritis. This is an inflammation of the costal cartilage, which joins the ribs to the sternum, and can cause severe pain in the sternal area. There can also be radiation of the pain and it can be reproduced with palpation. However, there is no nausea, vomiting, or dyspnea.

Other common causes of chest pain include pericarditis, cardiomyopathy, pneumonia, cholecystitis, gastroesophageal reflux, rib fraction, and anemia. A differential diagnosis needs to be made quickly to rule out conditions such as aortic dissection, acute ischemic heart disease, tension pneumothorax, or pulmonary embolus, which can all lead to severe complications or even death. Acting quickly at the first complaint of chest pain is vital, but a coolheaded assessment of the patient and his symptoms is key to finding its cause and effective treatment.

SUGGESTED READINGS

Aroesty JM, Kannam JP. Patient information: Chest pain. UpToDate for patients. Available at: http://www.uptodate.com/patients/content/topic.do?topicKey=hrt_dis/11827. Accessed August 8, 2008.

Pope BB. What's causing your patient's chest pain? *Crit Care Insider*. 2006;21–24.

Wisniewski A. Taking a closer look at costochondritis. *Nursing*. 2006;36:11.

REMEMBER THAT WOMEN ALSO GET HEART DISEASE, BUT OFTEN PRESENT WITH ATYPICAL SYMPTOMS

JEANNIE SCRUGGS GARBER, DNP, RN

WHAT TO DO: ASSESS

Heart disease has historically been perceived as a disease that primarily affects older men; however, heart disease is the number one killer of women. It is also widely published that women's symptoms may differ from men's and are many times labeled as "atypical." Fogoros (2008) speculates that "since more women are dying from heart disease than men these days, it may be statistically more correct to consider men's symptoms as the ones that are atypical."

Using the information from the National Center on Health Statistics (2002), National Heart, Lung, and Blood Institute and American Heart Association's 2002 Heart and Stroke Statistical Update, the National Coalition for Women with Heart Disease compiled the following summary regarding women and heart disease statistics:

- 8,000,000 American women are currently living with heart disease.
- Heart disease is the leading cause of death of American women and kills 32% of them.
- 267,000 women die each year from heart attacks, which kill six times as many women as breast cancer.
- Women who smoke risk having a heart attack 19 years earlier than nonsmoking women.
- Women with diabetes are two to three times more likely to have heart attacks.
- 38% of women and 25% of men will die within 1 year of their first recognized heart attack.
- Women are almost twice as likely as men to die after bypass surgery.
- Women are less likely than men to receive β-blockers, ACE inhibitors, or even aspirin after a heart attack.
- More women than men die of heart disease annually, yet women receive only:
  - 33% of angioplasties, stents, and bypass surgeries
  - 28% of inplantable defibrillators
  - 36% of open-heart surgeries
- Women comprise only 25% of participants in all heart-related research studies.

Considering these statistics, women and healthcare providers have much to learn about preventing and treating heart disease in women.

Although it is commonly reported that women's symptoms are different from men's, it remains difficult to articulate just "how" different they might be. Women sometimes do not have chest pain, but may have back pain, arm pain, a hot or burning sensation, and perhaps a perceived tenderness to touch on the chest or back. Fogoro also reports that "when women have heart attacks, they are often misdiagnosed as having gas or stomach problems." Other possible symptoms that are more commonly reported in women include extreme fatigue, gastric discomfort, uncontrollable belching, and sleep disturbances. It is also widely reported that women minimize their symptoms. One possible reason for underreporting or minimization of symptoms is embarrassment. The most useful advice women can follow is that "no one ever died of embarrassment" (M. Johnson, personal communication, 2002). There are many speculations as to why women might delay treatment, but minimal research has been done on the topic. Healthcare providers must be aware of the potential "atypical" presentation of cardiac symptoms in women to diagnose and treat efficiently and effectively. Merz et al. (2004) write "Better understanding of gender differences in manifestation and detection of myocardial ischemia is a critical initial step to improve outcomes for women."

SUGGESTED READINGS

American Heart Association. *Heart Disease and Stroke Statistics—2008 Update*. Dallas, Tx: American Heart Association; 2008.

Fogoros RN. Cardiac symptoms in women: Cardiac symptoms in women often differ from what the textbook says. About.com. Available at: http://heartdisease.about.com/od/chestpain angina/a/women_symptoms.htm. Accessed June 18, 2008.

Hope Heart Institute. Healthy heart resources. Available at: http://www.hopeheart.org/resources/signs_symptoms.cfm. Accessed June 18, 2008.

Merz N, Bonow R, Sopko G, et al. Women's ischemic syndrome evaluation: current status and future research directions: Report of the National Heart, Lung and Blood Institute Workshop. *Circulation*. 2004;109:805–807.

Do not use an AED on a person who is speaking to you

Alice M. Christaldi, RN, BSN, CRRN

WHAT TO DO: IMPLEMENT

The Automated External Defibrillator (AED) was developed in the1980s as a means for treating ventricular fibrillation outside of the hospital setting. Emergency medical technicians needed portable defibrillators that were easy to use and accurate. Today, AEDs can be found in many public areas such as airplanes and gyms and are used by laypeople in their homes.

Hospitals also have benefited by their availability. Over 500,000 cardiac arrests occur in hospitals yearly. The primary lethal arrhythmias are ventricular fibrillation and pulseless ventricular tachycardia. Not all hospital personnel are trained in EKG interpretation and seconds matter when attempting to save a life. With an AED on each nursing unit, simple-to-use equipment is immediately available at the bedside and can be used by all levels of personnel including those with minimal training.

Just when do you use an AED? And more importantly, when do you not? An AED is placed on the person who is unresponsive, pulseless, and not breathing. It would not be appropriate for a person complaining of chest pain nor for routine cardiac monitoring. When the person is discovered to be unresponsive, pulseless, and not breathing in the hospital setting, a code blue should be initiated, which provides for additional staff, expertise, and equipment. Basic life support should be initiated until the arrival of the AED. It should be a goal for health care providers to defibrillate within 3 min of collapse.

The AED is applied to the person with pads that have an adhesive backing. It may be necessary to dry the area of the chest first, shave off any excess hair, and avoid placing the AED pads over permanent pacemakers, automated implantable cardioverter-defibrillators (AICD), or EKG leads. In addition, medication patches and intravenous devices such as Port-A-Caths should be avoided during placement. Burns may occur under the patch and block the energy of the charge. One pad is generally placed at the second intercostal space to the right of the sternum and the second pad is placed to the left of the nipple at the midaxillary line.

AEDs have microprocessors that analyze the EKG and detect lethal nonperfusing shockable rhythms. They are especially useful in departments of the hospital that contain personnel who are not familiar with EKG rhythms. When a shockable rhythm is detected, the AED advises the personnel that a shock is needed. This is done with voice prompts, text messages across the monitor face, and flashing lights. More importantly, it recognizes when there is no shock needed.

Asystole is not a shockable rhythm. Contrary to popular television dramas that always show patients who have a flat line on their EKG receiving multiple shocks, defibrillation is ineffective in asystole. Indeed, studies have shown that there is a trend toward a worse outcome for interrupting chest compressions to shock for asystole.

All hospital personnel should be familiar with AED use. Seconds do count, and in large hospitals, it may take precious minutes for emergency personnel to arrive on the scene. Staff should be proficient in basic life support. They should also feel comfortable applying and using their AEDs. Training programs need to stress the importance of quick action and a 3-min goal for shocking the patient who has collapsed.

Personnel need to be prepared for these emergencies and have equipment that is readily available and well maintained. Equipment should be checked daily. The equipment should be plugged in immediately when brought to the bedside. Check expiration dates for pads; they tend to dry out as they age. Always have a supply of monitor paper available. Staff should be encouraged to handle emergency supplies frequently. Often they fear this equipment, when they actually need to view it as a life saver.

AEDs are a welcome addition to today's nurse station. Just remember they are used on the unresponsive, pulseless, nonbreathing individual. If they are sitting up telling you about it, rethink the type of equipment you should be using.

SUGGESTED READINGS

2005 American Heart Association Guidelines for Cardiopulmonary Resuscitation and Emergency Cardiovascular Care, Part 5: Electrical Therapies. *Circulation.* 2005;112:IV-35–IV-46; Published online before print November 28, 2005, doi: 10.1161/CIRCULATIONAHA.105.166554. Available at: http://circ.ahajournals.org/cgi/content/full/112/24_suppl/IV-35? maxtoshow=&HITS= 10&hits=10&RESULTFORMAT=&fulltext=aed+use&searchid=1&FIRSTINDEX=0&volume=112&issue=24_suppl&resourcetype=HWCIT. Accessed August 8, 2008.

KNOW WHERE YOUR EMERGENCY EQUIPMENT IS AND HOW TO USE IT

KATHERINE M. PENTURFF, RN, CAPA

WHAT TO DO: IMPLEMENT

Sudden cardiac arrest (SCA) is a leading cause of death worldwide, claiming more than 300,000 lives annually in the United States alone. Expert guidelines advocate defibrillation within 2 min after an in-hospital cardiac arrest caused by ventricular arrhythmia, but a recent American Heart Association study of 6,789 patients with in-patient SCA found that defibrillation was delayed in over 30% of patients. Studies have shown that for each minute of untreated cardiac arrest, the probability of successful rhythm conversion decreases by 7% to 10%.

Unfortunately, defibrillator user errors are not uncommon. Common user errors include attempting to shock ventricular fibrillation in synchronized mode, inattention to lead selection, failure to properly maintain and check devices resulting in uncharged batteries, mismatch of cables with specific defibrillators, and holding the defibrillator in a charged state too long, leading to an automatic discharge that requires recharging for actual use. Two probable causes for variation in the quality of resuscitation efforts are infrequent practice of resuscitation skills training by hospital staff and the requirement of providers to immediately function as a team with others with whom they have not rehearsed.

One method of preventing user error related to equipment inexperience and unfamiliarity is to require checks of the equipment daily, or per shift, in high-use areas. While most facilities require this to maintain the equipment, it may be even more important to ensure that the staff is likewise prepared. Since performing this checklist is a way of familiarizing staff with the device, as many potential rescuers as possible should be taught to perform these inspections. An additional step toward minimizing user error is to utilize a checklist system for assessing the readiness of the equipment and in its operation. Such checklists are a proven tool in such industries as aviation, where a highly complex set of equipment must function correctly with essentially no tolerance for error. When possible, defibrillators should be standardized within institutions to avoid equipment confusion and the mismatching of cables and other disposable supplies. By incorporating these strategies into daily practice, resuscitation equipment can become both familiar and safe, and cardiac arrest treatment can be approached with greater confidence by all members of the hospital team.

SUGGESTED READINGS

Abella BS, Edelson DP. Resuscitation errors: A shocking problem. Agency for Healthcare Research and Quality's WEB M&M July/August 2007. Available at: www.webmm.ahrq.gov/case.aspx?caseID=155#figureback.

Chan PS, Krumholz HM, Nichol G, et al. Delayed time to defibrillation after in-hospital cardiac arrest. *N Engl J Med* 2008;358(1):9–17. Available at: http://content.nejm.org/cgi/content/short/358/1/9.

Thom T, Haase N, Rosamund W, et al. and the American Heart Association Statistics Committee and Stroke Statistics Subcommittee. Heart disease and stroke statistics—2006 update. *Circulation*. 2006;113:e85–151. Epub Jan 11, 2006.

Patients develop heart failure from structural problems with their heart, and the nurse can often help identify the etiology

Anthony D. Slonim, MD, DrPH

Congestive heart failure (CHF) is a major condition, which is one of the leading causes of acute hospitalization for adults. CHF often presents with acute decompensation including shortness of breath, hypertension, and occasionally chest pain. An analysis that considers the contributors to CHF by evaluating each of the components of the heart allows the differential diagnosis to be readily available. While the clinical providers are busy treating the patients for their acute symptoms with medications like diuretics, antihypertensives, and inotropic support, a search for the etiology is important and can often be identified through readily available diagnostic techniques.

CHF occurs from a number of structural problems of the heart, and a quick review of those is important in understanding the etiology. The most common underlying reason for acute heart failure in the adult is ischemia. Patients with ischemic cardiac failure often have a predisposing history of coronary artery disease or a prior myocardial infarction. They present with a complaint of chest pain in addition to their complaints of dyspnea, orthopnea, and fluid overload. The identification of ischemia can be performed with a 12-lead EKG and substantiated with cardiac enzyme analysis.

In addition to ischemia, patients with CHF can present with valvular problems that have become decompensated. Aortic stenosis, mitral regurgitation, and stenosis can present with signs of left-sided CHF. These problems may be detected from physical examination by the presence of a murmur and can be substantiated through echocardiography.

Arrhythmias are another common reason for CHF and are readily recognized by the nurse through the evaluation of pulses for their regularity and end organ perfusion. The cardiac monitor provides a readily available tool that can assist the nurse in identifying the problem.

Finally, the patient with CHF can have cardiac muscle problems; while this is most often related to the presence of ischemia, myocarditis can sometimes be implicated. Patients present with signs of overt failure and shock and may require mechanical support for their failing heart.

SUGGESTED READINGS

Hunt SA, Abraham WT, Chin MH, et al. ACC/AHA 2005 guideline update for the diagnosis and management of chronic heart failure in the adult. *Circulation.* 2005;112:1825–1852.

REMEMBER THE OTHER ARTERIAL VESSELS AFFECTED BY ATHEROSCLEROSIS

ANTHONY D. SLONIM, MD, DrPH

WHAT TO DO: EVALUATE

Atherosclerosis is a major contributor to coronary artery disease and the subsequent development of both acute myocardial infarction and chronic cardiac failure. While considerable attention of the nurse may be focused on the examination of the heart during an acute event, it is important to remember that there are a number of other large vascular structures that can also cause important diseases and lead to major problems for patients.

The abdominal aorta is an important vascular structure that delivers blood from the heart to the organs of the abdomen, pelvis, and legs. Atherosclerotic disease of the aorta is manifested through problems leading to dilation and weakening of the aortic wall, making it prone to rupture. Ruptured abdominal aortic aneurysms can present with nonspecific symptoms such as abdominal pain, dyspepsia, nausea, pallor, or leg pain since the abdominal aorta supplies the iliacs and femoral vessels of the legs. When the abdominal aorta is ruptured, the patient can quickly deteriorate and develop shock or death. Abdominal aneurysms are usually identified through a physical examination of the abdomen and are recognized as a pulsatile mass. Serial observations at regular intervals are usually considered using ultrasound or CT scanning. When the size of the aneurysm expands beyond approximately 6 cm, intervention is often required to prevent an unexpected rupture. Awareness of this condition in the patient who presents with shock can be important to avoid missing a potentially deadly condition.

The carotid arteries are another important vascular structure that carries blood from the aortic arch to the brain. These arteries often experience atherosclerosis and lead to diminished blood flow to the brain. The most common symptom associated with this disorder is a transient ischemic attack (TIA). These episodes are brief periods of weakness and are sometimes considered a sentinel sign of potential cerebrovascular accidents. Patients with carotid disease usually have other manifestations of vascular disease, including hypertension and coronary artery disease. A bruit may be found on examination of the carotids, but the nurse should avoid palpation of the carotid for fear of stimulating a vagal response and bradycardia.

An evaluation of large arteries is necessary when a patient with coronary artery disease presents for treatment. Evaluating the abdominal aorta and carotids should be included in the cardiac examination of these patients.

SUGGESTED READINGS

Isselbacher E. Thoracic and abdominal aortic aneurysms. *Circulation.* 2005;111:816–828. Available at: http://circ.ahajournals.org/cgi/reprint/111/6/816?maxtoshow=&HITS=10&hits=10&RESULTFORMAT=&fulltext=abdominal+aortic+aneurysms&searchid=1&FIRSTINDEX=0&resourcetype=HWCIT. Accessed August 8, 2008.

Moore WS, Barnett HJM, Beebe HG, et al. Guidelines for carotid endarterectomy: A multidisciplinary consensus statement from the ad hoc committee. American Heart Association. *Circulation.* 1995;91:566–579. Available at: http://circ.ahajournals.org/cgi/content/full/91/2/566?maxtoshow=&HITS=10&hits=10&RESULTFORMAT=&fulltext=carotid+insufficiency&searchid=1&FIRSTINDEX=0&resourcetype=HWCIT. Accessed August 8, 2008.

ALWAYS CLOSE THE STOPCOCK OF AN ARTERIAL LINE AFTER DRAWING BLOOD AND FLUSHING THE LINE

FRANCINE B. YATES, RRT, RN, BSN

WHAT TO DO: EVALUATE

Many patients in the intensive care unit (ICU) setting have arterial lines that, when maintained properly, continually measure blood pressure and allow blood gases to be drawn without subjecting the patient to multiple punctures for lab draws. After accessing the line, the nurse should review the monitor to ensure that the waveform has returned to baseline.

Arterial lines are relatively simple to maintain and facilitate patient care by reducing the number of lab sticks and continually monitoring blood pressures. When fluctuations in blood pressures arise, they are attended to immediately, before the patient becomes symptomatic. However, due to the invasive nature of the arterial line placement, it raises the patient's risk of a blood infection or hemorrhage.

When monitoring the arterial line, the first thing to examine is the quality of the waveform, which can vary from patient to patient. If the quality of the waveform has declined and the line has just been accessed for a blood draw and flushed, make certain the stopcock is in the appropriate position. If the stopcock is turned the wrong way, the patient could bleed excessively or even hemorrhage. A nurse can draw blood and flush the line and assume the stopcock and connections are closed without

being fully attentive to a dampened or nonexistent waveform on the monitor. A short time later, the bed can be saturated with the patient's blood because the patient bled out of the line.

It is also important to check the arterial line for blood backflow. If present, determine if all the stopcocks are in the correct position, make sure all the connections are tight, and flush the catheter. Check to be certain that the pressure bag is inflated to 300 mm Hg. Also, arterial lines should be leveled and zeroed at least once a shift. If the line does not flush properly, check for kinks in the line, ensure that the position of the arm is correct if it is a radial line, and consider placing an armboard to maintain adequate readings and properly flush the line.

Arterial lines are a beneficial part of critical care. Education on properly maintaining the arterial line and complications that can occur should be an integral part of critical care orientation.

SUGGESTED READINGS

Carlson KK, Lynn-McHale D, Weigand DJ. Arterial catheter insertion (assist), care and removal. In: *AACN Procedure Manual for Critical Care*. 5th Ed. St. Louis: Saunders; 2005, pp. 451–464.

Kaur A. Caring for a patient with an arterial line. *Nursing*. 2006;36(4):64.

RADIAL ARTERIAL LINES AND BP CUFFS DO NOT BELONG ON THE SAME ARM

FRANCINE B. YATES, RRT, RN, BSN

WHAT TO DO: PLAN

Blood pressure is one of the most important hemodynamic parameters measured in the intensive care unit (ICU). Blood pressure can be measured invasively by an arterial line or noninvasively by a blood pressure cuff. It is important that both methods be as accurate as possible since many decisions regarding patient care depend on blood pressure monitoring.

In the ICU setting, a patient may be placed on an intravenous drip of vasopressors due to hypotension, may be postoperative, or may become hypertensive and require a vasodilator. These medications require constant and consistent monitoring of the systolic, diastolic, and mean arterial pressures. This constant monitoring provides the nurse with the parameters for the necessary titration of these medications to ensure the patient's hemodynamic stability.

It is imperative that the arterial lines read appropriately. If the blood pressure from the arterial line reading is low, it should be checked with the blood pressure cuff applied to the arm. If the cuff is reading significantly higher, then all the connections and stopcocks on the arterial line should be checked and an appropriate waveform should be verified. If the waveform is dampened, ensure that the line has been leveled and zeroed. Examine the line for kinks in the tubing or air bubbles in the line, which could cause underdampening

or emboli. Make certain that the patient's wrist or leg is straight and consider the use of an armboard if a radial arterial line is being used. The pressure bag should be checked to ensure that it is accurately inflated.

An arterial blood pressure can be compared to a noninvasive blood pressure with a cuff. If the arterial reading is inaccurate, it should first be ascertained that the cuff is not on the same arm as the radial arterial line. If this happens, when the cuff inflates, the waveform will dampen or flatten. At times, a patient will be admitted to the ICU with the cuff on the same arm as the arterial line. The first step should be to move the cuff to the opposite arm to ensure accuracy of the arterial line readings.

Maintaining an arterial line is a complex process requiring several steps. Extensive training on maintaining and trouble shooting an arterial line is required during critical care orientation and re-evaluated through competencies. Only nurses who have had proper training and have displayed and maintain competency in managing A-lines should participate in caring for these patients.

SUGGESTED READINGS

Carlson KK, Lynn-McHale D, Weigand DJ. Arterial catheter insertion (assist), care and removal. In: *AACN Procedure Manual for Critical Care*. 5th Ed. St. Louis: Saunders; 2005, pp. 451–464.

Kaur A. Caring for a patient with an arterial line. *Nursing*. 2006; 36(4):64.

ENSURE SAFE PATIENT TRANSFERS OF CRITICALLY ILL PATIENTS

JEANNIE SCRUGGS GARBER, DNP, RN

WHAT TO DO: PLAN

Intrahospital patient transfers are necessary for diagnostic testing and to place patients in the most appropriate clinical setting for their severity of illness. Critically ill patients are frequently transferred from the nursing unit to radiology units, invasive procedure areas, and operating rooms. The decision to transfer a critically ill patient from one unit to another is based on an analysis of the benefits and risks to the patient. Intensive care patients have altered physiology, require invasive monitoring and organ support, and may experience instability during transfer. Developing practices to reduce or minimize this necessary risk represents a potentially important area of patient safety research.

Transferring patients within a hospital is defined as intrahospital and is usually done for diagnostic tests or patient relocation to a different unit. Interhospital transfer refers to patient movement between facilities. Stabilizing the patient before any transfer, either intra- or interhospital, is the most important priority; however, it may not always be possible. Ensuring adequate ventilation, oxygenation, and hemodynamic stability are often the most crucial processes that need to be maintained during transfer. The nurse, respiratory therapist, anesthesiologist, or other provider must work together to develop the best plan for the patient to minimize risk and improve safety. There is almost always additional equipment associated with transferring critically ill patients, so safeguards must be in place to transfer the equipment and maintain the function as much as possible.

The ideal transport would be performed by highly specialized transport teams who perform these tasks over and over, day after day. Consistency in process, familiarity with equipment, and expertise may provide a safer environment for transfer.

According to Martins and Shojanai, there are two major categories that describe adverse events during patient transportation of the critically ill: "mishaps related to intensive care and physiologic deteriorations related to critical illness." They describe the most common "mishap" problems as equipment malfunction or accidents such as extubation or tubing disconnects. They describe the physiologic problems as most likely low or a change in blood pressure and low oxygen saturation.

The literature describing or explaining adverse events as a result of patient transportation is sparse. The studies reviewed by Martins and Shojanai were very small, mostly descriptive and did not allow for comparisons due to variation in conceptual definitions. While significant progress has been made in the past several decades to address provider education, transport monitoring, and portability of clinical equipment, the bedside nurse who deals with these patients every day needs a checklist of tasks to ensure that every patient gets the care he or she needs before, during, and after the transport. These advances are surely improving outcomes and decreasing risks, yet more research is needed to verify the outcomes.

SUGGESTED READINGS

Martins S, Shojanai K. Safety during transport of critically ill patients. In: Wachter RM, ed. *Making Health Care Safer: A Critical Analysis of Patient Safety Practices*. Archived EPC Evidence Reports. 2001. Available at: http://www.ahrq.gov/clinic/ptsafety/chap47.htm. Accessed June 19, 2008.

Wallace PGM, Ridley SA. ABC of intensive care: Transport of critically ill patients. *Br Med J*. 1999;319:368–371.

AN UNDERSTANDING OF ARDS IS IMPORTANT FOR THE NURSE TO EFFECTIVELY PLAN CARE FOR THE CRITICALLY ILL PATIENT

JEANNIE SCRUGGS GARBER, DNP, RN

WHAT TO DO: PLAN

Acute Respiratory Distress Syndrome (ARDS) is a lung condition that can be life threatening. Most patients who develop ARDS are hospitalized and experience critical illness, disease, or trauma. Nurses in critical care units need to understand the etiology, pathophysiology, and treatment of ARDS, so that they can prioritize appropriate care, limit complicating factors, and educate families on this condition. ARDS is a syndrome of inflammation and increased permeability that allows fluid into the alveoli instead of air, which prevents oxygen transfer into the bloodstream. This lack of oxygen creates systemic complications within a short period of time.

Patients diagnosed with this disease meet the following criteria:

- Identifiable associated condition
- Acute onset
- Pulmonary artery wedge pressure less than 18 mmHg or absence of clinical evidence of left atrial hypertension
- Bilateral infiltrates on chest radiography
- Acute lung injury (ALI) is present if Pao_2/Fio_2 ratio is less than 300
- ARDS is present if Pao_2/Fio_2 ratio is less than 200

According to Moses (2008), other common characteristics of ARDS patients are:

- Symptoms present within 12 to 24 h of antecedent event
- Patients are intubated within 72 h
- ARDS diagnosis is associated with a high mortality rate (ICU: 37%, overall: 42%)

Moses (2008) also indicates that there is a better prognosis for patients who survive the first 2 weeks, who are below 55 years, and who have trauma-related ARDS. He also suggests a poor prognosis for those who are above 70 years, who are immunocompromised, and who have chronic liver disease or increased dead space fraction.

The most common clinical conditions associated with ARDS are:

- Pneumonia
- Aspiration of gastric contents
- Inhalation injury
- Near drowning
- Pulmonary contusion
- Fat embolism
- Reperfusion pulmonary edema post lung transplantation or pulmonary embolectomy
- Sepsis
- Severe trauma
- Acute pancreatitis
- Cardiopulmonary bypass
- Massive transfusions
- Drug overdose

Clinical management of the patient with ARDS is focused on obtaining adequate oxygenation, preventing infection, maintaining fluid and electrolyte balance, and providing adequate nutrition to promote healing. The nurse needs to prioritize these efforts to ensure that the patient has the best chances for improving his or her survival. According to the National Heart, Blood and Lung Institute (2007), ARDS treatment has improved, and the survival rate is increasing. About 190,000 people in the United States are diagnosed with ARDS each year and approximately 7 out of 10 people who get timely treatment survive. ARDS research is ongoing to work toward better understanding of the disease and to create a continued improvement in patient outcomes.

SUGGESTED READINGS

American Thoracic Society. What is acute respiratory distress syndrome? 2007. Available at: http://www.thoracic.org/sections/education/patient-education/patient-education-materials/patient-information-series/ards.html. Accessed July 15, 2008.

Medical Criteria.com. Diagnostic criteria for adult respiratory distress syndrome. 2007. Retrieved on July 15, 2008 from http://www.medicalcriteria.com/criteria/uti_ards.htm.

Moses S. Acute respiratory distress syndrome. *Family Practice Notebook*. 2008. Available at: http://www.fpnotebook.com/Lung/Failure/ActRsprtryDstrsSyndrm.htm. Accessed July 15, 2008.

National Heart, Blood and Lung Institute. What is ARDS? 2007. Available at: http://www.nhlbi.nih.gov/health/dci/Diseases/Ards/Ards_WhatIs.html. Accessed July 15, 2008.

Surgical-tutor.org (n.d.). Acute respiratory distress syndrome. Available at: http://www.surgical-tutor.org.uk/default-home.htm?core/ITU/ards.htm~right. Accessed July 15, 2008.

DIC REQUIRES SPECIAL NURSING CONSIDERATIONS

JEANNIE SCRUGGS GARBER, DNP, RN

WHAT TO DO: ASSESS, IMPLEMENT, AND EVALUATE

Disseminated Intravascular Coagulation (DIC) is a syndrome of deranged blood coagulation that results in a complex response of simultaneous clotting and hemorrhage. There are a number of causes for DIC, including trauma, surgery, critical illness, malignancy, liver disease, sepsis, and large-volume transfusions. This condition is very difficult to treat and has a high mortality rate. The major treatment for DIC is a treatment of the underlying etiology. Patient outcome is directly dependent on early diagnosis and treatment.

The bleeding associated with DIC may start suddenly and become excessive in a very short period of time. The bleeding occurs from a number of sites. If there has been a recent operative or invasive procedure, incisions or puncture sites may bleed. The gastrointestinal and genitorurinary systems may also experience bleeding from indwelling catheters. The sputum from ventilated patients may become blood tinged, and the patient may experience a spontaneous intracranial hemorrhage. Intravenous and central venous catheter sites may also begin to bleed. Blood loss can be rapid, resulting in shock.

If DIC is severe, the patient needs attention to the As, Bs, and Cs to ensure adequate tissue oxygenation and perfusion. The administration of fluid and targeted blood products can be specified through laboratory testing including hemoglobin, hematocrit, platelet count, fibrinogen, prothrombin and partial thromboplastin times, and fibrin degradation products.

Early diagnosis and intervention is critical to patient survival.

According to Dressler (2007), the most commonly ordered treatments for DIC include

- Packed red blood cells (warmed)
- Fresh frozen plasma
- Cryoprecipitate
- Platelets
- Low molecular weight heparin (in some cases)
- Other drugs that impact clotting factors

The most important assessments during the acute treatment phase of DIC are coagulation studies (about every 4 h) and evaluation of neurologic, cardiovascular, respiratory, and renal systems. Care should be taken to minimize any invasive procedures or any procedures that would exert pressure of any kind on any body part. Even bathing should be done with caution. Another priority is the patient's comfort, both physically and emotionally, while paying close attention to the effects of pain medication on blood pressure. Family support is also very important during the diagnosis and treatment phases of DIC. There is usually great uncertainty surrounding both the diagnosis and the effectiveness of treatment, and families need to be informed of the process and expected outcome for the patient.

SUGGESTED READINGS

Dressler D. DIC: Coping with a coagulation crisis. *Nursing*. 2004. Available at: http://findarticles.com/p/articles/mi_qa3689/is_200405/ai_n9377065/pg_3?tag=artBody;col1. Accessed July 16, 2008.

CARING FOR THE PATIENT WITH SHOCK

JEANNIE SCRUGGS GARBER, DNP, RN

WHAT TO DO: IMPLEMENT

"Shock" is a commonly used term that means very different things to the general public and medical professionals. The general public uses the word "shock" to describe how individuals react to a traumatic or stressful situation, and in the medical community, "shock" is defined as inadequate delivery or use of oxygen and substrate by the tissues and cells of the body in sufficient enough amounts to sustain their viability. When there is minimal or no blood flow to vital organs, their function is compromised, and organ failure and death may result if blood flow is not restored quickly. Shock requires immediate attention to maximize the possibility of recovery.

The major types of shock are:

- Cardiogenic shock (related to heart function)
- Hypovolemic shock (related to low blood volume)
- Anaphylactic shock (related to allergic reaction)
- Septic shock (related to infection)
- Neurogenic shock (related to insult to the nervous system)

Any condition that reduces blood flow can lead to shock. Some of the most common conditions associated with shock include myocardial infarction, congestive heart failure, bleeding, severe allergic reactions, trauma, and infection. It is important to consider other potential causes of shock that may be more subtle. Shock related to fluid volume can occur from dehydration resulting from excessive vomiting and diarrhea, heat exposure, high fever, or diabetic ketoacidosis. Shock from excessive bleeding can occur as a result of a situation other than trauma, such as bleeding from the gastrointestinal system, the uterus, cancer, and medications.

The treatment of shock depends on the cause. Table 156-1 summarizes some of the common causes of shock and common treatments.

TABLE 156.1.	COMMON CAUSES AND TREATMENTS OF SHOCK
CAUSE OF SHOCK	**TREATMENT OF SHOCK**
Hemorrhagic shock—excessive bleeding	Stop source of bleeding and fluid replacement
Hypovolemic shock—dehydration	Fluid replacement
Cardiogenic shock—reduced cardiac output	Medications to support vital signs, consider mechanical support of the heart
Neurogenic shock	Fluid and medications to increase vascular tone

The signs and symptoms of shock may include: hypotension, anxiety, agitation, confusion, clammy skin, pale color, blue-colored lips and nail beds, little or no urine output, tachycardia, weak pulse, respiratory difficulties, chest pain, and loss of consciousness. Treatment of patients experiencing shock is emergent and includes interventions such as oxygen administration or intubation, insertion of invasive monitoring lines to aid in diagnosis, urinary catheters, constant blood pressure and cardiac monitoring, laboratory analysis, fluid replacement and blood transfusion if indicated, and intravenous medications to support blood pressure.

The recovery period from a shock experience may include long-term care and rehabilitation. Permanent changes in major organ functions may occur as a result of shock, and the recovery may be slow and incremental. Early intervention and treatment are necessary to minimize long-term implications.

SUGGESTED READINGS

Wedro B. Shock. *e-MedicineHealth-Practical Guide to Health.* 2008. Available at: http://www.emedicinehealth.com/shock/page10_em.htm. Accessed July 29, 2008.

TRANSDUCER LEVELING IS CRITICAL FOR ENSURING APPROPRIATE INTERVENTIONS

LEA E. LINEBERRY, RNIII, BSN, CCRN, CPN

WHAT TO DO: EVALUATE

Invasive catheters are frequently used to monitor hemodynamic pressures and to calculate hemodynamic indices for cardiac, respiratory, and neurologic functioning in critically ill patients. The transducer system allows the conversion of pressure signals within the vasculature to produce dynamic electric responses that can be visualized on the monitor. The management of fluids, medications, and critical interventions depends on the pressure readings obtained by the use of these invasive monitoring devices. By understanding the basic principles of this commonly used system of continuous monitoring, correct pressure measurements, subsequent treatment interventions, and evaluation of the patient's response to selective therapies can be more accurately performed by the nurse.

The pressure transducer is a device used to change physiologic pressure into an electric signal that is displayed on a monitor. Calibration, balancing, and leveling of the transducer to the monitor are required before accurate readings can be obtained. The positioning of the transducer must be above the pressure source. This will vary according to the type of pressure reading needed, that is, blood pressure, central venous pressure, or intracranial pressure.

Changes in body position affect the hydrostatic pressure at the level of the tricuspid valve. This valve, therefore, becomes the reference point for cardiac pressure measurement and the point at which the transducer must be aligned or leveled. The area on the body that corresponds to this valve is known as the phlebostatic axis and is found at the fourth intercostal space and one half the anterior–posterior diameter of the chest. The measurement of pressure within the skull can be managed by the insertion of a ventricular catheter and the use of intracranial pressure monitoring. Transducer placement for intracranial pressure is maintained at the level of the foramen of Monro, which is correlated to the tragus of the ear. In some critically ill patients, both these systems will be hemodynamically monitored, so transducer management is vital to proper treatment. Since the difference in leveling for intracranial pressure and the various cardiac pressures lies in the place of anatomy, placement of the transducer holder is crucial. If technical errors occur, as with improper transducer placement, up to one third of readings may be off by less than 4 mm Hg. It should be noted that two different transducer holders should always be used when intracranial pressure and cardiac pressure are being monitored.

Transducer leveling in all types of pressure monitoring is the responsibility of the nurse. Errors in pressure readings can be avoided by knowing the proper anatomic areas for calibration and leveling and changing the transducer position if the patient's position is changed.

SUGGESTED READINGS

deBoisblanc BP, Brierre SP. Common pitfalls in the use of the pulmonary artery catheter. 2006. Available at: www.chestnet.org/education/online/pccu/vol20/lesson13. Accessed June 3, 2008.

Kinney MR, Dunbar SB, Brooks-Brunn JA, et al. *AACN Clinical Reference for Critical Care Nursing*. St. Louis: Mosby; 1996.

PRESSURE BAG FOR INTRACRANIAL PRESSURE MONITORING? NO!

LEA E. LINEBERRY, RNIII, BSN, CCRN, CPN

The pressure exerted by the cranium on the brain tissue, cerebrospinal fluid (CSF), and the brain's circulating blood volume is called intracranial pressure (ICP). Activities such as exercise, coughing, straining, Valsalva, arterial pulsation, and respiratory cycle affect the ICP. Normal ICP is 5 to 15 mm Hg at rest, for both adults and children. Changes in ICP occur as volume changes occur within the cranium. Cerebral compliance, cerebral blood flow, and cerebral metabolism are integral to intracranial dynamics. An understanding of the relationships between the intracranial components is necessary to understand problems that occur with dynamic changes in ICP.

The skull functions like a rigid box. Any increase in the contents of that box, that is, blood, CSF, or brain size, causes an increase in ICP. Increased ICP requires critical care management and may require the insertion of a ventricular catheter to assist in decreasing ICP by draining CSF. ICP measurements can be obtained by placing a monitor in the cerebral ventricles. Ventricular pressure measurements are the most accurate and also allow for the draining of CSF.

The policy for ICP monitoring varies by institution following the insertion of a ventricular catheter. Some require a setup using a fluid-filled syringe, transducer, and tubing. Others use a flush system setup that is attached to the pressure line. This fluid is used by the nurse or physician to flush the external system, and never the ventricular system. This system is always clamped and never set up with a pressure bag in place. The pressure bag is used for other pressure line systems and places a pressure of 300 mm Hg to the system. This allows a continuous pressure infusion of 3 mL/h. A pressure bag applied to an intracranial flushing system would increase the volume within an already compromised intracerebral space, and the compliance would be lost. When this compliance is lost, there is risk of brain herniation.

Increased ICP is caused by a change in one or more of the cranial vault components. This pressure decreases cerebral perfusion and significant neurologic injury can occur. Correct setup and proper management of the ICP monitoring system is the responsibility of the registered nurse in most intensive care units. Knowing how to establish and maintain the ICP monitoring system appropriately is one of the many competencies of the critical care nurse.

SUGGESTED READINGS

Kinney MR, Dunbar SB, Brooks-Brunn JA, et al. *AACN Clinical Reference for Critical Care Nursing*. St. Louis: Mosby; 1996.

Logan P. *Principles of Practice for the Acute Care Nurse Practitioner*. Stamford: Appleton & Lange; 1999.

ENSURE THAT THE WAVEFORM IS NOT DAMPENED PRIOR TO READING

NANCY F. ALTICE, RN, MSN, CCNS, CNS-BC

WHAT TO DO: EVALUATE

Invasive hemodynamic monitoring can provide valuable information in situations where noninvasive parameters and physical assessment findings still leave questions about clinical status. However, the most sophisticated monitoring equipment can yield totally erroneous results if the clinician fails to recognize a dampened waveform. A dampened waveform tends to underestimate the systolic pressure and overestimate the diastolic pressure, without significantly affecting the mean pressure.

A dampened waveform occurs when there is a dynamic response artifact. The most common source of these artifacts is air in the pressure tubing or transducer. The amount of air can be as small as a tiny air bubble. Air bubbles will often cling to the ports of the stopcocks or the transducer. Another source of damping is blood in the transducer system. Maintaining the flush system at a pressure of 300 mm Hg will prevent backflow of blood into the pressure tubing. This will also help prevent blood from clotting on the tip of the catheter which may also contribute to a dampened waveform and inaccurate pressure reading. Anything that obstructs the tip of the catheter can also cause a dampened waveform. Catheter position can migrate forward, especially in the case of pulmonary artery catheters, leading to obstruction of a smaller pulmonary artery branch and a distorted waveform that does not reflect accurate pressures. The tip of the catheter can also lie against the arterial wall without migrating forward. This can obstruct the tip of the catheter, resulting in a distorted waveform. A leak in the system or a loose connection can also cause a damped waveform.

Remember to always assess the configuration of the waveform before deciding whether or not to accept the pressure readings obtained from invasive monitoring

lines. If there is no clear dicrotic notch and if the waveform appears wide and slurred, the monitoring system is most likely overdamped, and the readings will not be accurate and could result in inappropriate treatment decisions. When this type of waveform is encountered, carefully examine the tubing for evidence of small air bubbles. These often cling to the transducer and the sides of stopcock ports. Even if no air bubbles are seen, it is worth opening a stopcock to air and flushing the transducer using the fast flush device on the pressure line to attempt to uncover hidden bubbles. You may have to work your way down the line from the bag to the patient, flushing each stopcock port. Obviously, if blood is seen in the line, this should also be thoroughly flushed until only clear fluid remains in the line. Be sure to tighten all connections and replace all caps on the stopcock ports to maintain a fluid-filled, air-free pressure line. If these procedures do not improve the appearance of the waveform, the physician or mid-level provider should be alerted to assess for possible catheter migration which could be remedied by repositioning the catheter. Occasionally, changing the patient's position may alter the position of the catheter tip enough to see an improvement in the waveform. This would add further support that the catheter needs to be repositioned.

After a normal waveform is obtained, compare the new readings to previous readings. If the systolic or diastolic pressures have changed by more than 1 to 2 mm Hg, alert the physician or mid-level provider that this change may be due to a more accurate reading rather than a change in the patient's condition.

SUGGESTED READINGS

Dietz B, Smith, T. Enhancing the accuracy of hemodynamic monitoring. *J Nurs Care Qual.* 2002;17:30–38.
Frazier SK. Hemodynamic monitoring. In: Moser DK, Riegel B, eds. *Cardiac Nursing: A Companion to Braunwald's Heart Disease.* St Loius: Elsevier-Saunders; 2008.

Do not forget to relevel the transducer when the patient's position changes

Nancy F. Altice, RN, MSN, CCNS, CNS-BC

WHAT TO DO: IMPLEMENT

Sophisticated hemodynamic monitoring systems provide information that can lead to enhanced diagnosis and improved management of the critically ill patient. To maintain accuracy of the readings, the provider must remember to level the transducer each time the patient's position is changed. Leveling removes the effect of hydrostatic pressure created by the fluid-filled pressure line.

The transducer should be level with the patient's phlebostatic axis. The phlebostatic axis is at the intersection of the fourth intercostal space and the midaxillary line. This is approximately the location of the right atrium of the heart. Marking the phlebostatic axis on the patient's skin will aid each provider to use the same reference point when leveling the transducer. When the air–fluid interface of the transducer is 1 inch above the phlebostatic axis, the reading will be falsely decreased by 2 mm Hg. When the transducer is below the phlebostatic axis, readings will be falsely elevated to 2 mm Hg for each inch of variation. When measuring a pressure such as a pulmonary capillary wedge pressure, which has a normal range of 4 to 12 mm Hg, a 2 mm error is significant. Accurate leveling is best achieved with either a carpenter's level or a laser level. Visual estimation without the use of one of these tools is frequently inaccurate.

Historically, the supine position with no elevation of the head of the bed was used to obtain the most accurate readings of cardiac and arterial pressures. Often, the readings are obtained at least hourly, and repositioning the patient leads to disrupted sleep, increased discomfort, and potentially deleterious effects on pulmonary function and intracranial pressures.

For this reason, multiple nurse researchers sought to identify the limits of positioning that would still yield accurate pressure readings. Supine positioning with the head of the bed elevated up to 60° provides accurate pressure readings as long as the air–fluid interface of the transducer is accurately positioned at the level of the phlebostatic axis. Results for lateral positioning of the patient have varied and should be studied further before routinely using readings obtained in this manner.

Remember to relevel the transducer each time the patient's position is changed. Frequent patient repositioning is crucial for comfort and prevention of complications. Even if the bed position has not been altered, check to ensure that the patient's phlebostatic axis has not moved due to sliding down in the bed. Remember that each inch of position change can result in a 2 mmHg error.

SUGGESTED READINGS

Dietz B, Smith T. Enhancing the accuracy of hemodynamic monitoring. *J Nurs Care Qual.* 2002;17:30–38.

Frazier SK. Hemodynamic monitoring. In: Moser DK, Riegel B, eds. *Cardiac Nursing: A Companion to Braunwald's Heart Disease.* St Loius: Elsevier-Saunders; 2008.

FOR INTRA-AORTIC BALLOON PUMP TIMING OR TRIGGERING, PICK AN EKG LEAD WITH A TALL R WAVE

NANCY F. ALTICE, RN, MSN, CCNS, CNS-BC

WHAT TO DO: IMPLEMENT

Intra-aortic balloon pump (IABP) therapy requires advanced knowledge and skill. The technology available with today's IABP reduces the risk of errors with the timing of balloon inflation and deflation. The pumps have sophisticated, computerized algorithms, which detect various aspects of the EKG and the arterial and balloon waveforms to assist in maintaining appropriate timing.

Most IABPs allow a variety of triggers to be selected. When the trigger is detected, the intra-aortic balloon will inflate. It will remain inflated for the time period indicated by the timing that has been set using the arterial waveform. The most common trigger is the QRS waveform of the electrocardiogram. Most pumps will use height, width, and slope to recognize the QRS. This works so well that clinicians may assume that this small aspect is infallible. However, there is occasionally a patient for whom the QRS has very low voltage and the T wave is tall and peaked. The potential exists for the IABP to mistake the taller T wave complex for the QRS. This could cause the intra-aortic balloon to inflate later than intended. The main consequence of this

timing or triggering error is that the desired effect is not achieved. Late deflation will miss the opportunity to increase coronary artery perfusion. There is also a chance of late deflation, although most IABPs have built-in safety mechanisms to prevent this. Late deflation can be dangerous because the left ventricle will have to build up much more pressure than normal to open the aortic valve against the increased pressure that exists in the aorta during balloon inflation. This would greatly increase the myocardial oxygen demand of the left ventricle and could be extremely detrimental.

Always evaluate the timing of balloon inflation and deflation by looking for the hallmarks of optimum balloon timing. When the waveforms do not indicate optimum timing, make sure the trigger being used is appropriate. Choosing an EKG lead that has a QRS waveform with more voltage than the T wave will assist the pump to accurately identify the QRS.

SUGGESTED READINGS

Arrow International. ACAT I plus intraaortic balloon pump: Timing, triggering and troubleshooting. 2005. Available at: http://www.arrowintl.com/products/education/.

Metules T. IABP therapy: Getting patients treatment fast. *RN*. 2003;66(5):56–64.

DO NOT CONFUSE FAILURE TO CAPTURE AND FAILURE TO SENSE

NANCY F. ALTICE, RN, MSN, CCNS, CNS-BC

WHAT TO DO: ASSESS

Temporary invasive pacing is a lifesaving procedure that often confuses even experienced critical care nurses. Temporary invasive pacing includes both transvenous and epicardial approaches. Both approaches can provide cardiac electrical stimulation when the patient's own intrinsic pacemaker or conduction system fails to maintain an adequate heart rate. However, the instability of the patient's condition can lead to variations in pacing and sensing thresholds. The critical care nurse must be vigilant in recognizing problems with the pacing response.

The two most commonly encountered problems in temporary invasive pacing are failure to capture and failure to sense. If either of these malfunctions is sustained, the evidence on the electrocardiogram becomes obvious, and the patient's clinical condition may also indicate a crisis is occurring. But more often, the pacing or sensing thresholds will be close enough to the pacemaker settings that only an occasional problem is seen on the electrocardiogram. This requires that the nurse understand the potential danger that lurks behind each single pacing artifact that is noncaptured or fired at the wrong time (failure to sense).

Failure to capture simply means that the pacemaker fired an electrical stimulus but the patient's heart did not respond. The expected response to an electrical stimulus from the pacemaker is that the patient's heart will conduct the paced electrical stimulus through the cardiac chamber where the pacing catheter is located (atrium or ventricle) producing a P wave or QRS wave, respectively. Because these artificially stimulated impulses may travel through cardiac muscle cells without following the normal pathway of electrical conduction, the P waves and QRS waves produced are wider than normal. But when failure to capture occurs, the pacemaker spike is not followed by a P wave or QRS wave. The most common reason this occurs is that the pacemaker output setting is too low. This can be quickly fixed by adjusting the output, which is measured in milliamperes, to a slightly higher setting. The amount of electrical output needed to adequately stimulate the heart may change over time due to ischemic changes, electrolyte imbalance, change in patient position, or simply the buildup of fibrin around the tip of the catheter.

Failure to sense means that the pacemaker fails to recognize that the patient's heart has an adequate intrinsic heart rate. Typically, the pacemaker will be set at a rate similar to what the patient's baseline heart rate should be under the current state of illness. If, for example, this rate was set at 75, most pacemaker modes would allow the patient's heart to control the rate and rhythm as long as the patient's own rate is at least 75. If the patient's heart rate slows down below 75 for even one beat, the pacemaker should immediately fire to maintain the rate at 75. But the pacemaker senses only what it is programmed to sense. It is important to understand that what the pacemaker senses is the strength of the electrical impulse and not the visual configuration that is seen on the ECG. The sensitivity is set to recognize a specific amount of electrical activity measured in millivolts. Turning the setting to the smallest number of millivolts makes the pacemaker very sensitive. It will sense even the slightest amount of electrical stimulation. At the other extreme of possible settings, the sensitivity can be set so that only the strongest electrical stimuli are recognized. This could result in the pacemaker continuing to fire despite an adequate intrinsic rhythm as long as that intrinsic rhythm's electrical strength is less than the number of millivolts designated on the pacemaker. This is never a desired situation because the pacemaker may fire during the ventricular refractory period represented by the ST segment and T wave on the ECG. Stimulating the heart at this point in the cardiac cycle could precipitate a ventricular dysrhythmia such as ventricular tachycardia or ventricular fibrillation. Recognizing failure to sense is as simple as recognizing the beat-to-beat heart rate rather than relying on the overall one-minute heart rate displayed on the monitor. Each time the heart is stimulated by either the intrinsic or an artificial pacemaker, the artificial pacemaker should begin to watch for the next intrinsic beat within the number of milliseconds necessary to maintain the exact cycle length between two beats. Remember that milliseconds can be measured on standard ECG graph paper by dividing the number of little blocks between the beginning of one wave and the beginning of the next (QRS to QRS) into 1,500 units which is the number of little blocks that represents 1 min. So if the pacemaker rate is set at 75, divide 75 into 1,500. The result is 20 which is the number of little blocks which should exist between the beginning of one QRS and the next pacemaker spike. Each time the intrinsic pacemaker fires, the artificial pacemaker should reset its timing to look for the next intrinsic electrical stimulus within 20 little blocks. If none occurs, the artificial pacemaker should fire. Under no circumstance should the pacemaker fire sooner than 20 little blocks if the rate is set at 75. If a pacemaker spike is seen earlier than the 20th little block, it indicates failure to sense. Even if this happens only once, the potential exists for the next time to occur during a refractory period possibly stimulating a lethal ventricular arrhythmia. In some cases, when this occurs, the timing of the pacing spike is early enough in the refractory period that the heart is unable to conduct that beat.

This represents both failure to sense and failure to capture. In this situation, be thankful that capture did not occur! Adjust the sensitivity setting to ensure that all intrinsic beats are sensed, and the failure to capture resulting from poor timing in this case will resolve itself.

SUGGESTED READINGS

Overbay D, Criddle L. Mastering temporary invasive cardiac pacing. *Crit Care Nurse.* 2004;24(3):25–32.

KNOW HOW TO MANAGE THE PATIENT WITH OBSTRUCTIVE LUNG DISEASE ON A VENTILATOR

ANTHONY D. SLONIM, MD, DRPH

WHAT TO DO: IMPLEMENT

Mechanical ventilation is one of the most important supportive technologies available in the modern intensive care unit (ICU). Nurses in this setting must understand the fundamental aspects of the equipment, how to troubleshoot problems, and the application of mechanical ventilation to different disease processes. ICU nurses become very familiar with the care of patients with respiratory failure requiring mechanical ventilation. The nurse spends considerable time obtaining and responding to arterial blood gas samples with acute and chronic evidence of respiratory acidosis, but it is important to recognize how the management of patients with obstructive disease on a ventilator differs from that of other patients requiring this treatment.

Arterial blood gases provide evidence of both oxygenation and ventilation for acutely ill or injured patients. The pH on the blood gas provides evidence of the acid base status; the pCO_2 provides evidence of the ventilatory status; and the pO_2 provides important evidence about oxygenation. The pCO_2 will rise for a number of reasons indicating poor alveolar ventilation. When pCO_2 rises and the pH is in the acidotic range, a respiratory acidosis is present. For the patient on mechanical ventilation, this usually leads to a response of increasing minute ventilation either by increasing the respiratory rate or tidal volume. However, for the patient with either chronic obstructive pulmonary disease (COPD) or asthma, the increase in minute ventilation may be exactly the wrong thing to do. These diseases are characterized by obstruction in airflow. In severe condition, air trapping occurs and only worsens with an increase in respiratory rate. These patients often have a prolonged expiratory phase of the respiratory cycle.

Therefore, the appropriate approach is to actually reduce the respiratory rate to allow for a more complete exhalation and reduction in air trapping.

Another common problem in patients particularly with COPD is that they have a chronically elevated pCO_2. The presence of an elevated pCO_2 alone is not an indication for making any ventilatory adjustments either in the COPD patient or other patients with respiratory failure. The nurse should be guided by hypercarbia and the presence of acidosis on the arterial blood gas before adjusting the ventilator.

Permissive hypercarbia is an important strategy for mechanical ventilation in respiratory failure that reduces mechanical support, allows pCO_2 to rise, prevents lung injury, and improves mortality. If the pCO_2 rises to the point when acidosis occurs, then the clinicians need to have a discussion about the most appropriate approach to the patient.

Knowing the interaction between various parameters of the arterial blood gas, the pathophysiology of the mechanical ventilator, and the pathophysiology of the patient's condition allows the nurse to know what to do to manage aberrant results. The application of a "one-size fits all approach" simply does not work in the critically ill patient with obstructive lung disease.

SUGGESTED READINGS

Burns SM. Mechanical ventilation of patients with acute respiratory distress syndrome and patients requiring weaning: The evidence guiding practice. *Crit Care Nurse*. 2005;25(4):14–23. Available at: http://ccn.aacnjournals.org/cgi/content/full/25/4/14. Accessed August 16, 2008.

Jubran A, Tobin MJ. Mechanical ventilation in acute respiratory failure complicating COPD. Available at: http://www.uptodate.com/patients/content/topic.do?topicKey=~f3G34pnXNueef. Accessed August 16, 2008.

REMEMBER THAT THE PATIENT'S CARDIOVASCULAR AND PULMONARY SYSTEMS WORK TOGETHER...DYNAMIC HYPERINFLATION REQUIRES ACUTE TREATMENT WITH INTRAVENOUS FLUIDS

ANTHONY D. SLONIM, MD, DRPH

WHAT TO DO: IMPLEMENT

The human body is a complex interplay of cells, organs, and systems that work together to ensure homeostasis. Two of the most integrated systems are the cardiovascular and pulmonary systems. The interactions between these two systems are apparent in normal physiologic functioning. Air goes in and out, oxygen is transferred from the lungs to hemoglobin in the red blood cells, and the heart then pumps the oxygenated blood to distant cells and tissues through a complex network of arteries and arterioles only to have byproducts, including pCO_2 returned to the lungs for exhalation.

Acutely ill patients have these normal relationships deranged. Even though the modern intensive care unit (ICU) provides sophisticated physiologic support for many failed organ systems, the equipment and providers in the ICU can never provide the sophisticated support that comes naturally when the body is working in a state of health. As a result, providers are left to account for not only the problems associated with the disease of interest but also the effect of the disease and therapies on the other related organ systems and their functioning.

Patients with obstructive lung disease have a prolonged expiratory phase of the respiratory cycle. The patient manages this through pursed lip breathing and trying to remain calm. Mechanical support can also provide support in the chronic phase to "stent" airways and allow for improved exhalation. However, when these patients develop respiratory failure and require mechanical ventilation, the effects of this obstruction on their cardiovascular system need to be considered.

During intubation, patients require positive pressure ventilation while the sedation and anesthesia take effect. The ventilation is often robust because providers forget about the need to allow for full exhalation. As a result, the patient's lungs, which are already hyperinflated from the disease, develop even further hyperinflation because higher and higher lung volumes are being delivered prior to full exhalation. The hyperinflated lung begins to impose on the cardiovascular system. Importantly, the patient may also experience barotrauma from this hyperinflation, like a pneumothorax, but this may go undetected since breath sounds are usually difficult to auscultate. Venous return is impeded and patients develop acute hypotension and a shocklike condition. Hypotension may be the first sign of these problems.

Regardless of their etiology, the first step in the treatment of hypotension occurring from hyperinflation is isotonic intravenous fluid. This should be administered quickly and in sufficient volume to restore intravascular volume. Although this approach does not solve the problem, it provides temporary relief. The next step is to ensure that the ventilator rate is reduced and the patient is given an ample opportunity for exhalation.

Dynamic hyperinflation is an insidious complication of respiratory failure in obstructive lung disease. The nurse needs to know that it exists, recognize and treat it, and correct the underlying causes.

SUGGESTED READINGS

Kohlhaufl M. Dynamic hyperinflation in patients with COPD. Available at: http://www.uptodate.com/patients/content/topic.do?topicKey=copd/7619. Accessed August 16, 2008.

Myles PS, Madder H, Morgan EB. Intraoperative cardiac arrest after unrecognized dynamic hyperinflation. *Br J Anaesth.* 1995;74(3):340–342. Available at: http://bja.oxfordjournals.org/cgi/content/abstract/74/3/340. Accessed August 16, 2008.

REMEMBER THAT AN INTRAVENOUS FLUID BOLUS IS THE FIRST STEP IN RESUSCITATION FOR THE PATIENT WITH SHOCK

ANTHONY D. SLONIM, MD, DRPH

WHAT TO DO: IMPLEMENT

Shock is a clinical syndrome that leads to inadequate perfusion of the cells and tissues of the body. It can be classified as hypovolemic, resulting from the loss of fluid or blood; distributive, resulting from sepsis, neurologic trauma or anaphylaxis; cardiogenic, resulting from problems affecting the cardiac structures; or obstructive, occurring from obstruction to the delivery of substrate. The therapeutic approach to the patient with shock includes a strategy that identifies and treats the underlying cause. However, the underlying cause is not always immediately identified and the patient requires support while the search continues.

Cardiac output is determined by the relationship between the heart rate and stroke volume. Patients compensate for a reduction in stroke volume by increasing their heart rate. Stroke volume has three components including the preload or amount of intravascular fluid, contractility or the force of myocardial contraction and afterload or the force against which the heart can contract to maintain blood pressure. The classification of shock corresponds to one of these physiologic disruptions in stroke volume. Hypovolemic shock is considered a problem with preload, cardiogenic shock, a problem with contractility, and distributive and obstructive shocks, a problem with afterload. This is important since it helps not only with diagnosis and classification but also with treatment.

Patients with preload problems are often treated with intravenous fluid or blood to restore intravascular volume if it is the cause of shock. Problems with contractility can be addressed by the administration of inotropic agents. Afterload problems can be addressed by vasodilators if excessive afterload is the cause of shock or vasopressors if reduced afterload is the cause of shock. Despite these highly specific recommendations, often the etiology is unclear when patients first present with acute hypotension. The nurse should not worry about needing to deliver specific care acutely. Regardless of the etiology, the first step in the therapy should be the administration of an isotonic fluid bolus to restore intravascular volume status.

Often precious time is wasted trying to make a specific diagnosis for the etiology of shock in the critically ill patient, when the patient needs acute intervention with an intravenous fluid bolus, regardless of the etiology.

SUGGESTED READINGS

Diehl-Oplinger L, Kaminski MF. Choosing the right fluid to counter hypovolemic shock. *Nursing*. March 2004. Available at: http://findarticles.com/p/articles/mi_qa3689/is_200403/ai_n9405325. Accessed August 16, 2008.

Intravenous Fluid Resuscitation. Available at: http://www.merck.com/mmpe/sec06/ch067/ch067c.html. Accessed August 16, 2008.

Martin GS. An update on intravenous fluids. Available at: http://www.medscape.com/viewarticle/503138. Accessed August 16, 2008.

166

KNOW HOW TO MANAGE GLUCOSE LEVELS IN PATIENTS WITH DIABETES

MONTY D. GROSS, PhD, RN, CNE

WHAT TO DO: IMPLEMENT

Diabetes is a serious health issue in the United States. The 2007 Center for Disease Control's report for prevalence of diagnosed and undiagnosed diabetes is 23.6 million people or 7.8% of the population. A total of 17.9 million have been diagnosed with 5.7 million people at risk, but undiagnosed. In 2006, diabetes was reported on death certificates frequently enough to make it the seventh leading cause of death in the United States.

As new evidence regarding blood glucose levels for patients with and without diabetes has emerged, tighter control of blood glucose levels is now the goal. These lower glucose levels contribute to a reduction in mortality and infection rates in patients with blood glucose levels tightly controlled less than 110 mg/dL compared with patients whose levels were between 110 mg/dL and 150 mg/dL.

Particular glucose levels for patients may vary from the intensive care unit (ICU), non-ICU, or particular patient conditions. Often in ICUs, insulin drips are used with hourly monitoring of glucose levels. As the patient moves to a step down unit or discharge, the patient is transitioned to subcutaneous injections.

There are five types of insulin: rapid-acting, short-acting, intermediate-acting, mixtures, and long-acting. It is important to know the onset, peak, and duration of each type of insulin (Table 166.1). Shaking the insulin bottle damages the insulin molecules. It is recommended that the bottle be turned end-to-end (top to bottom) several times to get the insulin into suspension.

TABLE 166.1	INSULIN TYPES AND THERAPEUTIC ACTIONS (MIN/H*)		
TYPES	ONSET	PEAK	DURATION
Rapid-acting Humalog (Lispro) Novolog (Aspart)	5–15 min	60–90 min	3–5 h
Short-acting Novolin R Humulin R	0.5–1 h	2–4 h	5–7 h
Intermediate-acting Humulin N (NPH) Novolin N (NPH)	1–2 h 2 h	6–12 h 6–8 h	16–24 h 16–22 h
Mixtures Humulin 70/30 (70% NPH, 30% Regular) Novolin 70/30 (70% NPH, 30% Regular) Humulin 50/50 (50% NPH, 50% Regular) Humalog 75/25 (75% lispro protamine suspension, 25% lispro)	30 min 15 min	2–12 h 1 h	24 h 24 h
Long-acting Lantus (glargine)	4–6 h	No peak	24 h

* The time of insulin may vary significantly in different patients and in the same patient at different times.
Insulin is biologically engineered through the process of recombinant-DNA technology. Insulin is produced by different companies who use different names for short-, intermediate-, or long-acting forms of insulin or their mixtures.
NPH = neutral protamine Hagedorn
(From Smith S, Duell D, Martin B. Parenteral medication administration. In: *Clinical Nursing Skills: Basic to Advanced Skills.* Upper Saddle River, NJ: Pearson; 2008, p. 611.

Short- and intermediate-acting insulin may be mixed, but long-acting insulin (Lantus) should not be mixed with other types of insulin or solutions.

It is important to educate the patient and his or her family members on this goal of tightly controlled blood glucose. Family members, in an attempt to make the patient feel better, may bring in concentrated sweets for the patient's consumption. Elevated glucose levels require a more frequent dosing interval and higher doses of insulin to bring the glucose levels within the target range.

There is a considerable amount of information for the patient and family members to learn about diabetes and its management. While the nurse is a useful resource for education on glucose monitoring, medications and administration, and how to deal with this illness, a nutritionist can be a helpful resource for dietary information. The more the patients understand about how to manage diabetes the better their blood glucose levels and the fewer the complications they could experience.

SUGGESTED READINGS

Camp RK. Etiology and effect on outcomes of hyperglycemia in hospitalized patients. *Am J Health Syst Pharm.* 2007;64:S4–S8.

Centers for Disease Control and Prevention. 2007 National Diabetes Fact Sheet. Available at: from http://www.cdc.gov/diabetes/pubs/estimates07.htm#1. Accessed June 29, 2008.

Hassan E. Hyperglycemic management in the hospital setting. *Am J Health Syst Pharm.* 2007;64:S9–14.

Smith S, Duell D, Martin B. Parenteral medication administration. In: *Clinical Nursing Skills: Basic to Advanced Skills.* Upper Saddle River, NJ: Pearson; 2008, p. 611.

DIABETICS NEED TO MAINTAIN NORMAL BLOOD SUGAR OF 60–100 MG/DL

BONNIE L. PARKER, RN, CRRN

Diabetes is a disorder of insulin production or action in the body and is a growing epidemic with an estimated 20.8 million people in the United States living with the disease. Diabetes can be divided into two categories: Type I, sometimes referred to as juvenile onset diabetes, and Type II, also referred to as adult onset diabetes. Type I diabetes is an autoimmune disorder in which very little or no insulin is produced by the cells in the pancreas. Due to the lack of insulin production, the patient requires daily subcutaneous injections of insulin. Type I diabetes is most frequently diagnosed during childhood, hence the name "juvenile" diabetes, but it is more appropriate to call it "insulin dependent" diabetes. Unstable Type I diabetes is often referred to as "brittle diabetes" and is marked by radical changes of blood glucose levels from high to low. In addition to insulin, the treatment for Type I diabetes includes diet and exercise. Several different types of insulin are available to treat the diabetic, from short-acting aspart to long-acting glargine. Different types of insulin have different onsets and different half-lives, causing them to remain active for different periods of time. A patient may be prescribed several different types of insulin to give a better coverage for his individual situation. Type I diabetics need to be very conscientious about following a diet regimen and maintaining a health diet and exercise to prevent wide swings in blood glucose levels. With attention to their disease, diabetic patients can lead normal lives.

Type II diabetes is the result of a combination of ineffective insulin uptake and reduced insulin production. The majority of patients diagnosed with diabetes have Type II diabetes, also known as an adult onset disease since it usually occurs with increasing age. However, there has been a growing number of children diagnosed

with this disease, thought once to affect only adults. Type II diabetes occurs more often in the obese, sedentary, and in the elderly. The younger a person is at diagnosis, the higher the risk of developing complications such as blindness, renal failure, neuropathy, and coronary artery disease, and requiring limb amputations.

Symptoms of high blood glucose levels include increased urination, excessive thirst, hunger, fatigue, weight loss, and blurred vision. Due to the progressive onset of Type II diabetes, patients may not exhibit the cardinal symptoms; however, Type I diabetics develop symptoms more rapidly, and the onset may be more acute and emergent.

Normal blood glucose levels range from 60 to 120 mg/dL. A glucose level less than 50 mg/dL is considered an emergency. Not treating a low blood sugar can lead to hypoglycemic coma. Signs of a low blood sugar include weakness, headache, confusion, dizziness, double vision, lack of coordination, drowsiness, convulsions, or unconsciousness. A patient who has had Type I diabetes for many years may not experience or exhibit these signs and symptoms of hypoglycemia as readily as a newly diagnosed patient, tolerating even a glucose levels in the 20s or 30s. It is important that this patient be assessed and treated to prevent a further drop in his or her level. A delay in treating these low levels may result in brain damage or even death.

SUGGESTED READINGS

American Diabetes Association. Available at: http://www.diabetes.org. Accessed April 26, 2008.

American Diabetes Association. Consensus statement: Type 2 diabetes in children and adolescents. *Diab Care*. 2000;23(3): 381–389.

Mauk K. *The Specialty Practice of Rehabilitation Nursing*. Glenview, IL: Association of Rehabilitation Nurses; 2007.

Medical Encyclopedia: Diabetes Medline Plus. U.S. National Library of Medicine and the National Institutes of Health. Available at: http://nlm.nih.gov/medlineplus/ency/article/001214.htm. Accessed April 26, 2008.

WITH DIABETIC PATIENTS, BE AWARE OF PREEXISTING MEDICAL CONDITIONS THAT CAN INFLUENCE THE OUTCOME OF INVASIVE PROCEDURES AND SURGERY

JULIE MULLIGAN WATTS, RN, MN

WHAT TO DO: ASSESS

With the number of older adults rising in the United States, hospitals are seeing a sharply rising number of admissions of adults with chronic illnesses. It is important for nurses to be aware that most illnesses that arise in the aging population will arise against a backdrop of multiple coexisting health problems.

Because diabetes is becoming more common in the United States, it is an excellent example of when nurses must be alert to the sequelae of a chronic disease. From 1980 through 2005, the number of Americans with diabetes increased from 5.6 million to 15.8 million. People of 65 years and above account for approximately 38% of the population with diabetes. In 2005, about 15% of the adults with diabetes reported having had diabetes for more than 20 years. This means that the total number of people coming into hospitals with diabetes has risen and it also means that many have long histories of diabetes.

Among adults discharged from hospitals, who were discharged with diabetes as any listed diagnosis, the top five categories of first-listed discharge diagnoses include circulatory diseases, diabetes, respiratory diseases, digestive diseases, injury, and poisoning. Circulatory diseases (ICD-9-CM Codes 390–459) represented 1,595,000 discharges and accounted for approximately one third of all discharges. Among hospital discharges with diabetes as any listed diagnosis, the number of discharges with a lower extremity condition as a first-listed and as a secondary diagnosis more than doubled from 1980 through 2003. The lower extremity conditions included neuropathy, ulceration, or peripheral arterial disease.

Because people with diabetes are at higher risk for stroke, kidney failure, cardiovascular disease, and peripheral arterial disease than the average person, nurses must be alert for the presence of these conditions, which accompany patients who are admitted for surgeries and other procedures. Nurses should assess patients with a history of diabetes for the effects of vascular disease in places throughout the patient's body such as the kidney, brain, and legs. Note heart or kidney medications and any history of procedures to treat vascular disease. Ask about neuropathy, vision changes due to diabetes, and limited physical activity due to claudication.

For diabetic patients undergoing radiologic procedures, be aware that many agents used as contrast media can be toxic to the kidney, especially when there are preexisting renal changes. Assess renal function by looking at the blood urea nitrogen (BUN), creatinine, and presence of protein in the urine. Radiocontrast-induced renal toxicity is a leading cause of hospital-acquired acute renal failure and may be preventable with hydration or use of other studies that do not require contrast media. Be aware of other drugs that can be nephrotoxic such as antibiotics, especially the sulfonamides and aminoglycosides. Nonsteroidal anti-inflammatory drugs (NSAIDS) and cox-2 inhibitors as well as lithium can cause renal toxicity.

Diabetic patients entering the healthcare system for a variety of tests and procedures need to be identified as patients who are at risk for renal toxicity from a variety of medications. Nurses should be cautious when administering nephrotoxic drugs and should know the toxicities of the drugs they are giving. Nurses should also be attentive to the patient's history of diabetic problems and communicate any concerns to the medical team.

SUGGESTED READINGS

Cohen M. Contrast media posing renal risks. *Nursing.* 2006; 36(7):14.

Department of Health and Human Services, Center for Disease Control and Prevention. Diabetes data and trends. Available at: http://apps.nccd.cdc.gov/ddtstrs/. Accessed May 11, 2008.

Toprak O, Cirit M. Risk factors and therapy strategies for contrast-induced nephropathy. *Ren Fail.* 2006;28:365–381.

WHEN TEACHING ADOLESCENTS NEW INFORMATION ABOUT DIABETES MANAGEMENT, MAKE SURE ALL MEMBERS OF THE HEALTHCARE TEAM ARE WORKING TOGETHER TO MOTIVATE THE PATIENT AND AVOID INCREASING FEAR AND ANXIETY

JULIE MULLIGAN WATTS, RN, MN

WHAT TO DO: IMPLEMENT

A diagnosis of Type 1 insulin dependent diabetes mellitus (IDDM) in a preteen adolescent is a time of crisis within the family. Parents and caretakers, as well as the child, will have concerns about how to manage the disease, long-term care needs, and complications. Feelings of anxiety, fear, and guilt may arise and exhaust the family's ability to cope. In this time of crisis, parents and caretakers may feel physically and emotionally stressed in their supportive role. The adolescent needs to be able to learn the skills to manage IDDM and express feelings about long-term management and coping methods.

One of the major tasks of a nurse with a newly diagnosed patient with IDDM is to work with a team to provide the knowledge and skills to the patient and family/caretakers. This is a team effort that requires a smooth process in order to achieve appropriate goals and outcomes. The patient, family, and other caretakers need information about the disease, insulin therapy, dietary requirements, blood sugar and urine monitoring, exercise and activity, and health promotion. The amount of information and skills that the patient and family are required to learn can be overwhelming, especially in a hospital setting and over a short period of time. Outcome criteria include that the clients verbalize understanding of IDDM, demonstrate correct monitor use, insulin injection, nutritional management, and physical activities.

Learning is an internally controlled process that is mainly controlled by the learner. The learning is affected by the person's motivation, knowledge, skills, and insight. Adolescent learning requires engagement and motivation, as well as interaction with the nurse–teacher team and action or practice of the skills that need to be learned. Adolescents will learn when they are able to apply the skills and discuss the use of the skills in "real-life" situations. The adolescent engages and becomes motivated to learn when the topic is relevant to his or her situation. Also, learning is enhanced when adolescents use previously learned information or life experiences along with the new information and skills. Strategies for the healthcare team that is providing patient education for the adolescent and family include:

- Encouraging the adolescent to take some responsibility for his or her own care by monitoring his or her own progress and understanding;
- Supporting parents and caretakers in allowing the adolescent some control over the disease and treatment;
- Providing teaching in an environment where there is privacy and where interactions can be relaxed and open;
- Pacing the practice of psychomotor skills according to the desires of the adolescent and parents;
- Providing a safe, supportive environment where the team members value input and ideas;
- Use of multiple strategies to acquire, integrate, and apply new knowledge;
- Providing information in ways that are challenging, new, and relevant to their own lives; and
- Minimizing feelings of fear and embarrassment.

Adolescent patients with a chronic disease report that addressing the following factors would help in their learning: ensuring that they receive the knowledge and skills they need by assessing and teaching them what they feel they need to learn; providing teaching in a location conducive to learning; making the education personal and appropriate to the adolescent's developmental level and cognitive abilities; avoiding medical terms; providing emotional support; allowing for two-way communication; and making sure that written information is geared toward the adolescent. Optimizing the patient education experience by teamwork is critical for adolescent patients with IDDM and their families and caretakers. As with other chronic diseases, education is a first step in helping lead adolescents to a lifetime of good habits and effective control of their IDDM.

SUGGESTED READINGS

Beamon G. Supporting and motivating adolescent thinking and learning. 2001. Available at: http://www.phschool.com?eteach?professional_development/adolescent_thinking_learning/essay.html. Accessed May 15, 2008.

Kyngas H. Patient education: Perspective of adolescents with a chronic disease. *J Clin Nurs*. 2003;12:744–751.

Luxner K. *Delmar's Pediatric Nursing Care Plans*. 3rd Ed. Clifton Park, NY: Thomson Delmar Learning; 2005.

Know how to assess diabetic foot ulcers

Jeannie Scruggs Garber, DNP, RN

WHAT TO DO: ASSESS

Diabetic foot ulcers are not uncommon. Approximately 15% of diabetic patients will experience foot ulcers, resulting in approximately 6% being hospitalized. A percentage of those patients will end up with an amputated limb. These statistics are alarming considering that research in this area indicates that foot ulcers can be prevented. According to the American Podiatric Medical Association (APMA), certain ethnic groups, older men, insulin users, those with kidney, eye, and heart diseases, obesity, and alcohol and tobacco use are more susceptible to diabetic ulcers. The ulcers develop as a result of decreased peripheral circulation, pressure, friction, and injury. Other compounding factors include vascular disease and unstable blood glucose levels. Early treatment of foot ulcers decreases the risk for infection and the potential for surgical intervention. The APMA identifies the following as key factors in treating the diabetic foot ulcer and preventing infection:

- Taking the pressure off the area, called "off-loading"
- Removing dead skin and tissue, called "debridement"
- Applying medication or dressings to the ulcer
- Managing blood glucose and other health problems
- Keeping blood glucose levels under tight control
- Keeping the ulcer clean and bandaged
- Cleaning the wound daily, using a wound dressing or bandage
- Avoiding walking barefoot

The Wound, Ostomy, and Continence Nurses Society also published guidelines related to appropriate assessment, prevention, and treatment of diabetic ulcers. A partial listing of additional interventions identified by this group includes

- Perform risk and nutritional assessments
- Assess for history of prior ulcer and presence of current ulcer
- Use turning or lift sheets or devices to turn or transfer patients
- Avoid vigorous massage over bony prominences
- Turn and reposition frequently
- Use pressure-reduction surfaces
- Avoid using foam rings, donuts, and sheepskin for pressure reduction
- Use pressure-relief devices in the operating room
- Reposition chair-bound individuals every hour if they cannot perform pressure-relief exercises every 15 min
- Relieve pressure under heels by using pillows or other devices
- Establish a bowel and bladder program for patients with incontinence

- Use incontinence skin barriers as needed to protect and maintain skin integrity
- Reduce friction and shear
- Cleanse the wound at each dressing change with a non-cytotoxic cleanser, minimizing trauma to the wound
- Evaluate the need for operative repair for patients with Stage III and IV ulcers who do not respond to conservative therapy
- Implement measures to eliminate or control pain
- Educate patients, caregivers, and healthcare providers involved in the continuum of care about prevention, treatment, and factors contributing to recurrence of pressure ulcers
- Monitor vigilantly for recurrence of any pressure ulcers

As with many health issues, prevention should be the focus rather than treatment after the fact. Patients need to be educated on how to minimize their risks and how to assess their feet on a routine basis. They must also be reminded of the importance of properly fitting shoes and socks. The most significant patient-education topics for prevention of diabetic foot ulcers include

- Wash and inspect feet and toes daily
- Minimize the use of lotions
- Maintain appropriate weight
- Avoid smoking and alcohol use
- Cut toenails straight across
- Exercise
- See your physician regularly for a foot exam
- Wear shoes and socks that fit
- Avoid going barefoot
- Do not wear clothing that is constrictive around the legs
- Seek medical assistance when calluses, warts, and corns need to be removed

The healthcare provider and the patient are partners in preventing diabetic foot ulcers and their complications. Whether the patient is being monitored as an outpatient or an inpatient, the assessment, prevention, and treatments listed above are relevant. Prevention of diabetic ulcers is achievable.

SUGGESTED READINGS

American Podiatric Medical Association, Inc. Your podiatric physician talks about diabetic wound care. 2008. Retrieved on July 9, 2008 from http://www.apma.org/s_apma/doc.asp?CID=182&DID=

Guideline for Prevention and Management of Pressure Ulcers. Glenview, IL: Wound, Ostomy, and Continence Nurses Society (WOCN); 2003, p. 52. Available at: http://www.guideline.gov/summary/summary.aspx?ss=15&doc_id=3860&nbr=3071#s2. Accessed July 9, 2008.

COULD YOUR PATIENT WITH NONSPECIFIC SYMPTOMS BE HYPOTHYROID?

SAM HARVEY AND ANTHONY D. SLONIM, MD, DrPH

WHAT TO DO: IMPLEMENT

Hypothyroidism is a condition caused by a deficiency in the thyroid hormone thyroxin. Hypothyroidism is most often caused by an autoimmune disorder known as Hashimoto thyroiditis. Other causes of the disease include radioactive treatment of the thyroid or a thyroidectomy. Many patients who have been diagnosed with head or neck cancer may be at an increased risk for hypothyroidism. The demographic most susceptible to hypothyroidism are women between the ages of 30 and 60. In fact, women are five times as likely to develop the disorder as men (Fig. 171.1).

Few symptoms are present for early hypothyroidism. Some of the most common symptoms include extreme fatigue, hair loss, brittle nails, and dry skin. Variations in the voice causing huskiness and hoarseness may be indicators of the onset of hypothyroidism. As the disease progresses, inordinate weight gain and swelling of the skin (myxedema) may occur. At advanced stages, neurologic function decreases and the patient may appear sullen or apathetic. Speech may become slow or slurred and the extremities may swell. The patient may become cold in a warm environment.

The primary treatment for hypothyroidism involves the replacement of thyroxine using synthetic solutions such as Synthroid or Levothroid. However, several complications can occur due to the alteration of metabolic function when the thyroxine is introduced. Long-term hypothyroidism often results in elevated cholesterol levels, atherosclerosis, and coronary artery disease, placing a patient at severe risk for heart disease. If a patient has remained undiagnosed for a long period of time, it may be appropriate to begin preventative treatment for cardiac dysfunction. A sudden increase in thyroxin may also elevate blood glucose, necessitating insulin adjustment for diabetics with hypothyroidism. Other adverse medication interactions occurring alongside thyroxin administration include amplification of glycosides, anticoagulant agents, and indomethacin. Bone loss and osteoporosis are also side effects of thyroid therapy.

As a hypothyroid patient experiences extreme fatigue, it is important to prevent immobilization complications by requiring regular exercise in a treatment plan. Hypothyroid patients are also often immensely sensitive to cold and should be provided with adequate blankets and clothing to prevent discomfort. Heating pads and electric blankets are not recommended due to vasodilation and subsequent loss of body heat. Due to the physically and mentally altering symptoms of hypothyroidism, counseling should be available for patients experiencing emotional stress. Depression is also common even after treatment is successful. As most treatment for hypothyroidism occurs at home, it is important to continue to monitor patients under emotional duress once home administration of thyroxin is achieved.

SUGGESTED READINGS

American Association of Clinical Endocrinologists (AACE) Thyroid Task Force. AACE medical guidelines for clinical practice for the evaluation and treatment of hyperthyroidism and hypothyroidism. *Endocr Pract.* 2002;8(6):457–469.

Smeltzer S, Bare B, Hinkle J, et al. *Textbook of Medical-Surgical Nursing.* Philadelphia, PA: Lippincott Williams & Wilkins; 2008.

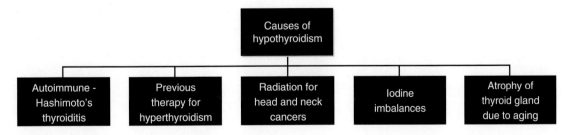

FIGURE 171.1. The causes of hypothyroidism.

EVALUATING FOR HYPOPARATHYROIDISM IN PATIENTS AFTER NECK SURGERY

EDWARD HUMERICKHOUSE, MS, MD

WHAT TO DO: EVALUATE

Hypoparathyroidism occurs in 1% to 2% of patients undergoing neck surgery and needs to be evaluated in the postoperative period. The parathyroid system is concerned with managing the body's calcium. At the system's core are four very small glands approximately of the size of a pencil eraser. These four glands are immediately posterior to the four corners of the thyroid gland. They each have a single blood vessel that feeds them. Parathyroid hormone (PTH) is the principal mechanism of these glands for regulating blood calcium levels. The basic idea is that when blood calcium levels get low, the parathyroid glands secrete more PTH. This mobilizes calcium from bones, decreases calcium loss from the urine, and stimulates Vitamin D to increase absorption from food. When there is no PTH to coordinate this activity, blood calcium levels fall.

The most common cause of low parathyroid hormone involves manipulation of the tissue surrounding it. Total and subtotal thyroidectomies are the usual culprits due to the proximity of these small and inconspicuous glands to the bulky goiter that is being removed. They can also be removed during neck dissections for various cancers in the area as they look very similar to the lymph nodes. Unless all the four glands are removed or their fragile blood supply destroyed, the glands are generally able to recover their function over a period of weeks after the surgery. In the meantime, calcium levels can become dangerously low, and it is important for nurses to recognize the signs and symptoms of hypocalcemia.

Luckily, the effects of hypocalcemia are fairly consistent and easily recognizable. Usually, the postoperative course has been uncomplicated with prompt extubation in the OR and uneventful stay in the postoperative area. As the anesthesia begins to wear off, patients may begin to complain about tingling of the lips, vague symptoms like abdominal pain and generally feeling unwell. At later stages, the patient involuntarily flexes his wrist and cries out in pain (Trousseau sign) when the blood pressure cuff is used. Seizures may be the presenting sign. The diagnosis is made with an ionized calcium level and the treatment is with IV calcium gluconate. The patient's symptoms resolve as soon as the calcium infusion is complete.

Hypocalcemia is common after surgery of the thyroid and parathyroids. Nurses can help identify these patients early through appropriate assessments and evaluation and the routine monitoring of the ionized calcium level.

SUGGESTED READINGS

Algus Z. Clinical manifestations of hypocalcemia. Uptodate Online Version 16.2, October 2006. Available at: http://www.uptodate.com/patients/content/topic.do?topicKey=~fTMU ErxAXkcXM&selectedTitle=2~149&source=search_result. Accessed August 18, 2008.

Algus Z. Etiology of hypocalcemia in adults. Uptodate Online Version 16.2, April 2008. Available at: http://www.uptodate.com/patients/content/topic.do;jsessionid=DFE178D5D93DE7AB52 2EF0E32CF52AB7.1103?topicKey=~cYPyJHUC2sB2c&selecte dTitle=6~42&source=search_result. Accessed August 18, 2008.

KNOW THE IMPORTANT ASPECTS OF INSULIN PHYSIOLOGY

EDWARD HUMERICKHOUSE, MS, MD

WHAT TO DO: PLAN

Insulin dosing is confusing, but it is necessary for all healthcare professionals to know. Which insulin to use, when to give it, and when to hold it must all be considered carefully. Insulin is a necessary protein hormone exclusively produced by the pancreas. It is required for sugar in blood to be transported into the cells where it is used. There are two basic situations when insulin needs to be given: (1) the pancreas stopped producing insulin and (2) the amount of insulin produced by the pancreas is not enough to meet the body's needs. The most recognizable cause of total loss of insulin production (1) is Type I (juvenile) diabetes; however, this can also happen with patients who suffer from chronic pancreatitis or who have "burnt out" their pancreas after years of Type II (adult) diabetes. Insulin insufficiency (2) is almost exclusively found in Type II diabetics who, for various reasons, have become insensitive to the effects of insulin.

The best way to approach insulin is to divide it into categories based on length of action. There are essentially four categories: (1) long, (2) intermediate, (3) short, and (4) very short. The application of the different types of insulins is based on which category the insulin falls into.

There are basically two long-acting insulins. The first is Lantus (glargine). It lasts between 18 and 24 h, so it is usually given just once a day (traditionally at night). The other is Levemir (detemir). It lasts between 12 and 18 h, so it can be given once or twice daily. These are used to provide "basal" insulin needs. In other words, these insulins keep patients from being hyperglycemic even when they are fasting. Since they cover only the baseline needs of the body, they generally need to be supplemented with short- or very short-acting insulin for prevention of hyperglycemia. This results in a LOT of shots. But, on the other side, there is no real "peak" of insulin activity; therefore, they are generally less likely to cause hypoglycemia if patients miss a meal. This sort of insulin dosing is making its way into hospital protocols.

The only intermediate-acting insulin is NPH. This insulin will last about 8 to 12 h, and it is also generally used to provide a basal insulin usually on a twice-a-day schedule. However, this insulin DOES have a peak and can cause significant hypoglycemia in patients who miss meals. It is usually given in combination with short- or very short-acting insulin as a premixed solution. The most recognizable premix is 70/30 that contains 70% NPH and 30% short acting. This insulin is given at breakfast with the general idea that it will peak in time to cover lunch with the climb to the peak covering the time between the two meals. The trend down from the peak covers the afternoon. It is then given a second time before dinner. If you think about it, this puts the second peak at bed time, hence the "HS snack." When mixed with short-acting insulin, the short-acting part covers breakfast and dinner. As you can see, NPH gets really complicated in the hospital and is generally avoided in patients who are prone to miss meals due to sickness or testing (essentially everyone in the hospital). On an outpatient who has well-scheduled meals with appropriate snacks, every meal can be covered with just two shots of premixed 70/30 insulin, a pretty good deal when compared to the alternative.

The short-acting insulin is "regular" insulin. This was the first insulin and was initially taken from pigs before modern technology allowed for commercial laboratory production. It is used quite often in the hospital as "sliding scale" insulin. Regular insulin is not a "clean" drug. It starts to work between 15 and 30 min; it peaks between 2 and 4 h, and lasts between 5 and 8 h. As with NPH, there is starting to be a move away from routine use of regular insulin as there are safer alternatives. On the other hand, it is really the only insulin for IV use. It is frequently needed in the ER or ICU setting where it is given IV as a drip (DKA) or as a bolus (correction of hyperkalemia). In the outpatient setting, it is useful in patients with insulin pumps or as part of premixed combinations with 70/30 insulin.

There are three ultra-short-acting insulins. These are Apidra (glulisine), NovaLog (asparte), and HumaLog (lispro). All the three have fairly dependable times to onset (5–15 min), times to peak (45–75 min), and lengths of action (2–4 h). They are rapidly becoming the first choice for correcting (sliding scale) and preventing (premeal) hyperglycemia in the hospital and at home. To compare with regular insulin, your pneumonia patient needs premeal insulin. Regular insulin is ordered and is given 30 min before meal time so that it will hopefully start working when the meal starts and reach its peak as the meal is digested. The patient gets nauseated and misses the meal.... Now what? If the patient had an ultra-short-acting insulin ordered, the dose could be scheduled during or even immediately AFTER the meal.

As you can see, insulin can get quite complicated in the hospital, and it is important for nurses to have a basic understanding of which insulin they are giving and why. Patients in the hospital are constantly out of schedule with meal times and even missing meals. As an integral part of the healthcare team, nurses can help ensure that glycemic control is assured and that symptomatic periods are adjusted with changes in the insulin regimen.

SUGGESTED READINGS

Campbell KB, Braithwaite SS. Hospital management of hyperglycemia. *Clin Diab*. 2004;22:81–88. Available at: http://clinical.diabetesjournals.org/cgi/content/full/22/2/81. Accessed August 15, 2008.

McCulloch DK. General principles of insulin therapy in diabetes mellitus. Uptodate Online Version 16.2. October 26, 2007. Available at: http://www.uptodate.com/patients/content/topic.do?topicKey=~ssBBBTKCaCWIU5n&selectedTitle=5~150&source=search_result. Accessed August 15, 2008.

McCulloch DK, Inzucci SE. Management of diabetes mellitus in the acute care setting. Uptodate Online Version 16.2. January 18, 2008. Available at: http://www.uptodate.com/patients/content/topic.do?topicKey=~LZbL0IhVAV2lvR5&selectedTitle=2~150&source=search_result. Accessed August 15, 2008.

INSULIN: KNOW WHEN TO GIVE IT AND WHEN NOT TO

EDWARD HUMERICKHOUSE, MS, MD

WHAT TO DO: IMPLEMENT

One of the primary problems with insulin dosing in the hospital revolves around when you should think twice about giving it. Hypoglycemia is a fairly common problem in acutely ill patients who require hospitalization and can be difficult to recognize due to medications that diminish the common symptoms of diaphoresis, tachycardia, and general nervousness. It is of utmost importance that it be correctly prevented while being aware that an improperly held dose can put a Type I diabetic into diabetic ketoacidosis very rapidly. A couple of scenarios can help with clarifying this problem.

Your Type II diabetic is on insulin glargine (Lantus) daily as a basal insulin with premeal aspart (NovoLog) as well as a correction dose (sliding scale) aspart. It is breakfast time, and your ordered premeal accucheck shows a fasting glucose of 75. The patient clearly does not require a correction dose, but you wonder if it is safe to give his premeal rapid acting and his scheduled Lantus. The answer is "yes" to the aspart, but call the doctor about the Lantus. The basal insulin will theoretically take care of his body's needs even if he does not eat all day. The premeal insulin is designed to keep his sugars from spiking from the meal. Right now, the patient is not hypoglycemic, but actually normoglycemic for a fasting state. But in general, it is better to let diabetics run a "little sweet" in the hospital. Current recommendations suggest a fasting glucose of around 100 and a postmeal peak of less than 180. This means that his Lantus dose is maybe just a little too aggressive. Hopefully, his premeal insulin is enough to cover his breakfast.

What if the same patient above had a fasting sugar of 190 instead of 75? What insulin would you give then? You would give the patient's scheduled basal glargine, his premeal aspart, AND however much correction insulin he is written for on his sliding scale. The patient is hyperglycemic. The premeal insulin will not be enough to keep his sugar in check after his meal when he is starting off high. Make sure that the hyperglycemia as well as how much correction insulin you gave is documented as it will help the patient's primary physician adjust the glargine dose up to the goal.

Your patient in the ICU is on an insulin drip for diabetic ketoacidosis (DKA), but his accuchecks are now approaching normal range. You look through the chart, but there are no parameters about what to do when the patient's glucose normalizes. You call the physician asking for a verbal order to d/c the insulin drip, but he tells you to draw a BMP (basic metabolic panel) and start a dextrose infusion instead. What is going on? In this case, the insulin is not there to correct the patient's sugar as much as it is to turn off the process that is causing his body to create acid. The BMP will allow the physician to measure the amount of acid remaining in the blood. The drip must remain on until all acid is gone from the BMP even if that means giving sugar at the same time.

You have another patient in the ICU who is intubated and on an insulin drip for strict glycemic control while he recovers from severe pneumonia. You receive orders to turn off his continuous tube feeding at midnight as he is going to have a tracheostomy in the morning. The nurse who was covering you for your break turned off the feeding 15 min ago, but the insulin is still running as there was no hold order on it. In this case, you would turn the drip off immediately BEFORE trying to page the physician. You would also need to repeat an accucheck every 3 to 4 h to ensure hypoglycemia does not occur. Remember that most insulin drips are with regular insulin which can stay in the body for up to 8 h.

You have a patient on the regular medical floor who was admitted for pneumonia and has a long history of poor diabetes control as an outpatient. The physician has ordered capillary glucose monitoring before every meal, at bedtime, and at the nurses' discretion. The patient has basal and premeal insulin ordered with a regular insulin sliding scale. At 9 PM, the patient's glucose was 310, which by his sliding scale means that he gets 5 units of regular insulin SC. Your floor requires documentation of outcomes after a nursing intervention, so you reassess his glucose in 1 h and it is 295. As it is still high, another 4 units of regular insulin is given from his sliding scale order. An hour later, his sugar is 253 and another 4 units is given. On the next check, his sugar is finally down to 130, and you breathe a sigh of relief because your nursing goal has been met, and you do not have to wake the patient up to stick his finger until breakfast. At 3 AM, the patient calls you to the room. He is diaphoretic and complaining of loss of function of his right hand. He is tachycardic and his blood pressure is up a little. As one of your colleagues calls the physician, you complete an accucheck...his sugar is 45. He is awake so you give glucose gel per protocol. In 10 min, all of his symptoms are gone and his glucose is 85. You just stepped into the regular insulin sliding scale trap. Remember, it takes at least 30 min for REGULAR insulin to even start working and another 2 to 4 h before it reaches its peak effect. Then, it stays in the system for up to 8 h from the last dose. This patient needs to be given small meal and be checked on regularly the rest of the night. This case also highlights one of the very frightening effects of hypoglycemia: transient paralysis that mimics stroke in otherwise normal people.

These brief cases highlight some of the more common insulin-dosing questions that come up in hospitalized patients. There is no doubt that insulin can be a very difficult medication to manage, and it is not expected of you to know exactly what to do when questions arise. As you can see, it is hard to tell when to hold insulin and when to give it. Never be afraid to call the treating physician with questions, and do not hesitate to check a random glucose in people who you are suspicious may become hypoglycemic.

SUGGESTED READINGS

Campbell KB, Braithwaite SS. Hospital management of hyperglycemia. *Clin Diab*. 2004;22:81–88. Available at: http:// clinical.diabetesjournals.org/cgi/content/full/22/2/81. Accessed August 15, 2008.

McCulloch DK, Inzucchi SE. Management of diabetes mellitus in the acute care setting. Uptodate Online Version 16.2. January 18, 2008. Available at: http://www.uptodate.com/patients/content/ topic.do?topicKey=~LZbL0IhVAV2lvR5& selectedTitle=2~15 0&source=search_result. Accessed August 15, 2008.

KNOW WHAT TO TELL INFERTILE COUPLES ABOUT THEIR CONDITION

ANTHONY D. SLONIM, MD, DrPH

WHAT TO DO: PLAN

Infertility affects approximately 5 million couples in the United States and approximately 14% of reproductive age women. Despite elaborate workups, nearly 20% of infertility remains unexplained. Approximately 60% of infertility is related to the problems experienced by women and 20% are related to men. Nearly 50% of female infertility is due to ovulatory dysfunction of which there is a variety of causes, but the major cause results from hypothalamic or pituitary dysfunction, and 30% relates to polycystic ovarian syndrome. The other causes of female infertility include tubal defects (40%) and endometriosis (10%). The majority of male cases of infertility are of unknown etiology. Primary hypogonadism accounts for approximately 30% to 40% and disordered sperm transport for another 15%.

There are a number of diagnostic tests that can be performed to test the endocrine system of the female. The use of ovulatory stimulants may help improve the chances of ovulation and hence fertilization. Tubal disease is diagnosed using hysterosalpingography, although tubal reconstruction is limited as a treatment modality.

For endometriosis, laparoscopic resection or surgery may be helpful. Beyond diagnosing and attempting treatment by conventional means depending upon the nature of the condition, the nurse dealing with the infertile couple also needs to know about assistive technologies to improve the odds of a successful fertilization including in vitro fertilization. These procedures are not without risk and should be prescribed by those who understand their risks, benefits and alternatives.

The nurse is often an important participant in the care of the infertile couple. The nurse hears their concerns, gets involved in the emotional aspects of the condition, and grieves with the couple as failed fertilization attempts occur. The nurse needs to be a knowledgeable partner who can explain diagnostic studies, encourage the couple when treatment options appear limited, and be able to assist in monitoring side effects of the treatment. For many nurses, infertility treatment is a challenging and rewarding career that is very satisfying.

SUGGESTED READINGS

Hall JE. Infertility and fertility control. In: Kasper DL, Braunwald E, Fauci AS, et al., eds. *Harrison's Principles of Internal Medicine*. 16th Ed. New York: McGraw Hill; 2005, pp. 279–283.

KNOW HOW TO TALK ABOUT PERFORMANCE-ENHANCING DRUGS

ANTHONY D. SLONIM, MD, DRPH

WHAT TO DO: ASSESS

Today's society is more competitive than ever before. This competition transcends almost every compartment of the society including academic life, work life, school life, and even social life. In no other area is the need to be bigger, better, and faster more evident than in sports and athletics. Here, there is a "win at all costs" mentality for some that have the potential for long lasting physical and emotional consequences. The nurse is positioned to identify the use of these drugs, by virtue of their physical effects but is also in a position to counsel against their use.

Performance-enhancing drugs come in a number of categories and include steroids, diuretics, growth hormone, and erythropoietin products. Many of these are used for medical indications, but when available in the underground market these drugs can be administered to young athletes in unsafe conditions in the locker room without adequate monitoring of their side effects.

Anabolic steroids enhance the bulk, mass, and power of muscles. These agents are usually synthetic compounds of testosterone and allow athletes to perform better and recover faster from aggressive workouts. While they have medical indications for men with testosterone deficiency, their use to enhance physical performance is illegal. The doses used to enhance performance are usually considerably higher than for medical uses and the side effects seen include acne, behavioral and mood changes, hirsutism, balding, increased appetite and reduced fat, and increased lipids. Importantly, when injected, the risks of illnesses like hepatitis and HIV increase, since these are usually performed in unsterile conditions.

Creatine is a natural compound found in proteins that release adenosine triphosphate (ATP), the energy packets of cells. These agents enhance the ability of muscle for quick bursts of activity. The side effects include nausea, vomiting, diarrhea, and muscle cramping when taken in excess.

Stimulants are drugs that are used to reduce fatigue and enhance performance. These agents work by enhancing the activity of the central nervous system and increasing alertness. They are commonly used to maintain alertness and reduce drowsiness during driving. Agents in this category include caffeine, Dexedrine, and other stimulants that reduce appetite and increase alertness. The complications include weight loss, anxiety, palpitations, headaches, and problems with the vascular system.

Finally, erythropoietin agents are compounds that enhance the production of red blood cells (RBCs). RBCs carry oxygen and are of use for long distance runners and bikers where oxygen-dependent activity of the muscles enhances their performance. When taken in high levels, too many RBCs can be produced, and the patient's risk of clotting disorders increases.

There are a number of ethical concerns about the use of performance-enhancing drugs in competitive sports. Regardless of these ethical dilemmas, the nurse is well positioned to share concrete information about the short- and long-term health risks of these products for athletes young and old.

SUGGESTED READINGS

Botrè F, Pavan A. Enhancement drugs and the athlete. *Neurol Clin*. 2008;26(1):149–67, abstract ix.

Laos C, Metzl JD. Performance-enhancing drug use in young athletes. *Adolesc Med Clin*. 2006;17(3):719–31, abstract xii.

MayoClinic.com. Taking performance-enhancing drugs: Are you risking your health. Available at: http://www.mayoclinic.com/health/performance-enhancing-drugs/HQ01105. Accessed August 31, 2008.

NOT ALL ABNORMALITIES IN THYROID HORMONE REQUIRE TREATMENT

ANTHONY D. SLONIM, MD, DRPH

Nurses are often faced with laboratory results and are responsible for transmission of the results for appropriate action. As the intermediary, it can often become difficult to wonder why something may not need to be done when a result is outside of the normal range. Thyroid hormones are particularly important in this regard since thyroid hormones have long half-lives. Increasing the dosage of thyroxine is not likely to affect the laboratory results for some time. It is important to know not only the laboratory result, but also what is going on with the patient so that an appropriate decision can be made on potential interactions and underlying causes for the deranged results.

The nurse needs to remember that the thyroid is an intricate endocrine organ that receives stimulation from the hypothalamic pituitary axis through the action of thyroid stimulating hormone (TSH). Acute illness can affect the levels of circulating TSH and thyroid hormones, even when there is no significant thyroid disease. Some would argue that the testing of thyroid function during hospitalization is a waste of time unless the thyroid is strongly suspected as the culprit in the presenting illness. Nonetheless, providers often order these tests and are then often left trying to figure out what to do with the results. The nurse needs to know what aspects of treatment can alter thyroid hormone levels and when it is perfectly alright not to worry about it.

Sick Euthyroid Syndrome is a condition that accompanies serious illness and results in normal T4 and TSH while the T3 is low. The patients are not symptomatic and do not require thyroid hormone replacement. In addition, the nurse has to be aware of how other aspects of treatment can affect the laboratory values. For example, the administration of steroids, dopamine, amiodarone, and cortisol can lead to wide variations in the TSH, but these changes are not reflective of a change in the patient's condition and do not require treatment.

Finally, illnesses involving other organ systems can affect the results on a given test. The inability of the liver to produce thyroid binding globulin alters the free thyroid hormone levels, but since the patient is unaffected and the reason for the change in the levels is easily understood by the underlying disease, no treatment is necessary.

Thyroid is a complicated organ that is often tested during hospitalization. The nurse needs to know when it is as important not to treat for a given laboratory test as when to treat.

SUGGESTED READINGS

Jameson JL, Weetman AP. Disorders of the thyroid gland. In: Kasper DL, Braunwald E, Fauci AS, et al., eds. *Harrison's Principles of Internal Medicine*. 16th Ed. New York: McGraw Hill; 2005, pp. 2104–2127.

Think about secondary adrenocortical insufficiency in your patients taking steroids long term... You may save a life

Anthony D. Slonim, MD, DrPH

WHAT TO DO: IMPLEMENT

Steroids are very useful agents for a variety of diseases ranging from asthma to systemic rheumatologic disorders. While there are a number of side effects associated with these medications, their value in these diseases outweighs their risks and contributes to improved life for patients that would have otherwise died. These risks include hyperglycemia, obesity, and skin and visual changes including cataracts. Perhaps one of the most important side effects is the resulting adrenocortical insufficiency that develops through the administration of these medications. These drugs provide negative feedback through the hypothalamic pituitary axis (HPA) to shut down the production of adrenocorticotrophic hormone (ACTH) since the body perceives that there is an ample supply of these hormones already present. The problem is that at times of stress, like an operative intervention or critical illness, the patients may experience a relative adrenal insufficiency because their HPA is lying dormant and has not been restarted.

Patients with adrenal insufficiency experience a low baseline rate of endogenous steroid production. These patients have a low level of circulating blood cortisol and ACTH. Ultimately, these patients will recover the function of their HPA access and begin to produce ACTH and cortisol appropriately, but it may not be for weeks to months. If exogenous steroids are not ordered and tapered during this interval, the patients can become symptomatic because their adrenal gland is atrophic.

One rule of thumb is to supply exogenous steroids for anyone who has taken steroids within the last 6 months who is undergoing a surgical procedure or critical illness. The complications and side effects from the short administration of steroids are safer than the unrecognized adrenal insufficiency that may go undetected.

Adrenal insufficiency can be a silent condition. The nurse is in a position to reconcile the medication list and highlight the need for steroids to be ordered if it is not recognized by the physician. By doing so, the nurse may save a life.

SUGGESTED READINGS

Arafah BM. Hypothalamic pituitary adrenal function during critical illness: Limitations of current assessment methods. *J Clin Endocrinol Metab*. 2006;91(10):3725–3745.

Cunningham SK, Moore A, McKenna TJ. Normal cortisol response to corticotropin in patients with secondary adrenal failure. *Arch Intern Med*. 1983;143(12):2276–2279.

Williams GH, Dluhy RG. Disorders of the adrenal cortex. In: Kasper DL, Braunwald E, Fauci AS, et al., eds. *Harrison's Principles of Internal Medicine*. 16th Ed. New York: McGraw Hill; 2005, pp. 2142–2143.

NOTHING IS EVER AS SIMPLE AS IT SEEMS... PARTICULARLY WHEN THE ENDOCRINE SYSTEM IS INVOLVED

ANTHONY D. SLONIM, MD, DRPH

WHAT TO DO: ASSESS AND EVALUATE

The nurse is often put in the position of being presented with a condition, a lab finding, and a diagnosis at admission that provides a "label" for what to expect of a patient. The nurse then incorporates their understanding of this disease into the care of this patient. However, patients do not read the textbooks and it is rare that they present with a singular condition. Certainly, all of us have seen the 20-something diabetic with diabetic ketoacidosis, who, by virtue of their young age, come in gravely ill and are discharged home within 24h on a tailored insulin regimen. But this is not the norm, particularly for diseases of the endocrine system, and nurses need to consistently assess and evaluate for findings that affect more than one endocrine organ since these diseases often occur together.

Polyglandular autoimmune syndromes occur when immune dysfunction of two or more endocrine glands is present simultaneously. There are two types: Type I occurs in children and Type II occurs in adults. Type I patients present with candidiasis, hypothyroidism, adrenal insufficiency, hepatitis, and hypoparathyroidism. They can live for long periods of time, and ongoing evaluation for endocrine abnormalities is required. Type II disorders include adrenal insufficiency, hypothyroidism, Graves disease, hypogonadism, and diabetes. Both these conditions usually present over time with slowly progressive adrenal insufficiency. Screening measures are often helpful when there is concern, but the nurse who sees a patient with adrenal insufficiency should consider coexisting illnesses of the endocrine system caused by this autoimmune disease.

Another group of endocrine diseases known as the multiple endocrine neoplasias (MEN) syndromes are also genetic in origin and consist of multiple endocrine abnormalities. For these patients, parathyroid abnormalities are usually the disease that should trigger further investigation. MEN syndromes are classified as MEN 1, which consists of (1) Hyperparathyroidism, which presents as hypercalcemia, (2) pancreatic islet cell tumors, (3) pituitary neoplasms, and (4) adrenal or thyroid involvement. MEN II syndromes are divided into two types, MEN 2A and MEN 2B. Both these have pheochromocytoma and medullary carcinoma of the thyroid as major components. Patients with 2B also have mucosal neuromas.

Patients with one endocrine disorder often have another. There are several well-described endocrine associations. The nurse needs to be aware of the associations and continue to assess and evaluate for abnormalities that do not fit a specific pattern of disease.

SUGGESTED READINGS

Berger JR, Weaver A, Greenlee J, et al. Neurologic consequences of autoimmune polyglandular syndrome type 1. *Neurology*. 2008;70(23):2248–2251.

Callender GG, Rich TA, Perrier ND. Multiple endocrine neoplasia syndromes. *Surg Clin North Am*. 2008;88(4):863–895.

López-Jornet P, García-Ballesta C, Pérez-Lajarín L. Mucocutaneous candidiasis as first manifestation of autoimmune polyglandular syndrome type I. *J Dent Child (Chic)*. 2005;72(1):21–24.

Sherman SI, Gagel RF. Disorders affecting multiple endocrine systems. In: Kasper DL, Braunwald E, Fauci AS, et al., eds. *Harrison's Principles of Internal Medicine*. 16th Ed. New York: McGraw Hill; 2005, pp. 2231–2238.

Topaloglu AK, Yuksel B, Yilmaz M, et al. Coexistence of common variable immunodeficiency and autoimmune polyglandular syndrome type 2. *J Pediatr Endocrinol Metab*. 2001;14(5): 565–566.

WATCH FOR THE ENDOCRINE CHANGES ASSOCIATED WITH SPECIFIC CANCERS

ANTHONY D. SLONIM, MD, DRPH

WHAT TO DO: ASSESS AND EVALUATE

Malignancies can cause a number of problems related to the unencumbered growth of cells. Usually, these are manifested by mass effects, obstruction, and other symptoms related to the organ in which the cancer arose. However, there are a number of cancers that have some very well defined effects distant from the site of the tumor. The effects are often endocrine in nature but may affect the hematologic or neurologic systems as well. It is important for the nurse to have an awareness of these symptoms and their occurrence with particular types of cancers.

Hypercalcemia of malignancy is a commonly occurring paraneoplastic syndrome that occurs in approximately 5% of patients. There are two major ways in which it occurs. First, it is associated with the production of a parathyroid hormone-related protein that binds to parathyroid hormone receptors and creates a hyperparathyroid like state. The second method is through the production of 1, 25 dihydroxyvitamin D that enhances calcium absorption from the gastrointestinal tract. These patients often have a squamous cell tumor of the head and neck, lung, breast, or gastrointestinal tract or a lymphoma. The major treatment strategy is hydration, excretion, and binding of the calcium.

The syndrome of inappropriate antidiuretic hormone (SIADH) or ectopic vasopressin production occurs in small cell and squamous cell cancer of the lung.

These patients experience hyponatremia and the associated symptoms, including weakness, confusion, and nausea. The treatment is fluid restriction. Demeclocycline may need to be used while the treatment for the cancer takes place.

Finally, Cushing syndrome from ectopic adrenocorticotrophic hormone (ACTH) production occurs in a number of cancers, including small cell carcinoma of the lung, thymus, pancreas, and thyroid. These patients experience symptoms of cortisol excess, including hypertension, fluid overload, hyperglycemia, and metabolic alkalosis. Patients can be treated with ketoconazole or metapyrone to block steroid synthesis, which is often the most practical solution.

Paraneoplastic syndrome is yet another thing that cancer patients and their providers need to worry about. These syndromes are associated with annoying and life limiting symptoms and require treatment that is beyond that of the primary malignancy.

SUGGESTED READINGS

Biller BM, Grossman AB, Stewart PM, et al. Treatment of adrenocorticotropin-dependent Cushing's syndrome: A consensus statement. *J Clin Endocrinol Metab.* 2008;93(7): 2454–2462.

Cho S, Ra YJ, Lee CT, et al. Difficulties in diagnosis and management of ectopic Cushing syndrome. *J Thorac Oncol.* 2008;3(4):444–446.

Jameson JL, Johnson BE. Paraneoplastic syndromes: Endocrinologic/hematologic. In: Kasper DL, Braunwald E, Fauci AS, et al., eds. *Harrison's Principles of Internal Medicine.* 16th Ed. New York: McGraw-Hill; 2005, pp. 566–571.

FOOD CONSISTENCIES ARE REALLY DIFFERENT AND CAN AFFECT A PATIENT'S ABILITY TO SWALLOW

ALICE M. CHRISTALDI, RN, BSN, CRRN

WHAT TO DO: ASSESS

Swallowing difficulties are a very common problem in today's healthcare environment. Dysphagia is a general term to describe an obstruction of the passage of food or liquids from the mouth down through the esophagus. The causes can be mechanical such as congenital defects, strictures, or tumors, and diseases of the cerebral cortex and brainstem such as dementia, stroke, encephalopathy, brain injuries, Parkinson disease, and neuropathy. There might be esophageal mechanical dysphagia caused by wall defects, webs and rings, and tumors or an esophageal motor dysphagia characterized by diseases of the smooth muscle or a diffuse esophageal spasm.

Swallowing is a complex act involving a coordinated effort of the tongue, pharynx, and esophagus. People generally swallow once every minute or 1,000 times a day. One classifies dysphagia by the affected swallowing phase. The "oral" phase occurs when the tongue presses against the hard palate and transfers food that has been chewed to the back of the throat. The "pharyngeal" phase starts when the soft palate closes against the wall of the pharynx to prevent regurgitation into the nose. At the same time, the larynx rises up and vocal cords close to keep the food from advancing into the lungs. The throat muscles constrict to move food bolus into the esophagus. Finally, the "esophageal" phase occurs as food moves through the esophagus into the stomach.

When a person presents with swallowing difficulties, generally, he will be evaluated to determine the underlying causes. A speech therapist may be consulted to complete a swallowing assessment and make recommendations for an appropriate diet. Detailed histories are necessary and provide guidance as to the etiology of the problem. A barium swallow or esophagoscopy may be ordered.

A number of diets are available to assist with the mechanics of swallowing. A soft diet is easy to chew and digest and contains foods such as plain custards, mashed potatoes, smooth cooked cereals such as grits, and fruit nectars. Mechanically altered diets consist of foods that have been chopped, such as ground up meats, cut up pasta, and cut up cooked vegetables. Pureed diets contain foods that have been placed in a blender and made smooth. They therefore require minimal chewing or bolus formation.

Liquids can be thickened to assist in swallowing. Nectar thick liquids include apricot nectar and are thicker cream soups. They are easily pourable. Honey thickened liquids are slightly thicker and less pourable from a spoon. Pudding consistency items hold their shape and cannot be poured but must be eaten with a spoon. This category includes applesauce or pudding. There are several commercial thickeners available, and several of them are provided with small cups with nectar- or honey-thickened liquids already prepared which can be kept in the refrigerator. Thickened liquids taste better when cold. Tomato juice has formally been thought to be nectar thick, but in reality, it needs to have a thickener added to make it so.

Another strategy to assist the patient with swallowing is to have the patient tuck his or her chin, which aids the passage of food. However, knowing what foods to avoid is also important. Ice should not be added to drinks that must be thickened since it will dilute them. "Juicy fruits" that are heavy in water content, such as oranges and watermelon, should be avoided since choking on the thinner juices is a real possibility. Suction should be readily available and in working order. The patients should be sitting up when they are eating or drinking and alcoholic beverages should be avoided since they interfere with effective swallowing and impair the cough and gag reflexes.

Small food particles that can be found in foods such as rice, peas, or nuts should be avoided as should sticky foods, including peanut butter and honey. A chin tuck can be very helpful in managing to swallow liquids or foods.

Since the thickening of liquids alters their taste, patients prefer to attempt mechanical means first, such as the chin tuck or double swallow method. Remember to provide the correct food consistency for your patient and, in case of difficulty, be prepared with emergency suction equipment.

SUGGESTED READINGS

Logemann JA. Medical and rehabilitative therapy of oral pharyngeal motor disorders GI motility. GI Motility Online.2006. doi:10.1038/gimo50. Available at: www.nature.com/gimo/contents/pt1/full/gimo50.html. Accessed April 3, 2008.

MAINTAIN A ROUTINE BOWEL REGIMEN FOR YOUR PATIENT

MONTY D. GROSS, PhD, RN, CNE

WHAT TO DO: ASSESS AND IMPLEMENT

Bowel management is an important responsibility of healthcare providers. When patients enter the hospital, their diet changes, activity decreases, and medications are often ordered that increase the risk of constipation. Monitoring bowel routines and preventing constipation is important and considerably better than dealing with problems including fecal impaction.

Constipation is defined as having less than three bowel movements per week. Having hard dry stool or having to strain >25% of the time spent passing stool is also considered constipation. Constipation causes abdominal and rectal pain, nausea, vomiting, and discomfort. Feelings of anorexia, restlessness, and confusion can also result. Having a bowel movement every other day is recommended to avoid constipation. Frequency, consistency, and volume of the stool should be assessed.

The nurse needs to assess for the risk factors that could cause constipation and implement interventions to address the identified risks. Pay attention to the patient's diet and activity level. Is the patient receiving enough fiber? Is the patient ambulating or at least getting into a chair? Peristalsis is enhanced with ambulation and physical activity. Consider the patient's privacy. If the patient is self conscious, like most healthy people, he or she may ignore the desire to defecate in a bedpan or room where others will experience the odor.

Interventions to prevent constipation should start before signs and symptoms of constipation manifest. Assess the patient daily for bowel pattern. Ensure patient privacy and adequate nutrition with fiber. Ensure they are receiving adequate fluids. Encourage the patient to use the bathroom if possible. Offer assistance as needed. If the patient cannot use the bathroom, provide a bedside commode or bedpan. If the patient does have a bowel movement, do your best to help the patient feel like it was not an imposition or that they should be embarrassed. Otherwise, they would be more likely to suppress their need to have a bowel movement in the future, hence increasing their risk for constipation.

Generally, stool softeners can be used on a short term basis to relieve constipation. Colace or Docusate capsules or liquid can be given once or twice a day. They work by softening stool to make it easier to pass through the colon and rectum. Stimulant laxatives are used to treat constipation. They work by increasing the peristaltic movement in the bowel. Stimulant laxatives come in many different forms, including liquids, powders, granules, tablets, and suppositories. Bisacodyl, Dulcolax, and Senokot are examples of laxatives. Bulk forming laxatives, such as Metamucil or FiberCon, are used to treat chronic constipation and take several days to work. It is important to take bulk laxatives with a generous amount of fluids to prevent obstruction. Osmotic laxatives work by drawing water into the bowel. Examples of osmotic laxatives include lactulose and sorbital. These laxatives can take 1 to 3 days to work. A stimulant laxative should be administered with osmotic laxatives if there is reduced bowel motility.

More invasive approaches include suppositories, digital stimulation, and enemas. Remember, if a patient has a spinal cord injury, to watch for signs of autonomic hyper-reflexia. These signs include goose pimples, pounding headache, hypertension, and perspiration above the level of the injury. If these appear, discontinue digital stimulation.

Osmotic enemas are the most powerful and fastest acting laxatives. A variety of choices are available, including simple soap suds, tap water, and saline. Remember that it is much easier to prevent constipation than to have to resort to these alternatives. Assess your patient daily for bowel pattern and intervene appropriately.

SUGGESTED READINGS

Coggrave M, Burrows D, Durand M. Progressive management in the bowel management of spinal cord injuries. *Br J Nurs.* 2006;15(20):1108–1113.

Ross H. Constipation: Cause and control in an acute care hospital setting. *Br J Nurs.* 1998;7(15):907–913.

Smith S, Duell D, Martin B. *Clinical Nursing Skills: Basic to Advanced Skills.* Upper Saddle River, NJ: Pearson; 2008.

TUBE FEEDING INTERRUPTIONS

MONTY D. GROSS, PhD, RN, CNE

WHAT TO DO: IMPLEMENT

We often take nutrition for granted. Generally, we consume food and beverage three times a day to provide the nutrients our body needs to function, stay healthy, or recover from injury. When a person is ill or injured and requires hospitalization, the importance of nutrition is given a low priority and, at times, simply overlooked. At a time when the body's cells are craving nutrients to replenish energy or repair tissue, healthcare providers interrupt meals, discontinue tube feedings, or fail to provide the proper diet. Approximately only 59% to 87% of prescribed formula is actually delivered during hospitalization.

A major factor resulting in interruption of tube feedings is unintentional extubation. This can occur when the patient becomes confused or restless. The caregiver can also accidentally dislodge the tube while providing care.

A variety of procedures and tests, such as central line placement and X-rays, are performed during mealtime. The patient may start to eat but is interrupted so that he or she may be taken to another area of the hospital to have the procedure or test performed. By the time he or she returns to the meal, it is cold and less appealing than it was at first. Offering to microwave the food frequently leaves the meal tough to chew.

Tube feedings are stopped so that they do not interfere with the absorption of some medications. The drug administration information for Phenytoin, for example, states that tube feeding should be stopped 1 h before and be left off for 1 h after the drug's administration to improve absorption. Although the number of calories may take into account this interruption, the actual time during which the feeding is withheld may be longer than ideal due to the nurse being distracted by taking care of other patients and not being able to return to resume the feeding on schedule.

Patients are kept NPO while physicians debate a plan of care or are awaiting a consult. Does the patient need a surgery or a procedure that requires the patient to be NPO? The decision is not always forthcoming. Laboratory results need to arrive and discussions weighed. These are just several possible reasons the patient may not receive adequate nutrition.

What can be done to minimize interruptions to the tube feeding and ensure the delivery of the prescribed amount of nutritional calories? First, educate the patient on the need for the tube and ensure that the tube is secured. If the patient is confused or restless, regularly reorient to the environment. Encourage family members to monitor the patient and keep the patient from pulling out the tube. If the tube is removed before intended, do not waste time getting it reinserted. Remember to check for proper placement before restarting the nutrition or administering medication.

To prevent unnecessary interruptions from medication administration or procedures, plan accordingly. If tube feedings must be stopped an hour before or after a particular medication, set an alarm or use another strategy to remind yourself to restart the feeding as soon as possible. Consult with a pharmacist for alternative medications that would not require the stoppage of the tube feeding and work with diagnostic departments to minimize tube feeding interruptions.

SUGGESTED READINGS

Morgan L, Dickerson R, Alexander K, et al. Factors causing interrupted delivery of enteral nutrition in trauma intensive care unit patients. *Nutr Clin Pract*. 2004;19:511–517.

Whelan K, Hill L, Preedy V, et al. Formula delivery in patients receiving enteral tube feeding on general hospital wards: The impact of nasogastric extubation and diarrhea. *Nutrition*. 2006;27(10):1025–1031.

STOP THE TPN BEFORE OBTAINING LABS FROM THE CENTRAL LINE

BONNIE L. PARKER, RN, CRRN

WHAT TO DO: IMPLEMENT

Total parenteral nutrition (TPN) is the supplemental nutrition administered through an intravenous line to patients who are unable to take adequate nutrition through the gastrointestinal tract. TPN is composed of dextrose, carbohydrates, proteins, lipids, electrolytes, and trace elements. Due to its potential to cause tissue damage, TPN is usually administered through a central venous line.

Because of its composition, TPN is a perfect breeding ground for bacteria and must be handled carefully to reduce the risk of infection. The container or bag should be inspected before hanging and discarded if any leaks are noted. Typically, TPN infusions are hung daily with enough volume in the container to last for 24 h. The line is only accessed when the bag and tubing are changed. Many hospitals do not allow TPN tubing to be accessed or other infusions to run through the same port as the TPN so that the risk of contamination and incompatibility of fluids is minimized.

It is important to assess the patient's nutritional level while on TPN and labs, such as blood urea nitrogen (BUN), complete blood count (CBC), and prealbumin and electrolyte levels, are typically drawn daily. Many patients who require TPN are also the patients who are very difficult to obtain blood samples on. Hence, the central venous line becomes the only choice for drawing these labs.

To reduce the risk of infection and damage to the line, and to obtain the proper specimen, the correct technique must be followed. The blood specimen should be obtained by an RN credentialed to draw blood from a central line; complications can include occlusion, thrombosis, and infection. Not following correct procedure for the lab draw could yield incorrect lab results that could lead to improper and even dangerous treatment for the patient.

If any intravenous fluids are infusing at the time the labs are to be drawn, they must be stopped for at least a minute prior to drawing the blood even if they are infusing through a port other than the one intended for the lab draw. In a multilumen catheter, fluids infuse out of the lumens at slightly different angles but are still close enough that a blood draw through the central line has the potential for aspirating the infusing fluids. Neglecting to stop the infusion of TPN during a lab draw could provide erroneous lab results for glucose or electrolyte levels. To treat a patient based on these results would be harmful, even potentially fatal.

After discontinuing the fluids for one minute and using good hand hygiene, the nurse should put on gloves and clean the port with alcohol using a scrubbing motion. The line should first be flushed with at least 10 mL of normal saline and then using a 10 mL syringe, gently aspirate 5 to 10 mL of blood as waste. This blood will contain any fluids that were in the lumen that would invalidate the results. Drawing too forcefully can cause the lumen of the catheter and the vein to collapse. After wasting the first 10 mL, another syringe should be used with the same technique and the required amount of blood should be obtained for submission to the laboratory. After obtaining the blood specimen, the line should be flushed with at least 10 mL of normal saline and the TPN restarted. It is vital that strict aseptic technique be used throughout the procedure.

SUGGESTED READINGS

Arrow International. Arrow multi-lumen central venous catheter care, catheter maintenance, blood sampling. 12/94. pp. 105–111.

Guenter P. Monitoring total parenteral nutrition therapy in the elderly. *The Consultant Pharmacist.* Available at: www.ascp.com/public/pubs/tcp/1999/apr/monnut.shtml. Accessed May 13, 2008.

IS IT JUST CONSTIPATION OR IS IT SOMETHING MORE SERIOUS?

EDWARD HUMERICKHOUSE, MS, MD

WHAT TO DO: ASSESS, IMPLEMENT, AND EVALUATE

Constipation is an exceedingly common complaint both in the hospital and in the outpatient setting. An astute nurse will not only recognize constipation early in a hospitalization and therefore be able to provide great relief for a distressing patient concern, but he or she will also be the first in line in recognizing when benign constipation converts to the potentially deadly obstruction.

A key component to winning a patient over on a personal level by minimizing distress is to keep their bowels running smoothly. The last thing a patient under stress in the hospital needs is for hemorrhoids to get clotted from straining to move his bowels. A quick assessment question on presentation to the unit about bowel health will provide a nurse the ability to be proactive about keeping patients regular by making sure that the doctor knows that the patient has been taking miralax over the counter daily to maintain bowel regularity. Another place to advocate for your patients is to confirm that anyone who is on narcotics is also written for scheduled or PRN stool softeners. As always, the documentation of the color and consistency of stool in the flow sheet is just as important as timing and amount.

When a patient is not forming or passing stool appropriately, it is important to assess for additional details. Is this a chronic problem or did it just happen during admission. Is the stool that has been passed very hard and difficult to move? Has there been any blood? Has it been thin like a pencil, but soft? Has there been any abdominal pain? Most importantly, has there been any fever, distension, or change in vital signs? An identification of the stool quality, quantity, associated symptoms, and chronicity can assist the nurse and the multidisciplinary team in designing a bowel regimen that meets the patient's needs.

One of the most dangerous forms of constipation is the acute intestinal obstruction. This can be caused by a variety of pathologies, but one of the most common in the hospital setting is in the first few weeks after an abdominal surgery. These patients have a propensity to form adhesions within the bowel and may develop herniations through the operative incision sites. In certain subtypes, the obstruction can lead to very high intraintestinal pressures and resultant loss of blood flow to the bowel. The patient will complain of intermittent crampy abdominal pain that can be quite severe. Nausea with vomiting is almost always present. On examination, you may note a distended abdomen, fever, tachycardia, and hypotension. This is a surgical emergency that is unlikely to present itself during the physician's 15 min of direct patient contact that day.

Other causes of acute intestinal obstruction include fecal impaction from constipation (look for narcotics on the medication list), tumors both inside and outside of the gastrointestinal (GI) tract, diverticulitis, inflammatory bowel diseases, gall stones stuck in the intestine, or telescoping of the intestine inside itself (intussusception). These are all exceedingly dangerous as any complete obstruction of the GI tract carries with it an overall mortality of 10% to 20%.

Aside from the complete mechanical bowel obstructions described above, there is also the potential for an adynamic ileus. In this situation, the bowel basically becomes paralyzed by an irritating substance. This can range from hydrochloric acid from a perforated peptic ulcer to local inflammation caused by a kidney stone. These patients usually have a constant discomfort from distension rather than the off-and-on pain from obstruction. This usually resolves when the primary problem resolves.

A pseudo-obstruction is a general slowing of the GI tract and is usually related to narcotics. It can result in severe constipation from fecal impaction with resultant obstruction, so it should be treated fairly aggressively. Also, it is important to remember that this condition can largely be prevented with stool softeners.

There is much more to constipation than a verbal order for an enema. While not always a medical emergency, constipation can have important long term complications. New constipation should always be investigated. If the patient is experiencing severe crampy pain and tenderness, the urgency increases. Constipation should be prevented when there is a high likelihood of its occurrence. Always keep in mind that it is just as important for nursing to clearly document what comes out of a patient as what is put in!

SUGGESTED READINGS

Gearhart S, Silen W. Acute intestinal obstruction. In: Fauci AS, Braunwald E, Kasper DL, et al., eds. *Harrison's Principles of Internal Medicine*. 17th Ed. McGraw-Hill; 2008, pp. 1912–1914.

KNOW THE MANY PRESENTATIONS OF BLOOD IN THE STOOL

EDWARD HUMERICKHOUSE, MS, MD

WHAT TO DO: ASSESS

The color and texture of stools should be documented in the patient's record since blood in the stool can have a variety of presentations and etiologies. Understanding the history and character can assist in identifying the most likely diagnoses.

Hemorrhoids are common in our older patients but also occur very frequently in younger adults who have had natural child birth or chronic constipation. The straining during child-birth or stooling has caused the veins surrounding the anus to stretch and push up to the surface so that only a little skin separates them from the outside world. A quick look at the patient's anus confirms your suspicion and a stool softener and some soothing antiseptics will usually take care of the problem.

Diverticulae are small out-pouchings of the colon wall where the wall has gotten thin and bubbled out usually from years of straining at stool. These can become infected as in diverticulitis or a blood vessel can rupture, causing a very brisk but usually self-limiting bleed. Since the bleeding is deeper in the colon, it will usually have time to clot some and mix with the stool. These usually present with a large amount of dark blood with some clots or bright blood MIXED with a small amount of brown stool. Usually the bleeding is painless.

Upper GI bleeding can result from an ulcer or gastritis. When given time to digest, the iron from the blood turns the stool dark black and may be the first sign of trouble in an otherwise asymptomatic patient. Brisk upper GI bleeds from an ulcer or esophageal varices may present first as lower GI bleeding. Blood is an excellent cathartic and a large amount in the stomach will quickly turn into a large amount in the colon, sometimes without any vomiting. This is a medical emergency and should be considered as a possibility in any patient with large volume of bloody stool.

Nurses are often the first in line in recognizing that patients have bleeding in their GI tract and the color and character of the stool can help to identify the source. The first thing always is to stabilize the patient, which requires attention to the As, Bs, and Cs of resuscitation. Large bore intravenous catheters and intravenous fluid should be established. Patients should be supine, particularly if they have orthostatic symptoms or vital signs. It is important to have an understanding of where the bleeding is coming from and how severe it is. This begins with a nasogastric tube to determine the location of the bleeding, a hemoglobin and hematocrit to assess the extent of blood loss, and a type and crossmatch to prepare blood for resuscitation as needed.

SUGGESTED READINGS

Laine L. Gastrointestinal bleeding. In: Fauci AS, Braunwald E, Kasper DL, et al., eds. *Harrison's Principles of Internal Medicine*. 17th Ed. McGraw-Hill, New York; 2008, pp. 259–260.

SAVE THE STOOL AND SEND IT TO THE LAB WHEN INDICATED

EDWARD HUMERICKHOUSE, MS, MD

WHAT TO DO: ASSESS

The most important part of evaluating a patient with diarrhea is to understand if the stool needs to be sent to the laboratory for evaluation. The duration, character, and symptoms of diarrhea can often be some of the most helpful parts of this evaluation. Has it been present for several months or did it occur during this admission? Does the patient or physician already know of the problem and diagnosis? Is there abdominal pain, fever, or blood in the stool? There is a considerable difference in daily diarrhea that occurs after eating in a patient who has had gastric bypass or who has chronic pancreatitis versus a toxic diarrhea appearing in an otherwise healthy child who had a hamburger at the family reunion on Saturday. The laboratory can perform some common tests that can assist with identifying the cause. These include fecal leukocytes (must be a very fresh sample), stool cultures, stool occult blood, and toxin assays. It is unusual for an antidiarrheal medication to be administered in the hospital without assurance that the stool was free from invading bacteria. Some common etiologies of diarrhea are provided here.

Clostridium difficile (*C. difficile*) colitis can occur in a variety of situations and may occur several months after completing antibiotics. Patients have massive, dark green, watery, and incredibly foul smelling stool that may be associated with crampy abdominal pain, low grade fever, and perhaps incontinence in a previously continent patient. A nurse suspecting *C. difficile* should prompt isolation precautions until it has been ruled out. A *C. difficile* toxin assay can help with the diagnosis. The treatment consists of oral Flagyl and IV fluids.

Staphylococcal or bacillus toxin diarrhea is very short lived, but horribly symptomatic. These spores are ingested from spoiled food. Patients become nauseated very quickly, vomit, appear pale, become tachycardic, and then proceed to have large volumes of watery stools with some food in it. The administration of intravenous fluid, increased monitoring, and the disposal of the contaminated food are all in order.

Nursing staff is the key to recognizing acute changes in patient status, and new diarrhea in the hospital is one of those cases that have a number of causes. By collecting some background information and describing the stool, nursing staff can help to ensure that the proper laboratory studies are obtained and appropriate medications started.

SUGGESTED READINGS

Camilleri M, Murray J. Diarrhea and constipation. In: Fauci AS, Braunwald E, Kasper DL, et al., eds. *Harrison's Principles of Internal Medicine*. 17th Ed. McGraw-Hill, New York; 2008, pp. 247–249.

KNOW WHAT, WHEN, AND HOW TO FEED PATIENTS WITH PANCREATITIS

EDWARD HUMERICKHOUSE, MS, MD

WHAT TO DO: IMPLEMENT

Pancreatitis is a fairly common admission diagnosis in the acute care setting. The pancreas is a digestive and endocrine organ that is located just inferior and posterior to the stomach. It produces potent digestive enzymes that are secreted into the first part of the intestine through the same duct as bile from the liver. It also secretes the insulin necessary to make use of the materials it digests. Pancreatitis is quite simply the inflammation of that organ and can range in severity from mild abdominal pain to spillage of large amounts of digestive enzymes into the abdominal cavity with ensuing death.

There is a very broad list of causes of pancreatitis (about 30) with the most common being ingestion of alcohol. This is related to direct toxic effects of the drug over time (not common in occasional random binge drinkers). Next on the list is gall stone pancreatitis where small stones from the gall bladder block the exit of pancreatic enzymes. A third common cause is very high triglycerides where it is thought that the free fat in the bloodstream triggers hypersecretion of lipase. Regardless of the start, the end result is various degrees of self-digestion.

The primary treatment of pancreatitis is to solve the cause and prevent further pancreatic stimulation. The first part is fairly simple in most cases: stop the alcohol, open the duct that drains the pancreas, or give medication to lower triglycerides. The more difficult problem to tackle is preventing the stimulation of pancreatic enzyme formation. Unfortunately, stopping the secretion usually means bowel rest followed by cautious refeeding.

"When do I let my patient eat?" The most straightforward answer is "When they are hungry." Pancreatitis causes tremendous pain with nausea and vomiting. Generally, patients are not keen on eating until the pain is diminished, and they feel fairly confident that ice chips will not make the pain come back. The general rule for mild pancreatitis is to start with sips of clear liquids when the pain is tolerable. Simple sugars are easily absorbed by the stomach and intestine with little need for assistance from the pancreas. If tolerated, patients can advance to a little more robust diet with more complex carbohydrates but still avoiding fats and proteins. Most hospitals have a "pancreatic" diet that is over 50% carbohydrates.

For patients with severe pancreatitis (usually denoted by their presence in the ICU), feeding is started much earlier since the body has a high demand for nutrients in critical illness. In the past, these patients were provided with total parenteral nutrition via a central line. However, recent studies have demonstrated improved outcomes with the placement of feeding tubes inserted past the first part of the small intestine. By physically bypassing the pancreas and providing nutrients that do not require further digestion, patients are able to obtain the nutrition that they need without causing additional damage. As patients with severe pancreatitis recover, they would follow the same guidelines as above in resuming oral intake.

The pancreas also secretes insulin. A damaged pancreas may not be able to secrete enough insulin to cover the body's needs and represents another major pitfall to the treatment of pancreatitis. Ensuring that blood sugars are tracked and insulin is administered for hyperglycemia is an important part of treatment.

SUGGESTED READINGS

Corley D. Acute pancreatitis. In: Wachter RM, Goldman L, Hollander H, eds. *Hospital Medicine*. 2nd Ed. Philadelphia, PA: Lippincott Williams & Wilkins; 2005, pp. 849–858.

Vege SS, Chari ST. Pathogenesis of acute pancreatitis. Uptodate Online. Version 16.2. February 14, 2007. Available at: http://www.uptodate.com/patients/content/topic.do?topicKey=~TOqYJgCS2oB9c&selectedTitle=1~100&source=search_result. Accessed August 18, 2008.

WHO SHOULD BE NPO AND WHY

EDWARD HUMERICKHOUSE, MS, MD

NPO is a VERY common order in the inpatient setting. The term is based on the Latin "nulla per orem" and literally means "nothing by mouth." The primary points of confusion are: "How long should my patient be NPO? Is it really NPO or can the patient take ice chips? Should I also hold his medications?" These are all excellent questions that need to be clarified. One of the most basic reasons for NPO status is the risk of aspiration in nonsurgical patients who cannot protect their airway during swallowing. Two common scenarios are acutely ill patients in the ICU and recent stroke victims. In these cases, NPO means NPO. No meds, no sips, and no ice chips. If nutrition is needed, it should be through a feeding tube or a central line. All medications should be IV or, if an enteral tube is present, liquid. Your pharmacist can help make recommendations for comparative medications that are available in suspension form. Help your stroke victims by making sure that there is a speech therapy consultant available. Do not try a bedside swallow evaluation on your own!

Next on the list of NPO orders is the pre-op patient to prevent aspiration during intubation and vomiting during and after surgery. These patients should be devoid of food and fluids for approximately 8 h before the case. Numerous cases are postponed because patients have had a cup of coffee in that preoperative period. However, the other cause of case delay is strict NPO. Patients need to take there blood pressure medications before the surgery, especially if they are on a "β-blocker" such as metoprolol. If there is ANY question, page the surgeon or the anesthesiologist on the case to find out what medications should or should not be given during this preoperative fasting period.

Patients who will be receiving planned conscious sedation should be 8 h NPO except medications. Some common examples include cardiac catheterizations, liver biopsies, and removal of complicated skin tumors. Any one of these procedures may result in acute cardiac or respiratory failure from the procedure itself or an adverse reaction to the sedation medications. Some of the sedating medications can cause nausea and vomiting which are dangerous in a semiconscious patient.

The degree of NPO status must also be ascertained in patients who are scheduled for endoscopy. Since the procedure is relatively short with minimal recovery time, most medications can be administered after the procedure.

Six hours without eating is generally enough to ensure that the stomach is empty for complete viewing. Colonosopy requires a more prolonged and detailed order. These patients usually need to have clear liquids for supper which will then be washed out by the gastroenterologist's laxatives of choice. Call the gastroenterologist specifically to ask about any medications that need to be given before the procedure as well as the preferred time to give them.

There are a variety of noninvasive procedures that also require an empty stomach. Studies designed to evaluate the gall bladder require that the gall bladder be full. Food causes the gallbladder to empty, so patients should be without sustenance for several hours before abdominal ultrasounds and HIDA scans. Studies of esophageal and stomach mobility also require NPO status, so avoid breakfast in patients who have barium swallows or gastric emptying studies ordered. These studies are also fairly short, so check with the physician to hold meds until after the procedure.

A common medical illness that will lead to an NPO order is pancreatittis. In these cases, the NPO should be a true NPO. Even the slightest stimulation of the GI tract can cause severe pain and potentially prolong illness. Make sure that you have appropriate IV fluids and medications ordered to cover the patients' chronic medical conditions as well as their pain. As a general rule, NPO status should be maintained until the patient feels ready to try some sips of clears. If it is a severe or complicated case, the patient may require enteral feeding, in which case, medications should be ordered in liquid or suspension form (no one likes a clogged Dobhoff). Along the same line, acute cholecystitis and flairs of inflammatory bowel disease (Crohn colitis and ulcerative colitis) can also result in severe pain should the patient receive food. In all of these cases, the nausea and anorexia associated with the illness will usually result in the patients making themselves NPO.

The NPO order is commonly placed in the hospital and the preprocedure setting. Advocate for the patient's needs and get orders clarified in cases where the patient might need medications. Just as importantly, make sure that there is an order to resume the patient's diet when the procedure, test, or pathology is resolved.

SUGGESTED READINGS

Kramer FM. Patient perceptions of the importance of maintaining preoperative NPO status. *AANA J.* 2000;68(4):321–328.

Maziarski FT, Simonson D. NPO status prior to surgery: Two different approaches. *CRNA.* 1994;5(2):59–62.

NURSES NEED TO KNOW HOW TO ADMINISTER SEDATION SAFELY TO PATIENTS IN THE GI SUITE

ANTHONY D. SLONIM, MD, DrPH

WHAT TO DO: ASSESS, IMPLEMENT, AND EVALUATE

The gastrointestinal (GI) suite has become an important location for care as endoscopic strategies have improved screening approaches for patients with GI malignancies and have provided improved therapeutic strategies for patients with problems ranging from acute GI bleeding to polyp resection. The nurse has been pivotal in the growth of this area, bringing special skills to care for these patients. One of the most important aspects of this care is the delivery of sedation to these patients.

Sedation is used to provide anxiolysis and amnesia for patients and to facilitate the performance of the GI procedure. The provision of medications in the benzodiazepine and narcotic classes has been used safely for years for just this purpose. However, it is important for nurses to know how to prepare for sedation in patients undergoing GI procedures to perform it safely.

Regardless of the medication used, the nurse should ensure that the room has been prepared to perform not only the GI procedure but also the sedation. This often requires the availability of suction, electrocardiographic and oxygen saturation monitoring, and the availability of appropriate antidotes as needed to reverse medications if the patients' oxygen level deteriorates or they experience other complications of the medications. Resuscitation equipment should be available including oxygen and bag valve mask support, with medications for emergency resuscitation. The patient also needs preparation beyond the GI preparation. An assessment of the airway, whether or not the patient has obstructive apnea, whether the patient is obese, or whether the patient has any denture or any other coexistent medical problems that will be adversely affected through the selection of medications should be done.

Nurses should know the standard doses of commonly used medications. Midazolam and lorazepam, two members of the benzodiazepine group of medications,

have been used with some success. In addition, morphine, fentanyl, and meperidine from the narcotic class of medications can also be used. While these medications provide analgesia, they also have sedative properties that allow them to be used to accommodate the procedure.

From a monitoring perspective, it is usually the nurses' role to monitor the patient while the endoscopist focuses on the procedure. This monitoring requires the assessment of the patient's vital signs, oxygen saturations, and level of consciousness. Medications during these procedures are usually titrated to effect and it is important to have current vital signs readily available so that appropriate assessments regarding redosing can be done.

Finally, the recovery period is essential. The patients need to be monitored until they recover from the sedative medications and to meet the preestablished objective of discharge criteria and are discharged to an adult who can drive them home and be responsible for them during this recovery period.

The nurse is an essential member of the GI suite team. Apart from preparing for the GI procedure, the nurse is often responsible for monitoring the patient's sedation, which can be considered a separate procedure itself. Clarity around the requirements and expectations is important for the nurse to appropriately carry out these functions.

SUGGESTED READINGS

Froehlich F, Milliet N. Propofol sedation during endoscopic procedures in private practice: The case for capnography to make 1-nurse endoscopy acceptable. *Gastrointest Endosc.* 2008;67(6):1008.

Külling D, Orlandi M, Inauen W. Propofol sedation during endoscopic procedures: How much staff and monitoring are necessary? *Gastrointest Endosc.* 2007;66(3):443–449.

Moos DD. Obstructive sleep apnea and sedation in the endoscopy suite. *Gastroenterol Nurs.* 2006;29(6):456–463; quiz 464–465.

SGNA Practice Committee. Statement on the use of sedation and analgesia in the gastrointestinal endoscopy setting. *Gastroenterol Nurs.* 2008;31(3):249–251.

BE ABLE TO RECOGNIZE THE WARNING SIGNS FOR EATING DISORDERS

ANTHONY D. SLONIM, MD, DrPH

WHAT TO DO: ASSESS

The nurse is in an important position among members of the healthcare team to be able to identify eating disorders. Eating disorders represent a class of disorders that are associated with a number of serious complications. The nurse who appropriately identifies the patient and facilitates appropriate counseling may be able to save a life.

Eating disorders fall into two major categories: anorexia nervosa and bulimia. While these disorders are rather different, there is occasionally an overlap between the two. Demographically, while both disorders can occur at any age and in either gender, they are typically considered as disorders of adolescent and young adult female patients. While many disorders have a predisposition for lower socioeconomic classes, these eating disorders have a propensity for middle-class Caucasians.

Anorexia nervosa is heralded by severe weight loss that is grounded in a problem with the patients' perception of their body. These patients, despite significant loss of weight, often perceive the image of their body to be overweight. As a result, they limit their nutritional intake, use diet pills and laxatives extensively, exercise vigorously, and may substitute meals with water. These patients exhibit signs of significant weight loss, malnutrition, and other signs and symptoms related to the malnutrition such as dry skin, amenorrhea, and dehydration.

Bulimia is a similar condition in that the patient's body image is impaired, but the symptoms are different and the patients are usually overweight. These patients often experience "binge-purge" episodes where their hunger and craving for food leads them to eat large quantities of food. This "binge" is often followed by a "purge" where forceful vomiting or excessive laxative or diuretic use is encountered. As a result, the patient experiences overt signs of vomiting or metabolic signs of purging. Examination of the teeth may reveal dental caries, particularly on the incisors, from the effects of hydrochloric acid from the repetitive vomiting. There may be abrasions or scars on the hands from the use of the fingers to incite vomiting through gagging. In addition, a metabolic alkalosis may ensue from this vomiting. Patients who abuse laxatives or diuretics will experience metabolic effects from the overuse of these medications including hypokalemic, metabolic alkalosis.

Patients with eating disorders may not present for medical care until late in the course of their disease. Therefore, the nurse should be aware of these problems in all patients who present for care. Assessment of a nutritional history and emotional concerns like depression, situational stressors, and body image can help the nurse become aware of a potentially undiagnosed problem. The treatment is centered on providing appropriate guidance for nutritional support and weight gain, the use of antidepressants if depression is present, and the treatment of the complications of the disease including dehydration and potassium and metabolic derangements.

SUGGESTED READINGS

West DS. The eating disorders. In: Goldman L, Ausiello D, eds. *Cecil Textbook of Medicine*. 22nd Ed. Philadelphia, PA: Saunders; 2004, pp. 1336–1338.

BE ABLE TO ASSIST YOUR PATIENT WITH APPROPRIATE WEIGHT REDUCTION STRATEGIES

ANTHONY D. SLONIM, MD, DRPH

Obesity has become a major epidemic in the United States with approximately 60% of the adult population being obese, defined as a body mass index $>30 \, kg/m^2$, and a considerable proportion of children also experiencing obesity. This is important since obese patients experience health problems to a greater extent and obesity is a major risk factor for hypertension, diabetes, coronary artery disease, hyperlipidemia, and cancer. Obese people also tend to exercise less. This inactivity also has problems of its own, including a predisposition to some of the diseases mentioned.

Nurses will often be in a position to assist patients who are interested in weight reduction programs. In collaboration with the physician, a multifaceted plan can be encouraged including dieting, a reduction in total calories, attention to appropriate nutrition that encourages the intake of specific foods that are healthier choices over others, and improvements in physical activity to assist in increasing the patient's metabolism and maintaining physical fitness. When these strategies are insufficient, the nurses may find that they are in a position to assist with any number of other efforts including operative procedures like gastric bypass or banding, medications, and other remedies.

For many patients, a plan that allows appropriate quantification of calories and exercise may be all that is needed. The patients, when motivated to lose weight, may only need to realize that they are relatively sedentary and consume too much food of the wrong type. A transition to increase physical activity and eat more fish, vegetables, and chicken in deference to complex carbohydrates may be helpful as a starting point. When the patients begin to notice changes in their weight, the motivation to continue with these strategies will be there. An assessment of weight should not occur more frequently than weekly. In addition, the nurse can help the patient keep track of important nutritional parameters including triglyceride levels, glucose levels, and other anthropometric measurements that allow for a better assessment of nutritional status.

The use of medications or the possibility for surgical solutions should be discussed with the patient's physician and an assessment of the patient's readiness to change be incorporated.

Nurses are well positioned to assist patients with weight problems. An understanding of the strategies that can be used will improve health and prevent complications for these patients while also improving their quality of life.

SUGGESTED READINGS

Jensen MD. Obesity. In: Goldman L, Ausiello D, eds. *Cecil Textbook of Medicine*. 22nd Ed. Philadelphia, PA: Saunders; 2004, pp. 1338–1346.

KNOW HOW TO MANAGE ACUTE GASTROINTESTINAL BLEEDING

ANTHONY D. SLONIM, MD, DRPH

WHAT TO DO: ASSESS, IMPLEMENT, AND EVALUATE

Gastrointestinal (GI) bleeding is a common presenting complaint for patients in the emergency department or in the inpatient setting. This condition has a variety of diagnoses associated with it and it is important for the nurse to know what to do to assist the patient while a diagnosis is being made.

The bleeding from the upper GI tract arises from any structure from the mouth to the Ligament of Treitz in the duodenum. This may present acutely with the patient vomiting blood or passing blood per rectum in some cases. The condition may also present subacutely with anemia, tarry stools, or heme positive stools. Depending on the circumstance, the nurse's response should be tailored.

For acute GI bleeding that presents with the vomiting of blood, the passage of blood per rectum, or the alteration in vital signs including tachycardia, hypotension, or orthostatic changes associated with position, immediate attention is required. In these circumstances, the patient should have attention to airway, breathing, and Circulation and have two large bore intravenous lines established. If symptomatic, IV fluid boluses can be given to restore intravascular volume. The nurse will need to establish the source of bleeding by placing a nasogastric tube and sending coagulation studies, a complete blood count, and a type and crossmatch to the laboratory. If the patient presents in the subacute phase, these steps are unnecessary and a strategy for further diagnostic testing can be developed.

Diagnostic testing can be performed depending on the patient's presentation. While an upper GI series, computerized tomography, and radionuclide scans can all be used depending upon the situation, in reality, upper GI endoscopy is often used to directly assess the gastric mucosa and provide a definitive diagnosis.

Regardless of the acuity, the diagnostic possibilities are very similar for upper GI bleeding. In these cases, gastritis, peptic ulcer disease, esophageal varices, and Mallory Weiss tears are all possibilities. Patients taking certain medications, including aspirin or anticoagulants, can experience a more brisk bleeding than those who are not taking these agents, so nurses should ascertain the medication list upon presentation of the patient.

The treatment of the patient with GI bleeding may involve direct endoscopic interventions like cauterization or sclerotherapy. Alternatively, the use of proton pump inhibitors, H2 blockers, and lifestyle modification including the reduction or elimination of alcohol, spicy foods, and late night meals should be encouraged. Specific therapy for *H. pylori*, if present, should also be included.

The patient with bleeding in the upper GI tract can present in casually or in extremis. The nurse should assess vital signs, provide supportive care depending upon the situation, facilitate diagnostic testing, and reevaluate as the condition warrants while the diagnosis is confirmed.

SUGGESTED READINGS

Bjorkman DJ. Gastrointestinal hemorrhage and occult gastrointestinal bleeding. In: Goldman L, Ausiello D, eds. *Cecil Textbook of Medicine.* 22nd Ed. Philadelphia, PA: Saunders; 2004, pp. 795–800.

ENCOURAGE APPROPRIATE SCREENING FOR CANCER OF THE LOWER GASTROINTESTINAL TRACT

ANTHONY D. SLONIM, MD, DrPH

WHAT TO DO: ASSESS

Nurses are an important component of the team that encourages healthy living. One part of these responsibilities is the encouragement of appropriate screening for malignancy. The gastrointestinal (GI) tract is an important location for malignancies and may be asymptomatic until late stages of disease. It is important for the nurse to be familiar with the common causes of GI cancers and what can be done to prevent their occurrence. Because of the number of organs in the GI tract, the nurse needs to have some familiarity with the assessment methods for cancer in each of these areas.

Cancers of the upper aerodigestive tract, including the mouth, oropharynx, and esophagus, are relatively uncommon. Cancers of the tongue and lips can occur but are usually predisposed by smoking and ethanol use. Good oral care including inspection and palpation of the oropharynx and cervical lymph nodes by a dental professional may be able to identify these cancers early. Patients should be encouraged to stop smoking, reduce alcohol intake, and seek medical treatment for any cancer sores or lesions that last more than a few days.

Cancer of the stomach is also rare, but when it occurs, it is quite serious and associated with a high mortality. Risk factors include smoking and alcohol use and in some cultures, the ingestion of large amounts of smoked fish. These patients have nonspecific symptoms including indigestion and belching until late in the course of disease when bloating, or early satiety and vomiting may appear.

Cancer of the small intestine is also rare. These cancers are often associated with predisposing conditions like the Crohn disease and the Peutz–Jeghers syndrome. Large intestine cancers are relatively common, however, occurring in 6% of patients and are the second leading cause of mortality. Of importance, cancers of the colon have screening tests available to identify them early and reduce the spread of disease. Fecal occult blood testing is one strategy for identifying blood in the GI tract that may be associated with colon cancer. While this test has a number of problems associated with it, it can also be quite valuable. Colonoscopy is a modality that allows direct inspection of the colonic mucosa, the identification and removal of polyps, and the recognition of early malignancies when they occur. Colonoscopy is recommended every 10 years in those patients more than 50 years old or more than 40 years old if there is a significant family history including familial polyposis syndromes.

Primary malignant cancers of the liver are rare. These hepatocellular carcinomas often occur in patients with preexisting Hepatitis B or Hepatitis C infection. More common than primary cancers, however, is the presence of cancers that metastasize to the liver from other organs. Among these are the breast, lung, colon, prostate, pancreas, and stomach. There are no effective screening measures for these cancers and the prognosis for metastatic liver disease is poor.

Pancreatic cancer is an indolent cancer with a high mortality. Patients will quickly progress from diagnosis to death. Part of the reason is that pancreatic cancer goes undetected until it becomes symptomatic. This usually presents with nonspecific abdominal pain, anorexia, malaise, and painless jaundice.

The nurse is in a good position to be able to assist in encouraging appropriate screening tests for patients at risk for GI malignancies.

SUGGESTED READINGS

DuBois RN. Neoplasms of the large and small intestine. In: Goldman L, Ausiello D, eds. *Cecil Textbook of Medicine*. 22nd Ed. Philadelphia, PA: Saunders; 2004, pp. 1211–1220.

Fallon M. Hepatic tumors. In: Goldman L, Ausiello D, eds. *Cecil Textbook of Medicine*. 22nd Ed. Philadelphia, PA: Saunders; 2004, pp. 1222–1226.

Rustgi AK. Neoplasms of the stomach. In: Goldman L, Ausiello D, eds. *Cecil Textbook of Medicine*. 22nd Ed. Philadelphia, PA: Saunders; 2004, pp. 1208–1211.

Tempero M, Brand R. Pancreatic cancer. In: Goldman L, Ausiello D, eds. *Cecil Textbook of Medicine*. 22nd Ed. Philadelphia, PA: Saunders; 2004, pp. 1220–1222.

REMEMBER THAT NOT ALL CHEST PAINS ARE RELATED TO THE HEART

ANTHONY D. SLONIM, MD, DRPH

WHAT TO DO: ASSESS

Chest pain is a common complaint among adult patients and a major reason for visits to the emergency department. However, not all chest pains are related to ischemic cardiac disease. While this is certainly important and needs to be ruled out, referred pain to the chest from the gastrointestinal (GI) tract is also important and may be more easily treated.

Nurses responding to patient questions about a symptom like chest pain are often put in the uncomfortable position of being asked what the patient should do. If the call is on the phone, there is relatively little that one can do except for asking some important questions to help differentiate the etiology of the pain. However, in the end, the nurse is obligated to having the patient evaluated immediately and more thoroughly, in person, either in the office or in the emergency department. While this may not be the most appropriate use of resources, the nurse needs to err on the side of safety.

Patients can experience chest pain because of a number of GI causes including esophagitis, gastritis, peptic ulcer disease, cholecystitis, and renal colic. The patient may also experience chest pain from cardiovascular conditions like aortic aneurysms and pulmonary conditions like pneumonia, pleurisy, and chest wall disorders. Recognizing the differences can assist the nurse in helping the patient seek out appropriate care.

When chest pain is cardiac in nature, there are often a number of associated symptoms including diaphoresis, shortness of breath, and nausea. Patients often describe the pain as pressure like and radiating to the arm, shoulder, or neck. It is not worsened with pressure to the chest wall and may be relieved with rest. Additional diagnostic testing including an electrocardiogram and cardiac enzymes may be necessary for improved diagnosis.

Pain from the GI tract, depending on its source, may also have associated symptoms, like nausea and diaphoresis, but often the pain is described as colicky or crampy and is more likely to radiate to the shoulder blades. There may be associated belching or a sour taste in the back of the throat from reflux. The condition may be made better or worse depending upon the patient's position and may be relieved with antacids, H2 blockers, or antireflux medications.

Overall, the type of pain and associated symptoms can assist the nurse in helping the patient seek appropriate care. Importantly, the nurse should refer patients to medical care when the condition is unclear or the patient needs to be evaluated in person.

SUGGESTED READINGS

Goyal RK. Dysphagia. In: Kasper DL, Braunwald E, et al., eds. *Harrison's Principles of Internal Medicine*. 16th Ed. Philadelphia, PA: McGraw-Hill; 2005, pp. 217–218.

RECOGNIZE THAT THE VARIOUS TYPES OF ANTICOAGULANTS CAN INCREASE THE RISK OF BLEEDING

JENNIFER BATH, RN, BSN, FNE, SANE-A

WHAT TO DO: ASSESS

Anticoagulants are used for a variety of reasons. Patients with a history of a stroke or prior heart attack are placed on anticoagulants to reduce the risk of a second episode. Inpatients who are bedridden are placed on anticoagulants prophylactically to prevent clot formation. Anticoagulants are also used in the treatment of conditions like atrial fibrillation and deep vein thromboses. Anticoagulants work by a variety of mechanisms including blocking platelet and clotting factors activity.

The three types of anticoagulants include thrombin inhibitors, antiplatelet drugs, and clotting factor inhibitors. Inhibitors of thrombin block the activity of thrombin; heparin is a thrombin inhibitor. Antiplatelet drugs block the platelets from aggregating into clots. Aspirin is one of the most common antiplatelet drugs available. Inhibitors of clotting factor synthesis are the third common type of anticoagulant. These drugs decrease the production of certain clotting factors of the liver; Coumadin is an example of this type of drug. Due to potentially serious side effects, most blood thinners require a prescription. Aspirin, however, can be obtained over the counter. However, even though it is available over the counter, its effects on bleeding can be severe.

All patients on these medications are at increased risk for bleeding problems and need to take care to avoid any injuries. They should avoid sports and hazardous activities. Falls or blows to the head need to be reported to their physician immediately since they may result in serious bleeding. Care with shaving and brushing/flossing their teeth is also important. These patients may also bruise easily. Drugs such as Coumadin and heparin are routinely monitored through lab testing to maintain a therapeutic level.

Patient education should include signs and symptoms of abnormal bleeding such as nosebleeds, bleeding gums, excessive amounts of bruising, heavy bleeding from wounds, heavy or unexpected menstrual periods, blood in the urine, cloudy or dark urine, black, tarry, or bloody stools, vomiting blood/coffee grounds, pain or swelling in the abdomen, severe and constant headache, weakness, or hemoptysis. Patients taking anticoagulants should be instructed to contact their doctor or seek medical treatment if they experience any of these conditions. Patients on anticoagulant therapy should be encouraged to wear a medical identification.

Knowing that the patient is being treated with an anticoagulant will increase a provider's index of suspicion when trying to diagnose the patient with an unusual or obscure condition. A thorough history is important with these patients. Many patients, particularly the elderly, may not recall the names of their medications or understand when asked whether they are taking anticoagulants. Anticoagulants provide a number of benefits but because of a narrow therapeutic window, these may cause adverse reactions as well.

SUGGESTED READINGS

Flanagan N. Anticoagulant and antiplatelet drugs. *Surgery Encyclopedia*. Available at: http://www.surgeryencyclopedia.com/A-Ce/Anticoagulant-and-Antiplatelet-Drugs.html. Accessed August 13, 2008.

Iyer P. Anticoagulants: A double edged sword. *Med League Support Services*. Available at: http://www.medleague.com/Articles/Newsletters/newsletter37.pdf. Accessed August 24, 2008.

ALWAYS FOLLOW THE CORRECT PROCEDURE WHEN ADMINISTERING PACKED RED BLOOD CELLS

ALICE M. CHRISTALDI, RN, BSN, CRRN

WHAT TO DO: IMPLEMENT

Throughout the world, approximately 75 million units of whole blood are donated each year. In the United States alone, more than 13 million units are transfused annually. The American Red Cross supplies almost half of all blood products. To administer blood safely, specific procedures must be followed to assure that patients are safe.

Whole blood is rarely administered; packed red blood cells (PRBCs), on the other hand, are commonly administered. PRBCs are the cells collected from whole blood in which the plasma and platelets are removed. They are administered for a variety of reasons. While a specific hemoglobin level should not be used to trigger a transfusion, most PRBC transfusions are provided when the hemoglobin is less than 6 to 8 g/dL.

After compatibility testing is completed by a type and cross match, the patient must be prepared to receive the blood. Blood may be administered though a peripheral or central catheter. Ensuring that the line is in place and patient before calling for the blood to be delivered to the nursing unit is a good practice. A No. 18 or No. 20 gauge needle is preferred and allows for a faster flow rate. A No. 22 gauge needle can be used, but the flow rate might be slower. There is a myth that the blood cells will be damaged by using a smaller gauge needle; it is not true.

Only after consent is assured and a working intravenous line is established, should the blood be delivered. Blood components can be fragile and it is important to minimize the time from removal of blood from the blood bank refrigeration to the administration of the blood to the patient. Optimally, blood should remain out of refrigeration for less than 4 h.

A filter is always used to administer blood. Its purpose is to remove clots or cellular debris that have developed during storage. Filters can only be used for 4 h, after which the risk of bacterial growth is increased. You should be familiar with your hospital's policy for specifics related to the administration of blood and blood components. Y type administration sets are often used for administering blood. In this case, one port is used for the administration of blood and the other for normal saline solution (0.9%), which is the only fluid that should be hung with blood products. Dextrose solutions should never be used since 5% dextrose solution is hypotonic and may cause red blood cells to lyse. Medications should never be given through the same line as blood products. A multilumen central line can be used to infuse blood, fluids, and medications if separate ports are accessed.

Prior to administering the blood product, the patient's temperature, pulse, respiration, and blood pressure need to be taken. A baseline assessment including auscultation of the lungs should be performed so that a baseline is available. The physician's order and current laboratory values should be verified. If the patient has received blood in the past, it would be helpful to know if he had any reactions. Two nurses will need to verify the patient's identity. Make sure the patient has a blood bracelet and that it matches the blood unit's information. Check expiration date of the blood, ABO/Rh label, unit number, and the type of blood component ordered and verify that this is the correct patient. Note the time when the blood transfusion is started. The two people verifying the unit and the patient should sign the transfusion record. Do not remove the tag applied to the unit of blood until the transfusion is completed. Check the unit of blood for any abnormal color or obvious clots. Also check to make sure that there is no leakage of blood from the bag.

The transfusion should be started slowly and the nurse should remain with the patient for a minimum of 15 min. Vital signs should be taken after the first 15 min. Your hospital may have more specific guidelines. Clinical symptoms such as itching or flushing might be noticed first before a change in vital signs, so close monitoring of the patient is necessary. Be prepared to stop the transfusion immediately should the patient develop symptoms of a reaction such as fever and chills, hives, dyspnea, or hypotension. When the transfusion is completed, another set of vital signs should be taken and appropriate documentation completed. The patient's response to the transfusion should also be documented.

SUGGESTED READINGS

Rosenthal K. Avoiding bad blood: Key steps to safe transfusions. *Nursing Made Incredibly Easy*. September/October 2004, pp. 21–28. Available at: http://www.nursingcenter.com/pdf.asp. Accessed August 24, 2008.

KNOW THE SIGNS AND SYMPTOMS OF A BLOOD TRANSFUSION REACTION

MELISSA H. CRIGGER, BSN, MHA, RN

WHAT TO DO: ASSESS AND EVALUATE

The signs and symptoms of a blood transfusion reaction can be more than an elevated temperature or change in blood pressure. Blood administration is a common procedure performed in the acute care setting. However, blood administration is a serious procedure that would lead to serious complications including febrile reactions, hemolytic reactions, anaphylaxis, and hypersensitivities to the product. Packed red blood cells (PRBCs) are used to treat severe anemia or blood loss. Careful monitoring is required to identify possible complications. There are four major types of reactions that can occur with blood administration. These include hemolytic, anaphylactic, febrile, and circulatory overload.

Hemolytic reactions are often the most deadly form of transfusion reactions. Luckily, they are also the rarest. Hemolytic reactions occur due to the administration of incompatible blood and are noticed within minutes of starting the blood product. Common complaints of the patient include back or chest pain, shortness of breath, fever, chills, nausea, and vomiting. If symptoms are allowed to progress, hypotension, oliguria, and symptoms of shock can occur. The nurse who is administering blood products must always remember to follow hospital protocol for the correct identification of the patient. This includes reading the armband and having a second person also verify the identity. Should a hemolytic reaction occur, the nurse must stop the transfusion and notify the physician immediately.

Febrile reactions are the most common transfusion reaction and occur in up to 2% of the time. Febrile reactions can occur after the transfusion is completed with the most common signs being increased fever, shaking, and chills. If the febrile reaction occurs during the administration of the blood product, the nurse should stop the transfusion and notify the physician immediately. The nurse also needs to refer to the hospital protocol for febrile reactions.

Anaphylactic reactions occur due to hypersensitivity to plasma proteins in the blood product. This is often seen in patients who have received numerous transfusions. Urticaria, wheezing, dyspnea, and hypotension within 30 min of starting the transfusion are the symptoms of anaphylactic reaction, but the cardinal symptom is a hive like rash. If discovered, the nurse should remember to notify the physician immediately and follow the hospital protocol. This could include immediately stopping the transfusion and administering epinephrine and steroids. In some cases, the patient may require emergency resuscitation depending on the severity of symptoms.

Circulatory overload is another complication that can occur with blood administration, especially in the elderly or debilitated patient. Symptoms of circulatory overload include chest pain, a cough, distended jugular veins in the neck, increased heart rate, and crackles and wheezes upon auscultation. Circulatory overload can occur at any time during the transfusion or several hours after the transfusion is complete. Should circulatory overload occur, the transfusion should be stopped immediately and the physician notified. The nurse may administer diuretics as per physician's order and oxygen for respiratory distress. The physician may decide to restart the transfusion at a much slower rate.

With blood administration, there are a number of symptoms that can occur that are related to transfusion reaction. The nurse must be aware of the possible signs and symptoms that can be associated with blood administration. Remember to stop the transfusion immediately upon identification of a reaction and notify the patient's physician while monitoring the patient and intervening for decompensation.

SUGGESTED READINGS

Linton AD. *Introduction to Medical–Surgical Nursing*. 4th Ed. St. Louis, MO: Saunders-Elsevier; 2007, pp. 578–581.
Williams LS, Hopper PD. Hematopoietic and lymphatic system function, assessment, and therapeutic measures. In: Williams LS, Hopper PD, Venes D, eds. *Understanding Medical Surgical Nursing*. 2nd Ed. Philadelphia, PA: F.A. Davis Company; 2003, pp. 372 374.

BLOOD COMPONENT THERAPY SHOULD ONLY BE PERFORMED WITH ISOTONIC SOLUTIONS OF 0.9% NORMAL SALINE

MARY S. WARD, RN, BS, OCN

WHAT TO DO: IMPLEMENT

Most nurses would not state that they work in a transplant setting. However, many nurses, particularly in the emergency department, operating room, critical care, orthopedics, and hematology/oncology departments, do work in a transplant setting. Red blood cells (RBCs), platelets, and plasma are all connective tissues of the body and any nurse who administers a transfusion to a patient is indeed a "transplant" nurse in a limited sense. The same risks that occur when a solid organ is transplanted, including organ rejection and organ system failure, can occur with a patient who is receiving a transfusion of a unit of a blood component.

Blood component transfusion therapy is an essential element of patient care but does carry many risks for the patient. Due to improved and sophisticated techniques of testing, transfusion therapy has advanced far beyond when little was known of antibodies and ABO or Rh compatibility. Transfusion therapy today is much safer than it was 50 years ago. There are still risks to patients, however, and many of these are due to clinician error rather than unpredictable causes. ABO and Rh incompatible RBCs should never be given to a patient. Errors can occur in the drawing of the cross match, labeling, in the lab itself, in labeling the unit, or in the administration of the wrong unit to the wrong patient. A double verification system should be in place at each step of the process to ensure that the proper identification is followed all the way through the process.

One additional potential error can be made in the administration of the unit of blood or blood component. Many facilities prime the IV tubing of the blood component with an isotonic solution. The same solution may also be used to infuse along with the unit of blood. The isotonic solution that is used is 0.9% normal saline that has the same osmolarity as blood and will not cause any fluid movement in or out of the individual blood cells. If a nurse accidentally hangs the blood or mixes the blood with a solution other than 0.9% normal saline, there is a risk that the RBCs will hemolyze. Dextrose, lactated ringers, and other common IV solutions have greater osmolarity than blood cells. These cause fluid to shift into the RBCs, forcing the cells to swell and eventually burst. The patient may exhibit symptoms of hemolytic reaction such as a reduced hematocrit, increased creatinine, and hematuria. With this hemolysis, the patient could go into kidney failure since the destroyed cells obstruct the renal tubules. It is also important to remember not to administer medication through blood administration tubing unless it has first been flushed with 0.9% normal saline. Medication that remains in the blood tubing without proper flushing will also cause rupture of the blood cells.

Nurses get busy, lines get attached in the wrong places, patients who are in a critical condition have a lot of medications and lines going to a lot of different places, and IV bags don't always get stocked in the same places. It is always the nurse's responsibility to look at what is being hung with the blood, the platelets, the plasma, the albumin, the cryoprecitpitate, or any other blood component and to be fully aware that not all precipitates will be seen before they enter the patient.

SUGGESTED READINGS

CDC. Hemolysis associated with 25% human albumin diluted with sterile water—United States, 1994–1998. *J Am Med Assoc*. 1999;281(12):1076–1077.

Lewis S, Heitkemper MM, Dirksen S. *Medical–Surgical Nursing*. St. Louis, MO: Mosby; 2007, pp. 782–783.

Martini FH. *Fundamentals of Anatomy and Physiology*. 4th Ed. Upper Saddle River, NJ: Prentice Hall; 1998, pp. 74–76.

THE NEUTROPENIC STATUS OF PATIENTS CAN ONLY BE DETERMINED BY THE COMPLETE BLOOD COUNT WITH DIFFERENTIAL AND NOT JUST THE WHITE BLOOD CELL COUNT ALONE

MARY S. WARD, RN, BS, OCN

WHAT TO DO: ASSESS

Patients undergoing cancer therapy such as chemotherapy, biotherapy, or radiation therapy are considered immune compromised when their circulating, infection fighting white cells, or neutrophils, are severely depleted. Any of the treatments for cancer has a varying degree of potential for causing neutropenia in patients. When a patient receives chemotherapy or biotherapy, the bone marrow is adversely affected, causing a decrease in production of white blood cells. The normal time for these cells to be produced and mature in the bone marrow is 10 to 14 days. A patient experiences the most significant drop in the white blood cell count, or nadir, about 7–14 days after a myelosuppressive chemotherapy treatment. This drop may last from a few days to a week before the marrow begins to recover. It is important for the nurse caring for a patient who has received cancer therapy to understand how an absolute neutrophil count (ANC) is calculated and be able to determine if these patients are neutropenic. Patients whose ANC falls <1,500/mm^3 are considered moderately neutropenic, <1,000/mm^3 are considered moderately neutropenic, and <500/mm^3 are considered severely neutropenic.

To determine the ANC, the patient must have had a complete blood count with a differential. For the calculation, the white blood count is multiplied by the percentage of neutrophils. This may show up in the differential as a combination of polys or segs and bands. In this case, these numbers are added together and this percentage is used. This number then represents the percentage of infection fighting white blood cells.

It is important for these patients to always calculate an actual ANC. A simple WBC number without a differential will not always give a true reflection of the patient's neutropenic condition. A patient may have a "normal" white count of 3,400/mm^3 but his bands and segs may only total 22/mm^3. Multiplying these figures out would give an ANC of 748/mm^3, showing that this patient is moderately neutropenic.

Patients with treatment induced neutropenia are at serious risk for infection. Patients for whom the ANC stays <1,000/mm^3 for greater than a week have a 50% chance of developing an infection, and the longer the patient remains in a neutropenic condition, the greater the risk of infection. Mortality for these patients remains >50% if their counts continue to fall.

In addition to the increased risk of severe infection, neutropenic patients are hospitalized more frequently, have more IV antibiotic therapy, and have significant quality of life issues, loss of productivity, economic loss for themselves and their families, and potential delays in treatment.

These patients need to be placed in reverse isolation for their own protection and should not be exposed to infectious diseases from staff or visitors. They should wear a mask when in group settings and good hand hygiene is crucial for everyone who comes into contact with them. Patients who are discharged with the potential for neutropenia or who are neutropenic on discharge MUST be taught to report any fever >100.3°F to their physician immediately. They should not take aspirin, acetaminophen, or NSAID containing products that may mask a fever. These patients develop sepsis quickly and may be at an increased risk for multiorgan dysfunction within just a few hours of developing a fever and require evaluation by a physician as soon as possible.

SUGGESTED READINGS

Cappozo C. Optimal use of granulocyte-colony-stimulating factor in patients with cancer who are at risk for chemotherapy-induced neutropenia. *Oncol Nurs Forum*. 2004;31(3):569–574.

Nirenbert A, Bush AP, Davis A. Neutropenia: State of the knowledge. Part 1. *Oncol Nurs Forum*. 2006;33(6):1193–1201.

Polovich M, White JM, Kelleher LO. *Chemotherapy and Biotherapy Guidelines and Recommendations for Practice*. 2nd Ed. Pittsburgh, PA: Oncology Nursing Society; 2005, p. 96.

KNOW THE METHODS TO REDUCE CHEMOTHERAPY ADMINISTRATION MEDICATION ERROR

MARY S. WARD, RN, BS, OCN

WHAT TO DO: IMPLEMENT

The Institute of Safe Medication Practices continues to place chemotherapy on its list of High-Alert Medications. This distinction is related to many factors including the low therapeutic index of cytotoxic drugs, individualized dosing based either on body surface area or renal function, occasional dose adjustments requiring a second dose calculation, and the narrow safety margin in which even a small error can cause significant toxicity or even death. Errors in chemotherapy can occur at all levels: prescribing, transcribing, mixing, and administration. All individuals involved in the process need to be knowledgeable of the risk factors and actively involved in measures that can reduce errors to a minimum for patient safety. Guidelines have been proposed by both the Oncology Nursing Society and the Association of Health-Allied Pharmacists to improve processes at all levels of chemotherapy administration. Following these guidelines will assist nurses who administer these high-risk drugs safely.

The first recommendation is chemotherapy education. Nurses who administer chemotherapy should be knowledgeable about the nature of the drugs, the regimens and diseases for which they are prescribed, side effects, the risks involved, and correct methods of dose calculations. Nurses who administer chemotherapy are responsible to know whether the drugs they are giving are within the established parameters for the diseases, routes, and protocols that they are using. Many drugs are given by different routes, with widely varying doses, and in multidrug protocols. It is important that the administering nurse be educated on how to calculate doses, how to locate references for regimens, and the safe administration routes of all drugs. Some drugs may safely be given by one route but may be lethal in another.

Because of the risks associated with chemotherapy administration, it is recommended that a system of double verification be established for nurses at each step of the noting and administration process, beginning with noting of the original order. All steps of the double verification process should be done as independent checks. First, the order with the BSA, the protocol, and doses should all be double-checked by two chemotherapy competent nurses. Second, each day that chemotherapy is to be administered, starting with day one, a separate double verification of each drug to be administered that day should be carried out and documented. The BSA, drug(s), and doses should be rechecked and compared to the original order. Third, each bag of chemotherapy to be administered should be double verified by two nurses just prior to the infusion. To complete this check, two patient identifiers should be used; the drug, dose, and diluent, if specified, should be checked against the original order. This verification should also be documented. When the chemotherapy is hung, the patient should be identified with the bag being used and the original order using two patient identifiers. At the initiation of the infusion, the infusion rate should also be double verified to prevent infusion rate error. In addition to all of these double verifications, good patient education will also help to reduce risk. Including the patient and/or patient's family as a stakeholder in the chemo administration process is an essential element in preventing error. Giving the patient permission to question the drug or the drug amount and encouraging the nurse to take a time out if there is any question about the process are important factors to emphasize on and may prevent an error from occurring.

Chemotherapy continues to stay on the list of the ISMP's list of High-Alert Medications. While double verification is time and labor intensive, the benefits of taking this time in increasing patient safety and reducing potential medication errors far outweigh the efforts involved. Including patients and caregivers in the process is also an essential element to reducing risk. Patient safety should always be at the top of every nurse's priority list.

SUGGESTED READINGS

Polovich M, White JM, Kelleher LO. *Chemotherapy and Biotherapy Guidelines and Recommendations for Practice.* 2nd Ed. Pittsburgh, PA: Oncology Nursing Society; 2005, pp. 63–78.

Schulmeister L. Ten simple strategies to prevent chemotherapy errors. *Clin J Oncol Nurs.* 2005;9(2):201–205.

Sheridan-Leos N. A model of chemotherapy education for novice oncology nurses that supports a culture of safety. *Clin J Oncol Nurs.* 2007;11(4):545–551.

PRACTICE SAFE HANDLING FOR ALL HAZARDOUS DRUG ADMINISTRATION—INCLUDING ORAL DRUGS

MARY S. WARD, RN, BS, OCN

WHAT TO DO: IMPLEMENT

If exposure to a drug has the potential to cause cancer, reproductive or developmental toxicity, or harm to organs, the National Institute for Occupational Safety and Health (NIOSH) classifies the drug as hazardous. Any person who comes into contact with the drug, the drug residue, or waste from the drug or the patient who has received the drug is at risk for occupational exposure. Guidelines for safe handling of hazardous drugs have been established by NIOSH, OSHA, the American Association of Health-System Pharmacists, and the Oncology Nursing Society with the goal of reducing exposure to a minimum. Drugs most often thought of in this category are chemotherapy drugs, but the list also includes many antibiotics, antivirals, contraceptives, drugs given for HIV, medications used as antirejection therapy after transplants, oxytocic drugs, estrogens, and gonadotropins. Not all of the drugs will cause cancer or organ toxicities, but the common element is that they all require special handling consideration.

The majority of the drugs on NIOSH's hazardous drug list are administered by infusion, and most are antineoplastics that are usually given in a very controlled environment in an infusion center or an inpatient setting by trained oncology nurses. It has been demonstrated that nurses who use personal protective equipment to administer chemotherapy, such as special chemotherapy gowns and gloves, significantly reduce their risk of exposure to the drugs.

There are a smaller number of drugs on the NIOSH list, however, that are oral drugs. Nurses administering these drugs need to be aware of their classification as hazardous drugs and follow specific handling guidelines to reduce the risk of occupational exposure. Patients and family members who assist them in taking their medicines at home also need to be taught how to safely handle these hazardous drugs.

The first guideline to follow with all hazardous oral drugs is to never cut or crush a pill or tablet outside a Biological Safety Cabinet. Patients who are unable to take whole pills should be given other options for their medications or the pills should be sent back to the pharmacy for compounding and individual dosing under the hood of the BSC. Cutting or crushing pills causes aerosolization of the pill and the powder from this is an exposure risk. Most hormone agents are coated pills indicating that the coating should be left intact. The coating acts as a protectant and reduces risk to the individual handling the pill. If a patient needs to cut a hazardous pill at home, he or she should be instructed to use a pill cutter separate from the one being used for other medications. For oral antineoplastic agents, additional handling precautions are needed. The person administering the drug should wear gloves when handling the medication. Any wrappers, pill bottles, paper cups, gloves, etc. are considered hazardous waste and should be disposed of in yellow hazardous waste containers. If a hospital unit has no hazardous waste container, the pharmacy can dispose of the waste.

Finally, it is important to note that patients taking oral antineoplastics will have contaminated waste products. Urine, feces, sweat, emesis, and blood are all considered hazardous while the patient is taking these medications and for 5 to 7 days after he has completed taking them. For incontinent patients, caregivers should always protect their own skin from exposure to body fluids, barrier cream should be applied to the patient's skin to protect him or her, and soiled linens should be washed separately from the rest of the family's linen in hot water. In institutions, the linen does not need to be separated, but universal precautions need to be emphasized.

SUGGESTED READINGS

Birner A. Safe administration of oral chemotherapy. *Clin J Oncol Nurs*. 2003;7(2):158–162.

Griffin E. AOCN, safety considerations and safe handling of oral chemotherapy agents. *Clin J Oncol Nurs*. 2003;7(2S):25–29.

NIOSH Alert. Preventing occupational exposures to antineoplastic and other hazardous drugs in health care settings. DHHS (NIOSH) Publication Number 2004-165. September 2004.

Polovich M, White JM, Kelleher LO. *Chemotherapy and Biotherapy Guidelines and Recommendations for Practice*. 2nd Ed. Pittsburgh, PA: Oncology Nursing Society; 2005, pp. 15, 71.

USE PERSONAL PROTECTIVE EQUIPMENT FOR CHEMOTHERAPY HANDLING FROM BEGINNING TO END

MARY S. WARD, RN, BS, OCN

Chemotherapy works by causing cell death by a variety of mechanisms. It is well known that healthcare workers, pharmacists, nurses, personal care aids, and even environmental service personnel who come into contact with these drugs and their waste products have an occupational health risk. The effects of these drugs can be exhibited by mutagenicity, developmental or reproductive side effects, and cancer. Exposure can come through a variety of sources, like the skin exposure, inhalation, or injection, but skin exposure is the most likely route.

Studies of preparation and administration areas reveal surface contamination in all study areas. There is no measurable amount of exposure that is considered "safe"; the goal is to reduce exposure for healthcare workers, caregivers, and family members to a minimum. Worker exposure has been tested utilizing a variety of mechanisms, one of which is to test active compounds of chemotherapy in the urine of workers in preparation and administration settings, and a surprising amount of chemotherapy drug has been found in the urine of these workers.

The National Occupation and Safety Health Administration, Occupational Safety and Health Administration, and the Oncology Nursing Society have developed guidelines for workers who handle chemotherapy from preparation to waste disposal. It has been shown that workers who follow these guidelines and wear the appropriate personal protective equipment at each stage of chemotherapy handling have reduced amounts of measurable drug in urine samples as well as a reduction in measured chromosome abnormality.

All chemotherapy preparations must be done under a laminar flow biological safety cabinet that directs the flow of air away from the practitioner. The nurse or pharmacist who prepares the chemotherapy must wear appropriate chemotherapy gown and gloves. When an infusion bag has been prepared, it should be spiked under the hood with tubing that has been primed with nonchemotherapy fluid and wiped with moist gauze. Studies have shown that vials of chemotherapy that come from the manufacturer may have large amounts of concentrated drug on the outside of the vials. When the preparer picks up the vial, he may inadvertently transfer the drug from the outside of the vial to the outside of the infusion bag, contaminating it with chemotherapy. Nurses who administer chemotherapy should handle all bags and syringes with gloves on, even if just checking the bag or taking it down once the infusion is complete. The bag and tubing should be considered contaminated at all times.

During IV administration, the nurse should wear chemotherapy gown and gloves for personal protection. After the infusion is complete, gloves should be worn to remove the bag and tubing and it should be placed in the hazardous waste. Gloves should also be worn when handling patient waste during chemo-infusions and for 48 h afterward. If there is a chance that clothes may be soiled, from an incontinent patient for example, then a gown should also be worn. Careful handwashing after the removal of any PPE is also necessary to reduce contamination risk.

Caring for a patient receiving chemotherapy brings many challenges. Routinely utilizing proper personal protective equipment will reduce the risk of exposure and allow the nurse to focus on the other aspects of care that the patient needs.

SUGGESTED READINGS

NIOSH Alert. Preventing occupational exposures to antineoplastic and other hazardous drugs in health care settings. DHHS (NIOSH) Publication Number 2004-165. September 2004.

Polovich M, Blecher CS, Glynn-Tucker EM, et al. *Safe Handling of Hazardous Drugs*. Pittsburgh, PA: Oncology Nursing Society; 2003.

Polovich M, White JM, Kelleher LO. *Chemotherapy and Biotherapy Guidelines and Recommendations for Practice*. 2nd Ed. Pittsburgh, PA: Oncology Nursing Society; 2005, pp. 53–62.

Carefully Monitor the Patients Receiving High Dose Methotrexate to Prevent Toxicities

Mary S. Ward, RN, BS, OCN

WHAT TO DO: EVALUATE

Methotrexate is an antimetabolite chemotherapy agent used in multiple chemotherapy regimens either as a single agent or in combination therapy. It is also utilized as a treatment in other diseases such as rheumatoid arthritis, psoriasis, and as an alternative treatment to surgical management of ectopic pregnancy. The dose ranges from 7.5 mg/week to 20 g/m^2 per cycle of chemotherapy in osteosarcoma patients. The drug can be administered orally, IM, IV, and intrathecally.

Standard IV doses of methotrexate are usually tolerated well by patients, although the drug carries some black box warnings including the potential for GI and pulmonary toxicities. However, when given in high dose regimens, the drug has the possibility of serious toxicities due to the accumulation of crystals in the urine, leading to the obstruction of the renal tubules and toxic systemic accumulation of the drug. With reduced renal clearance, the drug will have increased systemic toxicity, causing significant harm to the patient. The renal insufficiency may be preexisting or drug-induced.

Nurses who administer high dose methotrexate protocols must be aware of the potential toxicities and the nursing implications surrounding its administration. Failure to implement prevention strategies and monitoring protocols will put the patient at significant risk for methotrexate toxicity.

The initial requirement of therapy is that the patient must be well hydrated prior to the initiation of treatment, receiving at least 1 L of fluid over 6 h before initiation of the chemotherapy. Hydration should continue while the chemotherapy is infusing at a rate of at least 125 mL/h and for at least two days after infusion to assure proper renal function. The patient must be kept on strict I's and O's and any significant decrease in output must be brought to the physician's attention without delay.

Second, the patient's urine pH must be checked for alkalinity. The treatment should not be initiated until the urine pH is > 7 and the pH should be checked every 6 h during treatment. If the urine pH drops < 7.0, the patient should receive sodium bicarbonate either as part of the maintenance IV fluid or in oral form. Keeping the urine alkalinized will decrease the precipitation of crystals in the kidneys. The serum creatinine should be checked prior to the initiation of therapy and daily thereafter to monitor kidney function.

Methotrexate levels should be drawn 24 h after therapy has been initiated and daily thereafter. These drug levels are used to determine the length of leucovorin rescue therapy for the patient. Methotrexate is a folate antagonist; leucovorin is a folate precursor that replenishes the cells' folic acid. Leucovorin is started 24 h after the initiation of methotrexate and is given every 6 h after that until the methotrexate levels drop below a designated level. It is of critical importance that the ordered leucovorin be given as scheduled. Leucovorin may be given PO, IV, or IM.

High dose methotrexate can cause side effects such as neurotoxicities, leukoencephalopathy, focal or generalized seizures, stroke-like symptoms of confusion, hemiparesis, transient blindness, and coma. Other side effects include liver and pulmonary toxicities. Nurses caring for these patients must be vigilant for these side effects while monitoring the patient during the administration of methotrexate and leucovorin rescue. Though it is probable that the physician will remember to order all the monitoring parameters, it should not be assumed. Nurses who function proactively will make certain that the patient is carefully monitored during this drug regimen.

SUGGESTED READINGS

Polovich M, White JM, Kelleher LO. *Chemotherapy and Biotherapy Guidelines and Recommendations for Practice.* 2nd Ed. Pittsburgh, PA: Oncology Nursing Society; 2005, pp. 25.

Always confirm correct placement of a central venous access device that will not give a blood return before administering chemotherapy and blood products

Julie Mulligan Watts, RN, MN

WHAT TO DO: EVALUATE

Nurses should only use a central venous access device (CVAD) after tip placement has been confirmed. Immediately after the insertion of the CVAD, correct placement of the CVAD is determined radiographically. The optimal placement of the catheter tip is in the distal superior vena cava at, or near, the caval–atrial junction. When the CVAD catheter tip is not located there, there are higher rates of complications, especially thrombosis of the catheter. Nurses need to be aware that catheters inserted via the subclavian or jugular veins will move, on average, 2 to 3 cm toward the head after placement. Before administering any type of medication or blood product through a CVAD, a nurse should always evaluate proper functioning of the device. A common malfunction of CVAD is the inability to obtain a blood return through the catheter even though the nurse can infuse fluid and the catheter flushes easily. For the safety of the patient, a prudent nurse needs to initiate steps to evaluate the catheter.

There are several reasons that CVADs will flush easily but not give a blood return. Catheters can be fully or partially occluded with a thrombosis, precipitate, or blood. There are several factors that the nurse should assess including presence of a blood return, resistance felt when flushing the line, swelling in the upper chest area, and symptoms of superior vena cava syndrome. Thrombus formation accounts for approximately 60% of occlusions. Improper flushing technique may account for thrombus formation and precipitate occlusions from medications or blood. If the nurse meets resistance when flushing, force should not be used. Fibrinolytic agents may need to be used to dissolve a clotted catheter on the order of a physician. There are also agents that are indicated for dissolving medication and solution precipitate on the order of a physician. Measures to prevent thrombus formation and occlusion of the catheter include flushing between medications with normal saline, clamping the tubing as the last 0.5 mL is infused in order to maintain positive pressure within the catheter, or use of a positive pressure cap to maintain pressure and prevent back flow of blood into the catheter.

Catheters can develop a fibrin sheath along the length of the catheter that partially or fully occludes the tip when negative pressure is applied. The nurse should assess for a blood return and resistance to flushing.

A fibrin sheath may develop when catheters have been in place for a long time. The nurse should attempt to flush the catheter but not apply forceful pressure. If the catheter flushes easily but does not have a blood return, the nurse should have the patient change his or her position. Various positions have been described in the literature but none are well supported. Examples are turning on their sides, raising arms, and turning their head as blood aspiration is attempted. Proper flushing between medications and use of positive pressure may assist in preventing the development of fibrin sheaths. It is recommended never to administer vesicant drugs when a fibrin sheath or clot is present because it can cause backflow of the agent and extravasation. Use of a fibrinolytic agent may clear the problem.

The nurse should also assess for damage to the catheter. Catheters can become damaged and rupture if flushed using high pressures, which most often occurs when a small syringe is used for flushing. For this reason, it is recommended that these lines not be flushed with syringes smaller than a 10 mL size. Catheters can also become kinked, fractured (shear completely and break apart), or separated from implanted ports if not connected properly prior to insertion of a port. Symptoms include shoulder pain, burning at the site, inability to obtain a blood return, and chest pain and dyspnea if the catheter shears off. If these symptoms occur, the physician should be notified and fluoroscopy or venogram ordered.

Catheter placement between the clavicle and first rib can result in repetitive compression causing catheter weakness and pinching of the catheter. This has been called "pinch-off syndrome." Pinch-off syndrome usually occurs several months after the insertion of the catheter or port. It can be observed on chest-X-ray as compressed or indented under the clavicle. Pinch-off syndrome increases the risk of rupture and fracture. The CVAD likely needs replacement when pinch-off is evident.

For the safety of a patient, nurses should always avoid giving drugs through CVADs when a blood return is not present. Obtain a physician's order for placement verification with X-ray or dye studies. CVADs with catheter tips located in places other than the lower third of the superior vena cava or at the caval–atrial junction should be discussed with physicians and used cautiously and only with physicians' orders.

SUGGESTED READINGS

Arch P. Port navigation: Let the journey begin. *Clin J Oncol Nurs.* 2007;11(4):485–486.

Camp-Sorrell D. *Access Device Guidelines: Recommendations for Nursing Practice and Education.* 2nd Ed. Pittsburgh, PA: Oncology Nursing Society; 2004.

Infusion Nursing Society 2006. Infusion nursing: Standards of practice. *J Infusion Nurs.* 2006;29(1 S).

McIntosh N. Central venous catheters: Reasons for insertion and removal. *Paediatr Nurs.* 2003;15(1):14–17.

Registered Nurses' Association of Ontario. *Care and Maintenance to Reduce Vascular Access Complications.* Toronto, ON: RNAO; 2005.

Schulmeister L. An unusual cause of shoulder pain. *Clin J Oncol Nurs.* 2005;9(4):476–477.

ALWAYS USE CURRENT HEIGHT AND WEIGHT TO VERIFY CHEMOTHERAPY DOSES

JULIE MULLIGAN WATTS, RN, MN

WHAT TO DO: IMPLEMENT

For the oncology nurse, fundamentals of safe chemotherapy administration include knowledge of doses and scheduling, dose determination, and safety procedures to ensure a safely administered dose. The use of guidelines and practice recommendations from national nursing organizations is standard within adult, pediatric, and gynecologic oncology nursing practices.

A review and verification of the patient's data is the first step in the process. Data such as laboratory test results, allergy history, and weight should be verified. It is never appropriate to base chemotherapy orders on a weight that the patient verbally reports or on historical weight from a previous chemotherapy encounter. Patients may have a drastic drop in weight between the first and second course of chemotherapy and an overdose could be made if a stated weight is used rather than a current weight measurement.

Understanding if the patient is to receive a standard-dose therapy or a high-dose therapy is helpful in checking for accuracy in the physician's order. Research has demonstrated that patients receiving standard-dose treatment often receive lower than intended doses due to delays, reductions taken due to abnormal labs, and miscalculations. The reduced doses have proven clinically significant when comparing remission and survival of those receiving standard dose with those who have received dose reductions.

Understanding how and why a certain chemotherapy dose is determined and verifying that the dose is appropriate are important functions in the treatment phase. Doses may be modified based on laboratory data and use of combined modalities (e.g., concurrent chemotherapy and radiation therapy). A systematic approach to dose calculation is recommended. Although there has been some discussion about alternate methods of dose calculation, doses are currently determined based on the height and weight of the patient. The dosing procedure involves a calculation of the patient's body surface area (BSA or m2). Several methods exist for determining the BSA including formulas, calculators, and use of a nomogram, which is not currently recommended due to inaccuracy. Recalculation of the dose by at least two chemotherapy-trained healthcare professionals is recommended. The patient's BSA is multiplied by the recommended dose cited in a reliable source such as a chemotherapy book, protocol information, package insert from the chemotherapy being given, or articles from reliable journals.

It is understood that modifications may be made to the dose based on the patient's age, renal function, liver function, obesity, recent weight loss, drug interactions, and concurrent therapies. From the nurses' perspective, the best way to ensure accurate dosing is by starting with an accurate, measured height and weight.

SUGGESTED READINGS

Gurney H. Developing a new framework for dose calculation. *J Clin Oncol.* 2006;24(10):1489–1490.

Polovich M, White J, Kelleher L, eds. *Chemotherapy and Biotherapy Guidelines and Recommendations for Practice.* 2nd Ed. Pittsburgh, PA: Oncology Nursing Society; 2005.

Schulmeister L. Preventing chemotherapy errors. *Oncologist.* 2006;11:463–468.

ALWAYS VERIFY THAT CHEMOTHERAPY ORDERS ARE COMPLETE. THIS NEEDS TO INCLUDE THE APPROPRIATE HYDRATION, ELECTROLYTES, PREMEDICATIONS, PROCEDURES, AND FOLLOW-UP LABORATORY TESTS THAT SHOULD ACCOMPANY THE SPECIFIC CHEMOTHERAPEUTIC AGENT THAT IS ORDERED.

JULIE MULLIGAN WATTS, RN, MN

WHAT TO DO: EVALUATE

Methotrexate is a widely used therapy in adult and pediatric oncology, gynecology, and rheumatology. Besides a wide range of tumors, it is used to treat hydatidiform mole, psoriasis, and rheumatoid arthritis. Routes of administration include intravenous infusion or bolus, intrathecally, intramuscularly, orally, intraperitoneally, intra-arterially, and by intravesical instillation. Uses of high dose methotrexate (HDM) include acute lymphoblastic leukemia, primary CNS lymphoma, central nervous system prophylaxis in patients with leukemia, meningeal lymphoma, other high-risk lymphomas, breast cancer, head and neck cancer, gastric cancer, and osteosarcoma. It is an agent that has a wide dose range depending on the disease being treated. Regimens of methotrexate are termed high, intermediate, or low-dose therapies. HDM is usually considered to include doses equal to or over $500 \, mg/m^2$ and can range up to $33,000 \, mg/m^2$.

When given at high doses, the methotrexate dose is considered a lethal dose of chemotherapy and must be followed by a "rescue" drug, or antidote, called leucovorin. The leucovorin acts to stop the toxic effects of the HDM. Because methotrexate is cleared through the kidneys, HDM requires aggressive hydration before, during, and after the dose is given. In order for the drug to be successfully cleared by the kidneys, the urine must be adequately alkalinized; so IV hydration contains sodium bicarbonate and patients are given oral doses of bicarbonate as well to bring the pH of the urine up to a range of 6.0 to 7.0. By alkalinizing the urine, the methotrexate becomes five to eight times more soluble in the urine and is filtered out. Methotrexate-induced renal dysfunction is believed to be caused through precipitation of the drug in the renal tubules or by a direct toxic effect of methotrexate on the renal tubules. Even though these preventive measures are required, approximately 1.8% of patients with osteosarcoma treated in clinical trials develop renal dysfunction. When renal dysfunction occurs and the methotrexate is not cleared, the results are elevated and sustained plasma levels of methotrexate and an increase in other toxicities of methotrexate.

Drug interactions may decrease the renal clearance of methotrexate and result in increased toxicity. Drug interactions have been noted with aspirin, other salicylates, nonsteroidal anti-inflammatory drugs (NSAIDs), probenecid, penicillins, sulfonamides, and trimethoprim (Bactrim, Septra). NSAIDs should not be given during HDM and likely should be discontinued 24h prior to HDM and not restarted until 48h after the methotrexate dose.

In checking that a complete order is written for HDM, the order should contain IV hydration of 2.5 to $3.5 \, L$ of fluid per m^2 for 24h, beginning before the HDM infusion and lasting until 24 to 48h after the HDM. The hydration orders should include 40 to 50 mEq of sodium bicarbonate per liter of IV fluid prior to, during, and after the administration of HDM. Oral sodium bicarbonate may be added and orders for urine pH checks until the pH reaches 6.0 to 7.0 are included prior to HDM administration. Intake and output, urine specific gravity, urine osmolality, and BUN and creatinine are usually ordered. Urine output should be maintained at 700 to $2,000 \, mL/day$, depending on hydration orders.

In addition to orders related to renal function, complete orders should include plasma methotrexate concentrations and orders for leucovorin rescue. Elevated plasma levels of methotrexate at 24, 48, and 72h may indicate the development of renal toxicity and require aggressive pharmacokinetically guided doses of leucovorin. Complete orders to prevent renal toxicity with HDM include urine alkalinization, adequate urine output, monitoring renal function, leucovorin orders, and plasma methotrexate levels. Physician orders that do not consider all of these factors are inadequate for safe patient care.

SUGGESTED READINGS

Fischer D, Knobf M, Durivage H, et al. *The Cancer Chemotherapy Handbook*. 6th Ed. Philadelphia, PA: Mosby; 2003.

LaCasce A. Therapeutic use of high-dose methotrexate. UpToDate, Inc. 2008. Available at: http://www.uptodate.com/patients/content/topic.do?topicKey=chemagen/5867. Accessed August 13, 2008.

Polovich M, White J, Kelleher L, eds. *Chemotherapy and Biotherapy Guidelines and Recommendations for Practice*. 2nd Ed. Pittsburgh, PA: Oncology Nursing Society; 2005.

Widemann B, Adamson P. Pediatric oncology: Understanding and managing methotrexate nephrotoxicity. *The Oncologist*. 2006;11(6):694–703.

IN NEUTROPENIC ONCOLOGY PATIENTS WHERE THE BODY'S SECOND LINE OF DEFENSE IS GONE, IT IS A GOOD IDEA TO PROTECT THE FIRST LINE OF DEFENSE—THE SKIN

JULIE MULLIGAN WATTS, RN, MN

WHAT TO DO: IMPLEMENT

Prevention of healthcare-associated pressure ulcers (decubitus ulcers), along with actions to treat pressure ulcers, is an important part of care for all patients. In hospital settings, the incidence of pressure ulcers ranges from 2.7% to 29.5%. Some special populations may be at increased risk for the development of pressure ulcers, including quadriplegic patients, orthopedic patients, and cancer patients.

Hospitalized cancer patients can have multiple reasons for being at risk for pressure ulcers. At diagnosis, patients may have experienced weight loss and be experiencing protein-calorie malnutrition. At the time of diagnosis, many cancer patients have extensive surgical procedures that can further diminish protein stores and open up the skin to infection. Urinary catheters, IV sites, and surgical wounds are all avenues to infectious agents that further compromise skin integrity. Treatment with chemo or biologic therapy can cause neutropenia, skin reactions, and compromise protection by long-term IV access. Radiation therapy is known for causing skin reactions, although progress has been made over the past decades with tissue-sparing energy sources. Radiation also compromises skin integrity by requiring that patients be immobile during treatment. Fatigue and pain are conditions experienced by many oncology patients at some point after diagnosis, which can add to the risk for pressure ulcers by increasing immobility. Nonhealing of wounds is significantly higher in cancer patients when compared to noncancer patients. In general, cancer patients have more comorbid conditions and other factors that have the potential to impair wound healing.

Guidelines for prevention and treatment of pressure ulcers contain recommendations for assessment for those who are at risk, evaluation of the wound, education and development of a treatment plan, a nutritional assessment, management of tissue loads, ulcer assessment, management of infection, and care, education, monitoring, and evaluation. Most guidelines also contain a process for staging of wounds. A Stage I pressure ulcer is an observable alteration in intact skin. The ulcer appears as a defined area of persistent redness in lightly pigmented skin whereas in darker skin tones, the ulcer may appear with persistent red, blue, or purple hues. A stage II pressure is a partial thickness skin loss involving epidermis, dermis, or both. The ulcer is superficial and presents clinically as an abrasion, blister, or shallow crater. Stage III is defined as having full thickness skin loss involving damage to, or necrosis of, subcutaneous tissue that may extend down to, but not through, underlying fascia. The ulcer presents clinically as a deep crater with or without undermining of adjacent tissue. Stage IV exhibits full thickness skin loss with extensive destruction, tissue necrosis, or damage to muscle, bone, or supporting structures (e.g., tendon and joint capsule). Undermining and sinus tracts also may be associated with Stage IV pressure ulcers.

The nurse caring for a cancer patient with a pressure ulcer must relieve factors that have caused the ulcer including pressure, friction, shear, and moisture. Nurses also need to support the patient's mobility and nutritional status for healing to occur. In neutropenic patients, the wound must be kept clean, antibiotics should be prescribed, and debridement should be carried out to promote a clean wound bed that will heal. Removal of sources that keep the wound too moist is important. Barriers to protect the surrounding skin can be helpful, but antiseptics to reduce bacterial counts in the wound itself are usually not recommended.

Prevention of pressure ulcers is a key task in working with oncology patients who have prolonged periods of neutropenia. With neutropenia, the second line of defense against infection is already removed, so protection of the first line of defense is critical.

SUGGESTED READINGS

Hess C, ed. JCAHO adopts pressure ulcer prevention goal. *Adv Skin Wound Care*. 2005;18(6):293.

McNees P, Meneses K. Pressure ulcers and other chronic wounds in patients with and patients without cancer: A retrospective, comparative analysis of healing patterns. *Ostomy Wound Manage*. 2007;53(2):70–78.

National Library of Medicine. AHCPR supported clinical practice guidelines: Treatment of pressure ulcers. 1994. Available at: http://www.ncbi.nlm.gov/books/bv.fcgi?rid=hstat2.chapter5124.

Registered Nurses' Association of Ontario. Assessment & management of stage I to IV pressure ulcers. Available at: http://www.rnao.org/Storage/29/2372_BPG_Pressure_Ulcers_I_to_IV_Summary.pdf. Accessed August 13, 2008.

Registered Nurses' Association of Ontario. Risk assessment & prevention of pressure ulcers: Nursing best practice guidelines. 2005. Available at: http://www.rnao.org/Storage/12/638_BPG_Pressure_Ulcers_v2.pdf. Accessed August 13, 2008.

Always verify that a patient understands patient education prior to initiating cancer treatment

Julie Mulligan Watts, RN, MN

WHAT TO DO: EVALUATE

In today's fast-paced world when cancer diagnoses are made and treatment is initiated quickly, the nurse must make sure that the patient and the family understand what is happening and why it is happening. Cancer and the treatment for cancer are complex concepts to understand, so patient education is integral to oncology nursing practice. The education about a new diagnosis often takes place at a time of crisis when emotions run high and patients can be in a state of shock or denial. Learning will be diminished during periods of high anxiety and stress. A new diagnosis of cancer may mean a death sentence with pain and suffering to the average individual experiencing a new diagnosis. For oncology nurses, patient education is a rewarding part of oncology nursing care and every oncology nurse must provide excellent patient education as part of his or her everyday practice.

Verbal explanations are one of the most commonly used ways that nurses educate patients. Oncology nurses explain and answer questions regarding the diagnosis, treatment, side effects, self-care measures, and end-of-life issues. In both inpatient and outpatient settings, verbal instructions may be accompanied by written materials and other methods of education. Effective patient education requires that oncology nurses be aware of a patient's educational level, developmental level, preferences for learning, ability to read, and cultural and language characteristics. Also important are the factors that affect a patient's motivation to learn. The context in which learning takes place can affect the patient's motivation. A new mother may be more motivated to learn newborn care than a person with colon cancer learning colostomy care.

Use of medical terminology can present a challenge when oncology nurses are teaching patients. Nurses are used to hearing medical terminology in their work settings and often nurses use the same terminology in patient teaching. A woman that hears that her lymph nodes are positive may not understand that it means that the cancer has spread. A patient who is told that his diagnosis is myeloid leukemia may understand that the leukemia is mild rather than the aggressive cancer that it is. A patient with metastatic cancer may think that he or she has a new diagnosis of bone cancer when the physician relays information about bone metastasis. Cancer patients often do not understand the overall concept of therapy to decrease the tumor burden and lessen symptoms when advanced disease is present. The nurse or physician may be asked questions about why the cure remains unlikely even when a patient has a complete response to chemotherapy or radiation.

Excellent resources for patient education are available from the American Cancer Society, the National Cancer Institute, the Leukemia and Lymphoma Society, and many other agencies. Many publications are available in languages other than English. The ability to use printed materials for patient education depends on the patient's ability to read, the reading level of the publication, and the comprehension by the patient. About half of the population has low levels of literacy. These individuals may lack the ability to adequately understand complex health information. There is a correlation between low-literacy, income, and education levels. It is difficult to produce written materials that are easily understood when writing about cancer, chemotherapy, and other complex concepts. Many materials have been found to have a 12th grade or higher reading level, so nurses must use additional materials and explanations in their teaching.

Important steps in the patient education process include assessment for readiness to learn, preferred methods of learning, understanding of what is taught, and repetition of teaching to reinforce the desired outcome. Beneficial outcomes of patient education in the cancer population include the ability to manage side effects, identification of new problems, increased understanding about the disease and treatment, and improved coping abilities.

Reassessing and verifying the understanding of the patient are critical steps. Active listening by the nurse and asking questions to help assess the patient's learning are important. Keeping information clear and understandable is the key to successful oncology patient education.

SUGGESTED READINGS

Carroll-Johnson R, Gorman L, Bush N. *Psychosocial Nursing Care Along the Cancer Continuum*. 2nd Ed. Pittsburgh, PA: Oncology Nursing Society; 2005.

Foyle L, Hostad J. *Innovations in Cancer and Palliative Care Education*. Oxon, England: Radcliffe Publishing; 2007.

National Cancer Institute. Clear & simple: Developing effective print materials for low-literate readers. 2008. Available at: http://www.cancer.gov/cancerinformation/clearandsimple. Accessed August 13, 2008.

Potter P, Perry A. *Fundamentals of Nursing*. 6th Ed. St. Louis, MO: Mosby, Inc; 2005.

ALWAYS CHECK LAB VALUES PREOPERATIVELY FOR PATIENTS WITH LEUKEMIA WHO HAVE RECEIVED INDUCTION CHEMOTHERAPY WITH EXTENDED LENGTHS OF STAYS

JULIE MULLIGAN WATTS, RN, MN

WHAT TO DO: EVALUATE

An estimated 44,270 new cases of leukemia were diagnosed in 2008, with about 40% of those being acute leukemia. Leukemia is often thought of as a pediatric cancer but it occurs more often in adults. The usual treatment for acute leukemia is chemotherapy. Depending on the type of acute leukemia, a variety of cytotoxic drugs and biologic agents are employed to treat the leukemia. The immediate goal of therapy is to induce a remission.

Newly diagnosed patients with acute leukemia often have extended stays in the hospital due to the effects of the initial induction therapy. Almost all treatments for acute leukemia cause myelosuppression. Bone marrow recovery usually takes 14 to 21 days after the end of chemotherapy, and in acute myeloid leukemia, the time for complete recovery is 28 to 32 days. Multiple antibiotics and blood products are used during this time as supportive therapy. This period of time of prolonged hospitalization is very difficult on the patient due to the side effects of treatment that include pancytopenia and often, poor appetite, fever, weight loss, and diarrhea. Loneliness and depression may be experienced due to protective isolation, which is necessary to protect the patient from infection during periods of prolonged neutropenia. Daily CBC, platelet count, and differential are recommended during chemotherapy. Platelet counts are checked every day while in the hospital until the patient is platelet-transfusion independent.

Besides neutropenia, these patients experience thrombocytopenia, or decreased platelets. Clinical signs of decreased platelets include easy bruising, petechiae, and bleeding from the gums, nose, or other orifices. When platelet counts fall below $50,000 cells/mm^3$, there is a moderate risk of bleeding. When the platelet count falls below $10,000 cells/mm^3$, there is a severe risk of bleeding which may include fatal bleeding from the central nervous system, gastrointestinal system, or respiratory system. Platelet transfusions are required for the acute leukemic following a high dose of chemotherapy. Platelets are usually transfused prophylactically at a level of $10,000 cells/mm^3$ or less for stable patients. Patients who have bleeding, coagulopathies, sepsis, serious mucositis or cystitis, or drug-induced platelet dysfunction should receive platelets at higher levels.

Both acute myeloid leukemia and acute lymphoid leukemia patients have a risk of meningeal leukemia, with the acute lymphoid risk being about 35%. When meningeal leukemia occurs, the treatment is intrathecal or intraventricular chemotherapy. The chemotherapy can be given with a lumbar puncture or through an implanted Ommaya reservoir that allows the drug to be given directly into a ventricle in the brain. The reservoir is placed underneath the skin on the head with a small catheter extending into the ventricle. Even though there is a risk from the surgical procedure, many physicians prefer this route because there is a higher chance that therapeutic drug levels will be achieved in the ventricles with this route rather than through lumbar punctures.

Cancer patients who have thrombocytopenia often require invasive diagnostic or therapeutic procedures. Those with acute leukemia may require placement of a central venous catheter, placement of an Ommaya reservoir, bone marrow biopsies, and drainage and repair of abscesses. A platelet count of $40,000 cells/mm^3$ to $50,000 cells/mm^3$ is often cited as a standard for the level at which major surgery can be performed safely. Minor procedures such as a bone marrow aspirate and biopsy can be performed safely at platelet levels of $20,000 cells/mm^3$, but there is little data to support safety of other invasive procedures at counts of less than $20,000 cells/mm^3$.

When platelets are administered to thrombocytopenic patients prior to an invasive procedure, it is imperative that nurses assess a posttransfusion platelet count to be sure that the platelet count has reached the desired safe level. Prior to sending any patient to surgery, the nurse should verify that lab results are current. Checking for a current platelet count on a thrombocytopenic patient bound for surgery is critical.

SUGGESTED READINGS

American Cancer Society. *Cancer Facts and Figures*. Atlanta: American Cancer Society; 2008.

American Red Cross. *Practice Guidelines for Blood Transfusion: A Compilation from Recent Peer-Reviewed Literature*. 2nd Ed. Washington, DC: American National Red Cross; 2007.

Arnold D, Crowther M, Cook R, et al. Utilization of platelet transfusions in the intensive care unit: Indications, transfusion triggers, and platelet count responses. *Transfusion*. 2006;46: 1286–1291.

Henke-Yarbro C, Frogge M, Goodman M, eds. *Cancer Nursing: Principles and Practice*. 6th Ed. Sudbury, MA: Jones and Bartlett Publishers; 2005.

National Comprehensive Cancer Network, Inc. Acute myeloid leukemia. *Practice Guidelines in Oncology-v.1.2008*. 2007. Available at: http://www.nccn.org/professionals/physician_gls/PDF/aml.pdf. Accessed May 9, 2008.

Schiffer C, AndersonK, Bennett C, et al. Platelet transfusion for patients with cancer: Clinical practice guidelines of the American society of clinical oncology. *J Clin Oncol*. 2001;19(5):1519–1538.

BE AWARE OF DIFFERENT DOSING REGIMENS OF CYTARABINE

MARY S. WARD, RN, BS, OCN

WHAT TO DO: ASSESS AND PLAN

Cytarabine, also known as Cytosar or Ara-C, is an antimetabolite chemotherapy drug used principally in the treatment of hematological malignancies. It is one of the chief drugs used in the treatment of acute myelogenous leukemia (AML). AML treatment consists of two stages. In the first phase, or induction, Ara-C is given in combination regimens typically with an anthracycline. The second phase, or consolidation, is begun once the patient has gone into complete remission. This comprises three shorter cycles of treatment and frequently consists of Ara-C in single drug or multidrug regimen.

One reason chemotherapy drugs are high risk drugs is that some drugs have wide dosing ranges. Ara-C has two different dosing levels: standard dose and high dose. Standard dose Ara-C is 100 to 200 mg/m^2 given over 24 h as a continuous infusion and is used in induction AML. High dose Ara-C is usually prescribed in consolidation treatment, although it has been used in combination study in the induction phase. The dose range for high dose Ara-C is 1,000 to 3,000 mg/m^2 given over 1 to 3 h every 12 h for 8 to 12 doses. The shorter infusion time for the higher dose allows for cell recovery prior to the subsequent infusion. A risk for medication error exists with this drug since it is given for the same disease with the doses having exactly a tenfold difference. A misplaced decimal point is all that is needed for high dose Ara-C to be mistakenly prescribed, mixed, or given as a 24-h infusion in place of standard dose Ara-C.

Side effects for standard dose Ara-C include anemia, neutropenia, thrombocytopenia, mild to moderate nausea and vomiting, and hepatic dysfunction. About 20% to 50% of the serum concentration of Ara-C crosses the blood–brain barrier. The side effects for high-dose Ara-C consist of severe nausea and vomiting, stomatitis, diarrhea, GI bleeding, cerebellar and cerebral toxicities exhibited by ataxia, nystagmus, dysarthria, and tremors. The high level of concentration of the drug also causes it to be excreted in the tears and puts the patient at risk for developing drug-induced keratitis. Patients are prescribed prophylactic steroid eye drops to prevent this complication.

AML patients receiving Ara-C should be closely monitored for side effects. All doses of chemotherapy should be double checked and independently verified by two chemotherapy competent practitioners prior to hanging. Likewise, each bag should be verified against the original chemotherapy order by two chemotherapy competent RNs. Calculations should not be done quickly in the head but should be written out and checked on paper since it is easy to "lose" a zero while doing mental calculations.

Finally, the nurse should always be alert to the patient for any extreme adverse side effects that appear to be out of proportion to the dose being administered. A patient who is supposed to receive standard dose Ara-C with uncontrolled and unrelenting nausea, vomiting, and diarrhea should have his or her dose reverified. Likewise, if the patient develops stomatitis within a few days of the initiation of standard dose Ara-C, it may be an indication that the dose he or she is receiving is outside the standard dose range. Signs of cerebral or cerebellar toxicity clearly indicate an elevated dose of the drug.

Double nurse verification of the drug, dose, and bags is the key element to prevent medication errors with chemotherapy infusions. However, good assessment skills and critical thinking are also essential to quality patient care.

SUGGESTED READINGS

Drugs, supplements, and herbal information. MedlinePlus. Available at: http://www.nlm.nih.gov/medlineplus/druginfo/medmaster/a682222.html. Accessed August 24, 2008.

INVESTIGATE ANY CENTRAL VENOUS ACCESS DEVICE (CVAD) WITHOUT A BLOOD RETURN

MARY S. WARD, RN, BS, OCN

WHAT TO DO: EVALUATE

Central venous access devices (CVADs), including tunneled and nontunneled catheters and implanted ports, are indispensable medical devices for optimizing care for many patients. Central lines are required for infusions of drugs that would be harsh, irritating, or harmful to peripheral veins; drugs such as chemotherapy, total parenteral nutrition, and potassium chloride. These lines are also used for lab draws, saving patients' countless phlebotomy sticks.

As beneficial as these lines are, they hold high risk for the patient. Insertion of the line is a high risk procedure, dependent upon practitioner experience. Once inserted, the patient is at risk for infection, embolus, thrombus formation, vascular erosion, vessel penetration, stenosis, and line damage.

Catheter occlusion occurs in a large percentage of CVADs and can result from thrombus formation or a mechanical malfunction of the catheter. Catheter thrombus formation is the most common cause of catheter occlusion, occurring in approximately 33% to 59% of catheters, but other possible causes of catheter occlusion can develop and should be investigated. Factors that contribute to thrombus formation include endothelial injury, turbulence of venous flow, composition of the infusate, and disease process. Dehydration, hypotension, atrial fibrillation, malignancy, and mechanical vessel compression are risk factors. Medications that can also increase the risk of thrombus formation include chemotherapy, TPN, steroids, and Tamoxifen. Trauma to the vessel during insertion and the use of larger diameter catheters also increase risk.

Thrombus formation occurs with the formation of a fibrin sheath at the catheter tip, creating a one way "valve" over the opening, allowing flow of fluid into the catheter but preventing blood return. This may progress to intraluminal fibrosis which completely occludes the catheter. Occluded catheter lines place the patient at an increased risk for infection and must be addressed. Attempting to declot the catheter with prescribed tPA is the first step in addressing catheter occlusion. This may be repeated twice and must always be done with a 10 cc or larger syringe to control the amount of pressure on the catheter lumen.

Thrombus formation is not the only cause of catheter occlusion. Mechanical occlusion, catheter erosion, or split internal catheter lines may also cause malfunction. A central line that is inserted between the clavicle and first rib is prone to shearing forces of wear and could eventually wear through or rupture. This line will allow infusion of fluid but will have diminished or absent blood return. The patient is also at risk of foreign body embolism as the rupture causes the catheter to shear completely. Lines can also split internally, rendering an infusion that yields little or no blood return. In both cases, extravasation of fluid into interstitial tissue is almost certain. A malfunctioning implanted port should also be assessed for the possibility of catheter–portal disconnection. In this scenario, the fluid will infuse into the interstitial space around the port, causing a "port pocket" extravasation.

Nurses are responsible for assessing patency of CVADs, or at least checking for a blood return every shift. If a line does not yield a blood return, it is vital that it be investigated. If declotting the line is unsuccessful, a Doppler flow study should be performed to confirm line placement and patency.

At no time should a line of a multilumen catheter be taped or put "out of service" for occlusion without declotting procedures and investigation of the device integrity. To ignore one line because other functioning lines exist puts the patient at a risk for infection, extravasation, and foreign body embolus. CVADs have proven to be highly beneficial to the patient populations that require them, provided they are well managed and the risks that accompany them are properly addressed.

SUGGESTED READINGS

Abeloff M, Armitage JO, Niederhuber JE. Management of nonfunctioning catheters. In: *Clinical Oncology*. 3rd Ed. Philadelphia, PA: Elsevier Churchill Livingstone; 2004.

Kusminsky RE. Complications of central venous catheterization. *J Am Coll Surg*. 2007;204(4):681–696.

McKnight S. Nurse's guide to understanding and treating thrombotic occlusion of central venous access devices. *MedSurg Nurs*. December 2004. Available at: http://findarticles.com/p/articles/mi_m0FSS/is_6_13/ai_n17208028/pg_1?tag=artBody;col1. Accessed August 24, 2008.

PATIENTS RECEIVING ORAL CHEMOTHERAPY MUST STAY ON THEIR PRESCRIBED REGIMENS

MARY S. WARD, RN, BS, OCN

WHAT TO DO: EVALUATE

Chemotherapy is most often thought of as an intravenous medication given in an outpatient or controlled inpatient setting. Most facilities require special training for nurses who infuse these medications; these nurses are trained in the dosing and special handling of these hazardous drugs. Chemotherapy is a high risk category of medications because of the narrow therapeutic index of the drugs, individual dosing, complex regimens, and high toxicity profiles of the drugs. Oncology nurses become familiar over time with the intricacies of many of the more common intravenous regimens, but the field of oncology research is dynamic and new drugs and regimens are approved on an ongoing basis.

While chemotherapy infusions tend to be well addressed in most settings, oral chemotherapy is often overlooked. It is estimated that 25% to 30% of newly approved chemotherapy drugs in the next several years will be oral drugs. These medications have significant lifestyle improvements for the patients who take them; reducing and, in some cases, eliminating confinement to an infusion chair or hospitalization for multiple-day chemotherapy regimens. These oral drugs also offer significant manageability for many diseases and symptoms, improving quality of life. However, there are some concerns that these drugs raise. Many of the regimens are complex and the dosing of the drugs is similar to that of IV chemotherapy, i.e., the drugs are dosed individually rather than by standard dosing for all patients. This can lead to error either by a patient or a nurse who may not understand body surface area dosing or that drugs are given on certain days of a regimen and held on others. Sometimes, different strengths of drugs are used to achieve a therapeutic effect, alternating doses to achieve a total dose over the course of the regimen.

Another potential for error with these drugs may occur when a patient is admitted to the hospital or a skilled nursing facility and the staff may be unfamiliar with the drug and dosing schedule. Even many primary care physicians or consulting physicians, other than an oncologist, who admit a patient may be unfamiliar with these drugs. Besides, chemotherapy drugs are not only used for treating cancer but also used to treat rheumatoid arthritis and psoriasis, e.g., Methotrexate.

It is necessary for an admitting nurse to clearly understand the patient's medication regimen if he or she is taking an antineoplastic drug. Underdosing the drug by either stopping it or not administering the correct dose will drop the patient's therapeutic levels of the agent and make the treatment ineffective. Giving too much of the drug or giving the drug more often than the regimen calls for will cause toxicities and increased side effects, potentially very harmful to the patient. Side effects are agent specific but are the same as their IV counterparts in most cases: myelosuppression, alopecia, mouth sores, liver and renal toxicities, nausea, vomiting, and diarrhea.

If nurses or physicians have any questions about the specific drugs, dosing, schedule, or reason for the patient taking the drug, it is crucial that the ordering physician be contacted as soon as possible to clarify the information. Missing doses or doubling up on doses is not an option with these drugs.

Oral chemotherapy drugs allow patients to have an improved quality of life and more control over their disease process but they also give the healthcare team many challenges. The role of a nurse involves knowing the importance of keeping the patients on their prescribed regimen.

SUGGESTED READINGS

Birner A. Safe administration of oral chemotherapy. *Clin J Oncol Nurs*. 2003;7(2):158–162.

Griffin E. AOCN, safety considerations and safe handling of oral chemotherapy agents. *Clin J Oncol Nurs*. 2003;7(S6):25–29.

NIOSH Alert. Preventing occupational exposures to antineoplastic and other hazardous drugs in health care settings. DHHS (NIOSH) Publication Number 2004-165, September 2004.

Polovich M, White JM, Kelleher LO. *Chemotherapy and Biotherapy Guidelines and Recommendations for Practice*. 2nd Ed. Pittsburgh, PA: Oncology Nursing Society; 2005, pp. 15, 71.

Eliminate accidental and fatal intrathecal vincristine administration

Mary S. Ward, RN, BS, OCN

WHAT TO DO: IMPLEMENT

Vincristine is a vinca alkaloid chemotherapy agent used in combination therapy for many types of cancer, including acute lymphocytic leukemia, Hodgkin and non-Hodgkin lymphomas, sarcomas, and breast cancer. It is administered as an IV drug and may be given via IV push gravity or continuous infusion and it a vesicant with the potential to cause tissue damage upon extravasation. Several protocols in which vincristine is used also call for intrathecal administration of other drugs, such as methotrexate or cytarabine, through a lumbar puncture or directly into the fourth ventricle of the brain through a device known as Ommaya reservoir. However, if vincristine is accidentally given intrathecally, the patient will begin to experience motor and sensory nerve damage, encephalopathy, coma, and death. Patients with accidental IT vincristine administration are found to have demyelation of spinal nerves and severe damage to the cerebral tissue. These patients die a slow and painful death.

There have been 37 documented cases of accidental IT vincristine administration. Most drug protocols call for small amounts of drug to be infused, <3 cc. The least complicated method of infusion is IV push with a syringe. However, since many of these same protocols involve IT administration of another drug, there is increased risk for accidental IT vincristine administration. Syringes may get mixed up on the administration field, the vincristine syringe may be mistaken for an additional IT drug to be administered, it may be mislabeled, or a nurse unfamiliar with either the drug or the regimen may unwittingly hand it to the physician to administer.

The World Health Organization, Institute of Safe Medication Practices, and JCAHO have all made strong recommendations regarding the safe administration of vincristine. USP labeling requires all vincristine syringes to carry a label stating, "FATAL IF GIVEN INTRATHECALLY. FOR IV USE ONLY. DO NOT REMOVE COVERING UNTIL MOMENT OF INJECTION." In addition to the required label, other recommendations that have been made include writing the intrathecal chemo orders separately from all other chemo orders, having intrathecal chemo bagged and transported separately from all other chemo drugs, and taking a "time out" just prior to any IT administration. The most impacting suggestion for practice change, however, is to eliminate syringes altogether for vincristine administration. Instead of being administered by a syringe, WHO recommends that all vincristine be mixed in 50 mL infusion bags to be given over 5 to 10 min. This would significantly reduce the potential of accidental IT vincristine administration.

Several concerns have arisen as a result of this suggestion. The most significant concern relates to the question of whether there is more potential for the drug to extravasate if it is given by infusion over a longer period of time. Data appear to support that the incidence of extravasation is similar with infusion and IV push. The second concern raised is that of cost; preparation as well as nurse monitoring time. According to both ONS guidelines and ISMP's recommendations for vesicant infusion, the nurse should be present and visually observe the infusion for its entirety, although this is more time consuming than giving an IV push medication. The third concern relates to the increased amount of fluid in the infusion bags. This is a particular concern for pediatric patients, although the amount of fluid can be reduced by extracting fluid from the minibag prior to mixing.

Accidental intrathecal vincristine administration could be almost eliminated by adopting the recommendations of putting the drug in infusion bags versus infusing by syringes. Nurses and physicians who administer vincristine must consider patient safety above all when examining current practices and contemplating practice changes.

SUGGESTED READINGS

Institute for Safe Medication Practices. ISMP medication safety alert. December 1, 2005. Available at: www.ismp.org/Newsletters. Accessed August 13, 2008.

Polovich M, White JM, Kelleher LO. *Chemotherapy and Biotherapy Guidelines and Recommendations for Practice*. 2nd Ed. Pittsburgh, PA: Oncology Nursing Society; 2005, pp. 53–62.

Schulmeister L. Preventing vincristine administration error: Does evidence support minibag infusions? *Clin J Nurs.* 2006;10(2):271–273.

WHO warns about fatal errors with vincristine: FDA patient safety news. October 2007. Available at: http://www.who.int/medicines/publications/drugalerts/Alert_115_vincristine.pdf. Accessed August 24, 2008.

Choose carefully—Peripheral IV site placement for chemotherapy infusions

Mary S. Ward, RN, BS, OCN

WHAT TO DO: ASSESS

Chemotherapy is considered a hazardous drug category for many reasons: narrow therapeutic index, side effect profiles, high risk for toxicities, safe handling considerations, and extravasation potential. One of the most concerning aspect of chemotherapy administration is vesicant drug delivery. Not all chemotherapy drugs are considered vesicants, which are defined as drugs that have the potential to cause tissue damage or necrosis when they pass into the tissue, or extravasate. Many chemotherapy drugs could be classified as irritants rather than vesicants. These drugs cause aching, tightness, or phlebitis along the vein or insertion site without causing tissue necrosis.

Vesicant drugs work by one of the two mechanisms. The first, and most destructive, is the absorption of the drug by the local cells, uptake by the intracellular structures, such as DNA, and release into the surrounding tissue. The drug is then taken up by other cells and "passed on" in like manner. Extravasations of this nature cause severe damage as the cells transfer the destructive cytotoxic chemical and disseminate tissue destruction. The second mechanism of tissue damage is due to the solvents used in the drug formulations. These extravasations are more easily controlled and neutralized.

Because some cytotoxic drugs have the potential for severe tissue damage and necrosis, the placement of a peripheral IV site for chemotherapy administration is an issue that requires careful attention. It is estimated that extravasation can occur in up to 6% of patients receiving chemotherapy. To reduce risk and complications, the site must be carefully chosen and the insertion technique must be skillful. When choosing a site, begin in the distal forearm and move proximally. Avoid areas of flexion and the dorsum of the hand, the wrist, and the antecubital fossa. Damage from vesicant extravasation in these areas can cause significant tissue, tendon, and even joint damage and has lead to skin graft, limb dysfunction, and even amputation in severe cases. Areas of flexion allow for displacement of the cannula around the insertion site, which may cause leakage of the infusate, leading to tissue damage. Avoid any site of tissue or venous compromise, sites with edema, small tortuous veins, poor vascular integrity, or poor venous return. Areas of decreased sensation should also be avoided; the patient should be taught to notify the nurse for any sign of burning or pain which may not be noticed in areas of decreased sensation.

When inserting the cannula, a smooth technique is necessary. If a second attempt is needed, it is best to use the other arm. Insertion attempt sites above the IV site may leak vesicant drug, causing an extravasation site above the actual IV site when the drug is infusing.

When the chemotherapy is infusing, blood return in the IV site should be monitored frequently. If the patient has any complaints of pain or burning, the chemotherapy should be stopped and the site flushed with normal saline and assessed. The site should be changed if there is any sign of redness or leaking of fluid. If there is an extravasation of chemotherapy, the pharmacy should be contacted for antidote protocols.

Many chemotherapy regimens include vesicant and irritant drugs. Nurses preparing patients to receive chemotherapy need to assess the patient and take the necessary time to insert the IV and to monitor the patient throughout the infusion to reduce complications of therapy.

SUGGESTED READINGS

Fischer DS, Knobf MT, Durivage HJ, et al. *The Cancer Chemotherapy Handbook*. 6th Ed. Philadelphia, PA: Mosby; 2003, pp. 311–312.

Polovich M, White JM, Kelleher LO. *Chemotherapy and Biotherapy Guidelines and Recommendations for Practice*. 2nd Ed. Pittsburgh, PA: Oncology Nursing Society; 2005, pp. 74, 75, 78, 81.

Sani A, Berruti A, Sperone P, et al. Recall inflammatory skin reaction after use of pegylated liposomal doxorubicin in site of previous drug extravasation. *The Lancet Oncol*. 2006; 7(2):186–188.

TUMOR LYSIS SYNDROME IS A SERIOUS ONCOLOGIC EMERGENCY RELATED TO CHEMOTHERAPY ADMINISTRATION

MARY S. WARD, RN, BS, OCN

WHAT TO DO: ASSESS

Tumor lysis syndrome is a serious complication for patients receiving chemotherapy treatment, especially patients with hematological malignancies and high grade lymphomas. Patients with a large number of cancer cells, or high tumor burdens, and rapidly growing and dividing cells are at greatest risk. Tumor lysis syndrome develops as the cytotoxic effects of the chemotherapy operates on these actively dividing cancer cells. The cells are destroyed by the infusing chemotherapy and burst, expelling the intracellular contents into the systemic circulation. Potassium, phosphate, and uric acid from purine nucleic acid degradation increase in substantial amounts in the serum. Accompanying hyperphasphatemia is a corresponding drop in calcium concentration. Other patients who have increased risk factors are those with high white blood cell counts, dehydration, or decreased renal function. Prophylaxis and early detection are essential components to preventing life threatening complications for these patients.

Prophylaxis consists of intense hydration prior to and during chemotherapy treatment, up to three liters of fluid per day. Patients should maintain alkalinized urine, adding sodium bicarbonate if necessary either to the IV fluid or by mouth, to keep the urine pH above 7.0. This is to prevent uric acid crystallization in the kidneys, which occurs more readily in an acidic urine environment. Lab values should be monitored every 6h for hyperkalemia, hyperphosphatemia, hyperuricemia, and hypocalcemia. Vital signs should be noted every 4h and any abnormalities addressed. Intake and output are essential; any decrease in urine output should be assessed. The patient should be started on Allopurinol by mouth or Rasburicase IV infusion prophylactically to decrease uric acid levels. Tumor lysis syndrome is most likely to occur 12 to 72h after the initiation of chemotherapy infusion.

The signs and symptoms of tumor lysis syndrome are dependent upon the severity of the electrolyte abnormalities that accompany it. When the patient's lab values indicate a decline, the patient should be placed on a monitored unit, the electrolyte abnormalities treated with appropriate therapies, the patient kept well hydrated, and diuretics utilized to maintain kidney function. If the kidneys begin to fail, the patient may be placed on short-term dialysis treatment. The most severe complications of tumor lysis syndrome are renal failure and alterations in cardiac function.

Patients receiving chemotherapy for high tumor burden and rapidly proliferating tumor cells are at significant risk for developing this oncologic emergency. It can have a sudden onset, catching the nurse unaware. Prevention and early detection are essential interventions to warding off long-term complications for this patient.

SUGGESTED READINGS

Higdon M, Higdon J. Treatment of oncologic emergencies. *Am Fam Phys.* 2006;74(11):1873–1880.

Kaplan M. *Understanding and Managing Oncologic Emergencies: A Resource for Nurses.* Pittsburgh, PA: Oncology Nursing Society; 2006, pp. 285–304.

Zojer N, Ludwig H. Hematological emergencies. *Ann Oncol.* 2007;18(S1):145–148.

KNOW HOW TO ASSESS AND EVALUATE PATIENTS IN SICKLE CELL CRISIS

SAM HARVEY AND ANTHONY D. SLONIM, MD, DrPH

WHAT TO DO: ASSESS AND EVALUATE

Sickle cell anemia is one of the most severe forms of hemolytic anemia, affecting the erythrocytes in the blood. Sickle cell anemia is caused by the inheritance of the sickle hemoglobin gene. This defective hemoglobin gene interferes with the proper structure of erythrocytes, causing them to change from their normally pliable, disk shape to a rigid, sickle shape in the presence of low oxygen levels. In venous blood, oxygen levels can become low enough for the defective hemoglobin to crystallize and cause sickle cell anemia. The sickle cell can adhere to small vessels and result in painful clotting and oxygen deprivation to organ systems. These periods of ischemia and infarction are known as "sickle crises" and can induce extreme pain, fever, and swelling (Fig. 217.1).

In the adult population with sickle cell anemia, there are three types of sickle cell crises. The first is sickle crisis, where hypoxia and necrosis occur due to decreased blood flow to a specific region of the body. Pain is intense with this crisis. The second is aplastic crisis caused by infection with the human parvovirus. In this crisis, hemoglobin levels drop dramatically and the patient's marrow does not have enough time to replenish the supply to keep oxygen levels up. Therefore, oxygen deprivation leads to the formation of sickle cells and the onset of sickle crisis. Lastly, sequestration crisis occurs when specific organs pool the sickle erythrocytes. The spleen is the most common organ in children to pool the cells while adults suffer most commonly in the lungs and liver.

Sickle cell anemia is typically diagnosed at a young age due to the early onset of sickle crises at 1 or 2 years of age. Many infants with the disease die due to complication with opportunistic diseases. Treatment is limited for sickle cell anemia and the average life expectancy is only 42 to 48 years. Often, young adults affected develop severe and permanent complications in their early 20s. Sickle cell anemia is almost completely racially specific to people of African descent, though a select few of the cases occur in those of the Middle Eastern descent. Services such as genetic counseling are important for parents who carry the defective sickle cell gene but do not have symptomatic sickle cell anemia. Two carriers of the sickle trait are at a very high risk of bearing a child with sickle cell anemia. Pain management is an important aspect of the disease. Common drugs such as aspirin are very effective at limiting inflammation and potential thrombosis. Unfortunately, as a patient ages, chronic pain may develop. For nurses, it is important to educate patients about the limitations of treatment for chronic pain and the precarious balance between pain and functionality that chronic pain management requires.

SUGGESTED READINGS

Johnson L. Sickle cell disease patients and patient-controlled analgesia. *Br J Nurs*. 2003;12(3):144–153.
Smeltzer S, Bare B, Hinkle J, et al. *Textbook of Medical-Surgical Nursing*. Philadelphia, PA: Lippincott Williams & Wilkins; 2008.

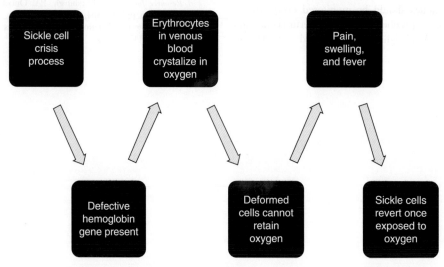

FIGURE 217.1. Periods of ischemia and infarction are known as "sickle crises" and can induce extreme pain, fever, and swelling.

THROMBOTIC THROMBOCYTOPENIC PURPURA CAN BE A CONFUSING CONDITION...KNOW HOW TO CONNECT THE DOTS...

SAM HARVEY AND ANTHONY D. SLONIM, MD, DrPH

WHAT TO DO: ASSESS

Thrombotic Thrombocytopenic Purpura (TTP) is a rare and dangerous thrombocytopenic disorder that involves the rapid aggregation of platelets in the blood that ultimately occludes arterioles and capillaries throughout the entire circulatory system. Approximately 1:1,000,000 people are affected, with women in their 30s being the most susceptible. As a thrombocytopenic disorder, TTP involves a severe decrease of platelets in the blood (<100,000 platelets/mm³). Thrombocytopenia below 50,000 platelets/mm³ greatly increases the chance of hemorrhage from minor injury or even common daily activity. As a purpuric disorder, TTP results in insufficient blood coagulation in normally functioning capillaries, which causes microhemorrhaging beneath the skin.

Two types of TTP exist: acute idiopathic TTP and chronic relapsing TTP (Fig. 218.1). Chronic TTP is an exceedingly rare condition that occurs most often in children. Regularly occurring bouts of TTP occur at approximately 3 week intervals but are usually very responsive to treatment. Acute idiopathic TTP is much more common and dangerous, with a 90% mortality rate if left untreated. The symptoms of TTP fall are identified as the "pathognomonic pentad": anemia, thrombocytopenia, neurologic abnormalities, fever, and renal problems. Not all of these symptoms need be present at diagnosis, but advanced TTP generally exhibits all of these symptoms eventually. Platelet aggregation and the formation of thrombi in the microcirculatory system also cause ischemia in the kidney, brain, and heart. Other less susceptible organs include the pancreas, spleen, and adrenal glands (Fig. 218.2).

The etiology of TTP is mysterious due to several interconnected factors present around its manifestation.

Recently, it has been found that the presence of von Willebrand factor in the blood, when the disease is diagnosed, could lead to the platelet aggregation. Cleavage of von Willebrand factor is important in preventing this aggregation and the metalloprotease responsible for cleaving the factor is deficient in most TTP patients. Additionally, IgG antibodies against metalloprotease have been identified, indicating that TTP may result due to an autoimmune disorder.

SUGGESTED READINGS

McCance K, Heuther S. *Pathophysiology: The Biologic Basis for Disease in Adults and Children*. Philadelphia, PA: Elsevier Mosby; 2006.

Nabhan C, Kwaan HC. Current concepts in the diagnosis and management of thrombotic thrombocytopenic purpura. *Hematol Oncol Clin North Am*. 2003;17(1):177–199.

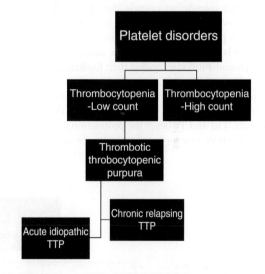

FIGURE 218.1. Classification of platelet disorders.

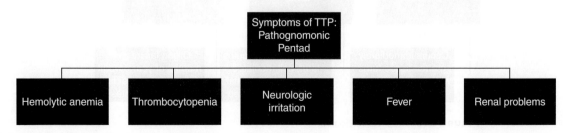

FIGURE 218.2. Classic symptoms of TTP.

TRANSPLANT REJECTION

SAM HARVEY AND ANTHONY D. SLONIM, MD, DrPH

WHAT TO DO: ASSESS

One of the many complicating factors that can occur after organ transplantation is an immune response to the foreign tissue. The most common immune response occurs against HLA antigens that are present on almost all donated tissues. There are three classes of transplant rejection characterized by the length of time before the onset of symptoms occurs. These classes are hyperacute rejection, acute rejection, and chronic rejection (Fig. 219.1).

Hyperacute immune responses are rare due to generally successful pretransplantation screening. To avoid these responses, it is important to screen the organ recipient for antibodies against the donor's HLA antigens. The most common symptom of hyperacute response is a white graft, where donated tissue immediately turns white instead of the usual pink color. The immune response stimulates striking inflammation as well as initiates the coagulation cascade that drastically reduces blood flow to the donated tissue. Women who have had multiple pregnancies and are receiving tissue from their husbands are the most common sufferers due to the presence of antibodies against their husbands' HLA.

Acute rejection is much more common than hyperacute rejection and has several of the same symptoms. Once the foreign tissue is detected by the immune system, Th1 and Tc begin the production of antibodies and stimulate macrophages to begin the inflammatory response. Then, symptoms similar to hyperacute rejection gradually begin to occur in increasingly higher severity.

Chronic rejection occurs due to a very minor histocompatibility against antigens on foreign tissue. This incompatibility results in the slow degradation of grafted endothelial tissue and continues until the damage is symptomatic.

The most effective way to preclude immune response is to prescreen recipients for suspected antibodies against donor antigens. A regimen of immunosuppressive drugs may be required to facilitate successful transplantation, but the risk of opportunistic infections increases their use. Therefore, if an immunosuppressive medication regimen is prescribed, extra care must be taken in monitoring the patient, either hospitalized or an outpatient. Regular check-ups should be scheduled to monitor organ recipients to prevent damage to the grafted tissue. An autoimmune response, if undiagnosed, can sometimes be severe enough to necessitate another transplantation that is costly and detrimental to the patient.

SUGGESTED READINGS

McCance K, Heuther S. *Pathophysiology: The Biologic Basis for Disease in Adults and Children*. Philadelphia, PA: Elsevier Mosby; 2006.
Ohashi PS, DeFranco AL. Making and breaking tolerance. *Curr Opin Immunol*. 2002;14(6):744–759.

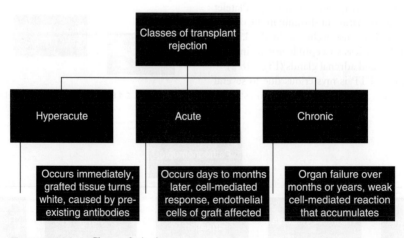

FIGURE 219.1. Classes of rejection.

EDUCATE ON CANCER PREVENTION

ANTHONY D. SLONIM, MD, DRPH

WHAT TO DO: IMPLEMENT

Cancer is a leading disease that is responsible for a considerable amount of healthcare resource use in its diagnosis and treatment. Further, cancer is responsible for a large number of deaths in the United States and adversely impacts families because of its emotional and financial burden.

Although cancer is a serious concern, there are several very well-known risk factors associated with cancer. The nurse provides an important service by counseling patients who are at risk from these conditions and providing direct and concrete advice on the methods in which patients can reduce their risk of developing cancer.

Smoking is an important contributor to a number of cancers including lung, colon, and breast and is a major contributor to cardiovascular diseases as well. Nurses are in a position to counsel patients against smoking initiation, particularly young adolescent patients who, by their nature, are unable to identify relationships between antecedent and consequent events separated in time. If patients have begun smoking, the nurse can provide guidance into how important it is to discontinue tobacco use and provide concrete mechanisms through which it can be accomplished.

Alcohol use is a contributor to cancers of the aerodigestive tract, breast, and pancreas. When combined with smoking, alcohol acts synergistically in the development of cancer. Further, the use of alcohol and cigarette smoking occur coincidentally in social situations. The nurse can assess the use of alcohol, counsel against it, and, if necessary, provide guidance and support to assist with eradicating its use.

Diets high in saturated fats predispose patients to the development of carcinoma of the colon. A diet that is moderate in its fat intake and also includes the use of appropriate fiber can be beneficial for oncologic and cardiovascular health.

Finally, the nurse has a role in identifying the establishment of risk for cancer related to occupational and environmental exposures. There are a number of risk factors from chemical, infectious, and physical agents that predispose patients to cancer. An understanding of the risk factors, family history, and personal habits allows the nurse to understand the patients' cancer risk profile and counsel them on ways in which they can reduce their risk.

SUGGESTED READINGS

Omenn GS. Cancer prevention. In: Goldman L, Ausiello D, eds. *Cecil Textbook of Medicine*. 22nd Ed. Philadelphia, PA: Saunders; 2004, pp. 1134–1136.

ENSURE APPROPRIATE SCREENING FOR CERVICAL CANCER

ANTHONY D. SLONIM, MD, DrPH

Nearly 13,000 new cases of cervical cancer and 5,000 deaths occur in the United States annually from cervical cancer. Cervical cancer is preceded by a variable period of dysplasia prior to becoming invasive. It is during this time that women at risk should be identified to ensure the best outcome. Since the majority of cervical cancers are asymptomatic, the best way to achieve an early diagnosis is through routine screening. The Papanicoulou (Pap) smear has been used to successfully reduce the mortality rate from cervical cancer in women and remains the dominant mechanism for screening. Futher, since the majority of dysplastic cancers are found to have a human papillomavirus (HPV) etiology, the use of a vaccine to prevent the disease is important for young women in particular.

Cervical cancer screening is currently recommended in sexually active women. A baseline screening should be performed at age 21 or if the woman is sexually active prior to this age, within 3 years of onset of sexual activity. For women who have had three negative Pap smears on an annual basis, remain free from disease, and are at low risk for cervical cancer, screening can be advanced every 3 years. If the woman develops dysplastic findings, HPV infection, or has other symptoms that place her at higher risk, the screening should be reduced to an annual level. Screening should continue till the age of 65 years.

SUGGESTED READINGS

Get the facts about HPV. Available at: http://www.gardasil.com/hpv/index.html. Accessed August 24, 2008.

Molpus KL, Jones HW. Gynecologic cancers. In: Goldman L, Ausiello D, eds. *Cecil Textbook of Medicine*. 22nd Ed. Philadelphia, PA: Saunders; 2004, pp. 1238–1242.

Protecting against HPV and the diseases it causes. Available at: http://www.gardasil.com/hpv/pap-test/index.html. Accessed August 24, 2008.

KNOW THE CONDITIONS THAT PREDISPOSE YOUR PATIENTS TO HYPERCOAGULABILITY

ANTHONY D. SLONIM, MD, DRPH

WHAT TO DO: ASSESS

The hypercoagulable syndromes have become more important to healthcare with improvements in the understanding of their pathophysiologic basis. The nurse is in a unique role to improve conditions that predispose patients to hypercoagulability but also needs to be able to recognize these conditions when they occur.

Hypercoagulable syndromes are classified as primary, which originate from problems in the coagulation system, or secondary, which arise as a component of another disease or condition. The secondary hypercoagulable syndromes are far more common in practice. Coagulation results from a delicate balance in the prothrombotic and antithrombitic characteristics of certain plasma proteins. When either the prothrombotic factors become increased (Factor V Leiden, prothrombin mutation, hyper-homocysteinemia, or Factors VIII, XI, IX, fibrinogen or fibrinolysis inhibitor) or antithrombotic factors (antithrombin III, Protein C or S) become decreased, the propensity for the patient to clot increases.

In addition to these specific defects, there are a number of secondary factors that increase the patient's propensity to clot. These include personal characteristics like immobility, venous stasis, and obesity. Disease- or condition-specific characteristics like pregnancy, cancer, trauma, nephritic syndrome, hyperlipidemia, and diabetes can also increase clotting. The postoperative state also contributes to this.

Clinically, a patient with these disorders usually presents with venous thrombosis, of which deep venous thrombosis and pulmonary emboli are the two most common forms. Some patients may experience arterial thrombosis. Patients may also become symptomatic during the administration of certain medications, like warfarin, that predispose them to skin necrosis. In other patients, repetitive miscarriages may be the characteristic that brings the patient to medical attention. It is not uncommon for a patient to be at risk and then experience a superimposed risk factor that causes them to be symptomatic.

The treatment for most hypercoagulable syndromes includes anticoagulation. The nurse has a role in ensuring that appropriate medications are administered in correct doses, that laboratory diagnostic testing is done appropriately, and that patients are mobilized appropriately during hospitalization and receive appropriate prophylaxis for deep venous complications.

Hypercoagulable states are important hematologic conditions. Nurses need to know how to identify patients at risk, reduce their risk, and treat those affected in an effective manner.

SUGGESTED READINGS

Schafer AI. Thrombotic disorders: Hypercoagulable states. In: Goldman L, Ausiello D, eds. *Cecil Textbook of Medicine.* 22nd Ed. Philadelphia, PA: Saunders; 2004, pp. 1082–1087.

KNOW WHAT CAUSES EOSINOPHILS TO BE ELEVATED ON THE DIFFERENTIAL COUNT

ANTHONY D. SLONIM, MD, DRPH

WHAT TO DO: ASSESS

Eosinophils are an important white blood cell (WBC) constituent with very specific functions. These cells are produced in the bone marrow and participate actively in inflammation. The eosinophil contains a number of preformed granules that allow it to work against specific microbes, but even more importantly, the eosinophil plays a pivotal role in inflammation due to its ability to be summoned to the site of specific activity and then through a number of mediators to further recruit specific cells to assist the host in fighting disease.

While the usual number of eosinophils in the circulating bloodstream is low (<450 µL), their call to action is usually for very specific purposes. Eosinophils become active in neoplastic and myeloproliferative diseases. The myeloproliferative diseases can affect numerous organ systems. Allergic conditions, including asthma, are a common cause for peripheral eosinophilia. Adrenal insufficiency represents another characteristic condition where eosinophils become important. Collagen vascular diseases and vasculitic and parasitic conditions make up the remainder of the major categories leading to eosinophilia. Finally, medications can increase the eosinophil count.

Eosinophilia, by itself, is the only one characteristic that because of its rarity may provide clinical clues to the diagnosis. More important though is the effect that eosinophils can have in the creation of inflammation, including angioedema, and the symptoms that can subsequently develop in the patient.

Eosinophils are an important part of the differential count of the complete blood count and have very specific diseases associated with their occurrence. The nurse should not only identify this trend when it occurs but also assist in the identification of the causative agent.

SUGGESTED READINGS

Weller P. Eosinophilic syndromes. In: Goldman L, Ausiello D, eds. *Cecil Textbook of Medicine*. 22nd Ed. Philadelphia, PA: Saunders; 2004, pp. 1104–1106.

Bone marrow transplantation is an important treatment modality for cancer, and nurses need to be aware of the types, reasons for their use, and complications

Anthony D. Slonim, MD, DrPH

WHAT TO DO: EVALUATE

The administration of hematopoietic cells from the bone marrow is a useful technique for many diseases including resistant cancers and generically is classified as bone marrow transplantation (BMT). Usually, the reintroduction of stem cells is preceded by high–dose chemotherapy. With its increasing use, the nurse needs to know what the different types of transplantation are, what diseases it is used for, and what the complications of the procedure, both short- and long-term, encompass.

Allogeneic BMT is differentiated from autologous BMT by the source of the administered cells. In "allo," the donor cells originate from a donor, usually a relative of the patient. In autologous BMT, the patient donates his or her own cells prior to ablative chemotherapy. "Auto" BMT has fewer risks related to mismatch of cells, thereby eliminating the occurrence of graft versus host disease, but this is tempered by the possibility that tumor cells may invade the graft.

There are a number of uses for BMT including solid tumors like breast, testicular, and ovarian cancers. Lymphomas, multiple myelomas, and leukemias are also frequent targets. A number of nonmalignant diseases are emerging for treatment with this approach including aplastic anemia, genetic disorders, and immunodeficiency syndromes.

The major complications after transplantation include infection, which initially include, bacterial and fungal infections and later involve viruses. Graft versus host disease is an important problem in the "allo" BMT setting and represents a response of the graft and affects the skin, gastrointestinal tract, and liver. It may occur in the acute setting or be more chronic in its nature. There are also toxicities of major organs from the ablative chemotherapies.

The nurse has an important role in supporting the patient after a BMT. Once the procedure is complete, ongoing problems often require rehospitalization. These patients are markedly immunosuppressed and often require medications like steroids that alter their immune systems even further. Strict attention to hand washing, the accessing of the patient's central venous access, assessing for the long-term complications of infection or medications is important during the nurse's assessment.

SUGGESTED READINGS

Pavletic SZ, Vose JM. Hematopoietic stem cell transplantation. Goldman L, Ausiello D, eds. *Cecil Textbook of Medicine.* 22nd Ed. Philadelphia, PA: Saunders; 2004, pp. 999–1002.

LYMPH NODES DO NOT ALWAYS INDICATE THAT CANCER IS PRESENT

ANTHONY D. SLONIM, MD, DrPH

WHAT TO DO: ASSESS

The nurse is often placed in the position of answering questions and concerns on the part of the patient. One of the most important concerns raised by patients involves the presence of lymph node (LN) swelling. LNs are located throughout the body and are the places where plasma gets filtered and presented to immunologically active cells. LNs enlarge as they process antigens and increase the cellular activity in response to those antigens. What is important for patients to know is that LNs enlarge for a number of reasons and not all of which are bad and not all of which are related to cancer.

LN enlargement needs to be considered within the broader context of the patient. The patient's age is important. Children often experience benign LN swelling as their immunologic system "learns" from the antigens that it is being exposed to. LN swelling that is accompanied by symptoms like fever, chill, and rashes can help with identifying a systemic problem as compared to a local problem. Specific organ problems in combination with LN swelling are also important. A chronic cough that produces blood associated with LN enlargement in the neck may represent an occult malignancy of the lung. Signs of local disease are also important. For example, unilateral LN swelling in the groin should prompt an inspection of the leg to determine if a local infection is the cause of the problem. The size, consistency, and tenderness of an LN also play an important role in determining the concern. Small (less than 1–2 cm), localized,

and minimally tender LNs usually represent reactive LNs in response to a local phenomenon. LNs present in a disseminated pattern that are larger and affecting multiple locations are important to evaluate.

The causes of LN swelling are diverse. While cancer is certainly on the list of causes, infections are often more common and may arise from any number of microbiological etiologies including bacterial, fungal, mycobacterial, and viral. Immunologic disorders including collagen vascular diseases and lupus may cause disseminated LN enlargement. Malignancies and their representation of metastatic disease are always a consideration.

The patient with LN enlargement will often require a thorough history and physical and laboratory testing including a complete blood count, organ function studies, and anatomic evaluation using radiographic tests such as chest X-rays, computerized tomography, or scanning. The possibility of an LN biopsy to obtain specific tissue is often an option to derive a definitive diagnosis.

LN swelling is common and can often lead to fear in the patient. The nurse should provide appropriate counseling, obtain necessary information, assist with appropriate diagnostic testing, and reassure the patient as the condition permits.

SUGGESTED READINGS

Armitage JO. Approach to the patient with lymphadenopathy and splenomegaly. In: Goldman L, Ausiello D, eds. *Cecil Textbook of Medicine*. 22nd Ed. Philadelphia, PA: Saunders, 2004, pp. 990–992.

226

USE PROPER PERSONAL PROTECTIVE EQUIPMENT WHEN CARING FOR PATIENTS WITH HEAD LICE

BETSY HARGREAVES ALLBEE, BSN, CIC

WHAT TO DO: PLAN

Pediculus humanus capitis, the head louse, is an opportunistic parasite whose only host is man. These pesky insects, often referred to as "cooties," establish residence in the hair, scalp, eyebrows, and eyelashes (Fig. 226.1). Most outbreaks of infestation, or pediculosis, occur among school-aged children at the beginning of the school year, but other patient types may also be affected.

Head lice are transmitted by direct head-to-head contact with an infested person's hair. Personal objects and items, such as combs, hats, scarves, helmets, hair ribbons, bedding, and stuffed animals, used by an individual with pediculosis can become infested, resulting in the indirect transmission to others. Fortunately, since head lice require human blood for sustenance, they can survive on inanimate objects only for a day or two. When hospitalized, patients with head lice should be placed in a private room whenever possible. Although the head lice are not capable of flying or jumping, when a private room is

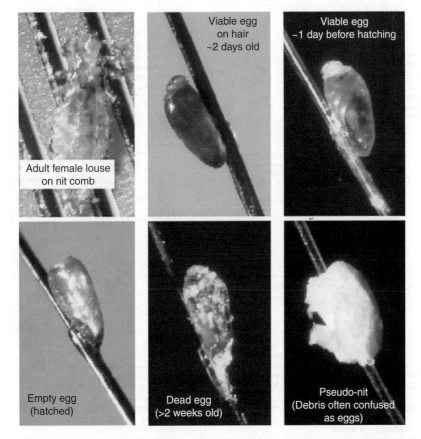

FIGURE 226.1. Images to assist in the identification of head lice and their eggs. (Available at: http://www.hsph.harvard.edu/headlice.html.)

not available, the general spatial rule of three feet between an infected and non-infected patient should be used.

When caring for a patient with head lice, it may be tempting to wear Level 3 Biosafety Personal Protective Equipment; however, contact precautions and the use of a gown and gloves is the current recommendation from the Centers for Disease Control and Prevention (CDC) when caring for patients with head lice (Fig. 226.2). Another component of contact precautions includes the dedication of patient care equipment to the patient in isolation. Other control measures include laundering of clothing, bedding, and other linens in hot water. Items that cannot be laundered should be placed in a plastic bag and sealed for 7 to 10 days. The duration

of isolation precaution is 24 h after treatment. However, head lice can be transmitted as long as the lice or eggs remain alive, suggesting that precautions should be continued as long as the patient is actively infested. Table 226.1 provides additional guidance for the prevention and control of pediculosis. Remember to check the patient's hair every 2 to 3 days after treatment and remove nits and lice. Also, observe whether the lice remain active, which may indicate a treatment failure. By understanding the transmission of infection, the life cycle, and the control measures such as contact precautions, you can more appropriately manage pediculosis in the hospital setting and alleviate the fear of infesting yourself or others.

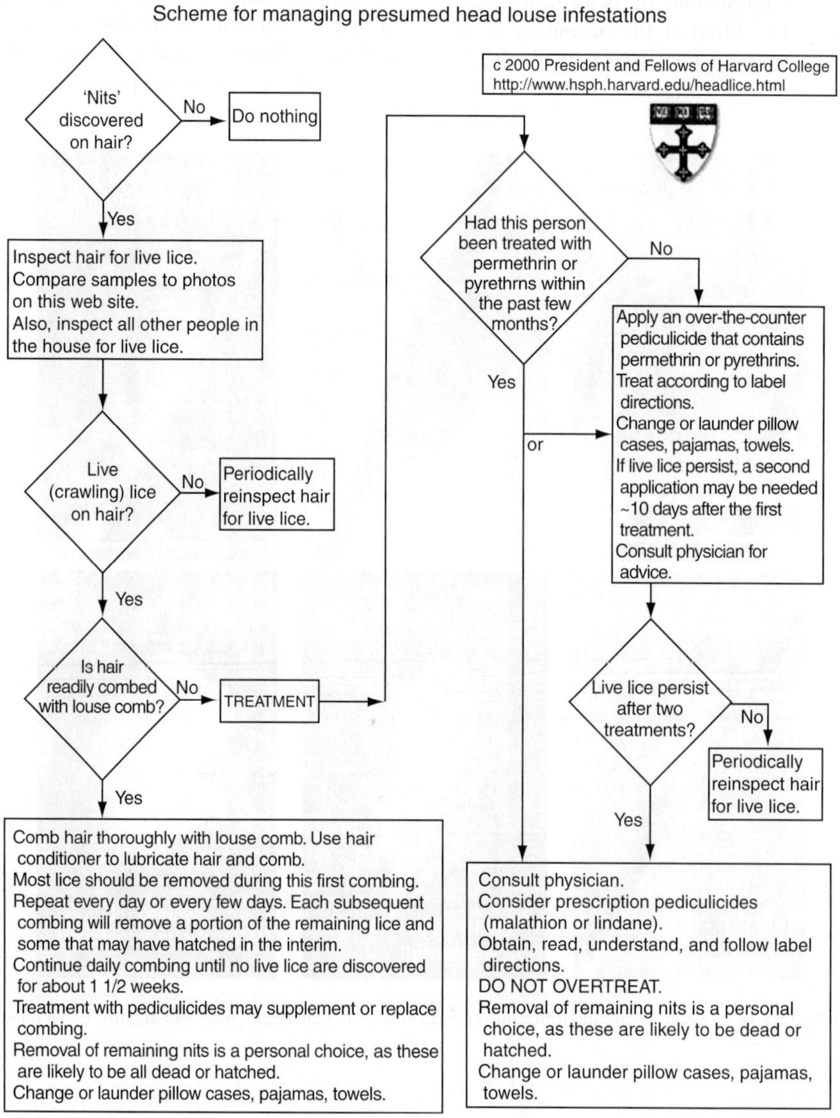

Scheme for managing presumed head louse infestations

FIGURE 226.2. Scheme for managing presumed head louse infestations. (Available at: http://www.hsph.harvard.edu/headlice.html. © 2000 Presidents and Fellows of Harvard College.)

TABLE 226.1	STAGE AND CHARACTERISTICS OF HEAD LICE

STAGE	CHARACTERISTICS
Egg-to-egg cycles last approximately 3 weeks.	
Egg (nits)	Nits are head lice eggs; nits may be confused for dandruff. Nits are laid by the adult female and adhere to the base of the hair shaft nearest the scalp. They are oval and usually yellow to white. Nits take 6–10 days (mean: 1 week) to hatch. Eggs cannot hatch at temperatures less than 72°F. Fortunately, most nits do not develop into lice.
Nymph	A nymph is released after the egg hatches. Nymphs are immature adult head lice. They are the size of a pinhead and are usually in dull yellow. Approximately 7 days after hatching, a nymph becomes an adult louse. To survive, nymphs must feed on blood.
Adult	Adult lice are about the size of a sesame seed. A louse has six legs with claws and is tan to grayish-white. To survive, adult lice need to feed on blood.

SUGGESTED READINGS

Harvard School of Public Health. Head Lice: Information and frequently asked questions. 2000. Available at: http://www.hsph.harvard.edu/headlice.html.

Heymann D. *Control of Communicable Disease Manual*. 18th Ed. Atlanta, GA: American Public Health Association; 2004, pp. 396–399.

Pickering LK, Baker CJ, Long SS, et al, eds. *Red Book: 2006 Report of the Committee on Infectious Diseases*. 27th Ed. Oak Grove Village, IL: American Academy of Pediatrics; 2006, pp. 488–492.

Siegel JD, Rhinehart E, Jackson M, et al. Guideline for isolation precautions: Preventing transmission of infectious agents in healthcare settings 2007. Available at: http://www.cdc.gov/ncidod/dhqp/pdf/isolation2007.pdf.

THERE IS NO NEED FOR MASS HYSTERIA OR MASS PROPHYLAXIS FOR ASEPTIC MENINGITIS

BETSY HARGREAVES ALLBEE, BSN, CIC

WHAT TO DO: IMPLEMENT

Meningitis is an infection of the meninges that surround the brain. The meninges consist of three separate layers of connective tissue that enclose the brain and spinal cord. The outer layer, the dura mater, is the thickest. The middle layer is called the arachnoid membrane, and the inner layer, closest to the brain, is called the pia mater. Cerebrospinal fluid (CSF) circulates in the arachnoid space, an area between the pia mater and the arachnoid. Normally, CSF is a clear, protective fluid which is produced in the brain. Meningitis occurs when the CSF and meninges are invaded by viruses or bacteria. Meningitis can be caused by either a virus or a bacterium. Viral meningitis generally causes mild illness and requires no treatment. Bacterial meningitis can be extremely debilitating and can result in brain damage or death. The symptoms of meningitis may appear rapidly or over a period of days, usually within 1 week of exposure. The symptoms include sudden fever, headache, stiff neck, and fatigue. Other symptoms may include rash, sore throat, nausea, and vomiting. Symptoms associated with viral meningitis can usually be relieved by over-the-counter medications and bed rest. Acute bacterial meningitis may progress to seizures, overwhelming systemic infection, and shock.

The majority of patients with meningitis present through the Emergency Department (ED) rather than being a direct admission. Because of the seriousness of bacterial meningitis, ED personnel should maintain a high index of suspicion when a patient presents with symptoms suggesting meningitis. In most cases, a spinal tap is performed relatively early in the visit. This procedure involves the insertion of a needle into the subarachnoid space of the lumbar region (lower back)

to obtain a sample of CSF for analysis (Table 227.1). Viral meningitis (also known as aseptic or nonbacterial meningitis) is caused by several viruses and is rarely serious. Cases of viral meningitis are reported worldwide, although outbreaks are unusual. In the United States, half of the diagnosed cases are caused by intestinal viruses, and the remaining half have no known etiology. The illness is more common in children and young adults. The incidence is not completely known since many individuals with the illness experience mild symptoms and often do not seek medical care.

It may be difficult to differentiate viral meningitis from partially treated bacterial meningitis in patients who have recently been treated with antibiotics. Since meningitis is spread by direct contact with secretions from the nose and throat of an infected person, proper hand hygiene is extremely important. If it is suspected that the patient has bacterial meningitis, precautionary measures such as droplet precautions should be initiated. It is at this stage of the diagnosis that many healthcare workers involved in the care of the meningitis patients become concerned about exposure. Only people who have been in close contact with the ill person need to receive prophylactic antibiotics. Close contacts are people who have exchanged respiratory or oral secretions with the ill person through activities such as kissing or sharing drinking glasses, eating utensils, cigarettes, or toothbrushes. These generally include household members, intimate contacts, and close friends. Healthcare workers who may have performed mouth-to-mouth resuscitation would be considered at risk.

Fortunately, the CSF cell counts, chemistries, and gram stain are often resulted quickly after collection and often provide important insights into the diagnosis (Table 227.1). Gram stain examination of the CSF

TABLE 227.1	CEREBROSPINAL FLUID (CSF) LAB TESTS FOR MENINGITIS		
	NORMAL	VIRAL MENINGITIS	BACTERIAL MENINGITIS
Color	Clear	Clear, hazy	Cloudy
White Blood Cells (WBCs/mm)	0–8	5–500	400–100,000
Protein mg/dL	12–60	30–150	80–500
Glucose mg/dL	40–70	Normal to low	<35
Differential percentage	PMNs: 0%–6% Monocytes: 94%–100%	Monocytes > 50%	PMNs > 90%

PMN: **polymorphonuclear** leukocytes (neutrophils); these cells are the first immune cells to arrive at a site of infection.

permits a rapid, accurate identification of the causative bacterium in 60% to 90% of patients with community-acquired bacterial meningitis, and it has a specificity of ≥97%. Unless there is a high suspicion for partially treated bacterial meningitis, these tests are reliable indicators of bacterial vs. viral meningitis. Mass prophylaxis with antibiotics is not necessary for personnel who collected demographic data such as admitting/patient access staff or healthcare workers who performed normal patient care activities such as a physical assessment, vital signs, medication administration, and even those who assisted with the spinal tap. Finally, remember that antibiotics are ineffective against viruses; therefore, if the CSF suggests viral meningitis, prophylactic antibiotics are not warranted.

SUGGESTED READINGS

Heymann DL, ed. *Control of Communicable Disease Manual.* 18th Ed. Atlanta, GA: American Public Health Association; 2004, pp. 357–359.

Pickering LK, Baker CJ, Long SS, et al, eds. *Red Book: 2006 Report of the Committee on Infectious Diseases.* 27th Ed. Oak Grove Village, IL: American Academy of Pediatrics; 2006, pp. 452–460.

Tunkel AR, Hartman BJ, Kaplan SL, et al. Practice guidelines for the management of bacterial meningitis. *Clin Infect Disease.* 2004;39:1268–1270.

KNOW HOW TO PREVENT INFECTION DURING YOUR PATIENT'S HOSPITALIZATION

SAM HARVEY AND ANTHONY D. SLONIM, MD, DrPH

WHAT TO DO: PLAN

Every year, approximately 2 million patients in the United States acquire infections while hospitalized. Infections that occur in the hospital are known as nosocomial infections and can usually be prevented by adhering to simple practices such as proper handwashing. Areas of the hospital, such as the intensive care unit (ICU), more prone to nosocomial infections, require health practitioners to be aware of their infectious potential when traveling from patient to patient. Healthcare practitioners should also be aware of the organisms most likely to cause a nosocomial infection, the symptoms associated, and the treatment required to minimize these infections should they occur.

Some microorganisms are very well adapted to the hospital atmosphere and take advantage of immunosuppressed or weakened individuals. Some of these specific organisms include *Clostridium difficile*, a gram positive bacterium that utilizes spores resistant to antimicrobial efforts to introduce toxins to the susceptible patient, and methicillin-resistant *Staphylococcus aureus* (MRSA). *S. aureus* is a skin colonizing bacterium that has evolved resistance to derivatives of penicillin and is often treated today with vancomycin. Due to its resistance to antibiotics and its presence on the skin of healthcare workers, it has become a feared nosocomial agent. Another prominent nosocomial bacterium is vancomycin-resistant *Enterococcus*, a bacterium common in the human intestines. When introduced into the bloodstream *Enterococcus* can cause significant patient infections. Unfortunately, *Enterococcus* adheres to the hands of healthcare workers and objects in the hospital and, when combined with its antibiotic resistance potential, can be a potentially dangerous organism.

The Hospital Infection Control Practices Advisory Committee in 1997 developed isolation procedures known as the Standard Precautions in an effort to educate healthcare workers about nosocomial infections and hopefully prevent their rapid spread. The Standard Precautions include safety requirements, such as glove use, eye protection, and gown use, for essentially any handling of objects that patients or personnel come in contact with. Specifically, handwashing is important to eliminate transient flora such as *S. aureus*. In order to be effective, hands must be washed for at least 10 seconds using antimicrobial soaps and specific areas such as the fingers and nails must be cleansed thoroughly. In areas, such as the ICU, where nosocomial infections are much more significant, alcohol, iodophors, or triclosan should accompany handwashing to augment the removal of transient flora.

The Standard Precautions also entail proper glove use, including replacement of gloves after each patient contact and handwashing after each glove removal. Flora grow easily in the warm, moist environment between the glove and the hand; therefore, simple replacement of gloves between each patient is not enough to prevent some infections. To avoid spray and splash exposure, barriers such as facemasks, goggles, and a gown should be worn.

Besides being an important factor in patient care, nurses should also be patient advocates. It is important that nurses monitor adherence to the Standard Precautions with all healthcare workers, such as lab workers, who come in contact with patients or patient material. It is only with effective coordination and agreement between healthcare professionals on the benefit and importance of preventing nosocomial infections that the number or such infections can be reduced.

SUGGESTED READINGS

Heymann, DL, ed. *Control of Communicable Disease Manual*. 18th Ed. Atlanta, GA: American Public Health Association; 2004, pp. 357–359.

Smeltzer S, Bare B. *Textbook of Medical-Surgical Nursing*. Philadelphia, PA: Lippincott Williams & Wilkins; 2000.

KNOW HOW TO PREVENT THE TRANSMISSION OF SHINGLES

BETSY HARGREAVES ALLBEE, BSN, CIC

Shingles, also known as herpes zoster or zoster, is a painful skin rash caused by the varicella zoster virus (VZV). VZV is the same virus that causes chickenpox, but not the same virus that causes genital herpes, a sexually transmitted disease. Approximately 25% of people develop shingles during their lifetime, with the majority of cases occurring in those over 50 years of age. In the United States, there are approximately 1 million cases of shingles per year. The complications from shingles include uncomfortable rash, eye and skin problems, scarring, nerve paralysis, pneumonia, encephalitis, and death. Excruciating pain from postherpetic neuralgia (PHN) can last for months or years. In Italy, shingles is called St. Anthony's fire, a fitting name for this virus since it can cause intense pain. It is no wonder that healthcare workers caring for patients with shingles are concerned about exposure.

Shingles is a localized infection due to the reactivation of the dormant varicella virus and occurs only in people who have had chickenpox in the past. After a person recovers from chickenpox, the varicella virus remains in the body, usually without causing any problems; however, the virus can reappear years later, causing shingles. The risk of getting shingles increases as people age. Other populations at risk for shingles are those who have medical conditions that alter the immune system (e.g., cancer, leukemia, lymphoma, and human immunodeficiency virus), people who take immunosuppressive drugs (e.g., steroids and drugs after organ transplantation), and newborns. An individual must have already had chickenpox in the past to develop shingles. Contact with an infected individual does not cause another person's dormant virus to reactivate. However, the virus from a shingles patient may cause chickenpox in someone who does not have immunity to the virus (e.g., no history of varicella or vaccination against the varicella virus). Therefore, a person exposed to a patient with shingles will not get shingles, but under certain conditions (e.g., lack of immunity) may get chickenpox. Although adults make up fewer than 5% of chickenpox cases in the United States, they account for half of the deaths from the disease.

The first sign of shingles is often a tingling feeling on the skin, itchiness, or a stabbing pain. During this preeruption stage, the diagnosis may be difficult and, depending on the affected nerve, the sign can be mistaken for more serious conditions such as a heart attack. Once activated, the virus travels along the path of a nerve to the skin's surface. After several days, a rash appears, beginning as a band or patch of raised dots on the side of the trunk or face. It then develops into small, fluid-filled blisters which begin to dry out and crust over within a few days. When the rash is at its peak, symptoms can range from mild itching to extreme and intense pain. The rash and pain usually disappear within 3 to 5 weeks. The virus is present at the site of the rash and is contagious for a week after the appearance of lesions (blisters). The Centers for Disease Control and Prevention (CDC) recommends the use of Standard Precautions while caring for patients with shingles. A private room is unnecessary; however, placement with a non-immune patient should be avoided. It is also recommended to cohort staff. A cohort is a group of individuals with similar symptoms, or exposures to similar illnesses, who are separated from the general population in order to minimize exposure to others. The assignment of staff to the cohort should only include those healthcare workers who have not had chickenpox or two doses of the varicella vaccine, since other providers should not be providing care to patients with open lesions. If an employee is unsure of his or her immunity status, a blood test that provides titers is available to confirm immunity. Other prevention strategies include cleaning the room and patient-care equipment with a hospital-approved disinfectant.

Treatment was once limited to wet compresses and aspirin. Recently, a licensed herpes zoster vaccine, Zostavax, was developed. The immunization of all adults aged above 60 years, including those with a prior history of shingles, is recommended. The shingles vaccine is safe and effective in providing protection against shingles and associated chronic pain.

As a healthcare provider it is important to know your immunization status and past history of communicable diseases such as chickenpox. If you had a history of chickenpox, you may have an episode of shingles caused by a reactivation of the dormant virus, not as a result of exposure to a patient with shingles. If you have not had chickenpox, consult your primary care physician or a health department employee to discuss vaccination.

SUGGESTED READINGS

Heymann DL, ed. *Control of Communicable Disease Manual*. 18th Ed. Atlanta, GA: American Public Health Association; 2004, pp. 94–100.

National Center for Immunization and Respiratory Diseases. Vaccine and preventable disease: Shingles disease—questions and answers; 2006. Available at: http://www.cdc.gov/vaccines/vpd-vac/shingles/dis-faqs.htm. Accessed April 2, 2009.

Pickering Lk, Baker CJ, Long SS, et al., eds. *Red Book:2006 Report of the Committee on Infectious Diseases*. 27th Ed. Oak Grove Village, IL: American Academy of Pediatrics 2006; pp. 711–725.

DO NOT FORGET THE OTHER SIDE OF INFECTION CONTROL: EMPLOYEES AND VOLUNTEERS

BETSY HARGREAVES ALLBEE, BSN, CIC

WHAT TO DO: EVALUATE

Traditional hospital-based infection control programs involve prevention strategies which focus on the patient. The other side of infection control considers the non-patient population, for example, employees and volunteers, as possible reservoirs for infection. Healthcare workers who report to work with an infectious disease pose a risk to the patients and other employees. The healthcare setting also poses a risk to the healthcare worker. Those who work in healthcare settings are exposed more frequently than the general public to communicable diseases. Employees who perform direct patient care have the greatest risk of exposure.

In the United States, there are more than 9 million persons who work in the healthcare industry. Hospital-based personnel may acquire infections from or transmit infections to patients, other personnel, household members, or other community contacts. Developing educational programs that focus on principles of infection control, innovative and cost-effective infection control measures, self reporting of procedural variances that may increase the risk of infection, procedures for caring for exposed persons, outbreak control, and personal responsibility and accountability for the prevention of infection in the workplace should be a priority. In addition, immunization programs that encourage employees to receive vaccines such as influenza, pertussis, measles, mumps and rubella, and hepatitis B allow employees to actively participate in effective prevention and control strategies. All employees should be considered infection control liaisons. Observing for potential clusters or patterns of infection allows measures to be implemented promptly. Employees should be empowered to initiate infection control measures such as isolation precautions, even before a diagnosis is made, thereby allowing the healthcare worker to segregate a potentially infectious patient from others and spreading the disease.

Table 230.1 describes precaution recommendations for several common conditions. These symptoms

TABLE 230.1	CLINICAL SYNDROMES OR CONDITIONS WARRANTING EMPIRIC TRANSMISSION-BASED PRECAUTIONS IN ADDITION TO STANDARD PRECAUTIONS PENDING CONFIRMATION OF DIAGNOSIS	
CLINICAL SYNDROME OR CONDITION	**POTENTIAL PATHOGENS**	**EMPIRIC PRECAUTIONS (ALWAYS INCLUDES STANDARD PRECAUTIONS)**
Diarrhea Acute diarrhea with a likely infectious cause in an incontinent or diapered patient	Enteric precautions	Contact precautions (pediatrics and adult)
Meningitis	*Neisseria meningitidis* Enteroviruses *Mycobacterium tuberculosis*	Droplet Precautions for first 24 hrs of antimicrobial therapy; mask and face protection for intubation. Contact precautions for infants and children. Airborne precautions if pulmonary infiltrate. Airborne precautions plus Contact precautions if potentially infectious draining body fluid present.
Rash or Exanthems, Generalized, Etiology Unknown		
Petechial/ecchymotic with fever (general) If positive history of travel to an area with an ongoing outbreak of Viral Hemorrhagic Fever in the 10 days before onset of fever Vesicular Maculopapular with cough, coryza, and fever	*Neisseria meningitidis* Ebola, Lassa, Marburg viruses Varicella-zoster, *herpes simplex*, variola (smallpox), vaccinia viruses Vaccinia virus Rubeola (measles) virus	Droplet precautions for first 24 h of antimicrobial therapy. Droplet precautions plus Contact precautions, with face/eye protection, emphasizing safety sharps and barrier precautions when blood exposure likely. Use N95 or higher respiratory protection when aerosol-generating procedure performed. Airborne plus Contact Precautions; Contact Precautions only if herpes simplex, localized zoster in an immunocompetent host or vaccinia viruses most likely. Airborne Precautions

(Continued)

TABLE 230.1	CLINICAL SYNDROMES OR CONDITIONS WARRANTING EMPIRIC TRANSMISSION-BASED PRECAUTIONS IN ADDITION TO STANDARD PRECAUTIONS PENDING CONFIRMATION OF DIAGNOSIS—CONT'D	
CLINICAL SYNDROME OR CONDITION	**POTENTIAL PATHOGENS**	**EMPIRIC PRECAUTIONS (ALWAYS INCLUDES STANDARD PRECAUTIONS)**
Respiratory Infections		
Cough/fever/pulmonary infiltrate in an HIV-negative patient or a patient at low risk for human immunodeficiency virus (HIV) infection	*M. tuberculosis*, Respiratory viruses, *S. pneumoniae*, *S. aureus* (MSSA or MRSA)	Airborne precautions plus contact precautions Airborne precautions plus contact precautions use eye/face protection if aerosol-generation procedure performed or contact with respiratory secretions anticipated. If tuberculosis is unlikely and there are no AIIRs and/or respirators available, use droplet precautions instead of airborne precaution. Tuberculosis more likely in HIV-infected individual than in HIV negative individual.
Cough/fever/pulmonary infiltrate in any lung location in an HIV-infected patient or a patient at high risk for HIV-infection	*M. tuberculosis*, Respiratory viruses, *S. pneumoniae*, *S. aureus* (MSSA or MRSA)	
Cough/fever/pulmonary infiltrate in any lung location in a patient with a history of recent travel (10–21 days) to countries with active outbreaks of SARS, avian influenza	*M. tuberculosis*, severe acute respiratory syndrome virus (SARS_ CoV), avian influenza	
Respiratory infections, particularly bronchiolitis and pneumonia, in infants and young children	Respiratory syncytial virus, parainfluenza virus, adenovirus, influenza virus, human metapneumovirus	Airborne plus contact precautions plus eye protection. If SARS and tuberculosis unlikely, use droplet precautions instead of airborne precautions. Contact plus droplet precautions; droplet precautions may be discontinued when adenovirus and influenza have been ruled out.
Skin or Wound Infection		
Abscess or draining wound that cannot be covered	*Staphylococcus aureus* (MSSA or MRSA0, group A *Streptococcus* (GAS)	Contact Precautions Add Droplet Precautions for the first 24 hours of appropriate antimicrobial therapy if invasive Group A streptococcal disease is suspected

Source: Centers for Disease Control Isolation Precautions Guideline, 2007.

and conditions are frequently associated with infectious diseases. Once these measures are initiated, employees should ensure they are followed consistently by all involved in the delivery of care. Work restriction policies that include an employee furlough program should be developed. Included in these policies should be instructions for informing the employee not to report to work when experiencing vomiting, diarrhea, fever, unexplained rash (other than hives or an allergic reaction), pink eye, draining wounds, and productive cough. As part of the work-restriction program, employees should be assessed by Employee Health and/or

Occupational Medicine prior to returning to work. Other programs should ensure immunization requirements for direct patient-care providers and exposure follow-up programs. Vaccination against vaccine-preventable diseases should be offered free of charge to patient-care providers. Employees should be educated about situations that constitute an exposure and if an exposure occurs, the risk of acquiring a communicable disease. Providing information about how diseases are transmitted will not only greatly reduce fear and panic but also help the employee implement measures that limit exposure to others. Table 230.2 provides definitions

TABLE 230.2	CRITERIA FOR DETERMINING EXPOSURE TO COMMUNICABLE DISEASE
DISEASE	**DEFINITION OF EXPOSURE**
AIDS	Parenteral or mucous membrane exposure to blood or body fluids of a patient who is HIV positive or diagnosed as having AIDS
Hepatitis A	An eligible contact should be a person who has during a period of 15 days before onset of overt symptoms/during a few days after the development of jaundice. • Lived in the same household with the patient/employee • Had intimate sexual contact with the patient/employee • Incurred known exposure to fecal material or vomitus of nonisolated patient/employee if exposed individual has not followed good handwashing technique

(Continued)

TABLE 230.2	CRITERIA FOR DETERMINING EXPOSURE TO COMMUNICABLE DISEASE—CONT'D
DISEASE	**DEFINITION OF EXPOSURE**
Hepatitis B	Documented percutaneous or permucosal exposure to infective body fluids
Herpes (acute gingivostomatitis	Direct contact with the saliva of carriers
Measles	Direct contact with nasal or throat secretions or airborne by droplet spread by a person who has not had measles or immunization against measles
Meningitis (meningococcal)	Direct contact with respiratory secretions from nose and throat of infected person
Mumps	Airborne transmission or by droplet spread and by direct contact with saliva of an infected person by those who have not had mumps or mumps vaccine
Pediculosis capitus (head lice)	Direct contact with an infested person/indirect contact with their clothing, head gear, or linens
Rubella	Direct contact with nasopharyngeal secretions of infected people
Scabies	Direct contact with the skin of infected persons. Can also be acquired during sexual contact
Tuberculosis	Significant exposure to persons capable of generating aerosolized particles containing tubercle bacilli from the respiratory tract
Varicella zoster (chickenpox)	Direct contact, droplet or airborne spread of vesicle fluid or secretions of the respiratory tract of chickenpox cases, or of vesicle fluid of persons with herpes zoster (shingles)

Note: Significant exposures will be determined on an individual basis. Factors to be considered include the following:

• Etiology agent
• Mode of transmission
• Degree and method of contact
• Susceptibility

Source: Chin J. Control of Communicable Diseases Manual. Available at: http://www.cdc.gov/ncidod/dhqp/pdf/guidelines/Isolation2007.pdf. Accessed April 30, 2009.

of exposure for some common conditions seen in the healthcare setting. Healthcare facilities not only deal with the health and well-being of patients but also the employees who provide care to the patients. A healthy work force is a key component in the prevention and control of infections.

SUGGESTED READINGS

Bolyard EA, Tablan OC, Williams W, et al. Guidelines for infection control in health care personnel. *Am J Infect Control.* 1998;26(3):289–339.

Heymann, DL, ed. *Control of Communicable Disease Manual.* 18th Ed. Atlanta, GA: American Public Health Association; 2004, pp. 357–359.

TWENTY STUDENTS PRESENT WITH NAUSEA, VOMITING, AND DIARRHEA: DO NOT ASSUME IT IS FOOD POISONING

BETSY HARGREAVES ALLBEE, BSN, CIC

WHAT TO DO: EVALUATE

Hospital emergency departments (ED) are utilized by a variety of individuals such as college students, residents of long term care facilities, and others in the community. It is not uncommon for several patients to present with similar symptoms on any given day. In most situations, patients with similar symptoms present sporadically throughout the day, making it difficult to detect patterns, trends or clusters of disease. Identifying these clusters can be challenging in an ED that treats large numbers of patients per day.

Complaints of acute gastroenteritis (AGE), (e.g., nausea, vomiting, and diarrhea) are a frequent reason for patients to seek medical attention in the ED. When a group of individuals who reside in a common location (e.g. college students) present with similar symptoms, an obvious component of the assessment includes an inquiry about food (e.g., how soon after consumption did the symptoms begin? Was a meal from a fast food restaurant or food court eaten?). Depending upon the responses, a preliminary diagnosis of a foodborne illness such as *Salmonella* may be entertained. However, assuming that the symptoms are foodborne can result in the contamination of the facility if an infectious agent is the cause.

Symptoms associated with norovirus, also called Norwalk-like illness, usually begin 24 to 48 h after exposure, but can appear as early as 10 h after exposure. Symptoms usually include nausea, vomiting, diarrhea, and stomach cramping. Occasionally there is a low-grade fever, chills, headache, muscle aches, and a general sense of tiredness. The illness is usually brief, with symptoms lasting only one or two days. Symptomatic patients are contagious from the onset of symptoms up to two weeks after recovery.

The norovirus is found in the stool and vomit of infected people. People can become infected in several ways, including direct contact with a symptomatic patient, eating food or drinking liquids that are contaminated by infected food handlers, touching surfaces or objects contaminated with norovirus and then touching their mouth. Gastrointestinal illness, such as norovirus, is spread by fecal–oral contact. As a result, hand hygiene is a significant strategy for the prevention and control of additional cases. There is no specific treatment available for norovirus. Patients who become severely dehydrated often require rehydration therapy. Illness due to norovirus does not result in immunity to the virus.

Outbreaks caused by norovirus-like illnesses are becoming more and more common in institutional settings such as college campuses, hospitals, and long term care facilities. The virus was first identified in 1972 after an outbreak of gastrointestinal illness in Norwalk, Ohio. From October 1, 2006, through January 31, 2007, a total of 333 acute gastroenteritis outbreaks were reported in New York. Of these 333 cases, 272 (82%) occurred in long-term care facilities and 26 (8%) in hospitals. Of 216 healthcare facility outbreaks, a total of 7,907 patients and 4,317 staff members were affected. In order to prevent the spread of this highly infectious virus, facilities should initiate important recommendations for patient placement, visitors, employees, and housekeeping (Table 231.1). These recommendations include

Patient Placement:

- Designate a unit as the "gastroenteritis" unit (cohort patients and employees).
- Place patients with symptoms of gastroenteritis (>3 loose stools in a 24-h period; vomiting and diarrhea) on strict contact precautions.
- Maintain contact precautions until 48 hours after symptoms cease.
- Establish the routes for patient, visitor, and staff transport.
- Confine the patient to the room except for essential purposes (e.g., radiology tests, surgical procedures). Instruct or assist the patient in hand hygiene prior to leaving the room.
- Equipment should be dedicated to the patient, if possible. If equipment must be shared, it should be cleaned thoroughly with a 1:10 solution of bleach and water or bleach wipe prior to use on other patients.

Visitors:

- Instruct visitors to wash hands with soap and water after visiting a patient with gastroenteritis.
- Instruct visitors not to travel in other areas of the facility (e.g., visit other patients) after visiting a patient with gastroenteritis.
- Assess visitors for gastrointestinal-like symptoms. Restrict symptomatic visitors from entering the facility.

Employees:

- Prohibit staff from eating and drinking on the unit.
- Implement staff cohorting (assign staff to the "gastroenteritis" unit and do not allow staff to float to other units)

TABLE 231.1	RECOMMENDED MEASURES FOR THE PREVENTION AND CONTROL OF NOROVIRUS INFECTION

1. Practice good hand hygiene.

   - Wash hands frequently with soap and water.
   - Alcohol-based sanitizing hand gels (> ethanol content) may be used to complement handwashing with soap and water.

2. Disinfect contaminated surfaces with either of the following methods:

   - Use a chlorine bleach solution with a concentration of 1,000–5,000 ppm (1:20–1:10 dilution of household bleach (5.25%) for hard, nonporous surfaces.
   - Use disinfectants registered as effective against norovirus by the Environment Protection Agency (EPA)[*] in accordance with the manufacturers' instructions.

3. Do not return to work or school until 24–72 h after symptoms resolve and practice good hand hygiene after returning.

4. Additional measures for outbreaks in healthcare and long-term care facilities include the following:

   - Use contact precautions for preventing gastroenteritis.
   - Avoid sharing staff members between units or facilities with affected patients and units or facilities that are not affected.
   - Group symptomatic patients and provide separate toilet facilities for ill and well patients.
   - Instruct visitors on appropriate hand hygiene and monitor compliance with contact isolation precautions.
   - Close affected units to new admissions and transfers.

[*]List of EPA-approved products available at http://www.epa.gov/oppad001/list_g_norovirus.pdf. Evidence for efficacy against norovirus is usually based on studies with feline calicivirus (FCV) as a substitute for norovirus. FCV and norovirus have different physiochemical properties, and whether inactivation of FCV reflects efficacy against norovirus is unclear.
Source: Centers for Disease Control and Prevention, Atlanta.

- Instruct and encourage staff to report symptoms of gastroenteritis. Furlough symptomatic employees until they have been free of symptoms for 48 hours.
- Encourage hand hygiene, before and after patient contact, with soap and water. Instruct staff to increase the duration of handwashing.

Housekeeping:

- Until an isolation unit is established, rooms used by symptomatic patients should be cleaned after all other non-contaminated rooms.
- Instruct the staff to thoroughly clean the patient's room with a 1:10 solution of bleach and water or bleach wipe.
- High-touch surfaces (doorknobs, light switches, tables, counter tops, computer keyboards) should be cleaned and disinfected at least every shift.
- Patient servers should be emptied, the contents discarded, and thoroughly cleaned.

Norovirus is a major cause of viral gastroenteritis and has been associated with many close-contact outbreaks including those in hospitals, schools, cruise ships, and residential facilities. In order to prevent an internal outbreak, early identification, segregation, and strict adherence to established infection control practices are essential.

SUGGESTED READINGS

Centers for Disease Control and Prevention (CDC). Norovirus activity in the United States, 2006–2007. *Morb Mort Week Rep.* 2007;56:842–846.

Johnson CO, Qui H, Ticehurst JR. Outbreak management and implications of a nosocomial norovirus outbreak. *Clin Infect Dis.* 2007;45:534–540.

Quest Diagnostics Infectious Disease Update. October 2007; 14(8):71.

COMPLY WITH HAND HYGIENE GUIDELINES: WHAT YOU DO NOT SEE IS WHAT YOU OR YOUR PATIENT CAN GET

BETSY HARGREAVES ALLBEE, BSN, CIC

WHAT TO DO: IMPLEMENT

Hand hygiene is a general term used to describe the action of hand cleansing. Hand hygiene with soap and water has been advocated in the healthcare setting since 1847 when Ignaz Semmelweis discovered an association between care providers who performed handwashing and reduced infection rates. The significance of handwashing was misunderstood then and is still misunderstood today. In fact, it was not until the 1980s, 140 years after Semmelweis' correlation was made, that the first national hand hygiene guidelines were published.

Most hospital-acquired pathogens are transmitted from patient to patient via the hands of healthcare workers. Human skin is colonized with bacteria called normal flora. In the healthcare setting, workers can pick up microorganisms from the environment. These microorganisms are called transient flora. Transient floras are the causative agents in most hospital-associated infections (HAIs). Routine handwashing can easily remove transient flora from the skin. HAIs rates could be significantly reduced if all care providers performed handwashing.

A survey of approximately 200 healthcare workers revealed that 89% recognized handwashing as an important means of preventing infection; yet, compliance with hand hygiene among healthcare workers ranges between 16% and 81%. Handwashing is a basic, low tech method of infection prevention. Perhaps, in this high tech environment, basic handwashing is not considered an evidence-based practice and is not taken seriously. Several years ago a handwashing study among staff at a university medical center found that the more educated an individual was, the less likely he was to wash his hands.

Another obstacle to compliance suggests that employees are more likely to wash hands when their hands are visibly soiled. Most patient encounters, for example, history and vital sign assessment, do not result in the soiling of hands. However, hands can be contaminated even when not visibly soiled. Many communicable diseases are spread by the hands. Basing hand hygiene on visual contamination can lead to hospital-associated outbreaks of pathogens such as respiratory and gastrointestinal illnesses and resistant microorganisms. Healthcare workers frequently apply gloves when exposure to blood or body fluid is anticipated. It is the recommendation of the Centers for Disease Control (CDC) and the Occupational Health and Safety Administration (OSHA) that hands be washed after gloves

are removed. Healthcare workers who believe their hands are contaminated only when visibly soiled often do not wash their hands after glove removal and are placing themselves and their patients at risk.

Being able to see parasites, insects, and other pathogens might also be an incentive for staff to practice good handwashing. In support of this theory, consider the following situation observed by an infection control practitioner. There were two patients on the same unit, one with methicillin resistant *Staphylococcus aureus* (MRSA) and the other with head lice. Staff caring for the patient with head lice, wore personal protective equipment from head to toe (e.g., caps, masks, gowns, gloves, and shoe covers). Staff caring for the patient with MRSA wore no personal protective equipment. A possible conclusion, head lice are insects that are visible to the human eye, MRSA is a microorganism and cannot be seen, therefore, staff concluded that lice posed a greater threat.

Organizations such as the Centers for Disease Control and Prevention (CDC) and the World Health Organization (WHO), along with The Joint Commission acknowledged the effectiveness of hand hygiene by releasing guidelines on the subject. The Joint Commission included hand hygiene compliance as a National Patient Safety Goal and evaluates a facility's compliance rates during their surveys.

Hand hygiene is considered to be the most important measure for preventing the spread of pathogens in healthcare settings. Forty years ago, healthcare workers were instructed to wash hands with soap and water for 1 to 2 min before and after patient contact. Handwashing with soap, particularly antimicrobial soap, tends to cause skin dryness. Dry, cracked skin is not only painful, but also removes the body's natural defense to microorganisms, that of intact skin.

In recent years, new products, such as alcohol-based solutions, have been developed and approved for use in the hospital setting. Alcohol-based cleansers are an acceptable method of performing hand hygiene, and in 2002, the CDC released its Guideline for Hand Hygiene in Health-Care Settings recommending alcohol-based cleaners. Alcohol-based products contain emollients, making them less irritating to the skin. These products are also much more convenient to use because they do not require running water. When polled, 98% of employees preferred the alcohol-based products over soap and water. Most facilities stock regular liquid soap and an alcohol-based product. Patient-care areas have dispensers with both products, suggesting availability is not the reason for low hand hygiene compliance rates. It is likely that healthcare facilities will continue to stock both an alcohol-based product and liquid soap. While the CDC endorses the alcohol-based products, they recommend the use of soap and water when caring for patients with *Clostridium difficile*. There is some question as to whether the alcohol-based products are effective against spore-forming bacteria such as *C. difficile*.

Hand hygiene products have come a long way in the past 140 years. But no matter how expensive or convenient the product is, it must first be used in order to be effective.

SUGGESTED READINGS

Boyce JM, et al. Guideline for hand hygiene in health-care settings. Recommendations of the Healthcare Infection Control Practices Advisory Committee and the ICPAC/SHEA/APIC/IDSA Hand Hygiene Task Force. Society for Healthcare Epidemiology of America/Association for Professionsals in Infection Control/Infectious Diseases Society of America. *Morb Mort Week Rep.* 2002.51(RR-16):1–45.

Harris AD, Samore MH, Nafziger R, et al. A survey on hand-washing practices and opinions of healthcare workers. *J Hosp Infect.* 2000;45:318–321.

Pittet D. Improving compliance with hand hygiene in hospitals. *Infect Control Hosp Epidemiol.* 2000;21(6):381–386.

KNOW HOW TO MANAGE AN INFECTIOUS DISEASE'S OUTBREAK

BETSY HARGREAVES ALLBEE, BSN, CIC

WHAT TO DO: IMPLEMENT

Seasonal and incidental clusters of patients who experience similar symptoms are not unusual. However, occasionally, these clusters represent more than a coincidence and are an indication of an outbreak. Early identification of an outbreak is the key to preventing hospital associated infections.

An outbreak is an excess of disease over the expected level of disease. An outbreak can involve an infectious disease or biological agent and usually occurs within a given place (or population) for a given time. Typically, infectious agents affect a small number of patients and may result in periods of increase and decrease in cases. Infectious diseases and agents frequently associated with outbreaks include salmonella, norovirus-like illnesses, legionella, meningitis, measles, mumps, pertussis, and tuberculosis. Biological agents, on the other hand, will generally cause large numbers of illness and fatalities in a specific geographical area over a short period of time. Biological agents include a wide range of live biological organisms and their products (toxins and venoms), which are intended to kill, seriously injure, or incapacitate. These agents may be difficult to detect and identify. The biological agents most likely to be released include anthrax, plague, ricin, smallpox, tularemia, and viral hemorrhagic fever.

Infectious diseases and biological agents may enter the body by inhalation, ingestion, or through the skin. Although the confirmed diagnosis may not be readily available, a tentative diagnosis is extremely useful in determining the mechanism of transmission. Meticulous hand hygiene is the cornerstone of infection prevention and, in conjunction with adherence to isolation, precautions may be the only preventive measure available during an outbreak in which there is no readily available vaccine, prophylaxis, or treatment.

Transmission risk in healthcare (including hospitals, long-term care, and outpatient facilities) depends on the extent of the outbreak activity in the community and in the facility. Initially, the use of social distancing will limit the spread to others. Social distancing involves keeping a distance of at least three feet between infectious/contaminated and noninfectious/noncontaminated patients and personnel. Also included would be the establishment of "sick" and "well" waiting rooms and sections of the nursing unit by cohorting affected individuals. The response for escalating infection control measures will be based on the nature of the outbreak and the transmission risk. As the epidemiologic characteristics of the outbreak are more clearly defined, the Infection Control Department in conjunction with the local health department and the Centers for Disease Control and Prevention (CDC) will update infection control guidance. Below is a useful triage tool that can be utilized when front line staff are confronted with an influx of patients who may bear an infectious risk. (Figure 233.1).

The federal, state, regional, or local health authorities will establish a case definition based on the symptoms. The use of a standard case definition ensures that patients are appropriately and expeditiously triaged, cared for, and housed. It also assists in ensuring infection prevention and control measures by identifying those affected. Although a standard case definition is established, the definition may change over the course of the outbreak. The change in definition may alter other activities, such as laboratory testing, protocols, patient disposition, and vaccine and medication administration. Although the case definition may change, it is important to gather consistent information when assessing the patient. Details that should be gathered from the patient during the assessment should include:

- Date (time of onset)
- Place
- Symptoms
- Patient characteristics (gender, age, date of admission, underlying disease)
- Possible exposure (to other patients and staff)

This information should be communicated to the facility's Infection Control Department who will then communicate with the health department. Patient placement of potentially infectious patients is very important. It is not uncommon for private or isolation room availability to be limited. During the initial phase of the outbreak, room placement and cohorting should be based on the mode of transmission of the suspected causative disease (Table 233.1). The following is a guide to determine private room prioritization, in descending order of priority:

1. Airborne transmission (e.g., smallpox, measles, tuberculosis)
2. Droplet transmission (e.g., influenza, meningitis)
3. Contact transmission (e.g., norovirus illnesses, hemorrhagic fever).

Patients with infections spread by contact, which are noncompliant or cannot be contained, such as

- Diarrhea in incontinent patients, feces not contained by diapers
- Respiratory tract infections in children or incapacitated adults, unable to appropriately handle respiratory secretions
- Infected wound or skin drainage not contained by dressing

Other control measures include visitor restrictions, staff cohorting, and equipment and environmental cleaning. It may be necessary to restrict visitors for two reasons: (1) they may have been exposed but not be presently exhibiting signs or symptoms: and (2) they may not follow recommended infection control measures while visiting an infectious patient and then may visit other patients in the facility. During outbreaks in which there may be staff shortages due to illness (e.g., pandemic influenza), it may be necessary to utilize family members to perform activities of daily living. If visitors are permitted, they must be instructed to practice infection control measures. It is also advisable to establish travel routes for visitors to use when entering and departing a facility.

Cohorting involves grouping individuals with similar symptoms, or exposure to similar illness, together to minimize the exposure to others. Not only will the patients be cohorted, but the staff should also be cohorted. If the outbreak involves a vaccine-preventable disease, staff should be screened for immunization and communicable disease immunity status. Staff members who have been appropriately vaccinated, or have previously had a vaccine-preventable disease, are immune and can safely care for these patients.

Reusable, durable medical equipment (e.g., wheelchairs, infusion pumps, blood pressure monitors, and stethoscopes) that become soiled or contaminated with blood, body fluids, secretions, or excretions should be handled in a manner that prevents exposure to skin and mucous membranes, avoids contamination of clothing, and minimizes the likelihood of transfer of microbes to other patients and the environment. Thorough disinfection of patient care equipment and the environment should be performed even before a definitive diagnosis is made since a definitive diagnosis may not be available for hours or days. However, if a cluster or outbreak is suspected, notify the Infection Control Department for

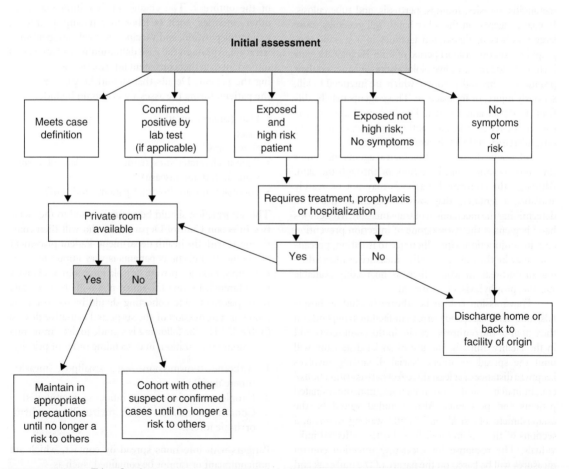

FIGURE 233.1. Triage flowchart.

TABLE 233.1	OUTBREAK MANAGEMENT QUICKCHART						
CONDITION (* = REPORTABLE)	TYPE OF PRECAUTIONS	DURATION OF ISOLATION/ PRECAUTIONS	HAND HYGIENE RECOMMENDATION	INCUBATION PERIOD	CLEANING	LAB TEST
Avian Influenza*	Airborne	Adult (7 days after resolution of fever) Child ≤ 12 y (21 days after onset of illness)	Alcohol-based or soap and water	1–3 days	Routine with tuberculocidal activity	Culture (nasal swab; aspirate; bronchoalveolar lavage) PCR; Antigen
Chicken Pox (Varicella)*	Airborne; contact	Until all lesions crusted	Alcohol-based or soap and water	14–28 days	Routine	Antibody
Hepatitis A*	Contact (Enteric)	Until 1 week after onset of jaundice	Alcohol-based or soap and water	28–30 days (range 15–50 days)	Routine	IgM antibody
Legionnaire*	Standard; person to person not documented	NA	Alcohol-based or soap and water	2–10 days; most often 5–6 days	Routine	Culture (sputum; lung, pleural fluid) Urine antigen
Measles (Rubeola)*	Airborne; contact	Until all lesions healed	Alcohol-based or soap and water	7–18 days	Routine	IgM antibody
Meningitis (Neisseria)*	Droplet	24 h after initiation of effective antibiotic	Alcohol-based or soap and water	2–10 days	Routine	Culture (blood, CSF)
Norwalk (Norovirus)*	Contact	Until 3 days after cessation of symptoms (virus may be shed for 2 weeks)	Soap and water may be more effective than alcohol-based (duration of handwash should be extended)	24–48h	Terminal (phenols and quats not reliable)	Culture (stool); PCR
Pertussis (Whooping cough)*	Droplet	Until 5 days after initiation of effective therapy	Alcohol-based or soap and water	6–20 days	Routine	Culture (nasopharyngeal); PCR
Salmonella*	Contact (Enteric)	Duration of illness	Alcohol-based or soap and water	6–72 h; usually 12–36 h	Terminal	Culture (stool)
Smallpox (Variola)*	Airborne; contact	Until all lesions healed	Alcohol-based or soap and water	7–19 days	Terminal	Culture (lesions); PCR
Strep Group (invasive)*	Contact	24 h after initiation of effective antibiotic; may extend duration until wound heals	Alcohol-based or soap and water	7–10 days	Terminal	Culture (blood and focal sites)

Routine use of standard precautions is essential with all patients. The most important means of controlling any communicable disease is prompt identification and isolation.
Airborne Precautions involves negative pressure room and use of N95 respiratory protection.
In all outbreak situations, commonly touched items such as doorknobs, handrails, and other environmental surfaces should be thoroughly disinfected.

prevention and control recommendations as soon as possible. Initiate the recommended precautions and ensure staff and visitors comply with these precautions. Early identification and prompt initiation of infection control measures will prevent the spread of illness in the hospital setting.

SUGGESTED READINGS

Checko PJ. Outbreak investigation. In: *APIC Text of Infection Control and Epidemiology*. Washington, DC: Association For Professionals in Infection Control; 2005, pp. 4–10.

Model Emergency Response Communications Planning for Infectious Disease Outbreaks and Bioterrorist Events. 2nd Ed. Washington, DC: Public Health Foundation; 2001.

Surveillance and Control of Communicable Diseases: Handbook for Health Providers in Georgia. 2004. Available at: http://www.popline.org/docs/1611/285676.html.

Ensure that Patient Care Equipment, Like Hoyer Lift Pads and Linens, are Laundered by the Hospital's Laundry and Not Taken Home by Staff for Laundering as a Nice Gesture

Betsy Hargreaves Allbee, BSN, CIC

WHAT TO DO: EVALUATE

A Hoyer lift is a mechanical device used to transfer the patient from one surface to another. The lift pad is a sling placed under the patient and then connected to a mechanical lift. These assistive devices are becoming more common in the delivery of care due to (1) an increasingly overweight patient population, (2) an increase in patients with mobility limitations due to age or illness, and (3) an aging nursing staff. These items are not only expensive, but also create a storage problem because they are bulky. As a result, most nursing units only stock one Hoyer lift and one or two lift pads.

The lift pads are made of a reusable, washable fabric and are sent to the laundry for cleaning. A patient with a communicable disease should have a lift pad dedicated to him or her and kept in his or her room to avoid use on other patients. Lift pads used on the general population must be laundered on a routine basis and when soiled with feces or other body fluids. Hospitals with a centralized laundry or which use contract services may experience problems with lost items or slow laundry turn-around-time, creating a shortage in lift pads. One possible solution could be to purchase a washer and dryer and launder these items in-house. However, there are several regulations which must be taken into consideration.

The American Hospital Association and the American Institute of Laundering have standards for handling "hygienically clean" textiles. These standards include temperature and processing requirements. For example, wash–water is to be 165°F and requires a dosage of chlorine bleach for heavily soiled items. A temperature of 120° to 140°F is acceptable with polyester/cotton blends. If a facility is only able to achieve a temperature of 110° to 120°F, an increased amount of chlorine bleach must be used in order to reduce the bacterial pathogens on the linen.

The Occupational Health and Safety Administration (OSHA) and the Centers for Disease Control (CDC) also have recommendations that must be followed. For example, areas processing contaminated textiles must have negative pressure airflow in relation to other areas of the facility. Sufficient space for separate areas designated for receipt of contaminated items and storage of clean items must be provided. Emergency eye wash stations or shower equipment must be readily available. Handwashing facilities must be conveniently located in the work area. These restrictions and recommendations make it impractical to install a washer and dryer in a storage area.

Although it might seem like a conscientious gesture and a cost saving solution to the problem, do not allow staff to launder lift pads or other patient-related linens at home. Compliance and quality control with wash–water temperature, detergent, bleach, and rinse cycles cannot be ensured; OSHA bloodborne pathogen standard violations may occur, and household members are at risk of exposure to a variety of pathogens. Contaminated textiles have been known to be a source of large numbers of pathogens. Recently, two resistant pathogens, methicillin-resistant *Staphylococcus aureus* (MRSA) and vancomycin-resistant *Enterococcus* (VRE) have been found to have an extended life expectancy on fabric. Researchers have discovered that MRSA was able to survive from 1 to 56 days on fabrics, and VRE survival was from 11 to 90 days. Although there has been no documentation about the life expectancy of *Clostridium difficile* (C-diff) and extended spectrum beta lactams (ESBL) on fabrics, these pathogens require isolation precautions and meticulous disinfection processes. Fabrics, therefore, should be considered fomites capable of harboring and transmitting microorganisms.

Foreign objects inadvertently left in the laundry pose additional safety issues. Items such as dentures, eye glasses, hearing aids, telemetry units, and needles have been found by laundry personnel. Not only is the presence of these items in the laundry an infection control issue, but they can easily result in injury or damaged appliances.

Key elements in the laundering process include appropriate water temperature, type of detergents, chlorine bleach, rinsing, and finishing. Home laundering of patient care equipment and linens is not appropriate, violates the OSHA bloodborne pathogens, and places patients, employees, and their families at risk.

SUGGESTED READINGS

Belkin NL. Laundry, linens, and textiles. *AJIC.* 2005; 103-1–103-8.

Centers for Disease Control and Prevention (CDC). Guidelines for environmental infection control in health-care facilties. *Morb Mort Week Rep.* 2003;52:27–28.

Neely AN, Maley MP. Survival of enterococci and staphylococci on hospital fabrics and plastic. *J Clin Microbiol.* 2000;38(2): 724–726.

THE JOINT COMMISSION IS HERE! WHAT'S OUR POLICY ON...?

BETSY HARGREAVES ALLBEE, BSN, CIC

WHAT TO DO: EVALUATE

The Joint Commission has been setting standards and surveying hospitals for compliance to these standards since 1951. While there have been many changes over the years (e.g., several name changes and survey cycle interval modifications), its main focus continues to be patient care. The mission of the Joint Commission is to continuously improve the safety and quality of care provided to the public through the provision of health care accreditation and related services that support performance improvement in healthcare organizations.

Recently, the Joint Commission began conducting random unannounced surveys across the nation. This survey process encouraged healthcare facilities to maintain compliance in a constant state of readiness. Prior to the introduction of random midcycle surveys, hospitals would operate as usual until 12 months before the expected survey. During the presurvey period, efforts were concentrated on the physical environment, policy manuals, and other documents. To ensure all elements of the Joint Commission standards would be met, existing policy manuals were revised and new policies developed. Those working on the policies were often knowledgeable, experienced personnel whose goals were well-intended and designed to meet the regulatory standards. While many of the policies were specific to a department, and the leaders of those departments were involved in the changes, during all the frenzy, front line workers did not receive notice of new or revised policies. Despite these flaws, healthcare facilities were able to maintain accreditation because those individuals interviewed were often the authors of the policy.

With a focus on patient safety, in 2002, the Joint Commission revised its approach to accreditation decisions with a new survey agenda. The new survey process became priority-focused using the patient tracer methodology. In 2006, the National Patient Safety Goals were announced to support a systems approach in order to prevent adverse events and caregiver errors from reaching the patient. The National Patient Safety Goals place a strong emphasis on quality and performance improvement activities and require a multidisciplinary team, including front line workers, to be actively involved. This new survey process allows the surveyors to follow the patient through the admission process, treatments, procedures, diagnostic tests, and when applicable, past discharge. The tracer methodology assesses a facility's credibility and actively engages all direct caregivers in the accreditation process. This shift in the survey process from table-top manual review and formal interviews to one of direct observation of the delivery of care provides an opportunity for the surveyors to analyse operational processes that may impact the quality and safety of patient care. During the tracer, a surveyor will interview healthcare personnel involved in the patient's care. Healthcare personnel are expected to: (1) be knowledgeable about the patient's plan of care, (2) provide quality care, and (3) maintain a safe environment.

Nursing personnel are often familiar with procedural protocols such as urinary catheter insertion, tracheostomy care, and medication administration. Personnel must also familiarize themselves with facility specific Safety, Emergency Management, and Infection Control policies. A surveyor tracing a patient isolated for Norovirus should be expected to challenge an employee's knowledge of safety-related policies. Be prepared to answer questions such as:

- How do you dispose of trash from an isolation room?
- What is your facility's plan for handling an influx of infectious patients?
- What type of isolation is appropriate for a patient with gastroenteritis?
- Is an alcohol-based hand cleaner effective?
- What is your facility's process for handling employee exposures?

In the past, these questions were addressed by Leadership, Safety, and Infection Control. Now, the surveyor will not only ask those involved in policy development, but also those who utilize the policy. Policies dealing with isolation precautions, bloodborne pathogens, hand hygiene, and regulated medical waste are tailored to meet the needs of a facility and should be readily available. Those responsible for Safety, Emergency Management, and Infection Control utilize evidence-based, nationally recognized guidelines from agencies such as the Occupational Health and Safety Administration (OSHA), the Centers for Disease Control and Prevention (CDC), the World Health Organization (WHO), the Environmental Protection Agency (EPA), etc as a resource. Because many of these guidelines provide rationale and evidence to support the recommendations, they are often too lengthy and therefore, impractical for most staff to consult. Facility-specific policies, developed by experts within the facility, are developed so they can be understood by all levels of staff.

The Joint Commission standards focus not simply on an organization's ability to provide safe, high quality care, but on its actual performance as well. Every year National Patient Safety Goals are revised, existing standards are refined, and new standards with a direct impact on the quality of care are added. While you may not be able to keep current with these changes, you should become familiar with your facility's policies. Don't wait until a surveyor is on your unit to read one of these documents. Know the experts in your facility and take advantage of their experience and knowledge when issues arise. The Joint Commission surveyors, along with all regulatory agencies, expect all personnel to have an understanding of a variety of safety-related issues and policies.

SUGGESTED READINGS

Bartley J. Accrediting and regulatory agencies. *Assoc Proff Infect Control Epidemiol.* 2005;10-1–10-10.

Friedman C. Infection control and prevention programs. *Assoc Proff Infect Control Epidemiol.* 2005;1-1–1-3.

The Joint Commission. Accreditation Process Overview. 2007.

KNOW THE BASICS OF INFECTION CONTROL

BETSY HARGREAVES ALLBEE, BSN, CIC

Eighty percent of all pathogens in the hospital and home environment spread through hand contact. The benefits of hand hygiene include a reduction in patient infections, hospital-associated outbreaks, transmission of multidrug resistant organisms, staff absenteeism due to infections, and cost. Handwashing is only one component of Standard Precautions, which are a set of practices designed to be used when caring for all patients regardless of their diagnosis or presumed infection status (Table 236.1). Standard precautions apply to blood, body fluids, secretions, and excretions. Included in Standard Precautions are other important control measures such as disinfection of patient equipment, handling of linen, the use of personal protective equipment, and patient placement recommendations.

Host factors such as diabetes and immunosuppressive disorders increase a patient's susceptibility to acquisition of infection. The extremes of life—infancy and old age—are also associated with a reduced resistance to infection. Patients with a chronic disease such as malignant tumors, leukemia, diabetes mellitus, renal failure, or the acquired

TABLE 236.1	STANDARD PRECAUTIONS

1. Handwashing

- Wash hands after touching blood, body fluids, secretions, excretions, and contaminated items, whether or not gloves are worn.
- Wash hands immediately after gloves are removed, between patient contacts, and when otherwise indicated to avoid transfer of microorganisms to other patients or environments. Wash hands between tasks and procedures on the same patient to prevent cross-contamination of different body sites.
- Use a plain soap or alcohol-based hand cleanser for routine handwashing.
- Use soap for handwashing when caring for patients with *C. difficile* or when hands are visibly soiled.

2. Personal Protective Equipment

Gloves

- Wear gloves (clean and nonsterile) when touching blood, body fluids, secretions, excretions, and contaminated items.
- Put on clean gloves just before touching mucous membranes and nonintact skin.
- Change gloves between tasks and procedures on the same patient after contact with material that may contain a high concentration of microorganisms.
- Remove gloves promptly after use, before touching noncontaminated items and environmental surfaces, and before caring for another patient. Wash hands immediately after removing gloves to avoid transfer of microorganisms to other patients or environments.

Masks, Eye Protection, Face Shields

- Wear a mask and eye protection or a face shield to protect mucous membranes of the eyes, nose, and mouth during procedures and patient-care activities that are likely to generate splashes or sprays of blood, body fluids, secretions, and excretions.

Gowns

- Wear a gown (clean and nonsterile) to protect skin and prevent soiling of clothing during procedures and patient care activities that are likely to generate splashes or sprays of blood, body fluids, secretions, or excretions or cause soiling of clothing.
- Remove a soiled gown as promptly as possible, taking care not to contaminate clothing, and wash hands to avoid transfer of microorganisms to other patients or environments.

3. Patient Care Equipment

- Handle used patient care equipment soiled with blood, body fluids, secretions, and excretions in a manner that prevents skin and mucous membrane exposures, contamination of clothing, and transfer of other microorganisms to other patients and environments.
- Ensure that reusable equipment is not used for the care of another patient until it has been appropriately cleaned and reprocessed. Single-use items are not reused and will be properly discarded.

4. Environmental Control

- Ensure that environmental surfaces, beds, bedrails, bedside equipment, and other frequently touched surfaces are appropriately cleaned.

(Continued)

TABLE 236.1	STANDARD PRECAUTIONS—COND'T

5. Linen

- Handle, transport, and process used linen soiled with blood, body fluids, secretions, and excretions in a manner that prevents skin and mucous membrane exposures, contamination of clothing, and avoids transfer of microorganisms to other patients and environments.

6. Patient Placement

- Place a patient who may have a suspected or confirmed infectious condition or who does not (or cannot be expected to) assist in maintaining appropriate hygiene or environmental control in a private room.

7. Employee Health

- Take care to prevent injuries when using needles, scalpels, and other sharp instruments or devices, when handling sharp instruments after procedures, when cleaning used instruments, and when disposing of used needles.
- Never recap used needles or otherwise manipulate them using both hands or any other technique that involves directing the point of a needle toward any part of the body.
- Do not remove used needles from disposable syringes by hand, and do not bend, break, or otherwise manipulate used needles by hand.
- Place used disposable syringes and needles, scalpel blades, and other sharp items in appropriate puncture-resistant containers located as close as practical to the area in which the items were used. Place reusable syringes and needles in a puncture-resistant container for transport to the reprocessing area.
- Use mouthpieces, resuscitation bags, or other ventilation devices as an alternative to mouth-to-mouth resuscitation methods in areas where the need for resuscitation is predictable.
- Report any exposure to blood or body fluids immediately. Follow facility policy for treatment and follow-up.
- Notify manager or designee if experiencing nausea, vomiting, diarrhea, jaundice, open wound, lesion or boil, unexplained rash, cough with productive sputum, or fever.

immunodeficiency syndrome (AIDS) have an increased susceptibility to infections with opportunistic pathogens. The early identification of an infection can improve patient outcome and reduce the spread of disease. The clinical features of infection include:

- Fever
- Elevated WBCs
- Unexplained changes in behavior
- Failure to thrive
- Worsening cognitive function
- Lethargy or agitation
- Loss of appetite

Infection may be difficult to assess in certain populations. Fever may be absent in the elderly and immunosuppressed populations. Long-term pharmacologic therapy such as antibiotics may mask fever and other symptoms. Symptoms often associated with infection may be attributed to underlying conditions.

The increased incidence of multidrug resistant pathogens in both the community and the hospital setting makes early identification and implementation of infection control measures important. Multidrug resistant organisms, also called problem pathogens, include methicillin resistant *Staphylococcus aureus* (MRSA), vancomycin resistant *Enterococcus*, *Clostridium difficile* (*c. difficile*), and extended spectrum beta lactam-producing organisms (ESBL). Patients may have an active infection with one of these organisms or may be colonized (the microorganism is present but not causing any symptoms). In most cases, a multidrug resistant organism is not the primary reason for admission. Patients may be admitted for conditions such as congestive heart failure and not be suspected of having a multidrug resistant pathogen. Limiting exposure to others and the environment by practicing standard precautions on all patients will reduce the risk of transmission of harmful pathogens to others.

Patient placement and isolation are essential elements in the control of infection. Patients with open draining wounds should, at a minimum, be segregated from fresh post-op patients. Patients with symptoms suggestive of tuberculosis, such as fever, cough, night sweats, and weight loss, should be placed in a negative pressure isolation room. Table 236.2 (p. 258) is a quick tool to use in making decisions about patient placement. Many microorganisms have the potential to survive in the hospital environment. Basic infection control measures such as hand hygiene, surface disinfection, and the careful placement of patients will significantly reduce the spread of microorganisms from patients to environmental surfaces.

SUGGESTED READINGS

Siegel JD, Rhinehart E, Jackson M, et al. Guideline for isolation precautions: Preventing transmission of infectious agents in healthcare settings. 2007.

World Health Organization. WHO guidelines on hand hygiene in health care. 2007.

World Health Organization. *Prevention of Hospital-Acquired Infections, A Practical Guide.* 2nd Ed. 2002, p. 2.

TABLE 236.2	LOCATION AND TRANSMISSION OF BACTERIA		
	ORGANISM	COMMON SITES	MODE OF TRANSMISSION
Gram positive aerobic bacteria	Methicillin-resistant staphylococci (MRSA)	Skin lesions, abscesses, impetigo, osteomyelitis, sepsis	Contact, autoinfection, fomites
	Vancomycin-resistant *Enterococcus faecium* (VRE)	Gastrointestinal tract, urinary tract infections, wound infections, bacteremia	Contact, autoinfection, fomites
	Streptococcus	Throat, skin, blood middle ear	Contact, droplet secretions
Gram negative aerobic bacteria	Extended spectrum beta-lactamase (ESBL)-producing GNRs	Urinary tract infections, wounds	Contact
	Pseudomonas aeruginosa and related GNRs	Urinary tract infections, wounds, pneumonia	Contact
Gram negative anaerobic bacteria	*Clostridium difficile* (C-diff)	Large intestine	Contact, fecal oral
Acid-fast Mycobacteria	Multidrug resistant (MDR) *Mycobacterium tuberculosis* (TB)	Lower respiratory tract, laryngeal, meningeal	Airborne (small particles less than 5 microns in diameter)
	Mycobacterium avium complex (MAC)	Lower respiratory tract, lymph nodes	Ingestion, skin lesions (noncommunicable)
Yeast and Fungi	*Candida* species	Mucocutaneous, skin	Endogenous, contact
Viruses	Human immunocdeficiency virus (HIV)	Skin	Sexual, percutaneous, exposure to blood or tissue
	Herpes simplex virus	Liver	Contact
	Hepatitis virus		Hepatitis A: ingestions, Hepatitis B: percutaneous and permucosal, exposure to blood or tissue, Hepatitis C: percutaneous and permucosal exposure to blood or tissue.

Source: Purdue. *Nosocomial Infections: A Multidisciplinary Approach to Management.* 2001.

KNOW THAT ISOLATION IS NOT A MYSTERY, BUT THAT THERE ARE CLEAR GUIDELINES

BETSY HARGREAVES ALLBEE, BSN, CIC

The basic concept of isolation involves the segregation of one patient from other patients to reduce the risk of transmission from patient to staff, staff to patient, and patient to patient. A study performed by a consulting group at a 150-bed facility in the mid 1990s found that the typical patient saw 50 healthcare workers in an average length of stay. This finding supports the importance of prompt segregation and early identification of a communicable disease.

An infectious disease is an illness resulting from the invasion of the body by bacteria, viruses, fungi, or parasites. The term "infection" refers to a condition caused by a pathogen. In contrast, a communicable disease is a disease which can be readily spread from one person to another under certain conditions. According to the World Health Organization (WHO), health care settings are an environment where both, infected persons and persons at increased risk of infection, congregate. Patients with infections or who are carriers of pathogenic microorganisms admitted to the hospital are potential sources of infection for patients and employees. Typically, many potentially communicable diseases are not confirmed until diagnostic tests such as cultures are obtained and results finalized. In many cases, the laboratory results are not finalized for 48 hours after collection of the specimen. With a shortage of private rooms, patients with unidentified resistant and/or communicable diseases are frequently roomed with other patients. Utilizing the concept of cohorting can simplify patient placement. A cohort is a group of individuals placed together to minimize exposure to other patients or personnel. Cohort isolation consists of two groups of people, an infected group and an uninfected group, who are separated from one another. The ideal mechanism of cohorting is placing individuals with similar diseases in an area physically separate from other patients. However, if unable to establish or designate a cohort area, patients can be separated by a minimum of three feet within the same area. In addition, every effort should be made to cohort staff. This involves designating certain personnel to care for patients with a communicable disease. There are two concepts to staff cohorting, (1) employees who may have already been exposed to the pathogen (i.e., staff who cared for a newly admitted patient prior to confirmation of a communicable disease), and (2) employees who have immunity to specific diseases (i.e.,

staff who previously had, or were vaccinated against, chicken pox should care for a patient with chicken pox). An effective cohort plan will minimize the risk of transmission of infection in a facility. To aid in a cohort program, many Infection Control practitioners have developed databases of patients with MRSA, VRE, and *C. difficile*. This database flags patients with a previous positive culture. Upon readmission, a notice pops up instructing personnel to initiate isolation.

Any communicable diseases can be spread via fomites. What are fomites? Fomites are objects, such as clothing, towels, and patient care equipment (i.e., indwelling urinary catheters, ventilators, wheelchairs, blood pressure cuffs, stethoscopes, etc.), that can harbor a disease agent or pathogen and are capable of transmitting the pathogen. It is important to consider these inanimate objects as mechanisms of transmission. The preferred handling of patient care equipment after use on a patient with a communicable disease is to dedicate the equipment to that patient. If a piece of equipment cannot be left in the isolation room, it must be disinfected, between patient use. A hospital-approved disinfectant or surface wipe is sufficient with most communicable diseases; however, diseases such as *C. difficile* and norovirus require disinfection with bleach. Sensitive electronic equipment has cleaning and disinfection recommendations listed in the operation manual. If an operation manual is not available, consult your Engineering, Infection Control, or Environmental Service Department(s) whenever cleaning guidance is needed.

Thirty years ago, the Centers for Disease Control and Prevention (CDC) developed isolation guidelines for specific diseases. Then, in 1992, the CDC revised the Isolation Precautions in an attempt to simplify the process. Those guidelines took into consideration the OSHA Bloodborne Pathogens Standard and incorporated Standard Precautions, formerly called Universal Precautions, into the recommendations. The 1992 CDC guidelines defined two basic categories: standard precautions and transmission-based precautions, with an emphasis on the practice of Standard Precautions when caring for all patients. Under the umbrella of Standard Precautions, healthcare workers are encouraged to practice hand hygiene and use personal protective equipment (PPE) prior to a diagnosis of a communicable condition. Transmission-based precautions are used with patients who have known or suspected infections that are highly contagious or more difficult to cure.

With the increased incidence of multidrug-resistant pathogens such as methicillin resistant *Staphylococcus aureus* (MRSA) and vancomycin resistant *Enterococcus faecium* (VRE), the resurgence of tuberculosis, and increased number of *Clostridium difficile* (*C. difficile*), the CDC issued new isolation precautions in 2007. The 2007 CDC Isolation Guidelines recommend five categories of isolation. These categories include:

- Contact Precautions
- Droplet Precautions
- Airborne Precautions
- Contact Enteric Precautions
- Protective Precautions

Precautions are assigned based on the mechanism of transmission. For example, microorganisms that contaminate the environment and are spread by the hands, patient care equipment, and other inanimate objects would require "contact" precautions. Table 237.1 is a quick guide to aid in deciding which category of isolation to utilize. Some patients may require isolation for the duration of the hospitalization. Others may be isolated due to a history of a condition or colonization. Patients can be "screened" to determine whether they remain colonized. Screening

TABLE 237.1	TRANSMISSION BASED PRECAUTIONS	
CONTACT	**AIRBORNE**	**DROPLET**
Designed to reduce the risk of transmission of microorganisms by direct or indirect contact.	Designed to reduce the risk of airborne transmission of small-particle infectious agents. Airborne transmission occurs when airborne droplet particles are suspended in the air and can be inhaled by a susceptible host.	Designed to reduce the risk of transmission of large-particle droplets which are spread when a patient sneezes, coughs, talks, or during certain procedures. These particles may enter a susceptible host through the mucous membranes in the eyes, nose, or mouth.
Patient Placement and Personnel Protective Equipment (PPE) Requirements		
A private room; however, patients with the same microorganism can be cohorted (share a room). Gloves and Gown. Mask for those illnesses marked with an * **Equipment**: dedicate the use of equipment such as BP cuffs, stethoscopes, thermometer, bedside commode.	A private, negative pressure room. Keep the doors closed at all times. Monitor negative pressure every day when in use. N95 mask (respirator)	A private room or in a room with a patient(s) who has active infection with the same microorganism (cohort). Special air handling and ventilation are not necessary. Isolation/surgical mask.
Examples Of Illnesses		
Hepatitis A	Measles	Haemophilus influenza (invasive)
Herpes simplex virus	SARS	Meningitis (bacterial)
Impetigo	Smallpox	Mycoplasma pneumonia
MRSA (methicillin-/oxacillin-resistant *Staphylococcus aureus*)	Tuberculosis	Pertussis
Pediculosis (head lice)	Varicella (chicken pox)—also requires contact precautions	Pneumonic plague
RSV (respiratory syncytial virus)		Streptococcal pharyngitis, pneumonia, scarlet fever
Scabies		Mumps
VRE (vancomycin-resistant *Enterococcus faecium*)		Rubella
Wounds: major (non-contained) abscesses, cellulitis, or decubiti; or in a patient with a recent hospital or nursing home stay in a facility where multidrug-resistant organisms are prevalent *		

CONTACT SPECIAL ENTERIC
Clostridium difficile (*C. difficile*); Diarrhea: acute diarrhea with a likely infectious cause or in an adult with a history of recent antibiotic use.

PROTECTIVE ENVIRONMENT
A fourth category called **PROTECTIVE ENVIRONMENT**. This is "protective" or "reverse" isolation for patients who are immunocompromised. A private room is preferred. No one with an infection may enter the room. Hands must be washed before **and after** patient contact.

involves obtaining a culture from the colonized site. Individuals with a history of MRSA infection can be colonized in a wound, the nares, and the axilla region. Individuals with vancomycin-resistant enterococcus are colonized in the gastrointestinal tract. A positive culture indicates the patient remains colonized and therefore should be maintained in isolation. A negative culture suggests that the patient is no longer colonized and, as a result, no longer requires isolation. For assistance with the decision to terminate isolation precautions in some commonly seen diseases, refer to Table 237.2. Standard precautions should be followed when caring for all patients. Additional specific precautions should be initiated for patients with known communicable diseases. By understanding the trans-

mission of infection, one can determine the appropriate precautions to apply. Promptly initiating infection control strategies such as cohorting and isolation improves healthcare quality and increases patient safety.

SUGGESTED READINGS

Association for Professionals in Infection Control and Epidemiology. Guide to the elimination of Methicillin resistant *Staphylococcus aureus* (MRSA) transmission in hospital settings. 2007;47–49.

Siegel JD, Rhinehart E, Jackson M, et al. Guideline for isolation precautions: Preventing transmission of infectious agents in healthcare settings. 2007.

World Health Organization. *Prevention of Hospital-Acquired Infections, A Practical Guide.* 2nd Ed. 2002.

TABLE 237.2	DISCONTINUATION OF ISOLATION		
CONDITION	**TYPE OF PRECAUTION**	**DURATION**	**COMMENTS**
Chickenpox (Varicella)	Airborne/Contact	Until the lesions are crusted and dry.	Susceptible (non-immune) healthcare workers and visitors should not enter room.
Clostridium difficile (*C. difficile*)	Contact (enteric)	Duration of illness.	*New admission:* If a patient has an Hx: of *C. difficile**, but no active symptoms (e.g., diarrhea and abdominal pain), may discontinue isolation. *Inpatient:* discontinue isolation if patient has been free of symptoms for 48 h.
Meningitis: Viral (Non-bacterial; Aseptic)	Standard		
Meningitis: Bacterial	Droplet	Until patient has received 24 h of appropriate antibiotic therapy.	After 24 h of appropriate/effective antibiotic therapy may discontinue isolation.
Methicillin-Resistant *Staphylococcus aureus* (MRSA)	Contact	Duration of illness.	*New admission:* If patient has Hx: of MRSA* (e.g., MRSA in wound), but no active infection or draining wound, obtain nasal culture for MRSA. If nasal culture is negative for MRSA, discontinue isolation. *Inpatient:* discontinue isolation if patient has been off appropriate/effective antibiotics for 72 hours and two cultures are negative for MRSA (culture original site of infection or colonization, or any openly draining site, and obtain a nasal swab).

KNOW THE BASICS OF MRSA AND HOW TO CARE FOR PATIENTS WITH THIS INFECTION

BETSY HARGREAVES ALLBEE, BSN, CIC

WHAT TO DO: IMPLEMENT

Staphylococcus aureus is a gram-positive bacterium that is part of the normal skin flora of healthy people. Approximately 25% to 30% of the population is colonized in the nose with staphylococci (staph) bacteria. Minor skin infections such as pimples and boils are often caused by a staph infection. When staphylococci become resistant to the antibiotics that were previously effective (e.g., methicillin, oxacillin, penicillin, and amoxicillin), the organism is referred to as methicillin-resistant *Staphylococcus aureus* (MRSA).

Both sensitive staphylococci and resistant staphylococci (MRSA) infections can be found in the community and in institutions such as schools, long-term care facilities, correctional facilities, and healthcare facilities. Along with skin infections, *Staphylococcus* can cause surgical wound infections, urinary tract infections, bloodstream infections, and pneumonia. Individuals can be colonized or infected with the organism. Everyone normally has many different bacteria on their skin and inside their bodies. When bacteria are present but not causing an infection, it is called colonization. There are no symptoms with MRSA colonization. MRSA can colonize an individual for months to years. Colonized individuals can spread MRSA to others by direct contact or indirect contact (via inanimate objects and surfaces). Basic control measures include (1) handwashing with either soap and water or an alcohol-based cleanser, (2) covering cuts and scrapes with a bandage or dressing until healed, (3) washing hands immediately after handling a bandage or dressing, and (4) avoiding sharing personal items such as towels and razors. In the healthcare setting, contact isolation is recommended.

Patients with MRSA can share a room with another patient with MRSA, but should not be roomed with a patient who does not have MRSA. In settings such as acute and long-term healthcare facilities, additional strategies may be beneficial (Table 238.1).

Studies on the duration of survival of MRSA on inanimate objects and surfaces showed that MRSA can be recovered from at least 1 day and up to 56 days after contamination. In addition, MRSA survived for 9 to 11 days on a plastic patient chart, a laminated tabletop, and a cloth curtain in a hospital. MRSA is believed to be spread by the hands of healthcare workers to these items, and then to the patient.

In 2007, the Association for Professionals in Infection Control and Epidemiology (APIC) performed a nationwide prevalence study to determine current rates of MRSA in the United States. Responses were received from facilities in all 50 states with 21% of all acute care hospitals (facility size includes <100 to >300 beds) and over 100 long-term care and rehabilitation facilities (n = 1,237 facilities) responding. The data showed that 46 out of every 1,000 patients in the survey were either infected or colonized with MRSA (34 infected, 12 colonized). This rate was between 8 to 11 times greater than previous MRSA estimates. The sites of infection or colonization included the skin and soft tissue (37%) and blood, lung, and urinary tract (63%).

In recent years, as the incidence of MRSA increased, particularly in healthcare settings, some healthcare providers have become complacent–as if it was inevitable that eventually everyone would develop MRSA. As a result, several guidance and regulatory agencies published infection control guidelines. A comparison of these recommendations is demonstrated in Table 238.2. The recommendations shown in Table 238.2 are the result of evidence-based findings. As demonstrated in

---

TABLE 238.1	INFECTION CONTROL MEASURES

- Implement a "flagging" system or alert to identify patients previously diagnosed with MRSA so that isolation may be initiated immediately on subsequent admissions.

- Develop a system for notifying receiving units and transport teams, to ensure proper management of MRSA within the hospital setting (hand-off communication).

- Develop a system for identifying MRSA-positive patients for receiving facilities and transport agencies outside of the hospital setting.

- Monitor adherence with hand hygiene and implement corrective actions as indicated.

- Monitor adherence with contact precautions and implement corrective actions as indicated.

- Monitor adherence to cleaning and disinfection recommendations

TABLE 238.1   METHICILLIN-RESISTANT STAPHYLOCOCCUS AUREUS RECOMMENDATIONS BY SELECTED AGENCIES

| AGENCY | GUIDELINE/ RECOMMEN- DATION DATE | PRECAUTIONS (ISOLATION) | | COHORT | DECOLONIZATION | ACTIVE SURVEILLANCE CULTURES | FLAGGING SYSTEM (READMITS) |
		STANDARD	CONTACT				
CDC (Centers for Disease Control and Prevention)	2006		Yes	Yes	Not routine; only during outbreaks	Yes	Yes
IHI (Institute of Healthcare Improvement)	12/06		Infected and colonized	Yes	Not routine; only during outbreaks	Yes	No recommendation
SHEA (Society for Healthcare Epidemiology of America)	2003		Infected and colonized	Yes	Not routine; only during outbreaks	Yes	Yes
WHO (World Health Organization)	2002		Yes	Yes	Not routine; only during outbreaks	Yes	Yes
APIC (Association for Professionals in Infection Control)	3/2007		Infected or colonized	Yes	Not routine; only during outbreaks (or specific pts)	Yes	Yes
Joint Commission (NPSG)	1/08*		Yes	No recommen- dation made	Yes	Yes	
VDH (Virginia Dept of Health)	11/07	Recommends following CDC MDRO Guideline, 2006 (above)	Not routine; only under rare circumstances	No recommen- dation made			
U.S. Senate House Bill S.2278 (Community and Health-care Associated Infections Reduction Act of 2007)	10/07		Proposed	Proposed	Proposed	Proposed	Proposed

*NPSG—National Patient Safety Goals.

the chart, all these agencies recommend contact precautions when caring for the patient with MRSA.

Precautions can be terminated by first determining whether the patient continues to be colonized or infected. This is achieved by obtaining a culture from the infected site, nares, or axilla. It is recommended to wait 72 h after the last dose of antibiotics before obtaining a culture. If cultures from all the sites tested are negative, isolation can be discontinued. If cultures from any of the sites are positive, isolation should be continued.

MRSA has become more prevalent in recent years. MRSA can survive on inanimate objects for extended periods of time. If MRSA becomes endemic to a unit or facility, it can be extremely difficult to eradicate. Control of MRSA requires prompt identification and initiation of aggressive infection control measures as well as strict adherence to the control measures.

SUGGESTED READINGS

Association for Professionals in Infection Control (APIC). *Guide to the Elimination of Methicillin-Resistant Staphylococcus aureus (MRSA) Transmission in Hospital Settings.* 2007.

Huang R, Mehta S, Weed D, Price C. Methicillin-resistant staphylococcus aureus survival on hospital fomites. *Infect Control Hosp Epidemiol.* 2006;27:1267–1269.

KNOW THE BASICS OF *CLOSTRIDIUM DIFFICILE* (*C. DIFFICILE*) TO PROTECT YOUR PATIENTS

BETSY HARGREAVES ALLBEE, BSN, CIC

WHAT TO DO: IMPLEMENT

Clostridium difficile (*C. difficile*) is a gram-negative anaerobic organism which can be part of the large intestine's normal flora. About 3% to 5% of normal healthy adults have *C. difficile* in their stool. *C. difficile* is a spore forming bacillus that produces a potent toxin. This toxin can cause an inflammation of the intestinal tract resulting in diarrhea and more serious intestinal conditions such as colitis, toxic megacolon, perforation of the colon, sepsis, and death. The most common antibiotics associated with *C. difficile* are clindamycin, ampicillin, and cephalosporins. Antibiotic-associated diarrhea is observed in 10% to 25% of patients on clindamycin and 5% to 10% of patients on ampicillin. Diarrhea is associated, although less frequently, with penicillins, erythromycin, sulfamethoxazole, tremethoprim, and tetracycline. A diagnosis of *C. difficile* should be suspected as a cause of diarrhea, especially in patients on antibiotics.

Clostridium difficile is shed in feces. Any surface, device, or material (e.g., commode, bath tub, and electronic rectal thermometer) that becomes contaminated with feces may serve as a reservoir for *C. difficile* spores. *C. difficile* spores are transferred to patients mainly by the hands of healthcare personnel who have touched a contaminated surface or item. Environmental cultures have shown extensive contamination of the environment in case-associated areas. Disinfection with a bleach solution has been shown to be the most effective method of cleaning.

The incubation period is usually 1 to 10 days after the initiation of antibiotic therapy (early onset) or occasionally 2 to 6 weeks after discontinuing the antibiotic (late onset). The severity of diarrhea ranges from mild diarrhea that resolves as soon as the inciting antibiotic is discontinued to a more serious diarrhea that can occur 20 to 30 times a day and last as long as 2 to 3 months without therapy.

Symptoms of *C. difficile* include:

- Watery diarrhea (at least three bowel movements per day for more than 2 days)
- Fever
- Loss of appetite
- Nausea
- Abdominal pain and/or tenderness

Patients who are at increased risk for *C. difficile* disease include those with:

- Antibiotic exposure
- Gastrointestinal surgery or manipulation
- Long length of stay in healthcare settings
- A serious underlying illness
- Immunocompromising conditions
- Advanced age

Prevention and control of *C. difficile*:

- Use antibiotics judiciously
- Use contact precautions for patients known or suspected to have *C. difficile* associated disease (until diarrhea ceases)
- Perform hand hygiene using soap and water. Instruct patient and visitors to wash hands.
- Dedicate the use of noncritical equipment such as blood pressure cuffs, stethoscopes, etc.
- Use gloves and gowns whenever entering room and during patient care activities or procedures
- Environmental cleaning with a bleach solution is recommended

SUGGESTED READINGS

Johnson S, Gerding DN. Clostridium difficile. *Hosp Epidemiol Infect Control.* 2004;623–631.

Tomiczek AC, Stumpo C, Downey JA. Enhancing patient safety through the management of clostridium difficile at Toronto East General Hospital. *Healthc Quart.* 2006;9:50–53.

KNOW HOW TO CARE FOR PATIENTS WITH VRE

BETSY HARGREAVES ALLBEE, BSN, CIC

WHAT TO DO: IMPLEMENT

Enterococci are gram-positive bacteria that are found normally in the gastrointestinal and female genital tract. Enterococci can also be found without causing infection along catheter sites and in the urine. Although enterococci are not always harmful or virulent, they can cause serious infections such as urinary tract infections, wound infections, and bloodstream infections. Vancomycin resistance in enterococci (VRE) is an emerging problem where these organisms demonstrate increased resistance to penicillin and aminoglycosides, thus presenting a serious challenge for physicians treating patients with infections due to these microorganisms. The only way to determine whether a patient has VRE is with a culture. Culture results usually take 2 to 3 days. Enterococci may be identified on laboratory reports by several different names such as *Enterococcus faecium*, *Enterococcus faecalis*, or *Enterococcus* species and it is important to remember that patients may be either colonized or infected.

- Colonization—the multiplication of microorganisms in a host without tissue invasion or injury.

- Infection—the multiplication of microorganisms in the tissues of a host (can be symptomatic or asymptomatic).

Everyone normally has many different bacteria on their skin and inside their bodies. When bacteria are present but not causing an infection, it is called colonization. There are no symptoms with VRE colonization. VRE can colonize an individual for months to years. Colonized individuals can spread VRE to others by direct contact or indirect contact (via inanimate objects and surfaces).

Certain patient populations have been found to be at increased risk for VRE infection or colonization. They include critically ill patients or those with severe underlying disease or immunosuppression, such as ICU patients or patients in the oncology or transplant wards; those who have had a major abdominal or cardiothoracic surgery, or invasive lines such as indwelling urinary or central venous catheter; and those who have had prolonged hospital stay or received multi-antimicrobial or vancomycin therapy.

Patients suspected or confirmed to have VRE should be placed in isolation. Table 240.1 provides the precautions that need to be taken with both colonized and infected patients.

TABLE 240.1	ISOLATION PRECAUTIONS TO PREVENT PATIENT-TO-PATIENT TRANSMISSION OF VRE

- Place VRE-infected or colonized patients in single rooms or in the same room as other patients with VRE.

- Procedures should be performed in the patient's room whenever possible. If the patient must leave the room for a procedure, instruct him to wash his hands. Cover wounds infected with VRE with an occlusive dressing.

- Wear gloves (clean nonsterile gloves are adequate) when entering the room of a VRE infected or colonized patient; extensive environmental contamination with VRE has been noted in some studies. During the course of caring for a patient, a change of gloves may be necessary after contact with material that may contain high concentrations of VRE (e.g., stool).

- Wear a gown (a clean nonsterile gown is adequate) when entering the room of a VRE infected or colonized patient if substantial contact with the patient is necessary or if the patient is incontinent, or has diarrhea, an ileostomy, a colostomy, or a wound drainage not contained by a dressing.

- Remove gloves and gown before leaving the patient's room, and wash hands immediately with an antiseptic soap. Hands can be contaminated with VRE (e.g., door knob or curtain) in the patient's room.

- Visitors should be encouraged to follow isolation precautions (gown and gloves). Visitors should be instructed not to visit other patients in the hospital after visiting a patient with VRE. If a visitor plans to visit other patients, he should visit patients with non-communicable diseases first.

- Dedicate the use of noncritical items, such as stethoscope, sphygmomanometer, or electronic rectal thermometer to a single patient or cohort of patients infected or colonized with VRE. If such devices are to be used on other patient(s), adequately clean and disinfect them first.

- Culture stools or rectal swabs of roommates of patients newly found to be infected or colonized with VRE to determine their colonization status and apply isolation precautions as necessary. Perform additional screening of patients on the ward at the discretion of the infection control staff.

Precautions can be terminated by first determining whether the patient continues to be colonized or infected. Obtain a culture from the infected site, rectum, axilla, or umbilical area. It is recommended to wait 72 h after last dose of antibiotics before obtaining a culture. If cultures from all the sites tested are negative, isolation can be discontinued. If cultures from any of the sites are positive, isolation should be continued.

The control of VRE requires prompt identification and initiation of aggressive infection control measures.

If VRE becomes endemic to the unit or facility, it can be extremely difficult to eradicate.

SUGGESTED READINGS

Centers for Disease Control and Prevention. Recommendations for preventing the spread of vancomycin resistance: Recommendations of the Hospital Infection Control Practices Advisory Committee (HICPAC). *MMWR*. 1995;44.

Maryland Department of Health and Mental Hygiene. *Epidemiology and Disease Control Program.* Baltimore, MD, September 1996.

241

DIALYSIS CATHETERS (VAS-CATHS) CONTAIN LARGE AMOUNTS OF HEPARIN

ALICE M. CHRISTALDI, RN, BSN, CRRN

WHAT TO DO: ASSESS

Many nursing units today can count on having one or two renal dialysis patients on them at any given time. The majority of the dialysis patients will have a mature fistula to use, but from time to time you will see a vas-cath. These catheters can be placed in the internal jugular vein, the subclavian vein, or femoral vein. Generally, they are inserted as a temporary measure until the arteriovenous (AV) fistula or graft matures.

AV fistulas or grafts are direct connections of an artery and vein made under the skin of a patient in surgery, which will be used for hemodialysis. This connection allows for an easily accessible route for the exchange of blood during dialysis treatments. Once established, they can last for many years, have large volumes for increased blood flows, and reduce the chances of infection. The downside is that they may take months to mature before they can be used. They are visible as they are often placed on the non-dominant forearm, and there may be bleeding from them after needles are removed.

Problems develop when the nursing staff is not aware that the patient has a vas-cath in place. Generally, catheter care is done by the staff at dialysis, and most place a large orange STOP sign over the insertion site warning other staff that it is indeed a dialysis catheter. Why the concern? Vas-caths contain several millimeters of heparin to keep the catheter patent. If the nurse is not aware of the heparin's presence, she may flush the catheter with normal saline without withdrawing the heparin first. This will cause the patient to receive a bolus of possibly greater then 10,000 units of heparin.

To reduce errors, staff members responsible for the care of these catheters need to be educated and feel comfortable with the many varieties of catheters available today. Staff members need to be aware of the differences between the devices, and especially what they contain. Assessments and use of any vascular access device should be documented properly. Notations need to be made both on the chart and on the nursing kardex.

Each company's catheter is different and may require different amounts of heparin to block the catheter. Blocking is the term for instilling the heparin back into the catheter after use. Again, most dialysis units will clearly mark the insertion site with the type of catheter and more importantly how much heparin is needed to block it and have it ready for its next use. The amount of heparin needed is also clearly marked on the side of the vas-cath generally on the blue or distal port.

Depending on hospital protocol, an RN may access the device after receiving instruction and becoming competent on its use. Generally, they are not accessed by nursing staff outside of dialysis unless there is no other venous access obtainable. Check your policy and procedures at your institution for details.

Remember that when the device is accessed, sterile procedure is maintained and the catheter/cap junction site is well cleansed. At least 3 mL is aspirated first, again checking the catheter wall itself for the volume of heparin that was used. Coagulation studies should never be obtained from a vas-cath, since heparin is used to block the catheter and accurate results may not be possible.

After each use, the dialysis catheter needs to be blocked with heparin. Again, check to see the exact amount of heparin needed and the correct concentration of heparin. This is not the time to be using a heparin flush, straight heparin is used (often 5,000 units per mL). The exact volume of heparin to instill must be known to prevent systemic heparinization of the patient. Make sure that the catheter cap remains on the catheter, and is kept clamped.

SUGGESTED READINGS

American Association of Kidney Patients. *Understanding Your Hemodialysis Access Options.* Available at: http://www.aakp.org/library/attachments/understanding%20your%20hemodialysis%20access%20options%20eng.pdf. Accessed May 27, 2008.

By BARD. *Patient's Guide.* Available at: http://www.bardaccess.com/pdfs/patient/pg-hemodialysis.pdf. Accessed April 2, 2008.

How to Care for your Bard Long-Term Polyurethane Hemo-dialysis/Apheresis Catheter Polyurethane Hemodialysis/Apheresis Catheter by Bard Access Systems. *Nursing Procedure Manual.* Available at: http://www.bardaccess.com/pdfs/nursing/ng-hemoglide hemosplit.pdf. Acccssed April 2, 2008.

POTASSIUM CAN BE LETHAL

MONTY D. GROSS, PHD, RN, CNE

WHAT TO DO: ASSESS

Potassium (K+) is the most abundant intracellular electrolyte. Because it plays a major role in maintaining the intracellular and extracellular homeostasis of electrolytes, it is very important for normal heart and nervous system function. The normal potassium range for adults in most labs is 3.5 to 5.5 milliequivalents (mEq) per liter. This range may vary slightly among laboratories. Potassium chemically balances sodium chloride. Potassium counters sodium's influence on raising blood pressure. Insulin moves K+ into cells. In metabolic conditions, such as diabetic ketoacidosis, where there are low levels of insulin, K+ will stay in the blood serum. Conditions of metabolic alkolosis will result in K+ moving into the cell resulting in a low serum K+ level. Although about 10% of K+ is excreted in stool, the majority is removed in urine.

High serum levels of potassium, known as hyperkalemia, can cause serious or lethal heart rhythms. Renal or adrenal disease, internal bleeding, or certain types of blood pressure medicines, such as ACE inhibitors and potassium-sparing diuretics, can produce hyperkalemia. These types of medicines cause the body to retain potassium. In conditions of hyperkalemia, these potassium retaining medications are held. Sodium polystyrene sulfonate in sorbitol can be given. It exchanges sodium for potassium, hence, sodium levels also need monitoring. The K+ is then excreted in the stool. In more severe cases, calcium gluconate or insulin may be used. The calcium gluconate is quick acting, but temporary. Insulin maybe administered followed by or simultaneously with a dextrose solution. The insulin pushes or takes the serum potassium into the cells. This approach will last for several hours.

Patterns of ECGs can change as potassium levels rise above normal. P waves may widen and flatten. T waves may become tall and have a sharp peak. As levels continue to rise, atrial activity is affected, producing atrial fibrillation. QRS complexes are wider than the normal 0.04 to 0.12 s. QT intervals increase. Fatal ventricular arrhythmias or asystole can develop.

Low levels of potassium, known as hypokalemia, can result from a disease of the renal, liver, heart, or adrenal system. Vomiting, diarrhea, excess sweating, medications such as diuretics like furosemide that cause the body to excrete potassium in the urine cause hypokalemia. Also, diets low in potassium may result in hypokalemia. Most hypokalemia result from excess urine output. Muscle weakness is experienced with hypokalemia. Potassium supplements either in oral or intravenous form are administered in small doses.

Unlike hyperkalemia, which is a good indicator of the higher than normal potassium levels, hypokalemia does not reflect in ECG recordings reliably. Hypokalemia can produce tachycardia and ventricular tachyarrythmias like Torsades de Pointes. Flat or inverted T and U waves, and ST segment depression can be seen.

Remember that monitoring and keeping potassium within normal range is critical for your patients. The earlier an abnormality is detected, the easier it is to correct it and avoid serious side effects, especially lethal arrhythmias. Know your patient's potassium level and act accordingly.

SUGGESTED READINGS

Hoye A, Clark A. Iatrogenic hyperkalemia. *Lancet.* 2003; 361:2124.

The Merk Manuals Online Medical Library. Disorders of potassium concentration. November 2005. Available at: http://www.merck.com/mmpe/sec12/ch156/ch156f.html. Accessed June 29, 2008.

Webster A, Brady W, Morris F. Recognising signs of danger: ECG changes resulting from an abnormal serum potassium concentration. *Emerg Med J.* 2002;19(1):74–77.

KNOW HOW TO DETECT URINARY RETENTION

MONTY D. GROSS, PHD, RN, CNE

WHAT TO DO: EVALUATE

Urinary catheterization is a common practice in hospitalized patients. Urinary catheters aid urinary drainage in patients who undergo surgery, who are severely immobilized, or who have urinary retention issues. However, the risk of urinary tract infections (UTI) is well documented. There is a strong trend in healthcare organizations to minimize the use of these catheters. Studies demonstrate that patients regain satisfactory voiding when intermittent catheterization is used instead of indwelling catheters. If indwelling catheters are needed, the goal is to remove them as soon as possible and promote natural voiding.

After the physician orders the catheter to be removed, the patient should void spontaneously within 6 h. If the patient does not void the bladder should be assessed for bladder fullness. Normally, the bladder cannot be palpated until it contains at least 150 mL. If the bladder is empty or nearly so, a hollow sound should be heard. Percussion that results in a dull or flat sound indicates that the bladder is full of fluid or distended. A distended bladder will feel firm and round when palpated. The patient's subjective sensations of fullness or needing to void is not reliable. It is important that you watch for spontaneous voiding and volume after a catheter is removed. Ask the patient to use a urinal to measure the volume and inform you when the patient voids. It is important to inform family members, so they do not empty a urinal without recording the volume.

If the patient is having difficulty voiding, assisting the patient to a sitting or standing position may facilitate voiding. Many patients need a quiet private environment to void. Ensuring the patient has such an environment can promote the patient's ability to urinate. The sound of running water has also helped some patients. Turning on a faucet and allowing water to run may help.

The use of urinary catheters is common in hospitals. Avoiding their use or discontinuing them as soon as possible decreases infection rates. However, when they are used and removed, ensure that the patient is voiding adequate amounts and not retaining urine.

SUGGESTED READINGS

Cavens D, Zweig S. Urinary catheter management. *Am Fam Phys.* 2000;61(2):369–375.

Smith S, Duell D, Martin B. *Clinical Nursing Skills: Basic to Advanced Skills.* Upper Saddle River, NJ: Pearson; 2008.

KNOW THE VALUE OF AN ANION GAP WHEN YOUR PATIENT HAS A METABOLIC ACIDOSIS

ANTHONY D. SLONIM, MD, DrPH

WHAT TO DO: PLAN

A metabolic acidosis occurs when the patient experiences either a gain in acid or a loss of bicarbonate. Acid can be administered directly for medicinal purposes in certain poisonings but can also occur when large amounts of total parenteral nutrition (TPN) are administered with chloride as the major ion for sodium, potassium, and other salts. Appropriate balance between the use of chloride and acetate in TPN solutions is essential to maintain the body's homeostatic mechanisms. The loss of bicarbonate from the body occurs either through the renal or gastrointestinal tract. In a series of disorders known collectively as the renal tubular acidoses, the kidney excretes excessive amounts of bicarbonate and reabsorbs chloride. These disorders are often referred to as hyperchloremic because it is the elevation in the serum chloride that usually brings them to presentation. Gastrointestinal losses of bicarbonate occur because of diarrhea or small bowel resections with large amounts of stool output. These losses tend to create an acidosis in the patient.

Metabolic acidosis is usually classified into either anion gap or nonanion gap metabolic acidosis. The hyperchloremic metabolic acidosis described above represents an example of the "nonanion gap" type. An anion gap is the difference between the serum anions and cations and is calculated as the [(sodium–chloride) + bicarbonate]. Many newer serum chemistry machines now calculate this value automatically. A normal value is 12 ± 2 or a range of 10 to 14. What is important about this type of metabolic acidosis is that it has a very narrow range of disorders associated with elevations in the anion gap and if they are diagnosed quickly, appropriate therapy can be provided for the patient before permanent damage occurs. Further, this type of metabolic acidosis should not be treated with serum bicarbonate. These "anion gap metabolic acidoses" are usually described by the mnemonic MUDPILES, the definitions of which are given in Table 244.1.

SUGGESTED READINGS

DuBose TD. Acidosis and alkalosis. In: Kasper DL, Braunwald E, Fauci AS, et al., eds. *Harrison's Principles of Internal Medicine.* 16th Ed. New York, NY: McGraw Hill; 2005, pp. 263–271.

TABLE 244.1	MUDPILES MNEMONIC AND THEIR ASSOCIATED CAUSES
"M"	Methanol
"U"	Uremia
"D"	Diabetic ketoacidosis
"P"	Paraldehyde
"I"	Iron, Isoniazid, Ischemia
"L"	Lactic acidosis
"E"	Ethanol, Ethylene Glycol
"S"	Salicylates

ACUTE RENAL FAILURE HAS MANY CAUSES, BUT RULING OUT AN OBSTRUCTED URINARY SYSTEM IS THE FIRST ORDER OF BUSINESS

ANTHONY D. SLONIM, MD, DrPH

WHAT TO DO: ASSESS AND IMPLEMENT

Acute renal failure is usually classified as prerenal, renal, or postrenal and is often represented by a recent elevation in the blood urea nitrogen (BUN), serum creatinine, or the fractional excretion of sodium (FENa). The FENa is calculated by calculating the ratio of the plasma creatinine × Urine Na to Plasma Na × Urine Creatinine × 100. It is important to remember that not all renal failures are due to a problem in the kidney, although the kidney often experiences the brunt of the derangements in other organs, particularly under severe physiologic conditions.

"Prerenal" acute renal failure is usually due to intravascular volume depletion. These volume losses may be due to true volume loss as occurs in dehydration and hypovolemic shock, but they can also be due to relative volume insufficiency as occurs in congestive heart failure, when the patient's heart is so ill that it cannot provide sufficient contractility. The result is that the kidneys experience a deficit in circulation. Preload problems often result in elevations in the BUN and creatinine in greater than a 20:1 ratio and have a FENa of less than 1%. These two markers assist in making the diagnosis. In addition, gastrointestinal bleeding can lead to "prerenal azotemia," because blood in the gastrointestinal lumen increases the nitrogen load and BUN out of proportion to the creatinine leading to a similar 20:1, BUN:Creatinine ratio. The treatment for prerenal acute renal failure is the restoration of intravascular volume, usually through the administration of isotonic (normal saline) intravenous fluids.

"Renal" acute renal failure occurs when the kidney itself experiences a derangement that results in the kidney failure. The causes of this may be medications, toxins, contrast agents, or ischemia following shock or cardiopulmonary arrest. The kidney is very sensitive to hypoxic injury but is also a pretty resilient organ when it is damaged. "Renal" acute renal failure is usually diagnosed by an elevated BUN:Creatinine ratio of 10:1, which is less than the ratio with "prerenal" failure. In this case, the FENa is usually greater than 1%. The treatment for "renal" acute renal failure is to restore the circulating blood volume and remove the offending agents. If the kidneys do not recover, either in the acute or chronic state, additional therapies including dialysis can be provided as needed to support the patient.

"Postrenal" acute renal failure is the type of renal failure that should not be missed since it is easily remedied. Postrenal renal failure is due to an obstruction that prevents the excretion of urine from the urinary tract. When this type of renal failure occurs, overcoming the obstruction prevents further damage to the kidneys. That is why many have recommended that all patients with acute renal failure should have a urinary catheter placed to ensure that postrenal obstruction is not the cause of the renal failure.

SUGGESTED READINGS

Brady HR, Brenner BM. Acute renal failure. In: Kasper DL, Braunwald E, Fauci AS, et al., eds. *Harrison's Principles of Internal Medicine.* 16th Ed. New York, NY: McGraw Hill; 2005, pp. 1644–1652.

KNOW WHAT TO DO FOR PATIENTS WITH NEPHROTIC SYNDROME

SAM HARVEY AND ANTHONY D. SLONIM, MD, DrPH

WHAT TO DO: IMPLEMENT

Nephrotic syndrome is an elusive condition due to the fact that it is not a specific glomerular disease but several symptoms combined (Figure 246.1). Consequently, diagnosis is often difficult.

The disease affects the glomerulus, the series of capillaries at the end of a kidney's tubule that filters proteins from the blood. Essentially, the glomerular membrane cannot retain the plasma proteins that pass through it. Nephrotic syndrome is often a secondary condition to other diseases such as diabetes mellitus and renal vein thrombosis that affect the glomerulus. Nephrotic syndrome is primarily a childhood disease, yet the elderly are often just as susceptible.

The primary clinical symptom of nephrotic syndrome is edema. The swelling occurs around the eyes, ankles, hands, and abdomen. Mood changes and headache are common as well. The primary means of diagnosis, however, is the presence of more than 3.5 g/day of proteinuria. Laboratory tests such as electrophoresis are often used to determine the type of proteinuria present. Complications of nephrotic syndrome include infection due to a weakened immune response and pulmonary emboli.

Management of nephrotic syndrome can be achieved in several ways. All attempt to preserve renal function while limiting complications (Figure 246.2).

Due to the diverse array of medications required to address the varied issues associated with nephrotic syndrome, it is important that a patient be educated as to each drug's effect as well as any special diet that is required. Due to the precarious balance of renal function such regimens achieve, the patient must also report any health changes immediately.

SUGGESTED READINGS

Brady HR, Wilcox CS. *Therapy in Nephrology and Hypertension,* 2nd Ed. St. Louis, MO: Elsevier Saunders; 2003.

Smeltzer S, Bare B, Hinkle J, et al. *Textbook of Medical-Surgical Nursing.* Philadelphia, PA: Lippincott Williams & Wilkins; 2008.

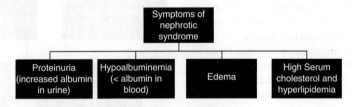

FIGURE 246.1. Symptoms of nephrotic syndrome.

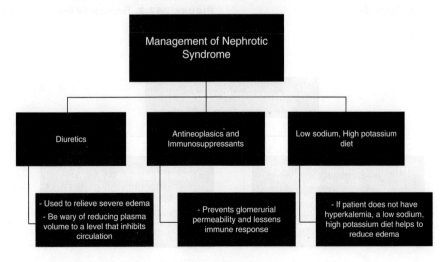

FIGURE 246.2. Management of nephrotic syndrome.

KNOW WHAT TO DO TO IDENTIFY AND CORRECT HYPOMAGNESEMIA

SAM HARVEY AND ANTHONY D. SLONIM, MD, DRPH

WHAT TO DO: ASSESS AND IMPLEMENT

Hypomagnesemia refers to a condition where magnesium serum levels are less than 1.3 mEq/L. Hypermagnesemia occurs when magnesium serum levels rise more than 2.5 mEq/L. Hypomagnesemia is much more common than hypermagnesemia because the kidneys are very efficient at removing magnesium from the bloodstream. Hypomagnesemia is most commonly caused by chronic alcoholism in the United States and is most problematic when treating symptoms of alcohol withdrawal. Magnesium is most commonly lost through the GI tract, where diarrhea and intestinal fistulas deplete the magnesium-rich fluid in the lower end of the tract. The symptoms of hypomagnesemia and hypermgnesemia are included in Figure 247.1.

Since neuromuscular symptoms are the most common signs of hypomagnesemia, several common ones include muscle weakness, tremors, and athetoid movements. Changes in mood are often observed with apathy and depression at the forefront. Magnesium imbalances are often closely related to potassium and calcium imbalances; therefore, some of the symptoms can be associated with all three mineral imbalances.

Mild to moderate magnesium deficiency can be easily relieved by simple changes in diet. Leafy vegetables containing chlorophyll as well as peanut butter and cocoa are an excellent source of magnesium. In severe hypomagnesemia, magnesium salts may be administered orally, or magnesium sulfate may be administered via infusion pump (Figure 247.2).

Since some of the most susceptible patients for hypomagnesemia are alcoholics, magnesium serum levels should be checked at least every 2 or 3 days. If magnesium sulfate is administered intravenously, it is important that calcium gluconate be readily available in the occurrence of hypermagnesemia. After care is administered, teaching is an important supplement in preventing hypomagnesemia in chronic alcoholics or cases of diuretic/laxative abuse.

SUGGESTED READINGS

Byrd R. Magnesium: Its proven clinical significance. *South Med J.* 2003;96(1):104–105.

Smeltzer S, Bare B, Hinkle J et al. *Textbook of Medical-Surgical Nursing*. Philadelphia, PA: Lippincott Williams & Wilkins; 2008.

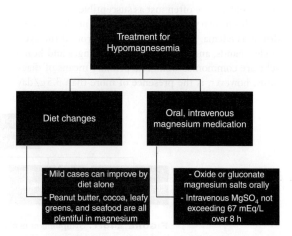

FIGURE 247.2. Treatment for hypomagnesemia.

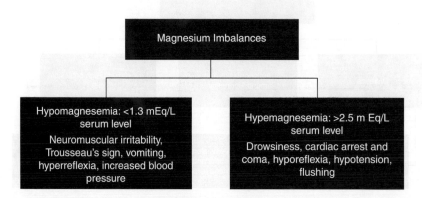

FIGURE 247.1. Symptoms of hypomagnesemia and hypermagnesemia.

KNOW WHAT TO DO TO IDENTIFY AND CORRECT HYPONATREMIA

SAM HARVEY AND ANTHONY D. SLONIM, MD, DRPH

WHAT TO DO: ASSESS AND IMPLEMENT

Hyponatremia refers to a serum sodium deficit and is generally classified as a specific electrolyte imbalance. A patient is in a state of clinical hyponatremia when serum sodium is lesser than 135 mEq/L, and it can occur for various reasons. The symptoms of this imbalance are listed in Figure 248.1. The symptoms of hypernatremia have been included in Figure 248.1 for comparison.

Because of the fact that these two imbalances often have similar symptoms, it is important to consider the important differences. Hyponatremia is characterized by elevated pulse yet low blood pressure. Hypernatremia is characterized by elevated pulse and high blood pressure. Differentiation is important because each is treated using opposite methods.

Once diagnosis of hyponatremia is complete, two methods of correcting the imbalance are available. Due to the osmotic chemistry of cellular sodium and water interaction, the cells of a patient with hyponatremia dilate. Consequently, at extreme levels (115 mEq/L or less), intracranial pressure elicits the neurological symptoms common to the imbalance. Treatment for hyponatremia includes both sodium replacement and water restriction to reverse the adverse cell swelling and consequent damage.

The treatment of choice should be water restriction primarily due to the high risk of administering hypertonic sodium solutions. It is recommended that hypertonic sodium solutions only be used to alleviate severe neurologic symptoms associated with hyponatremia up to a level of 125 mEq/L. The preferred treatment to return serum sodium level to normal, past 125 mEq/L, is water retention.

SUGGESTED READINGS

Eaton J. Detection of hyponatremia in the PACU. *J Perianaesth Nurs.* 2003;18(6):392–397.

Smeltzer S, Bare B, Hinkle J, et al. *Textbook of Medical-Surgical Nursing.* Philadelphia, PA: Lippincott Williams & Wilkins; 2008.

```
                    Sodium imbalances

Hyponatremia: <135 mEq/L sodium      Hypernatremia: > 145 mEq/L sodium
        serum level                           serum level

Nausea, vomiting, headache, dizziness,   Nausea, vomiting, extreme thirst,
muscle cramps and weakness, elevated     elevated temperature, hyperreflexia,
    pulse, low blood pressure            elevated pulse and blood pressure
```

FIGURE 248.1. Symptoms of hypernatremia.

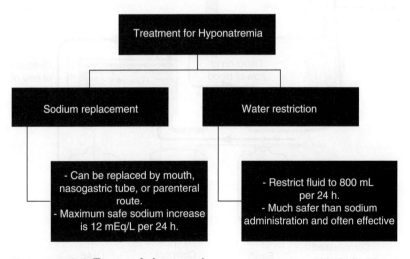

FIGURE 248.2. Treatment for hyponatremia.

KNOW WHAT YOUR DIALYSIS PATIENTS EXPERIENCE AND HOW TO HELP THEM

SAM HARVEY AND ANTHONY D. SLONIM, MD, DrPH

WHAT TO DO: PLAN

Currently, 280,000 Americans receive chronic hemodialysis via a dialyzer, an artificial semipermeable membrane that serves as a substitute for a functioning kidney. A dialysis routine is critical for patients with chronic renal failure to prevent the accumulation of waste in the circulatory system, and the treatment must usually be administered three times a week in 3 to 4 h treatment durations. A dialyzer is designed to remove nitrogenous toxins and excess water from the blood safely and efficiently, yet safety risks are an inherent part of the dialysis process. Due to the fact that a patient's blood is diverted to the machine and returned after filtration, there is an ever-present risk of infection, hemorrhage, and circulatory problems during the process.

A dialyzer utilizes three important principles when filtering the blood: diffusion, osmosis, and ultrafiltration. Each dialyzer contains thousands of artificial tubules that serve as a semipermeable membrane. Blood flows through the tubules in one direction while a fluid known as the dialysate flows in the other. The dialysate is composed of bicarbonate and other important electrolytes at ideal concentration. Using the principle of diffusion, the toxins in the blood at a high concentration pass to the dialysate at a low concentration. Excess water is removed from blood and passes to the dialysate through osmosis or more efficiently ultrafiltration. Most dialyzers today move water from pressurized blood to the low-pressure dialysate. The dialysate bath continually circulates as the blood passes through the membrane and replenishes the blood with necessary electrolytes and also contains the drug heparin, which prevents the blood from coagulating in the circuit (Figure 249.1).

Dialyzer manufacturers focus on both performance and biocompatibility during construction. Often, chronic hemodialysis produces neuropathy in the extremities, yet the condition can be delayed significantly if the dialysis process can be completed quickly. Today, dialyzers are capable of processing blood at a rate of 500 to 550 mL/min, a significant improvement over the first models. Hypersensitivity, allergic reactions, and other adverse conditions result from a dialyzer's poor biocompatibility.

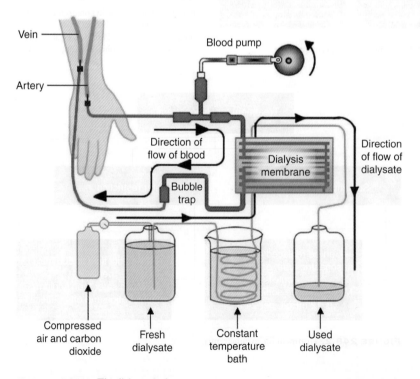

FIGURE 249.1. The dialysate bath.

Different materials are constantly tested to reduce the reactions the synthetic dialyzer may have on the blood exit and entry zones. Due to the complexity of the process, many dialyzers carry an enormous purchase and maintenance cost, and each requires rigorous federal regulations for use. Unsupervised dialysis is dangerous, and staff educated in the procedure should be available in the occurrence of a complication.

SUGGESTED READINGS

IvyRose Holistic. Kidney dialysis. 2008. Available at: http://www.ivy-rose.co.uk/Topics/Urinary_System_Kidney_Dialysis.htm. Accessed July 24, 2008.

Smeltzer S, Bare B, Hinkle J, et al. *Textbook of Medical-Surgical Nursing*. Philadelphia, PA: Lippincott Williams & Wilkins; 2008.

MY PATIENT IS NOT URINATING: INFORMATION TO GATHER BEFORE CALLING THE DOCTOR

EDWARD HUMERICKHOUSE, MS, MD

WHAT TO DO: ASSESS AND PLAN

There are a variety of reasons for patients to stop passing urine. Many of these can be diagnosed by a well-informed nurse and managed over the phone with the treating physician.

The primary cause of anuria is obstruction. The patient may complain of abdominal pain; there may be fever, and there can be either high or low blood pressure depending on the presence of infection. Urinary obstruction is usually (over 50%) caused by benign prostate hyperplasia. There are several other causes with the second leading cause surprisingly being constipation (about 7%). This is followed by prostate cancer, urethral strictures, kidney stones stuck in the urethra, prostate manipulation, stricture from previous infection or manipulation, prostate infection, cancer in the pelvis, or phimosis (penis foreskin constricts the urethra).

Other situations arise when there is not a physical blockage of the urethra, but there is paralysis of the bladder. This is usually caused by medications but can also be from acute bladder infection, immediate post-op status, loss of neural control (diabetes, multiple sclerosis, spinal cord compression), or a bladder muscle that is distended and/or weak at baseline and is then put on extra stress from IV fluids or medications.

Keep in mind that all these can and do happen to people who are already on dialysis. Contrary to popular belief, dialysis patients still make some urine although they may only need to pass it once a day. Many dialysis patients make as much urine (it just is not appropriately concentrated) as the general population. Keep this in mind when one of them complains of suprapubic pain.

Now that we have all of that down, let us go through a little exercise: as a well trained nurse, you notice on the flow sheet that your 73-years-old male patient has not urinated in the last shift despite scheduled IV lasix. You need to collect some information before you notify his physician at 3AM:

1) Why was the patient admitted?
2) Is the patient on dialysis and if so, is the low urine out normal?
3) Does the patient appear dehydrated or acutely ill?
4) Is the patient complaining of pain or fullness?
5) Does the patient have prostate problems (males only, of course)?
   a) Patient able to tell you?
   b) Listed in "Past Medical History"?
   c) Noted on physical exam?
   d) Flomax, terasozin/doxazosin, Avodart, etc. at home?
   e) "Weak stream" checked in "Review of Systems"?
1) When was his last bowel movement?
2) Does the patient have large volume on bladder scan?
3) Is the patient's blood pressure low or high?
4) Have there been any medications started today that might cause urine retention?
   a) Benadryl
   b) Sleeping medications
   c) Antidepressants
   d) Medications for overactive bladder (Detrol)
1) Is there a U/A on the chart and what did it show?
2) Has his serum creatinine been changing?

Through patient evaluation and directed chart review, you find out that the patient has a history of benign prostatic hypertrophy (BPH), but it was not symptomatic enough for the patient to be started on medications. He was admitted for a congestive heart failure (CHF) exacerbation and has been improving rapidly. He appears well, is afebrile, and his blood pressure is normal. He has been having some mild abdominal pain, but thought it was because he has not had a bowel movement since admission (he does not like moving his bowels unless at home so he was initially holding it). Bladder scan showed over 1,000 CC of urine. He has not been placed on any new medications in the last 24 h. His creatinine went up a little on this AM's labs, but his UA on admission was normal. You call the covering physician and tell her the above. She gives a verbal order for a large bore Foley catheter, flomax, and a bowel regimen. She also informs you that the patient's blood pressure may go down a little, and there may be some bleeding after the bladder is decompressed. She gives parameters to call her back and states that she will have the primary physician see him first thing in the morning.

A basic understanding of causes of anuria allowed you to anticipate what questions the average physician will have, provide the patient with rapid relief of his distress, and save his kidneys from unnecessary damage. By documenting the discussion and outcome in your nursing note, you help guarantee that the primary physician is also up to speed on his or her patient's condition.

SUGGESTED READINGS

Barrisford G, Steel G. Acute urinary retention. April 1, 2008. Uptodate Online Version 16.2. Accessed August 12, 2008.
Curtis LA, Dolan TS, Cespedes RD. Acute urinary retention and urinary incontinence. *Emerg Med Clin North Am.* 201;19:491.

FOLEY CATHETERS: DOES MY PATIENT REALLY NEED ONE?

EDWARD HUMERICKHOUSE, MS, MD

WHAT TO DO: IMPLEMENT

Foley catheters can either be a blessing or a curse for nursing staff. They limit calls for the bathroom; they keep the patient clean and dry; and they take the question out of the "O" part of monitoring "I's and O's." However, they also cause embarrassment, discomfort, and potentially important bladder infections. So, when should a nurse suggest a Foley to a physician?

There are several clear-cut indications for an indwelling urine collection system. First is the relief of a bladder outlet obstruction. The obstruction can be caused by a variety of pathologies with the most common being described in the case above: benign prostate hypertrophy. Another form of this indication may come to the nurse in the middle of the night via a very common medication. The patient who has mild complaints of a weak urine stream (check the review of systems on the chart) develops an itchy rash after antibiotics. You appropriately notified the physician on call who gave a verbal order for benadryl (diphenhydramine). Several hours later, the patient complains of pain in his lower abdomen and you note that he has not urinated. A quick bladder scan shows 550 mL of urine. The patient is experiencing a weak bladder from the benadryl and will need at least an "in-and-out" catheterization until the medicine wears off.

Second, another time to consider Foley catheter placement would be in the context of protecting broken-down skin. This can happen in several contexts, most of them involving debilitated patients with poor nutritional status and an inability to leave their bed. For example, an 88-year-old nursing home patient who had a small sacral decubitus on admission has been bedridden with pneumonia for the last week. She then gets *Clostridium difficile* colitis and a yeast infection of her perineum. Those areas need to be kept clean, dry, and away from the irritating effects of urine. In this case, a catheter may be the only real solution.

Third indication is for close monitoring of "ins and outs." This indication is mostly restricted to ICU or other patients who are too ill to assist in urine collection, but in whom fluid balance is critical to their improvement. An example would be a patient who presented with pulmonary edema from fluid overload. He was intubated, but responded to diuretics, so he was not placed on dialysis. He obviously cannot help with the critical process of urine collection.

Finally, indwelling urine drainage systems can also be used in a more palliative setting. An immobile patient with terminal lymphoma, who had hospice care at home but could not get adequate pain control now comes into the hospital for IV morphine, should be allowed a Foley. A patient with a neurogenic bladder from multiple sclerosis, who self-catheterizes every 6 h at home now comes to the hospital for high dose steroids from an acute exacerbation of MS, would be another example of when a Foley should be suggested by nursing staff.

Overall, Foley catheters are an exceptionally important armament in a nurse's fight against disease and suffering. Unfortunately, they can be placed in the wrong patients for the wrong reasons with at least patient discomfort and possibly infections, sepsis, and even patient death. As a patient advocate who can help a physician avoid some of the perils of this seemingly benign tool, nurses must ask themselves constantly: "Does this patient *really* need a Foley?" "Why does he or she need it?" "Should I ask the physician to remove it?"

While these examples are by no means a comprehensive list of *all* indications for Foley placement, if you have a patient with a Foley who does not have some form of one of these problems, find out (and document) why it is needed. Remember, often, the physician does not realize that it is still there.

SUGGESTED READINGS

Fekete T. Urinary tract infection associated with indwelling bladder catheters. 2008. Uptodate Online version 16.2. www. uptodate.com. Licensed by Carilion Clinic. Accessed August 11, 2008.

Griffiths R, Fernandez R. Policies for the removal of short-term indwelling urethral catheters (Cochrane Review). In: *The Cochrane Library*. 2007, Issue 1. Chichester, UK: John Wiley and Sons, Ltd; 2007.

Save the Stone for Your Renal Colic Patient...It May Provide the Diagnosis

Anthony D. Slonim, MD, DrPH

Nephrolithiasis or kidney stones are collections of crystals that accumulate in the urinary collecting system, causing significant pain and obstruction. They occur in approximately 12% of men and 5% of women in the United States. The composition of renal stones in descending order of frequency is calcium stones, uric acid stones, struvite stones, and cystine stones. Patients usually present acutely with pain in the flank region. This pain may be associated with nausea, vomiting, and hematuria. The major priorities include analgesia, adequate hydration, and diagnostic testing to confirm the diagnosis. When the stone passes through the urinary system, the pain is immediately resolved, but the urine should be filtered and the stone should be saved since these conditions often recur and an analysis of the stone may provide important clues that can be of significance in the diagnosis and therapy.

Stones often form when the solubility of certain products becomes super saturated, resulting in their precipitation out of solution. This usually begins with a "nidus" that initiates the adherence of the particles. There are a number of factors that can improve this crystallization. First, it is important that the patient maintains good urine flow, this is usually accomplished with fluid hydration. Second, urinary pH is also important. Depending upon the type of stone recovered, dietary and medication modification of the urine pH can assist with recurrence. Finally, the flow of certain electrolytes through the kidney, like calcium, can be improved with medications like thiazide diuretics.

Suggested Readings

Asplin JR, Coe FL, Favus MJ. Nephrolitihiasis. In: Kasper DL, Braunwald E, Fauci AS, et al., eds. *Harrison's Principles of Internal Medicine*. 16th Ed. New York, NY: McGraw Hill; 2005, pp. 1710–1714.

Ensure good control of your patient's blood pressure; the kidney may be the cause, but it is more likely that it will bear the brunt of uncontrolled blood pressure

Anthony D. Slonim, MD, DrPH

WHAT TO DO: IMPLEMENT

Hypertension is a major problem in the United States. Unfortunately, the cause of hypertension in the majority of patients is unknown. This is referred to as "essential" hypertension. When the cause of hypertension is known, it is referred to as secondary hypertension. Secondary hypertension is caused by a number of conditions including cardiovascular disease, as a side effect to medications, thyroid disease, adrenal tumors that drive the sympathetic nervous system, renovascular problems like renal artery stenosis, and chronic kidney disease. Hypertension also has a number of effects on end organs including the heart, the eyes, and the kidneys. Hence, the kidney plays pivotal role, being the cause and suffering some of the effects of hypertension.

There are a number of important steps the nurse can take to assist the patients with hypertension in improving their care. First, the nurse can provide nutritional support on methods to reduce sodium intake in the diet. Avoidance of canned fruits and vegetables and added sodium can help with this. Second, the nurse can ensure that the patients can do self-monitoring of their blood pressure. Ambulatory monitoring of blood pressure is easily taught and devices for home use are inexpensive. Patients can log their findings and ensure that they are effectively treated with their medications. Third, educate the patients on the importance of taking their blood pressure medication. Hypertension is usually asymptomatic and the patients do not realize the importance of non compliance. Fourth, encourage physicians to prescribe medications that patients can afford. There are a number of excellent antihypertensives in the market which are affordable. A selection that allows the patient to be compliant is most important. Finally, encourage the patients to have regular follow-up appointments and monitor their kidney function at regular intervals to determine if complications are beginning to occur.

The nurse is an important advocate for helping patients deal with hypertension and even more important for helping them avoid the complications of the disease.

SUGGESTED READINGS

Fisher NDL, Williams GH. Hypertensive vascular disease. In: Kasper DL, Braunwald E, Fauci AS, et al., eds. *Harrison's Principles of Internal Medicine*.16th Ed. New York, NY: McGraw Hill; 2005, pp. 1463–1481.

URINE INFECTIONS MEAN DIFFERENT THINGS TO DIFFERENT PATIENTS

ANTHONY D. SLONIM, MD, DRPH

WHAT TO DO: ASSESS

An infection of the urine is a common medical condition that requires treatment. However, not all urinary tract infections (UTIs) are created equal. The importance of the type of infection and the urgency for its treatment often depend upon the host. Patients at the extremes of age, including infants and the elderly, experience more difficult problems with infections, generally, and UTIs, specifically. For infants, concerns about a congenital malformation of the ureters into the bladder are important to reconcile if the infant has repeated infections. For the elderly, a UTI may, because of an inadequate immune system, quickly evolve to sepsis. Both these patient groups require therapy with antimicrobial agents and the identification of any predisposing issues, as in the case of the infant with reflux or the elderly patient with a catheter, needs to be considered.

Men, because of their long urethra, rarely get UTIs. However, women frequently experience UTIs either after intercourse or during the course of pregnancy. Women who experience postcoital UTIs may be self medicated, based upon appropriate guidance, when symptoms develop. Alternatively, pregnant women often need follow-up and testing since UTIs are a risk factor for premature labor and preterm delivery.

Patients with a history of immunosuppression, either from transplantation or the chronic use of medications such as steroids, may not be able to mount an immune response to the infectious agent and remain asymptomatic until late in the course. These patients require early diagnosis and treatment to prevent the bacteria from spreading. Patients with structural conditions of the urinary system are also predisposed to UTIs and early treatment, particularly if the patient has received a kidney transplant, needs to be considered.

UTIs can be classified into those of the "lower" or "upper" urinary tract. The differentiating factor is usually the involvement of the kidney. These patients, while they may still be treated as outpatients if they tolerate therapy appropriately, require close and consistent follow up to ensure that the condition is responding to treatment.

UTIs represent a spectrum of diseases that affect many patient types and occur in a variety of circumstances. The treatment approaches are as varied as the patient types and need to be appropriately managed to prevent long term complications.

SUGGESTED READINGS

Stamm WE. Urinary tract infections and pyelonephritis. In: Kasper DL, Braunwald E., Fauci AS, et al., eds. *Harrison's Principles of Internal Medicine*. 16th Ed. New York, NY: McGraw Hill; 2005, pp. 1715–1721.

PATIENTS WITH PROSTATE CANCER HAVE A NUMBER OF TREATMENT OPTIONS

ANTHONY D. SLONIM, MD, DrPH

Prostate cancer is an important diagnosis for men. There is a great deal of fear associated with a new or recurrent diagnosis. Most men do not even know where their prostate is or what it does, so the nurse is in an important position to assist the patient with this condition.

Prostate cancer affects approximately 250,000 men and leads to death in approximately 10%. Men may present for consultation because of urinary symptoms like nocturia, hesitancy, or dribbling of the urinary stream. In addition, digital rectal examination and prostate specific antigen screening have helped to improve the early detection of these cancers.

Men are not often clear on the difference between benign prostatic hypertrophy (BPH) and prostate cancer. It is true that both are enlargements of the prostate, but one is malignant and one is benign. Once a diagnosis of malignancy is made, the man will have several options available for treatment depending upon the extent and spread of the disease. These include radical prostatectomy, transurethral prostatectomy, castration, and robotic surgery. A major component of the treatment plan beyond surgery includes adjuvant treatment like chemotherapy, radiation, or hormonal therapy. Many prostate cancers require additional treatment with adjuvant therapies.

Rehabilitation is an important part of the recovery from prostate surgery. These patients will have questions about urinary and sexual function. It is important to provide educational materials to these patients. Responses in a direct and matter of fact manner will help the patient become comfortable with asking questions about erectile dysfunction and ejaculation. In addition, the nurse can also provide help to the sexual partner of the patient who may have a number of questions and concerns that are not being addressed. A comment like "it is not unusual for some sexual partners to have concerns about their relationship after a surgery like this. I would be happy to answer any questions for you or your wife, if you think I can be helpful" is often the opening a patient has been waiting for. Providing a number to follow-up appointments is often a great benefit for these men.

The nurse can help meet the needs of the newly diagnosed prostate cancer patients and their significant other. Direct and objective conversations about difficult topics such as urinary and sexual complications are often welcomed by these patients.

SUGGESTED READINGS

Scher HI. Hyperplastic and malignant diseases of the prostate. In: Kasper DL, Braunwald E, Fauci AS, et al., eds. *Harrison's Principles of Internal Medicine*. 16th Ed. New York, NY: McGraw Hill; 2005, pp. 543–553.

NOT ALL HEADACHES ARE CREATED EQUAL

JENNIFER BATH, RN, BSN, FNE, SANE-A

WHAT TO DO: ASSESS

Many patients present to the emergency department (ED) with complaints of a headache or migraine, but is it really a headache or is there something potentially worse going on? Patients with migraines often complain of headache, nausea, vomiting, visual disturbances, and sensitivity to light and noise. The pain is one-sided and usually near the eye on the affected side. The pain increases with exertion and usually hinders the patient's daily activities. Patients experiencing a migraine rarely complain of just a headache. They will have one or more of the symptoms listed above.

Migraines are classified as nonvascular or vascular. Nonvascular migraines are when skeletal muscles contract in the head and neck, which causes a steady, pulsatile pain. Because of the intensity of pain, the patient experiences limited range of motion in the jaw, head, and neck. The most common nonvascular migraine is the tension headache. Vascular migraines are a sudden intense and sharp pain described as piercing, pounding, or throbbing. Vascular migraines have three phases. The first phase is when the patient has an aura, usually visual in nature, but sometimes auditory or gustatory. The second phase is a period of cerebral vasodilation. The third phase is the recovery phase. Vascular migraines are usually associated with extreme temporal and cranial tenderness. Migraines tend to last between 4–72 h, but if untreated they can also last weeks.

Subdural hematomas (SDH) are much different than a migraine, since they usually have an associated mechanism of injury. An SDH occurs when vessels rupture and blood collects between the surface and the outer covering of the brain. This causes compression on the brain and may be life threatening. In the younger patient, it may take a significant impact to cause an SDH. However, the elderly patient requires less force to have an SDH and may experience this problem from a simple fall out of a chair. Use of blood thinners, alcohol abuse, and a seizure history also increase a patient's risk for SDH. There will usually be a clear mechanism of injury for this disorder; however, sometimes the injury occurs long before the patient presents and the patient may have forgotten the initial injury. Patients with an SDH will usually present with a temporary loss of consciousness. The bleeding is slow because the vessels leaking are veins rather than arteries. The patient may have other complaints such as a headache, weakness on one side, seizures, and changes in vision or speech and may gradually begin to lose consciousness. An acute SDH occurs within minutes to hours of the injury and, if not diagnosed and, treated, may lead to brain injury and death. Chronic SDH, occurs over weeks to months and develops signs and symptoms more slowly. The elderly are the most at risk for chronic SDH because their brain has atrophied due to age, which increases the amount of space available in the cranial vault to collect blood prior to becoming symptomatic. The treatment for an SDH is surgery. SDHs have a very high incidence of morbidity and mortality. It is important that a good history of any patient presenting with a headache be obtained to differentiate a migraine from a life threatening head injury.

SUGGESTED READINGS

Ignatavicius D, Bayne M. *Medical—Surgical Nursing: A Nursing Process Approach*. Philadelphia, PA: Harcourt; 1991, pp. 864–874, 925.

Sheehy S. *Emergency Nursing Principles and Practice*. 5th Ed. St. Louis, MO: Mosby; 2003, pp. 256–257, 519–521.

ENSURE THAT YOUR SPINAL CORD INJURY PATIENT KNOWS HOW TO CARE FOR BOWEL AND BLADDER CONCERNS

ALICE M. CHRISTALDI, RN, BSN, CRRN

WHAT TO DO: IMPLEMENT

There are approximately 200,000 spinal cord injury patients in the United States. Many of these are young males who, with the advent of rehabilitation medicine, have an improved life expectancy. Nurses expect to discuss the loss of mobility with the patients and their family, but bowel and bladder issues can be equally important for an acceptable quality of life and the prevention of complications.

There are two primary factors that affect bowel function in spinal cord injury, the level of injury and degree of completeness of injury neurologically. If the injury is above the T-12 level, bowel function is classified as a reflex neurogenic bowel or upper motor neuron bowel dysfunction. There may be no sensation that the rectum is full, and bowel movements will occur reflexively, when the rectum fills. There will be no control over bowel movements, leading to bouts of constipation and incontinence. These problems can be medically managed with suppositories or mini-enemas, or digitally at a planned time and place.

A spinal cord injury below T-12 may cause damage to the defecation reflex, which will relax the anal sphincter and thus the bowel will not respond to digital or chemical stimulation. This is called a flaccid or lower motor neuron neurogenic bowel dysfunction. Management of this type of dysfunction requires more frequent attention to emptying the bowel, usually through the manual removal of accumulated stool, which can often become hard and dry. This should be done on a daily or twice daily basis.

In reflexic neurogenic bowel, regularity and routine are the keys to success in maintaining continence. An every other day bowel program should be instituted at approximately the same time of day. This might be in the morning or at night and will greatly depend on lifestyle or personal preferences. An appropriate bowel program should be formulated early in the rehabilitation process of the spinal cord injury patient. Time for adequate training of the patient will allow for success in maintaining continence, decreasing constipation, and adding to the quality of their lives.

The good news is that with a successful bowel program, unplanned bowel movements, constipation, or diarrhea can be greatly reduced. There are a number of other factors and complications that should be discussed with the patient and family because of their influence on bowel and bladder continence. Some of these include medications, adequate hydration, avoidance of caffeine, appropriate amounts of dietary fiber, time commitment, and the possible need of assistance from others. These are essential elements to a successful bowel regimen.

SUGGESTED READINGS

Ash D. Sustaining safe and acceptable bowel care in spinal cord injured patients. *Nurs Stand*. 2005;20(8):55–64.

Hoeman SP. *Rehabilitation Nursing Process and Application*. 2nd Ed. St. Louis, MO: Mosby; 1996, pp. 465–471.

Valles M, Vidal J, Clave P, et al. Bowel dysfunction in patients with motor complete spinal cord injury: Clinical, neurological and pathophysiological associations. *Am J Gastroenterol*. 2006;101(10):2290–2299.

KNOW HOW TO CARE FOR THE PATIENT WITH STATUS EPILEPTICUS

ANTHONY D. SLONIM, MD, DRPH

A seizure is a result of a number of abnormal electrical discharges in the brain. When the seizure activity lasts more than 15 min or there are two or more repetitive seizures occurring without intervening consciousness, status epilepticus is said to exist. Status epilepticus is a medical emergency that requires the nurse be prepared to immediately care for the patients and protect them from their surroundings.

There are a number of causes of prolonged seizures including metabolic diagnoses, drug withdrawal and toxicity, and infections and tumors. Metabolic derangements including hypoglycemia, hyponatremia, and hypocalcemia can lead to refractory seizures until the underlying metabolic disturbance is corrected. Drug withdrawal for patients that have epilepsy and forget to take their prescribed medications is a common occurrence that can be identified through anticonvulsant levels. Withdrawal from alcohol is another common occurrence that can lead to seizures. Illicit drug use, for example cocaine, can cause seizures in patients. Infections are another common cause and include meningitis, encephalitis, or brain abscess. Finally, intracranial tumors or bleeding into the brain either from a tumor or trauma can cause refractory seizures.

Regardless of the cause, there are several things that the nurse must do to ensure the patient's safety. First, attention to the "As, Bs, Cs" of care is essential: ensuring that the patient's airway is maintained and suction is available if it becomes obstructed or the patient vomits, that there are adequate respirations, oxygen is administered to the patient, and that the circulatory system remains intact and intravenous access is established. If the underlying cause of status epilepticus can be readily identified and treated (e.g., hypoglycemia), this care should be instituted. If not, attention should be focused on controlling the seizures through the use of Fosphenytoin or another anticonvulsant agent, planning on acquiring intensive care resources, and planning the diagnostic approach to the patient.

SUGGESTED READINGS

Fagley MU. Taking charge of seizure activity. *Nursing*. 2007;37: 42–47.
Yamamoto L, Oldes E. Challenges in seizure management. *Topics Emerg Med*. 2004;26:212–224.

KNOW HOW TO CARE FOR THE POSTICTAL PATIENT WITH NEW SEIZURES

MELISSA H. CRIGGER, BSN, MHA, RN

WHAT TO DO: PLAN

Remember that the care of a patient with new seizures includes assuring safety and increasing the patient's knowledge of the condition. Seizure activity occurs when electric impulses that are generated in the brain occur in a chaotic manner. Seizures can lead to reduced oxygen and glucose supplies in the brain. Symptoms of seizures can include an aura, which provides a warning that a seizure is about to occur (e.g., visual changes, smelling a strange odor, or hearing an unusual sound). Symptoms usually correlate with the involved area of the brain. Seizures can be classified as partial or generalized. After a patient has a seizure, a recovery period occurs which is known as the postictal period. For those with generalized seizures, the postictal period can last half an hour to several hours. This includes a period of deep sleep with the patient complaining of symptoms such as headache, fatigue, and confusion.

When the nurse is caring for the postictal patient, she must remember that safety is the biggest concern. Since during active seizures the patients may strike their arms and legs against the siderail, the siderails should be padded to prevent or reduce injury. The patient should be placed on his or her side in the recovery position to prevent aspiration of vomitus. The nurse should also be prepared for further seizure activity. Suction should be readily available and restraints should be avoided because of their potential to cause injury. The nurses should implement the specific seizure precautions outlined by their institution.

During the postictal stage, the nurse should also observe for incontinence and monitor for alterations in neurologic status. The postictal patient can be confused and drowsy. During this period, the patient will usually sleep. The nurse must remember to document the characteristics of the seizure including any deviation of the eyes, the length of the seizure, associated symptoms, any activity that the patient was participating in at the time of the seizure, and the length of the recovery period.

Teaching is important for the post seizure patient. The nurse should remember that the patient will require education on the following topics:

1. Factors that trigger seizures, such as use of alcohol, failure to take prescribed antiseizure medications, fever, and stress;
2. For those that experience aura, to seek safety when an aura occurs;
3. Education of prescribed anticonvulsant medications including dosages, side effects, frequency, and when to notify the physician with any concerns;
4. The importance of not stopping anticonvulsant medications without directions from the physician;
5. The importance of wearing a Medic Alert bracelet which provides information regarding seizure disorder;
6. The symptoms of aura including dizziness, visual or hearing disturbances, pain, and perception of abnormal odor;
7. Those with poorly controlled seizures should be educated on the importance of not operating a motor vehicle;
8. Family education on what to do if a patient has an active seizure;
9. Importance of obtaining serum blood levels of anticonvulsant medications such as tegretol and depakote;
10. Limitations of activities like driving that may be mandated by law.

Each of the above-stated teaching topics is important for the patient diagnosed with seizures. The nurse must be prepared to provide safety, assess the patient, and provide adequate teaching for the postictal patient. With proper care, the seizure patient can be taught how to better prevent seizures and be protected from further injury and possibly death if they occur.

SUGGESTED READINGS

Linton AD. *Neurological Disorders: Introduction to Medical-Surgical Nursing.* 4th Ed. St. Louis, MO: Saunders Elsevier; 2007, pp. 435–438.
Williams LS, Hopper PD. *Nursing Care of Patients with Central Nervous System Disorders: Understanding Medical-Surgical Nursing.* 2nd Ed. Philadelphia, PA: F.A. Davis Company; 2003, pp. 843–845.

KNOW THE IMPORTANCE OF ENSURING THAT MYASTHENIA GRAVIS PATIENTS RECEIVE THEIR MEDICATIONS IN A TIMELY MANNER

MONTY D. GROSS, PhD, RN, CNE

WHAT TO DO: IMPLEMENT

Myasthenia gravis is an autoimmune disease that occurs when the nerve junctions have a deficit of acetylcholine, a neurotransmitter, resulting in increased weakness of the voluntary muscles. As the muscle is used, acetylcholine becomes diminished and does not produce enough stimuli for the impulse to travel down the axon contacting the muscle membrane to contract the muscle. The weakness decreases after a period of rest. This resting state allows the acetylcholine to reaccumulate to a functional level at the neuromuscular junction. The acetylcholine is reduced because antibodies destroy it or its receptors. Most often, muscles of the head are affected first, resulting in the so-called "bulbar signs" of diplopia, ptosis, slurred speech, and difficulty in swallowing and can later result in life-threatening breathing difficulty. The breathing can become so impaired that intubation and mechanical ventilation are required. Muscle groups of the arms and legs can become weak, resulting in difficulty with the activities of daily living such as eating and walking.

Myasthenia gravis occurs in all genders and ethnic groups. Although it can occur at any age, women below 40 years and men above 60 years are affected most commonly. It is not inherited or contagious.

The diagnosis is often delayed because muscle weakness can be a sign for other disorders. A medical history and general physical and neurologic examinations are obtained. Blood tests are ordered. Although not present in all cases, a subset of patients with myasthenia gravis has abnormally high levels of antibodies. An edrophonium test is also performed.

Edrophonium chloride (Tensilon) is a drug that temporarily stops the breakdown of acetylcholine and increases the levels at the neuromuscular junction.

Once injected into the patient with myasthenia gravis, the patient experiences a brief improvement in muscle strength and relief of symptoms. Electromylography (EMG) is also conducted to measure muscle fiber response to electric stimulation.

Pyridostigmine bromide (Mestinon) and neostigmine bromide (Prostigmin) are two medications that can be given to the patient to increase the levels of acetylcholine. Once given, they begin to work within 30 to 40 min and last for 3 to 4 h. If the prescribed dose is not administered on time, a myasthenic crisis could result.

Myasthenic crisis is a life-threatening condition that occurs when muscle weakness is so severe that breathing is impaired enough that airway intubation and ventilation are required. Infection and stress are two factors that can precipitate the crisis. Failing to administer the schedule medications on time can result in a crisis.

If responsible for ordering these medications or administering them, it is vital that these medications take priority over most other tasks. When these medications are delayed, the patient is at increased risk for experiencing a myasthenic crisis. The medications are routinely ordered as a pill. Difficulty swallowing is one of the first problems that will occur, making it more difficult to administer the medication. If the patient begins to experience a crisis and is unable to swallow, the problem will be compounded.

SUGGESTED READINGS

Mortensen Armstrong S, Schumann L. Myasthenia gravis: Diagnosis and treatment. *J Am Acad Nurse Pract.* 2003;15(2):72–78.

National Institute on Neurological Disorders and Stroke (n.d.). Myasthenia gravis fact sheet. Available at: http://www.ninds.nih.gov/disorders/myasthenia_gravis/detail_myasthenia_gravis.htm. Accessed July 1, 2008.

Tolle L. Myasthenia gravis: A review for dental hygienist. *J Dent Hyg.* 2007;81(1):12.

KNOW HOW TO MANAGE THE NONPHYSICAL ASPECTS OF TRAUMATIC BRAIN INJURY OF YOUR PATIENTS AND THEIR FAMILY

MONTY D. GROSS, PhD, RN, CNE

WHAT TO DO: PLAN

Traumatic brain injury (TBI) occurs in approximately 500,000 individuals a year. Brain injuries are a traumatic experience for both the patient and the family or significant other(s). On many occasions, the patient's behavior is temporarily or permanently changed. Family members may see behaviors they would never have expected. Healthcare providers need to educate and support these family members and significant others.

Patients with TBI can have disturbances in self-awareness and social cognition. They may be unaware of how their behavior may be seen as inappropriate. Their behavior and subtle social responses received from those present are not correctly interpreted by the patient. Therefore, family interactions are also inappropriate and unpleasant, and result in a stressful situation.

Although stressful, healthcare providers in trauma and neurologic injury settings find that this behavior is not uncommon for patients with TBI. Nurses have a key role in keeping the patient from injury to himself or others, educating, preparing, and supporting family members and significant others as part of the care they provide the patient. Providing families and significant others with information about what behaviors they may witness from their loved one after a TBI will help them prepare for their encounter(s) and help them prepare to offer better support instead of withdrawing. The duration of these behaviors is usually unclear since the recovery in TBI is often prolonged and uncertain. Nonetheless, there are a number of nursing interventions that can be of assistance to these patients and their families.

The priority is to provide a safe environment for the patient. Generally, a quiet, low stimulus environment is best. Remove any equipment or item in the room, such as pictures with glass in the frame, scissors or other sharp objects, or electrical cords that could trip the patient, that would pose a danger. Consider a low profile bed and floor pads if there is a possibility that the patient would fall out of bed.

Ensure psychologist and social workers are involved. Psychologist can assess and help determine more precisely what self awareness or social cognition issues exist. They can recommend strategies for the patient and family to improve or cope with issues. Social workers can help arrange out patient care needs. Patient's needs are often extensive.

Educate the family early and often. Let them know what to expect. If possible, discuss the potential behavior changes and/or physical limitations. Explain medications and diagnostic tests. This will help prepare them when interacting with their family member with TBI. Remember the more you and the healthcare team can support the family members and significant other(s) of a patient with TBI, the less stress they will perceive in dealing with the injury.

SUGGESTED READINGS

Bond E, Draeger C, Mandleco B, et al. Needs of family members of patients with severe traumatic brain injury: Implications for evidence-based practice. *Crit Care Nurse.* 2003;23(4): 63–72.

Centers for Disease Control and Prevention. Traumatic brain injury. 2003. Available at: www.cdc.gov/ncipc/factsheets/tbi.htm. Accessed June 28, 2008.

TRAUMATIC BRAIN INJURY VICTIMS REQUIRE HELP BEYOND THEIR PHYSICAL NEEDS

BONNIE L. PARKER, RN, CRRN

WHAT TO DO: ASSESS

A traumatic brain injury is a blow to the head that disrupts the function of the brain and can result in short- or long-term deficits with independent function. The principal causes are falls, motor vehicle accidents, sports, and physical assault. No two brain injuries are identical, and the effects of a brain injury are complex, multifactoral, and individual and are related to factors such as cause, location, severity, and age of the patient.

The brain is divided into several regions with individual regions controlling distinct functions including motor, cognitive, sensory, and autonomic function, and personality. The response to brain trauma varies dramatically from one individual to another in relation to the areas of the brain affected by injury. In addition, when spinal nerve tracts are damaged, the patient is unable to accurately process messages to the brain or from the brain to the muscles. This can result in changes in thought, motor coordination, personality, and behavior. Cognitive changes may lead to difficulties with memory, decision making, planning, judgment, attention, communication, and thought processes. Motor changes result in difficulties with muscle movement, coordination, sleep, hearing, vision, taste, smell, touch, fatigue, weakness, balanced speech, and seizures. Difficulty with social skills, emotional control and mood swings, depression, anxiety, anger management, irritability, agitation, and excessive laughing or crying can all arise from personality or behavioral changes associated with brain trauma.

While a head injury can result in a variety of symptoms, including seizures and motor dysfunction, some of the more common deficits that develop are with memory, problem solving, stress, emotional upsets, and outbursts of anger. A brain trauma may lead to profound mental and emotional changes and patients may have cognitive difficulties that lead to difficulties with multitasking. Over-stimulation often results in irritability; therefore, these patients respond better in a quiet, dimly lit environment that helps control their behavior. A brain injury not only affects the patient physically but also the way he interacts with everyone and everything around him. Making the environment as stimulus-free as possible is as important as other treatments that the patient receives. The treatment plan should include periods of active treatment interspersed with rest periods. Staff and visitors should be encouraged to speak in a calm, quiet voice, avoiding unnecessary chatter. Staff assignments should be made with a view to following a consistent pattern of activity for the patient, assigning him the same staff as much as possible and avoiding changes in the patient's routines. It is also important to bear in mind to avoid putting a patient in a position where he feels pressured to perform against his desires.

Caring for a patient with brain trauma can be a challenge that brings many rewards. Nurses who keep the special needs of these patients in mind are those with the greatest success.

SUGGESTED READINGS

Lew H, Cifu D, Sigford B, et al. Team approach to diagnosis and management of traumatic brain injury and its co morbidities. *J Rehabil Res Dev.* 2007;44(7):7–11.

Lux WA. Neuropsychiatric perspective on traumatic brain injury. *J Rehabil Res Dev.* 2007;44(7):951–962.

ENSURE THAT NEUROLOGICALLY IMPAIRED PATIENTS WITH AN EPIDURAL HEMORRHAGE ARE MONITORED EFFECTIVELY

KATHERINE M. PENTURFF, RN, CAPA

WHAT TO DO: EVALUATE

Neurologic patients admitted to the hospital due to trauma need careful monitoring at all times, no matter how alert and oriented they appear or how restless and fidgety they seem. While at times it can be a challenge to keep monitoring equipment in place on restless neuro patients, their condition can change quickly, and a change in vital signs may signal an otherwise subtle deterioration.

Epidural hemorrhage (EDH) is an easily treated form of head injury that is often associated with a good prognosis. Although in rare instances such hemorrhages can be spontaneous, most are caused by trauma to the head, most often in the temporal area. As many as 10% to 20% of all patients with head injuries are estimated to have an EDH, and approximately 17% of previously conscious patients who deteriorate into coma following a head injury have an EDH. Nearly 50% of the patients with EDH may present initially as clear and lucid. However, as the hemorrhage increases, the patient may develop increased intracranial pressure, reduced levels of consciousness, and the possibility of herniation syndrome. It is during the initial phase, when the patient has increased intracranial pressure, that monitoring of vital signs may herald a change of condition that is not yet detectable in a standard neurologic assessment. Increased intracranial pressure can lead to a Cushing triad, characterized by hypertension, bradycardia, and respiratory depression. The treatment of an EDH in a patient exhibiting neurologic deterioration is to relieve the pressure, either by Burr holes over the site of the hemorrhage or by more thorough surgical evacuation of the clot.

Vital sign assessment in the neurologic patient should include the basic vital signs: blood pressure, pulse, respirations, and temperature. It must be accompanied by a standard neurologic assessment, evaluating level of consciousness, orientation, memory, brainstem functions, cognition, papillary responses, and motor function. Further monitoring may include oxygen saturation and intracranial pressure monitoring. The initial assessment should be performed with subsequent assessments every 5 to 15 min for unstable patients and every 2 to 4 h for patients who are stabilized.

SUGGESTED READINGS

Acute and intermediate phase nursing in TBI. Neurological and other routine nursing interventions: Assessing vital neurological signs. Available at: www.calder.med.miami.edu/pointis/tbiprov/NURSING/neuro3.htm.

Epidural hemorrhage. Last Updated: Dec 11, 2007. Available at: www.emedicine.com/med/topic2898.htm.

Ikeda M, Matsunaga T, Irabu N, et al. Using vital signs to diagnose impaired consciousness: Cross sectional observational study. *BMJ*. 2002;325(7368):800–802. Available at: www.pubmedcentral.nih.gov/articlerender.fcgi?artid=128944.

Understanding the cushing reflex. Available at: www.jems.com/news_and_articles/columns/SMS/Understanding_the_Cushing_Reflex.html. Accessed July 10, 2007.

PATIENTS UNDERGOING CONSCIOUS SEDATION SHOULD BE CLOSELY MONITORED FOR PROLONGED EFFECTS OF MEDICATION, ESPECIALLY ONCE THE PROCEDURES ARE COMPLETED

KATHERINE M. PENTURFF, RN, CAPA

WHAT TO DO: EVALUATE

Conscious sedation is defined as an altered state of consciousness, induced by the administration of certain medications, which still allows the patient to respond to physical and verbal stimuli while protecting his own airway. The purpose is to produce a state of relaxation, relieve pain, and allay anxiety, usually for brief, but unpleasant procedures. Conscious sedation is most frequently accomplished through the administration of a combination of benzodiazepine and narcotic medications. Because of the potential for respiratory depression and loss of protective airway reflexes, patients receiving conscious sedation should be monitored continuously with the use of EKG, blood pressure, and oximetry during the administration of medications, during the procedure, and for a period of time after the procedure.

Midazolam, an anxiolytic, is one of the frequently used benzodiazepines for conscious sedation. Paradoxical reactions with midazolam use, including hyperactive or aggressive behavior, have been reported. It is a popular choice for sedation because of its fast-acting but brief sedative and amnestic effects when given intravenously. Patients achieve sedation within 1 to 5 min and effects peak within 30 min. The effects of midazolam, including amnestic effects, typically last from 1 to 6 h. Midazolam does not have any analgesic properties, and for this reason, it is usually given, with a narcotic.

Opiates, such as fentanyl, administered intravenously provide both analgesia and sedation. Fentanyl has a rapid onset of action, rapid clearance, and reduced incidence of nausea. Fentanyl also has a wider safety margin when compared with older opioids. The wider safety margin, relatively short duration of action, and minimal respiratory depression at analgesic doses observed for fentanyl have made it the preferred drug for intravenous anesthesia and sedation.

When these medications are used together for brief procedures, it is important to monitor the patient closely after the procedure. While the patient is being stimulated with a noxious stimulus, he may be awake and be able to converse with the staff; however, once the noxious stimulus has ceased, the patient may be prone to fall into a very deep sleep, even into a state of light anesthesia. Because the medications last longer than the sedation, patients may lose the ability to protect their airway.

SUGGESTED READINGS

Midazolam Hydrochloride Syrup, RxList. Available at: www.rxlist.com/cgi/generic/versedsyr_ids.htm.
Waring JP, Baron TH, Hirota WK, et al. Guidelines for conscious sedation and monitoring during gastrointestinal endoscopy. *Gastrointest Endosc.* 2003;58(3):317–322. Available at: www.guideline.gov/summary/summary.aspx?ss=15&doc_id=4141&nbr=3177.

KNOW HOW TO PREVENT NERVE COMPRESSION SYNDROMES

JEANNIE SCRUGGS GARBER, DNP, RN

WHAT TO DO: PLAN

Nerve compression syndromes are increasing in prevalence. While in daily life they may occur from overuse, it is important to remember that positioning of the immobile patient may lead to nerve compression in certain body parts. The nurse should remember the locations of nerve compression, the common signs and symptoms, and the use of appropriate padding and splinting to prevent or improve symptoms. The most common nerve compression syndromes include carpal tunnel, brachial plexus, and ulnar nerves. Patients will often present with signs and symptoms of numbness, tingling, and motor function changes.

Carpal tunnel symptoms include numbness and tingling in the hand, especially at night. Other possible symptoms include neck pain, a change in how one handles objects, or sharp pain that radiates from the wrist to the shoulder. The carpal tunnel is the part of the wrist where nerves, ligaments, and tendons pass to the hand. Carpal tunnel syndrome is most often diagnosed in middle-aged females. Physical assessment and possibly a nerve conduction test can be performed to determine the diagnosis of carpal tunnel syndrome. The treatment for carpal tunnel syndrome may first require rest or a brace and anti-inflammatory medications to help reduce swelling and pain. If conservative treatments are unsuccessful, surgery may be necessary.

Brachial plexus injuries may involve the shoulder, arm, or hand and is likely to result from traumatic injury such as sports or vehicle accidents or misappropriate positioning on an operative table. The symptoms of this type of injury may be paralysis, numbness, or tingling anywhere from the hand to the shoulder. These may occur from abduction of the arm during the operative procedure and need to be assessed in the postoperative setting.

The ulnar nerve is the nerve that provides feeling in the little finger, ring finger, and some of the muscles of the hand that starts at the side of the neck and joins three main nerves that travel down the arm to the hand. As it crosses the wrist, the ulnar nerve and artery run through the tunnel known as Guyon canal. After passing through the canal, the ulnar nerve branches out to supply feeling to the little finger and half the ring finger as well as the small muscles of the hand. The most common type of ulnar nerve compression results in numbness of the fingers and may cause hand muscle weakness. The most common treatment is immobilization or rest of the symptomatic area and surgery if conservative treatment is not effective.

SUGGESTED READINGS

Nerve compression syndromes. Available at: http://www.merck.com/mmhe/sec05/ch071/ch071d.html. Accessed August 16, 2008.

KNOW THAT THE STROKE PATIENT HAS A NUMBER OF NURSING NEEDS THAT CAN POSE SAFETY CONCERNS IF THEY ARE UNADDRESSED

ANTHONY D. SLONIM, MD, DRPH

WHAT TO DO: ASSESS

Acute stroke patients can be classified into those patients with ischemic stroke and those patients with hemorrhagic strokes. The ischemic variety makes up the majority of strokes accounting for nearly 85% of all strokes with the hemorrhagic making up the remainder. Patients presenting with the diagnosis of stroke, regardless of the type, present a number of challenges to care that, if unmet, can lead to important safety concerns.

Because of alterations in mobility, stroke patients are at risk for all the complications that are associated with immobility during hospitalization and beyond including pressure ulcers, deep venous thrombosis (DVT), and contractures. Hence, it becomes important to ensure that the patients are mobilized effectively, turned often, and receive appropriate splinting and DVT prophylaxis during their illness and through rehabilitation. Assist devices that help with ambulation may be an option, but represent safety concerns of their own.

Stroke patients often experience alterations in their speech and language processing and memory. A major part of the therapy for these problems may include speech therapy. In addition, swallowing is often affected and should be tested to ensure that the patient can accommodate the diet and does not experience aspiration. The inability to communicate and the loss of independence are often frustrating for the patients and their family and can be benefited by psychosocial support and intervention.

Activities of daily living including toileting and bathing are often compromised with a stroke. The patient may have retained urine or feces and experience complications including urinary tract infections and impaction with abdominal bloating as a result. Modesty may prevent the patient from asking for assistance with these activities and not attend to them or worse. The patient may attempt to be independent and fall during his or her effort of independence.

Stroke is a devastating clinical condition that is heavily reliant on nursing care to prevent complications and assist with restoring the patient to a physical condition and quality of life that is optimal.

SUGGESTED READINGS

NINDS stroke information page. Available at: http://www.ninds.nih.gov/disorders/stroke/stroke.htm. Accessed August 16, 2008.

AUTONOMIC DYSREFLEXIA DOES HAPPEN, KNOW HOW TO RESPOND WHEN IT HAPPENS TO YOUR SPINAL CORD INJURY PATIENT

ALICE M. CHRISTALDI, RN, BSN, CRRN

WHAT TO DO: IMPLEMENT

There are on average 11,000 spinal cord injuries a year. Forty-eight percent occur due to motor vehicle accidents and 23% due to falls. Eighty percent of all those injured are male. The degree of disability is determined by which level the injury occured, how it occurred, and the severity of the injury.

Cervical injuries are the most common type of spinal cord injury. A cervical injury may cause a partial or total paralysis of all four limbs (tetraplegia or more commonly referred to as quadriplegia), while injuries to the thoracic or lumbar area may cause a partial or total paralysis to the legs. A little more than half of all spinal cord injuries are quadriplegic.

A life threatening emergency that occurs among spinal cord injuries is autonomic dysreflexia, a big word to describe the effects of a noxious stimulus below the level of the injury. Autonomic dysreflexia occurs with spinal cord injuries above or at T6. To review some basic anatomy of the thoracic spine, the thoracic nerve innervates the chest, some of the muscles of the back, and parts of the abdomen. There are 12 vertebrae in the thoracic region. T1 innervates the medial side of the forearm. T2 to T4 injuries paralyze the legs and trunk and may cause a loss of feeling from nipples down. T5 to T8 injuries affect leg and lower trunk and may cause loss of feeling below the rib cage. T9 to T11 injuries cause leg paralysis and loss of feeling below the umbilicus. Below T12, there is paralysis and loss of feeling below the groin. The thoracic spinal cord is at a greater risk than the cervical or lumbar vertebrae because it is smaller than the other vertebrae.

Autonomic dysreflexia is an exaggerated sympathetic nervous response to noxious stimuli below the level of the spinal cord injury which leads to vasoconstriction and a hypertensive episode. Noxious stimuli can be a full bladder or need to empty the bowels, pain, pressure ulcer, pressure of any kind against the skin, or sexual excitation. Symptoms occur suddenly and can include severe hypertension, profuse sweating, flushing above the level of the injury, cold, clammy skin with piloerection below the injury, and a severe headache. Bradycardia may also be present.

Action must be taken quickly to prevent a stroke, cardiac arrest, intracranial hemorrhage, seizures, or even death. Quickly attempt to identify the cause of the event and remove it. Raise the head of the bed fully upright to attempt an orthostatic drop in blood pressure. Urinary distension is the number one cause of autonomic dysreflexia, so plan to perform straight catherization of the patient and use a lidocaine urojet to instill lidocaine into the urethral meatus to prevent any further exacerbation of symptoms. If the patient already has an indwelling catheter, it might be kinked or blocked, try irrigating the catheter.

If symptoms persist, continue the search for other possible triggers, which might be a fecal impaction. Possibly too tight lower extremity clothing or even wrinkled bed linens might be a cause. A change in position might be helpful. Medications will be used if the cause of the problem cannot quickly be identified and might include oral nifedipine or nitroglycerin ointment applied topically to control hypertension. Clonodine or Hyrdralazine may also be used.

Autonomic dysreflexia with all spinal cord injuries with involvement of the thoracic spine is an important topic to discuss. It is important to be aware of the signs and symptoms. Prevention, as well as quick action, is the key when symptoms present.

SUGGESTED READINGS

Krassioukov AV, Karlsson AK, Wecht JM, et al. Assessment of autonomic dysfunction following spinal cord injury: Rationale for addition to International Standards for Neurological Assessment. *J Rehabil Rese Dev.* 2007;44(1):103–112.

The Merck Manual of Diagnosis and Treatment Online Medical Library. Available at: http://www.merck.com/pubs/. Accessed April 1, 2008.

WATCH FOR RESPIRATORY FAILURE IN PATIENTS WITH GUILLAIN–BARRE SYNDROME

SAM HARVEY AND ANTHONY D. SLONIM, MD, DrPH

WHAT TO DO: EVALUATE

Guillain–Barre syndrome is an autoimmune disorder that attacks the myelin sheath of a victim's nervous system. Myelin is a special, insulating substance that covers nerves and facilitates improved conduction. The Schwann cell is the solitary production cell of myelin in the peripheral nervous system. Guillain–Barre syndrome results in a cell-mediated immune attack on the myelin sheath, starting in the lower extremities and progressing upward along a victim's nervous system. Fortunately, Guillain–Barre syndrome spares the Schwann cell, allowing for remyelinization during the recovery period. Approximately 65% to 75% of victims successfully recover from the disease.

Several theories exist for the etiology of the disorder, but the most prominent is the preliminary viral infection that occurs before the onset of the disease. Some viruses contain amino acid similar to the peripheral myelin protein, and in an attempt to respond to the infection, the immune system is unable to differentiate between the foreign viral amino acid and the myelin sheath. Several viruses connected to the development of Guillain–Barre syndrome include Epstein–Barr virus, HIV, cytomegalovirus, and *Mycoplasma pneumoniae*.

Guillain–Barre syndrome is characterized by muscle weakness and poor reflexes, initially in the legs. It is typical for the symptoms to ascend into the torso and even the head. Symptoms are specific to the region of the body affected. For example, once the demyelinization affects the optic nerve, blindness may result. Some of the most important concerns related to the disease occur when the disorder reaches the lungs and respiratory failure ensues. The demyelination ultimately results in complete muscle paralysis if the condition is left untreated. However, once the virus responsible for precipitating the disorder is treated, a full recovery is often expected. Sometimes this recovery can take as long as 2 years and occasionally permanent damage from the demyelinization process may result.

Guillain–Barre is a medical emergency due to its potential for rapid progression to the lungs or brain. Often the patient is placed on mechanical ventilation to preserve pulmonary function until recovery begins. The most common therapy for Guillain–Barre syndrome is intravenous immune globulin (IVIG), which successfully reduces the amount of myelin antibody in the bloodstream. Plasmapheresis is another option, but IVIG is usually selected due to a lower risk for complicating side effects. Once the disorder recedes to allow for relatively normal muscular function, therapy for the remediation of affected systems should be conducted (Figure 268-1).

SUGGESTED READINGS

Smeltzer S, Bare B, Hinkle J, et al. *Textbook of Medical–Surgical Nursing*. Philadelphia, PA: Lippincott Williams & Wilkins; 2008.

Winer JB. Treatment of Guillain–Barre syndrome. *Int J Med*. 2002;95(11):717–721.

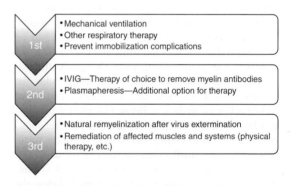

FIGURE 268.1. Guillain–Barre therapy process.

CREUTZFELDT–JAKOB DISEASE IS A RARE CAUSE OF PROGRESSIVE NEUROLOGIC DETERIORATION AND SHOULD BE CONSIDERED IN THE PATIENT DEMONSTRATING WORSENING STATUS

SAM HARVEY AND ANTHONY D. SLONIM, MD, DRPH

WHAT TO DO: EVALUATE

Creutzfeldt–Jakob disease (CJD) is a very rare neurologic disorder belonging to the class of diseases known as transmissible spongiform encephalopathies. Approximately one case occurs for every 1 million individuals. Two types exist, sporadic CJD and variant CJD. Variant CJD is essentially the human equivalent of bovine spongiform encephalopathy, also known as "Mad Cow Disease." The agent of infection in CJD is a prion, unique in the fact that, unlike bacteria and viruses, a prion has no nucleic acid. In CJD, the prion is the variant of a protein naturally found in the brain. There is no cure for CJD. The prion responsible for the disorder may lay dormant within the blood of an infected individual for years before neurologic deterioration begins (Figure 269.1).

A person becomes infected through direct contact with the CJD-prion. This can result from ingesting infected meat, exposure to contaminated instruments, or corneal implants. Once the prion enters into the brain tissue, the normal proteins present in the brain convert to abnormal structures and begin rapid brain tissue degeneration. Physiologically, empty vacuoles appear in the brain tissue and give it a "spongy" appearance. Specific symptoms of CJD are very distinct and occur with increasing severity as the disease progresses.

The prion responsible for CJD is folded in a very stable configuration, making it resistant to current proteases. Due to the fact that CJD does not have a nucleic acid to transmit infection, all the anti-infectious drugs have no effect. When a suspicious case of sporadic CJD presents itself, a brain biopsy must be obtained. Immunologic assessment of infected tissue indicates a protein kinase inhibitor that signals the presence of neuronal cell death. An electroencephalogram shows a characterized slowing of brain activity with periodic spikes followed by little to no activity later in the disease. Patients with variant CJD demonstrate hyperintensity in the thalamus on MRI scans. The prion associated with variant CJD also accumulates in the tonsils, allowing for tonsillar biopsy as well.

Care of CJD patients is similar to all end-of-life care as the disease is always fatal. To prevent blood-born infection, Standard precautions should be used with healthcare workers and family members. Infected objects must undergo extensive treatment for sterilization due to the tenacity of the infectious prion and its resistance to standard methods.

SUGGESTED READINGS

Belkin N. Creutzfeldt–Jakob disease: Identifying prions and carriers. *AORN*. 2003;78(2):204–208.

Smeltzer S, Bare B, HinkleJ, et al. *Textbook of Medical–Surgical Nursing*. Philadelphia, PA: Lippincott Williams & Wilkins; 2008.

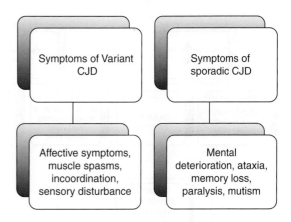

FIGURE 269.1. Symptoms of Creutzfeldt–Jakob disease (CJD).

UNILATERAL FACIAL SYMPTOMS MAY REFLECT EITHER BELL'S PALSY OR TRIGEMINAL NEURALGIA

SAM HARVEY AND ANTHONY D. SLONIM, MD, DrPH

WHAT TO DO: ASSESS

Several disorders exist due to improper cranial nerve function. The cranial nerves and brain stem preserve all the involuntary vital motor, sensory, and autonomic functions of the human body; therefore, disorders of the cranial nerve should be monitored very closely. Two closely related disorders are trigeminal neuralgia (tic douloureux) and Bell palsy. Each involves a specific cranial nerve: Bell palsy is disorder of the seventh cranial nerve while trigeminal neuralgia is a condition of the fifth cranial nerve. Each disorder affects a unilateral side of the face, although the symptoms are somewhat different. Each disorder lacks a specific etiology (Figure 270.1).

Each disorder requires different treatments as well. Bell's palsy's etiology could be viral or a type of pressure paralysis, but usually the only medical interventions necessary are moderate analgesics. Most patients usually recover in 3 to 5 weeks with no residual symptoms. The demographics most susceptible include the elderly as well as pregnant women in the third trimester. Trigeminal neuralgia usually appears in adults in the fifth or sixth decade of life and has much more serious consequences. As paroxysms occur with direct stimulation of the cranial nerve, many victims refrain from stimulating the facial muscles in any way possible. This includes avoiding chewing, washing the face, brushing teeth, etc. Episodes of neuralgia increase in frequency with age. Effective medications in controlling the involuntary spasms accompanying paroxysms include antiseizure agents, such as carbamazepine. Surgical intervention can also relieve trigeminal neuralgia and may offer extended relief in the future. Three effective procedures are included in Figure 270.2.

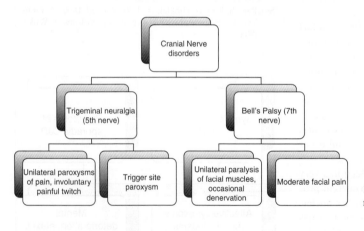

FIGURE 270.1. Classification of cranial nerve disorders.

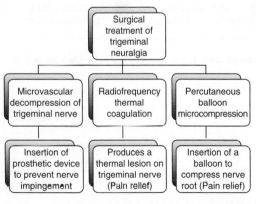

FIGURE 270.2. Surgical treatment options for trigeminal neuralgia.

Unfortunately, these surgical solutions have reportedly high instances of reoccurrence within 5 years, so at best, they offer temporary pain relief. It is essential that the patient be educated about the possibility of further medical or surgical therapy should reoccurrence of trigeminal neuralgia manifest.

SUGGESTED READINGS

Filipchuk D. Classic trigeminal neuralgia: A surgical perspective. *J Neurosci Nurs.* 2003;35(2):82–86.

Smeltzer S, Bare B, Hinkle J, et al. *Textbook of Medical–Surgical Nursing.* Philadelphia, PA: Lippincott Williams & Wilkins; 2008.

271

REMEMBER THAT ADEQUATE OXYGENATION IS CRITICAL TO OUR PATIENTS AND KNOWING WHEN THEY ARE GETTING INTO TROUBLE IS IMPORTANT FOR PREVENTING COMPLICATIONS

ANTHONY D. SLONIM, MD, DRPH

WHAT TO DO: ASSESS

Humans are heavily dependent upon oxygen for the functioning of cells, organs, and tissues. The respiratory system is primarily responsible for ensuring that gases, both oxygen and carbon dioxide, are exchanged appropriately. This is accomplished through the combined efforts of the upper and the lower respiratory system. The upper respiratory system is comprised of the structures from the nose and mouth down to the point where the trachea splits into right and left mainstem bronchi at the carina. From here, the lower respiratory system continues to divide into segmental and subsegmental bronchi and further into bronchioles, before ending in terminal units known as alveoli.

The delivery of air, which is made up of approximately 21% oxygen, from the nose to the terminal alveoli, where gas is exchanged, is crucial for survival. These structures represent the elements of the respiratory tree; however, it is important to remember that the actual exchange of gases, known as ventilation, depends not only on the tree itself but also on the muscles of the chest wall and elasticity of the lungs. When the air finally comes into contact with the alveolar capillary membrane, diffusion along its concentration gradient occurs from the alveoli into the blood. Oxygen is carried in the blood in two forms, dissolved and bound to hemoglobin. The majority of oxygen is carried in the bound state. Clinically, the dissolved oxygen is represented by the PaO_2 and the bound oxygen is represented as the oxygen saturation, SaO_2.

When patients experience hypoxemia, they manifest a number of clinical signs that are present not only in the respiratory system but also in other systems that are heavily dependent upon oxygen. These early signs can assist the nurses in understanding before it is too late that their patient may be getting into trouble. From a central nervous system (CNS) perspective, hypoxemia is often manifested as a change in behavior. Patients experience a range of behaviors from anxiety to restlessness and irritability to confusion and lethargy. It is important for the nurse to realize that these signs may not be willful changes in behavior on the part of the patient, but represent a physiologic problem that needs to be addressed. From a respiratory perspective, the patient's respiratory rate begins to increase, even at rest, and a feeling of breathlessness, known as dyspnea, occurs. As the hypoxemia progresses, the patients begin to use their accessory muscles of respiration and experience retractions in the intercostal spaces. These are very important signs for the nurse to notice since they represent increasing work of breathing. From a cardiovascular perspective, the patient's heart rate and blood pressure begins to rise up until the point when the heart becomes starved from oxygen, in which case dysrhythmias occur. It is important for the nurse to recognize these early signs of hypoxemia and intervene to establish normoxia.

Apart from the clinical examination, the nurse has a number of methods available to actually ensure that the patient is adequately oxygenated. Pulse oximetry provides a non invasive method for measuring the oxygen level in the blood. By measuring the wavelength of light in oxygenated and deoxygenated blood, the oximeter can assist in providing objective evidence of the patient's oxygen level. A more invasive method is an arterial blood gas (ABG). The ABG provides important information not only about gas exchange more generally but also about oxygenation specifically by providing estimates of both the PaO_2 and SaO_2. Together, these methods allow the nurse to have an objective measure to substantiate the patient's hypoxemia.

SUGGESTED READINGS

Nursing diagnosis: Impaired gas exchange, ventilation or perfusion imbalance. Available at: http://www1.us.elsevierhealth.com/MERLIN/Gulanick/Constructor/index.cfm?plan=23. Accessed August 20, 2008.

REMEMBER THAT THERE ARE A NUMBER OF SIGNS AND SYMPTOMS FOR RESPIRATORY SYSTEM PROBLEMS, BUT THERE IS ALSO CONSIDERABLE OVERLAP BETWEEN THESE SIGNS AND SYMPTOMS AND THE DISEASES CAUSING THEM

ANTHONY D. SLONIM, MD, DrPH

WHAT TO DO: ASSESS AND EVALUATE

The assessment of the respiratory system is critical to understand the challenges facing a patient's health. One of the more difficult and uncomfortable feelings for patients is the feeling of suffocation and having difficulty breathing. This is referred to as dyspnea, and while the nurse is unable to assess dyspnea directly, the patient can certainly share this feeling with the nurse during the assessment interview. Dyspnea may accompany many disorders of the cardiac and respiratory system including congestive heart failure (CHF), pneumonia, asthma, and exacerbations of chronic lung disease, but by itself is rather nonspecific, except allowing the nurse to focus on these two systems as a potential problem.

A number of other more specific signs are important for the nurse to assess. These include cough, wheezing, chest pain, and the coughing up of sputum or blood. Each of these is important for understanding potential underlying diagnoses of the cardiac and respiratory systems. It is important not only to recognize these symptoms but also to understand if there is a change from baseline. This is particularly helpful for patients that have these symptoms on a chronic basis.

Cough is a common symptom that can occur in all age groups. A cough may be either acute (hours to days) or chronic (weeks) and occurs as a manifestation of either an upper or lower respiratory system or cardiac problem. Coughs are characterized as "dry," in which case they may represent irritation or inflammation of the upper airway, "loose," if there are associated secretions, or "barky" in nature, which usually represents a problem in the area of the vocal cords as occurs with croup or epiglottitis. A cough will accompany pneumonia, CHF, and other problems of the upper airway. While being a general symptom, it often provides a clue to the underlying diagnosis.

When a cough is associated with the production of sputum or blood, the nurse learns more about the potential diagnoses. Usually, the sputum is characterized with respect to its character, color, amount, and odor. Normal sputum is thin and colorless. Sputum that is yellow in color may represent an infectious source, such as pneumonia or bronchitis, but patients with chronic lung disease and secretions from the upper airway may wake up with yellow sputum that clears during the course of the day. Patients with large volumes of yellow sputum that has changed in character and become thicker or foul smelling should be considered to have a lower respiratory tract infection. Patients with large amounts of frothy, pink sputum are often considered to have CHF in the right clinical setting.

The coughing up of blood (hemoptysis) can be a very important sign for evaluation since it represents a spectrum of disorders, some of which are a medical emergency. Hemoptysis can range from blood streaking to the production of large quantities of blood with coughing. The former can accompany bronchitis, pneumonia, or lung cancer while the latter can represent other infectious issues like tuberculosis, bronchiectasis, etc.

A wheeze is a high pitched whistling sound that can sometimes be audible to the patient and nurse without a stethoscope. Wheezes can occur from problems of either the respiratory or cardiac systems. Some patients with CHF will wheeze in what is occasionally called "cardiac asthma." More often, wheezing represents an alteration in the respiratory system that includes pneumonia, particularly if the wheezing is localized, and asthma when the wheezing occurs from bronchospasm and can be heard on inspiration and expiration or exacerbations of chronic lung disease like cystic fibrosis, emphysema, or chronic bronchitis.

Chest pain is a symptom that occurs from one of the components of the chest wall or internal organs. It is important to understand the nature of the chest pain, its characteristics, any radiation associated symptoms, and temporizing or exacerbating conditions. These characteristics will help the nurse distinguish between problems of the chest wall (injuries), pleura (Pleuritis), lung (pneumonia/empyema), or heart (ischemic cardiac disease).

The nurse needs to have an appreciation for the more common signs and symptoms of the respiratory system to provide a thorough assessment of the respiratory system and the potential underlying conditions of the patient.

SUGGESTED READINGS

Symptom: Cough. Available at: http://www.wrongdiagnosis.com/sym/cough.htm. Accessed August 20, 2008.

REMEMBER THAT AN ELEVATED PCO$_2$ ALONE IS NOT NECESSARILY AN URGENT PROBLEM FOR THE PATIENT

ANTHONY D. SLONIM, MD, DRPH

WHAT TO DO: EVALUATE

Acute acid–base disorders are some of the more common laboratory abnormalities encountered in hospitalized patients. The primary disorder is usually identified based upon the pH and the direction of either the PCO$_2$ or the bicarbonate of the arterial blood gas. The normal range of the pH is between 7.35 and 7.45. When the pH is below this range, the patient is described as acidotic. When the pH is above this range, the patient is described as alkalotic.

In the acidotic patient, it is important to describe the primary disorder as either respiratory or metabolic. A respiratory acidosis occurs when the PCO$_2$ rises above the normal range of 35 to 45. A metabolic acidosis occurs when the bicarbonate is reduced below the range of 20 to 24. Each of these is further subclassified as acute or chronic depending upon their duration and the degree of compensation. In the acute setting, the respiratory system is the primary compensatory mechanism. In the chronic state, the kidneys take over the compensation.

Any time when there is a reduction of CO$_2$ exhalation and a buildup of the pressure of CO$_2$ in the blood, a respiratory acidosis can occur. Several common causes of respiratory acidosis include exacerbations of obstructive and restrictive lung diseases including bronchitis, asthma, and emphysema. In addition, an acute respiratory acidosis can occur from obstruction to exhalation because of either acute airway obstruction or cardiac arrest. In these cases, the elevation of CO$_2$ is often accompanied by a reduction in pH which signals an acute acidotic condition. It is important to recognize this acute condition because intensive care unit (ICU) therapies including mechanical ventilation are available for these patients if they become severely ill. If the condition persists for more than a couple of days, the kidneys will begin to retain bicarbonate and the pH will normalize.

For patients with a more chronic condition, where the PCO$_2$ remains elevated for more than a few days, the kidneys have had an opportunity to compensate over a protracted period of time. In these cases, the patient may present to the hospital with an illness that does not consist of alterations in the respiratory system but has an elevated PCO$_2$ without an accompanying reduction in pH or acidosis. Clinically, these patients tend to be alert and without acute respiratory compromise. They may have a chronic underlying respiratory disease. Nonetheless, the alteration in their body's chemistry represents an important underlying metabolic abnormality, but one that does not require acute intervention because of the compensation provided by their kidney. You know this because the PCO$_2$ is elevated and the pH is normal.

There are a number of formulas and calculations to help determine whether or not the patient is appropriately compensated. In the acute setting, the bicarbonate rises by 1 for every 10 millimeters of mercury (mm Hg) elevations of the PCO$_2$. In the chronic setting, the bicarbonate rises by 4 to 5 for every 10 mm Hg elevations of the PCO$_2$.

An example helps to illustrate these points. An acute asthma patient admitted during your shift is in respiratory distress and has an arterial blood gas just performed that demonstrates a pH of 7.1, a PCO$_2$ of 60, a PO$_2$ of 100, and bicarbonate of 27. The patient is acidotic, and the disorder appears to be respiratory in origin since the PCO$_2$ is elevated. One can also see that the degree of compensation provided by the kidneys is nominal since the value is approximately 2 above a normal of 25. This indicates that the patient is suffering from an acute respiratory acidosis and needs immediate intervention to assist him or her during this acute illness. Another patient in the adjacent room is admitted with a cellulitis but happens to have a history of emphysema. An ABG done in the emergency department demonstrates a pH of 7.4, a PCO$_2$ of 75, and a bicarbonate of 38. Because of the chronic nature of this patient's disease, the patient's kidneys have been allowed adequate time to retain further bicarbonate and maintain a normal pH. This patient requires ongoing monitoring of his or her respiratory status during treatment for cellulitis, but does not require urgent respiratory support beyond his or her chronic medical regimen.

SUGGESTED READINGS

http://books.google.com/books?id=x9bvh6RyBwC&pg=PA7 8&lpg=PA78&dq=elevated+pco2+nursing&source=web &ots=ViG0uJyWfK&sig=WpKTrfH07tWGYsRW-4h- xhkRQJc&hl=en&sa=X&oi=book_result&resnum=5&ct= result#PPA79,M1. Accessed August 20, 2008.

REMEMBER THAT SOMETIMES WHAT YOU DO NOT HEAR IS MORE IMPORTANT THAN WHAT YOU DO HEAR

ANTHONY D. SLONIM, MD, DrPH

WHAT TO DO: ASSESS

The nurses spend a considerable amount of time learning the assessment skills that are necessary to assist patients in their care. A large focus during this training is on learning the "positive" signs and symptoms that accompany different conditions and disease entities. However, it is also important to recognize that sometimes the absence of a normal sign may be as if not more important to the clinical care of the patient. One of these so called "negative" signs is particularly relevant to the respiratory system.

Chest auscultation is a technique that allows the examiner to establish that air is entering and exiting the lungs. It also allows the examiner to listen to the lungs for normal and accessory sounds and to establish a presumptive list of diagnoses based upon the findings, their pattern, and the clinical condition of the patient. For one such condition, pneumothorax, the absence of breath sounds may be as important as the presence of breath sounds and needs to be noted.

A pneumothorax is a collection of air in the pleural space between the lung and chest wall. It often leads to a partial or total collapse of the lung. While often considered within the setting of trauma, it is important to recognize that a pneumothorax can occur without trauma from a variety of procedural interventions like mechanical ventilation or the placement of a central venous line or may occur spontaneously from a number of diseases including emphysema, asthma, *Pneumocystis carinii* pneumonia, alpha 1 antitrypsin deficiency, and others.

The astute nurse will not only attend to the presence of vesicular, bronchovesicular, and bronchial breath sounds but also recognize that the absence of appropriate breath sounds in a location, where they are supposed to be heard, may be as important to diagnose the patient's condition as the presence of accessory noises. The next step will be the integration of these findings with the clinical condition and the validation of other criteria like the patient's oxygen level and finally the request of a chest x-ray as needed.

SUGGESTED READINGS

Nursing bulletin notes on pneumothorax. Available at: http://www.slideshare.net/seigelystic/nursing-bulletin-notes-on-pneumothorax. Accessed August 20, 2008.

KNOW THAT STEROIDS ARE THE KEY TO UNLOCKING THE TREATMENT FOR ASTHMA

ANTHONY D. SLONIM, MD, DrPH

WHAT TO DO: IMPLEMENT

Asthma is an inflammatory disease of the lungs that affects patients of all ages and is responsible for a significant number of emergency department visits, hospitalizations, and deaths. While many patients with asthma live healthy and productive lives, acute exacerbations are disruptive and potentially dangerous if not managed aggressively, sometimes leading to sudden death. The National Institutes of Health has provided a "Stepwise Approach for Managing Asthma" that categorizes asthma into four levels of severity based upon the frequency of signs and symptoms and objective peak expiratory flow measurements. These guidelines have been useful in standardizing the chronic approach to asthma patients nationwide and have provided guidance about when care needs to escalate.

There are a number of triggers, both environmental and occupational, that can predispose patients to an acute asthma exacerbation. In addition, concomitant infections, smoke in the environment, and air pollution are major contributors. Asthma is characterized by episodic symptoms of cough, wheeze, and dyspnea with reversible airflow obstruction. Airway inflammation is the major pathophysiologic underpinning. This is important because airway inflammation will continue to worsen during the course of an acute exacerbation until aggressively managed. There are a number of medications available to assist patients with asthma including short and long acting bronchodilators, leukotriene modifiers, and inhaled and systemic steroids. While the delivery of inhaled steroids and bronchodilators may be helpful to maintain control on a chronic basis, during acute episodes, this care needs to escalate.

Patients experiencing acute asthma exacerbations benefit from having predetermined action plan with the steps written down for sequential activation as their condition begins to deteriorate. Despite the use of long acting bronchodilators and inhaled steroids, an exacerbation requires that the care be escalated by including additional therapies to the clinical situation. Most often, these include short acting beta agonists and steroids. While the short acting bronchodilators will assist with bronchospasm, it is the steroids that will treat the cause of the exacerbation, namely the inflammation. An antibiotic is not routinely necessary unless there are demonstrated signs of an infection.

Acute asthma exacerbations usually result from inflammation that leads to airway hyperresponsiveness and limitations in airflow. The treatment of the inflammation is the key to assisting the patient to recover.

SUGGESTED READINGS

Guidelines for the Diagnosis and Management of Asthma: Update on Selected Topics 2002. NIH Publications # 02–5074. Bethesda, MD: National Institutes of Health, National Heart, Lung and Blood Institute.

Kavuru MS. *Diagnosis and Management of Asthma*. 4th Ed. West Islip, NY: Professional Communications Inc; 2008.

KNOW HOW TO MANAGE YOUR PATIENT WITH A TRACHEOSTOMY

MONTY D. GROSS, PhD, RN, CNE

WHAT TO DO: PLAN

A tracheostomy is a surgical opening made in the trachea to allow for the insertion of a tube to maintain an open airway. Some reasons a tracheostomy may be required are the need for neck surgery for laryngeal cancer, emergency airway access, long-term ventilator use, or reduction of airway resistance by bypassing the oro-nasopharynx. The opening also provides access to suction secretions from the airway.

A sterile tracheostomy tube should be readily available to replace the patient's tracheostomy tube should it become dislodged or contaminated. Often, the new one is taped in a visible area, such as the head of the bed, to keep it visible and readily accessible should it be needed.

The upper airway heats, filters, and humidifies the air as it passes through the structures of the upper airway. Because a tracheostomy tube bypasses the upper airway, secretions become dry and thick. Suctioning is required to remove these secretions, maintain an open airway, and promote oxygenation. Before and after suctioning a patient, the patient should be hyperoxygenated and approximately one minute should pass before subsequent attempts at suctioning are performed to prevent hypoxemia. It is also recommended that the catheter used for suctioning be no larger than one-half the inner diameter of the tracheostomy tube. To determine the maximum size catheter to use, multiply the artificial airway two times. If the tube is 8 mm, multiply 8 × 2 and the result of 16 French is the largest catheter diameter that should be used to suction the patient. Set the suction regulator at 100 to 120 mm Hg. When suctioning, apply intermittent suctioning only when withdrawing the catheter and suction for no more than 5 to 10 s.

There is a risk for infection. Therefore, maintain sterile technique when suctioning. Remember to wash your hands before and after the procedure, and change gloves when you move from providing care from one part of the body to providing tracheostomy care. If the patient is on a ventilator, do not allow condensation in the circuit to drain into the patient's tracheostomy.

Speaking valves, such as the Passey–Muir, can be placed on the opening of the tracheostomy tube to enable the patients to use their normal airway to speak. The speaking valve closes at the beginning of expiration when air from the patient's lungs closes a one-way valve. This restores normal airflow through the oro-nasopharynx and allows speech production since the air flows out through the normal vocal cords. The valve opens during inspiration to permit fresh oxygen to reach the lungs.

When using a speaking valve, it is important to remember to deflate the cuff of the tracheostomy tube because if the tracheostomy tube is capped by the speaking valve and the cuff is inflated, the patient's airway is blocked. It is advisable to place a sign over the patient's bed reading, "Do not inflate cuff with speaking valve in place." The speaking valve should be removed at bedtime before the patient falls asleep. When not in use, place the speaking valve in a clean container with a lid at the bedside.

Tracheostomies are an essential tool for maintaining a patient's airway and are common in hospitals. Knowing how to safely manage the patient with a tracheostomy is an important skill. The key points to remember are to use sterile technique at all times, limit the duration of suctioning, and set the suction regulator <120 mm Hg. If a speaking valve is used, make sure the cuff on the tracheostomy is deflated.

SUGGESTED READINGS

Smith S, Duell D, Martin B. *Clinical Nursing Skills: Basic to Advanced Skills*. Upper Saddle River, NJ: Pearson; 2008.

WEAR A FACE SHIELD WHEN SUCTIONING

BONNIE L. PARKER, RN, CRRN

WHAT TO DO: PLAN

A tracheostomy is an opening, or a stoma, made into the trachea at the second, third, or fourth tracheal ring in which a tube is inserted to assist with a patient's breathing. It may be placed in critically ill patients who will require respiratory assistance longer than the recommended time that an endotracheal tube can remain in place. Patients who have a tracheostomy placed may also have an obstruction at or above the larynx, cancer of the throat, severe infection causing swelling, trauma to the mouth, or stenosis from prolonged intubation. Other patients who may require a tracheostomy are those who are unable to clear their secretions or breathe deeply enough to clear their airway including patients who have paralysis of their chest muscles and diaphragm, those with head injuries who are unconscious or semiconscious, and those with rib or chest fractures or who are in a drug induced coma. Patients who have suffered smoke inhalation or burns of the face and neck may also require a tracheostomy.

A tracheostomy provides excellent access to suction the airway to clear secretions that should be suctioned as often as necessary to maintain clearance. This may be as often as once every few minutes when the tracheostomy is first placed or every 3 to 4 h after it has been in place for several days. Patients who have had a tracheostomy for a while and are able to cough and clear secretions may not require suctioning at all. Patients who are able to clear their own secretions should not be suctioned to prevent trauma to the mucosa.

Suctioning a tracheostomy requires sterile technique using a catheter no larger than half the diameter of the inner cannula of the trach; the smallest size catheter possible should be used to prevent injury. The prepared nurse will don personal protective equipment prior to suctioning; sterile gloves may be adequate, but a face shield, goggles, or mask may be necessary since suctioning will stimulate a cough reflex and mucous can travel quite a distance when forcefully coughed from a tracheostomy. For the same reason, the nurse should avoid leaning over a patient while suctioning. The patient should be well oxygenated prior to suctioning which may be accomplished by supplying extra breaths with an artificial resuscitator bag or by asking the patient to take deep breaths while delivering oxygen through a trach collar for three breaths. Before turning on the suction, insert the catheter into the airway until resistance is met. Pull the catheter back by 1 to 2 cm to place it in the tracheobronchial tree and apply suction continuously while rotating and withdrawing the catheter, taking no more than 10 to 15 s. Assess the patient frequently during suctioning. Reoxygenate the patient between insertions of the catheter and after the procedure, and ensure that the patient's oxygen source is reapplied after suctioning.

Some patients may have a Passey–Muir valve inserted in the trach stoma. This device contains a one-way valve that allows the patient to talk. If one is in place when the patient requires suctioning, it will need to be removed and reapplied when suctioning is complete. Placing the device on the tracheostomy often causes movement of the cannula which can stimulate a cough reflex. Mucous coughed through the valve is finely aerosoled and spreads a large distance; therefore, any time the valve is being handled, a face shield and gloves should be used.

SUGGESTED READINGS

Butler T, Close J, Close R. *Laboratory Exercises for Competency in Respiratory Care*. Philadelphia, PA: FA Davis; 1998.

Endotracheal suctioning. Available at: http://www.umdnj.edu/rspthweb/rstn2250/et_suctioning.htm. Accessed August 13, 2008.

KNOW THE SIGNS AND SYMPTOMS OF PULMONARY EMBOLISM: THEY MAY BE NONSPECIFIC

MELISSA H. CRIGGER, BSN, MHA, RN

WHAT TO DO: ASSESS

Remember that the signs and symptoms of pulmonary embolism (PE) are not always classic. Pulmonary embolism occurs when a foreign substance is carried through the bloodstream to the pulmonary blood vessel. Emboli can either be thrombus, fat, air, tumors, blood marrow, or clumps of bacteria. Patients who have recently had surgery are obese and have been immobile, and those with clotting abnormalities are at higher risk for the development of emboli. The effects of the emboli depend on how much perfusion to the lung is restricted; hence, a smaller embolus may cause little damage when compared to a larger one that is obstructing a larger major pulmonary vessel.

The patient with PE may have few to no symptoms at all. Classic symptoms include complaints of sudden chest pain that worsens with breathing. The patient will also have increased respiratory rate (tachypnea) and dyspnea. Tachycardia, crackles heard upon auscultation, hypoxemia, and cough with hemoptysis might also occur. Nonspecific signs and symptoms, like apprehension and confusion, could also be observed in those patients with PE and require the nurse to have a high index of suspicion.

When caring for the PE patient, the nurse should remember to obtain an adequate health history including present illness, any complaints of pain and dyspnea, and any past medical conditions, especially recent surgeries. The nurse should also remember to complete a thorough assessment of the respiratory system, which includes:

1. General survey including appearance, facial expressions, speech, and signs of obvious distress
2. Vital signs and pulse oximetry monitoring
3. Lips for pursed-lip breathing and color
4. Breathing pattern and use of accessory muscles
5. Auscultation of lung sounds
6. Extremities for color, edema, clubbing, or Homan sign.

Besides performing a respiratory assessment, the nurse must also remember to auscultate heart sounds and observe for peripheral edema, since these are signs of heart failure. The nurse should always check the lab studies, especially the arterial blood gas results, which directly measure tissue perfusion. The nurse will also want to monitor anticoagulation studies such as the PT/PTT, since anticoagulants are used as a primary treatment.

Patients with PE may become anxious due to increase in respiratory distress and pain. The nurse must remember to remain calm and to explain each procedure that is being performed. The patient should be encouraged to ask questions. The patients receiving anticoagulants must be educated that they must report any signs of bleeding, such as hematuria, bruising, and active bleeding, immediately to their healthcare team. The patient should avoid the use of standard razors and opt for the use of an electric razor.

Pulmonary emboli are emergencies that must be treated quickly. Knowing both the classic and not so classic signs and symptoms can assist the nurse in assessing these patients quickly and intervening rapidly.

SUGGESTED READINGS

Linton AD. Acute respiratory disorders. *Introduction to Medical–Surgical Nursing*. 4th Ed. St. Louis, MO: Saunders-Elsevier; 2007, pp. 509–547.

Williams LS, Hopper PD. Understanding the respiratory system. *Understanding Medical Surgical Nursing*. 2nd Ed. Philadelphia, PA: F.A. Davis Company; 2003, pp. 457–459.

KNOW THAT EXCESSIVE OXYGEN THERAPY IN THE COPD PATIENT MAY LEAD TO RESPIRATORY FAILURE

ELIZABETH A. GILBERT, ADN, BA-CS

WHAT TO DO: EVALUATE

Chronic Obstructive Pulmonary Disease (COPD) is the fourth leading cause of death in Americans. Risk factors for COPD include smoking, pollution, second hand smoke, and longstanding respiratory problems. COPD refers to two different lung problems: chronic bronchitis and emphysema. These are characterized by airflow obstruction, chronic cough, increased mucus production, and shortness of breath. Patients report activity limitations and intolerance. The onset is gradual, and it is frequently ignored until irreversible damage occurs to the lungs.

Caring for the COPD patient can be challenging. Management is most often aimed at symptom control and the prevention of complications. Patients with a COPD exacerbation are frequently quite anxious and complain of shortness of breath. They are most often oxygen dependent and routinely use bronchodilator medications such as albuterol. They may also be on antibiotics and steroids to reduce bronchial inflammation. When confronted with a patient experiencing an acute exacerbation of COPD, the nurse must remain calm and attempt to reassure the patient. It is helpful if the nurse is able to anticipate the patients' needs and provide for them before the anxiety increases. Often,

explaining the steps of treatment and what you are doing to help the shortness of breath is reassuring.

One common reflexive pitfall for nurses is to increase the oxygen received by the patient in response to the patient's complaint of shortness of breath. The nurse needs to remember that the COPD patient tolerates lower oxygen saturations better than those without COPD and increasing the liter flow/minute of oxygen may actually do more harm than good by increasing the patient's PCO_2, leading to CO_2 narcosis. Of course, hypoxic patients that are symptomatic should be treated with carefully titrated oxygen dosages and monitored for respiratory failure so that appropriate interventions can be provided as needed.

This information needs to be communicated to support staff, particularly if they are to transport the patient to other areas of the hospital. The nurse should ensure that medications such as IV steroids and antibiotics are administered in a timely manner, and providing antianxiety agents may alleviate the patient's feelings of suffocation. Encourage the patient to quit smoking and provide support for the patient and family as needed.

SUGGESTED READINGS

American Lung Association. Chronic obstructive pulmonary disease fact sheet, August 2006.

KNOW THE RISK FACTORS FOR OBSTRUCTIVE SLEEP APNEA IN YOUR PATIENTS

KATHERINE M. PENTURFF, RN, CAPA

WHAT TO DO: ASSESS AND EVALUATE

Sleep apnea is a phenomenon defined as a pause in breathing for more than 10 seconds during sleep despite continued ventilatory effort. Obstructive sleep apnea (OSA) is defined as the occurrence of at least five apneas or hypopneas per hour in association with symptoms attributable to sleep-disordered breathing. The incidence of patients presenting for surgery with OSA has been estimated to be as high as 9%. Adverse surgical outcomes appear to be more frequent in patients with known OSA, highlighting the importance of identifying these patients early to allow the interventions that will improve postoperative outcomes. OSA is undiagnosed in an estimated 80% of patients, so it is necessary that anesthesia providers have adequate knowledge of the clinical presentation and diagnosis of OSA. Although a sleep study remains the gold standard for the diagnosis of OSA, it may not be always available. A presumptive diagnosis of OSA can be made based on abnormal breathing during sleep, such as loud snoring and witnessed apnea, frequent arousals, excessive daytime sleepiness, body mass index > 35, increased neck circumference > 17 inches for males and 16 inches for females, and the presence of comorbidities. The American Society of Anesthesiologists' practice guidelines recommend scoring patients on the following characteristics to determine if a patient is at increased risk of anesthetic complications:

- Severity of sleep apnea based on sleep study
- Invasiveness of the surgery and the anesthesia
- Need for post-op opioids

The perioperative risk is based on the total points given in each category. Patients with OSA are more likely to have upper-airway obstruction, difficult tracheal intubation, and postoperative respiratory depression and airway obstruction. Patients with significantly increased risk are not good candidates for ambulatory surgery. Postoperative complications include airway obstruction, oxygen desaturation, and the need for reintubation as well as hypertension, dysrhythmias, and possible inpatient admission. Recurrent hypoxemia may be better treated with continuous positive airway pressure (CPAP) along with oxygen rather than oxygen alone. CPAP administered during sleep at night is the current treatment of OSA in the nonsurgical setting and it is thought that the perioperative use of CPAP will reduce the risk of postoperative complications. Supplemental oxygen should be administered continuously to all patients who are at increased perioperative risk from OSA until they are able to maintain their baseline oxygen saturation while breathing room air. Adequate postoperative respiratory function can be documented by observing patients in an unstimulated environment, preferably while they appear to be asleep, to establish that they are able to maintain their baseline oxygen saturation while breathing room air.

SUGGESTED READINGS

Joshi GP. Are patients with obstructive sleep apnea syndrome suitable for ambulatory surgery? *ASA Newslett.* 2006;70(1). Available at: www.asahq.org/Newsletters/2006/01–06/joshi01_06.html. Accessed August 13, 2008.

Kaw R, Michota F, Jaffer A, et al. Unrecognized sleep apnea in the surgical patient: Implications for the perioperative setting. *Chest.* 2006;129:198–205. Available at: www.chestjournal.org/cgi/content/full/129/1/198. Accessed August 13, 2008.

Practice guidelines for the perioperative management of patients with obstructive sleep apnea: A report by the American Society of Anesthesiologists Task Force on perioperative management of patients with obstructive sleep apnea. *Anesthesiology.* 2006;104:1081–1093. Available at: www.asahq.org/publicationsAndServices/sleepapnea103105.pdf. Accessed August 13, 2008.

When Shaving a Ventilated/Intubated Patient, Always Ensure That the Balloon of the ET Tube or Tracheal Has Been Moved Out of the Way of the Razor

Francine B. Yates, RRT, RN, BSN

WHAT TO DO: IMPLEMENT

Patient safety is always a priority in a medical setting, particularly a critical care setting. During the past decade, attention has increased regarding the issues of patient safety and human error in the medical field where adverse events or incidents are used as an indicator of quality and safety in healthcare. Beckmann et al. (1996) defined Intensive Care Unit (ICU) incidents as any unintended event or outcome that could, or did, reduce the safety margin for the patient.

As a rule, patients that are admitted to the ICU usually cannot perform their activities of daily living (ADLs). A part of the role of the ICU nurse is to perform this routine care for these patients and ensure that they are bathed, had mouth care, and are shaved. Even when performing ADLs, patient safety can be an issue. A task as simple as shaving an intubated patient can lead to a sequence of events that could increase the time spent in the ICU and the total length of stay in the hospital. A large number of patients are seriously harmed as a result of adverse events that occur when routine duties are performed.

Unfortunately, incidents or adverse events occur on a daily basis. A study measuring the prevalence of unintended events that compromise patient safety in 205 ICUs worldwide was conducted, which revealed that out of 1,913 patients, 47 patients with an artificial airway had an obstruction, leakage, or loss of due to an unintended event. When the airway is compromised, whether the balloon to the ETT is cut during shaving or the ETT was accidentally dislodged, it is imperative for the nurse to know what actions to take and be fully aware of the complications that can arise from such an event.

The ABCs should always be kept in mind. First and foremost, airway; protect and maintain the airway. Have an ambu bag at the bedside at all times when the patient is intubated or has a tracheostomy. If the patient is trached, make sure there is another tracheostomy tube with the obturator at the bedside since there is always the chance that the tube can become dislodged or pulled out by the patient. The second priority is breathing; make sure the patient is breathing. If the airway is blocked by secretions or the tracheostomy is not functioning properly, the patient will not be able to breathe. Assist the patient with an ambu bag if necessary until another support arrives. Use suction to remove secretions or replace the tracheostomy tube if there is a blockage. The third priority is circulation; make sure the patient still has a pulse after a respiratory arrest. If not, CPR should be initiated. Always check the pulse when someone has a compromised airway; a rhythm on the monitor is not always an accurate indication of a pulse.

Patient safety is always the first priority. In the ICU setting, patients are severely ill and require a higher level of care that provides more opportunity for mistakes and unintended events. Nurses caring for these patients must strive to minimize these mistakes to optimize patient care.

SUGGESTED READINGS

Beckmann U, Baldwin I, Hart GK, et al. The Australian Incident Monitoring Study in Intensive Care: AIMS-ICU. An analysis of the first year of reporting. *Anesth. Intens. Care.* 1996; 24:320–329.

Patient safety in intensive care: Results from the multinational sentinel events evaluation study. Available at: http://dx.doi.org/10.1007/s00134–006–0290–7. Accessed August 13, 2008.

AIR IS YELLOW AND OXYGEN IS GREEN

JEANNIE SCRUGGS GARBER, DNP, RN

WHAT TO DO: ASSESS

Most hospitals have gas outlets set up as green for oxygen and yellow for air; however, even though this is a standardized approach, confusion and error exists when setting up oxygen and air systems. Oxygen and air flow meters are generally close in proximity, identical in shape and appearance, and are only differentiated by color. Although not all, but some organizations also label the flow meters in an attempt to prevent error. The outlets are usually located within inches of each other and are visibly easy to confuse.

The "Christmas Tree" adapters used are also yellow and green but function equally on either flow meter. This allows for the clinician to use either color adapter on either flow meter, which can add confusion and mitigates the use of color as a safety net.

Oxygen is used routinely and in emergency situations but compressed air is more likely to be used for scheduled respiratory treatments. Both oxygen and air flow meters may stay hooked up at all times to maintain availability of equipment, for convenience, and to improve efficiency.

The most commonly discussed safety concern regarding oxygen and air outlets is when the tubing is connected to air while it should have been connected to oxygen. This error can lead to patient harm if not corrected immediately, especially in life threatening clinical situations. The Veterans Administration Central Office (2002) published the following suggestions to minimize the potential for errors regarding this color confusion:

"Purchase clear adaptors and avoid green–yellow confusion. When appropriate purchase compressed air tubing that does not require 'Christmas Tree' adapters, so adapters are not needed for air. Consider removing air flow meters when not in use; this may require addressing informal norms through training, incentives. More prominently label air and oxygen outlets. Respiratory Therapy, Nursing, and Pharmacy must work together for the smoothest implementation of any redesign or training."

Education, awareness, and communication are the key ingredients to address the green–yellow confusion and create a safer patient environment.

SUGGESTED READINGS

VA Central Office (2002). Confusion between oxygen and compressed air wall outlet. Available at: http://64.233.167.104/search?q=cache:cNkS9yjkijIJ:www.va.gov/NCPS/curriculum/TeachingMethods/Work_Rounds_Modullette_Format/Material/Modulette1_O2_Air_Handout.doc+oxygen+is+green+air+is+yellow&hl=en&ct=clnk&cd=1&gl=us. Accessed August 12, 2008.

THE MULTIPLE FACES OF PNEUMOTHORAX

EDWARD HUMERICKHOUSE, MS, MD

WHAT TO DO: ASSESS

Pneumothorax is the presence of air between the lung tissue and the chest wall. Normally, this space is occupied by a thin layer of fluid that lubricates the lungs as they slide past the ribs and other structures. Air in this space is never normal and can make quite the dramatic presentation. Here are a few case examples and how they are managed from a nursing point of view.

The first case is a 57-year-old thin white male with a 250 packs/year smoking history. He has emphysema that requires continuous home oxygen. He is on your floor for the third time this year with an exacerbation of his COPD. He has improved steadily since admission with frequent nebs, oxygen, and IV steroids. He was converted to oral steroids today and the team is planning to send him home tomorrow. He calls you to the room complaining of SEVERE left-sided chest pain that came on after a hard cough. The pain is sharp and worse with deep breathing. You listen to his lungs and find that you don't hear much on the left side, which is a change from when you examined him at the start of the shift. You also note that in the few moments you have been with him, he has gotten much more tachypneic and is now in distress from shortness of breath. A closer look shows that his trachea is starting to drift to the right. You punch the "code blue" button and call a colleague to check his vitals. He is rapidly deteriorating with hypoxia, further deviation of his trachea, tachycardia, hypotension, and impending loss of consciousness. You realize that what you are looking at is a tension pneumothorax in a patient who has no pulmonary reserve. With no time to lose, the code team pulls an 18 gauge IV off the code cart and pushes it into the left intercostal space under the second rib. There is a whistle of air, and the patient starts to improve immediately. A chest tube is placed and the patient is transferred to the ICU in stable condition. This patient had rupture of an emphysematous bulla.

The second case is a 70-year-old white female who was just admitted to the ICU with septic shock secondary to a UTI. The ICU team just completed placing a central line in her internal jugular vein. It took several attempts, but they were finally able to find the vein after placing the patient in steep trendelenburg position. Moving on to the next admission on another floor, a STAT portable chest X-ray is ordered. About five minutes after the film is taken, the radiologist calls up to the floor to notify the team of a small pneumothorax on the

right. Still busy, you report to the ICU resident over the phone that the patient is saturating well and starting to perk up a bit after several liters of IV fluids. She is in no distress. Despite normal O_2 sats, he orders 100% face mask oxygen for the next 24 h with a follow up chest X-ray in the morning. You are instructed to keep a close eye on the patient and the resident will be by to see her in an hour. The morning X-ray shows complete resolution of the pneumothorax. The high oxygen content in the blood helped absorb the air outside the lung which is mostly nitrogen.

The third case is a 25-year-old white male smoker. He presents to the ER with sharp, right-sided chest pain stating "I think I have another pneumothorax." He is in mild distress from pain, is a little tachycardic, and has mildly elevated blood pressure. He is not short of breath and his O_2 sats are normal. A plain chest X-ray shows a small pneumothorax on the right. You administer oxygen as in the second case, but the patient is rather shocked when you tell him that he is going to be admitted for a fairly major procedure in the morning. "Last time they just gave me oxygen for four hours then sent me home after a second chest XRAY showed it wasn't bigger." This patient has recurrent primary spontaneous pneumothorax (PSP) and likely has a family history of it. Most cases of PSP occur in patients in their 20s and it is unlikely to be "primary" (no history of lung disease) in patients over 40. It can present fairly benignly in this case or with rapid progression to tension pneumothorax as in the first case. The problem is that it reoccurred. With a single occurrence, the risk of recurrence is up to 50%. After a second occurrence, interventions must be made to eliminate the space between the lung and the chest wall (pleurodesis). In general, pleurodesis can cut recurrence rates by 50%, with some types of pleurodesis reducing recurrence to just 5%. An important note is that smoking increases risk of pneumothorax regardless of previous history of lung disease. Smoking cessation is an important point of intervention for all members of the healthcare team.

These cases cover the range of common presentations of pneumothorax. It is important to note that any pre-existing lung disease increases the risk for secondary spontaneous pneumothorax. It must be stressed to caregivers that even the most benign appearing air pocket can develop into life-threatening tension pneumothorax in a matter of seconds. The onset of shortness of breath with unstable vital signs, a trachea that has shifted, and loss of breath sounds over a lung field are medical emergencies that must be dealt with swiftly and accurately. Tension pneumothorax is not a daily occurrence, but nurses must be aware of it … especially in pulmonary patients.

SUGGESTED READINGS

Light R. Primary spontaneous pneumothorax in adults. Uptodate Online version 16.2. June 6, 2008. Available at: http://www.uptodate.com/patients/content/topic.do?topicKey=~wtt3ricasnY9e/. Accessed August 20, 2008.

Light R. Secondary spontaneous pneumothorax in adults. Uptodate Online Version 16.2. September 21, 2001. Available at: http://www.uptodate.com/patients/content/topic.do?topicKey=~cZPcV7O4FMHBQw&selectedTitle=1~12&source=search_result. Accessed August 20, 2008.

KNOW HOW OXYGEN AFFECTS CO_2 IN PATIENTS WITH CHRONIC LUNG DISEASE

EDWARD HUMERICKHOUSE, MS, MD

WHAT TO DO: EVALUATE

There is a common notion among physicians and nurses that if you give oxygen (O_2) to patients with COPD, they will fall asleep and stop breathing. The basic idea behind this is that patients with chronic lung disease get accustomed to high carbon dioxide (CO_2) levels and so their drive to breathe is now based on low blood O_2. By that notion, if you give them O_2, they have no trigger to breathe. Without the trigger, CO_2 builds to levels of narcosis and death. While the physiology is mostly wrong, it is true that giving TOO MUCH O_2 to a patient with chronic hypercapnia (high blood CO_2) will cause an increase in CO_2. If the CO_2 goes above 90 to 100 in a chronic retainer, you will start to see some altered levels of consciousness.

There are three main ways that this occurs. The primary culprit is ventilation/perfusion mismatch. The lungs have a tidy little program where areas of the lung that do not provide O_2 (diseased areas) do not get blood flow. By giving high O_2 flow, there is enough stimulus to resume blood flow to these diseased areas, but no gas exchange takes place. You have perfusion (blood) with no ventilation (gas exchange). This results in the majority of CO_2 retention.

The second reason that CO_2 level rises during high flow O_2 therapy is in the blood cells themselves. In addition to binding O_2 for transport to tissues, hemoglobin in red blood cells also traps CO_2. The ability to bind CO_2 is decreased in the presence of O_2. This works to the body's advantage in healthy lungs; hemoglobin binds to O_2 which causes CO_2 to be released and exhaled. In diseased lungs receiving high flow O_2, the CO_2 is released directly into the blood stream. It stays in the blood longer than usual because of the effects of the ventilation/perfusion mismatch mentioned above.

The final contributor to CO_2 narcosis during O_2 therapy is the actual reduced rate of breathing. There are those who would argue that there is no such thing as the "hypoxic" drive and the decrease in respiration is from the narcosis caused by the first two. Regardless of this, it does happen and accounts for a significant minority of the total CO_2 increase.

Now that we know why CO_2 levels increase with high flow of O_2 in patients who have pulmonary disease, how does it affect our patients? CO_2 increases the amount of GABA (and other neurotransmitters) in the brain. GABA affects the brain in the same way as alcohol, benzodiazepines (valium), and barbiturates. As the CO_2 rises by about 20 mm Hg, the patient becomes drowsy but will cooperate with therapy and the CO_2 will go down back to baseline over the next 12 h. If the CO_2 rises by 30 mm Hg or more per hour, the patient will rapidly lose consciousness, stop breathing, and die unless appropriate intervention is made.

The prevention of CO_2 narcosis in the face of O_2 therapy revolves around the goal of O_2 saturation. In general, they need to be saturating at >87% but less than 92% to 93%. Any saturation greater than 93% does not increase tissue oxygenation; it only increases the effects of ventilation/perfusion mismatching and CO_2 unloading from hemoglobin. On the other side, tissue hypoxia at low O_2 saturations is unacceptable because just 4 to 6 min of brain hypoxia can lead to irreversible damage.

The best way to provide O_2 is through a venturi mask. It gives tight control over the O_2 percentage delivered with more guarantee that they are actually inhaling it. Increase the O_2 slowly while giving appropriate treatment to reopen the airways. Aim for a goal of 88% to 90% saturation. If the patient is starting to show signs of confusion or unresponsiveness, then transfer to the ICU for prompt intubation or noninvasive mask ventilation. Should you "inherit" a patient who has been on inappropriate levels of high flow O_2 and is getting somnolent, slowly decrease the O_2 flow. Stopping treated patient's O_2 will suddenly result in even lower O_2 sats than when they presented with little improvement in the CO_2 level.

Remember, do not withhold O_2 to people who need it. Hypoxia is far more dangerous than hypercapnia. Give O_2 slowly via venturi mask and titrate to a goal of 88% to 90%. If you are not able to reach that goal without causing somnolence, then the patient requires at least noninvasive mask ventilation and possibly intubation and mechanical ventilation. In the same regard, if your patient was already given high flow O_2 and is now showing high O_2 saturations and drowsiness, do not simply stop the O_2 but titrate it down.

SUGGESTED READINGS

Feller-Kopman D, Schwartzstein R. Use of oxygen in patients with hypercapnia. Uptodate Online vs 16.2. February 13, 2008. Available at: http://www.uptodate.com/patients/content/topic.do?topicKey=~vCpu.rbRZk&selectedTitle=2~143&source=search_result. Accessed August 20, 2008.

Panettieri R, Fisman A. Chronic obstructive pulmonary disease disorders. In: Fishman A, ed. *Fishman's Manual of Pulmonary Diseases and Disorders*. 3rd Ed. New York: McGraw-Hill; 2002, pp. 105–109.

PNEUMONIA CAN BE A BIGGER PROBLEM THAN YOU THINK: GET THE ANTIBIOTICS IN QUICKLY

ANTHONY D. SLONIM, MD, DRPH

WHAT TO DO: ASSESS

Pneumonia is one of the most common reasons for hospitalization and represents a constellation of findings. While usually considered a treatable illness, pneumonia can be devastating and can lead to mortality. Pneumonia is commonly classified as community acquired or hospital acquired depending upon very specific criteria.

From a clinical perspective, a patient with pneumonia may have fever, shortness of breath, dyspnea, chest pain, and may produce sputum. The patient will exhibit several signs on his or her physical examination including warm skin, wheezes, rhonchi, crackles, and perhaps dullness to percussion if there is the presence of a parapneumonic effusion. Diagnostic testing may reveal an elevated white blood cell count and an infiltrate on the chest X-ray. While these signs are typical, patients at the extremes of age or with an immunocompromised status may present in atypical ways. For example, infants and the elderly may have low white blood cell counts and be unable to mount a fever. The immunocompromised patient without neutrophils may be unable to produce sputum.

Patients with pneumonia can present in a number of different ways, but the management is important and should be provided in a timely manner. First, these patients need support of their airway and if it cannot be maintained, they require oxygen and monitoring of their oxygen saturations. If their circulation is becoming impaired and sepsis is becoming established, the support with IV fluids and vasoactive medications may be necessary. Finally, and most importantly, the patient requires the timely administration of antibacterial agents.

Antibacterial agents are often based upon an empiric trial of what is the most common offending organism based upon age and history. Well established guidelines help with the selection of antibacterials depending upon the most likely pathogen, but even the best agents will be useless if they remain in the pharmacy or pyxis machine.

Pneumonia is a common disease that requires prompt administration of antibacterial agents. Someone's life may depend upon it.

SUGGESTED READINGS

Mandell LA, Wunderink RG, Anzueto A, et al. Infectious Diseases Society of America/American Thoracic Society consensus guidelines on the management of community-acquired pneumonia in adults. *Clin Infect Dis.* 2007;44:S27–S72. Available at: http://www.journals.uchicago.edu/doi/pdf/10.1086/ 511159? cookieSet=1. Accessed August 20, 2008.

Misdiagnosis of Pneumonia. Available at: http://www. wrongdiagnosis.com/p/pneumonia/misdiag.htm. Accessed August 20, 2008.

IMPORTANCE OF PREOPERATIVE TEACHING FOR PATIENTS AND FAMILIES

JEANNIE SCRUGGS GARBER, DNP, RN

WHAT TO DO: PLAN

It is important to prepare the patient and family for the surgical and postoperative experience to minimize concerns and support expectations of recovery. The patient and family may have previous experiences with surgery that impact their beliefs and attitudes about the procedure. The nurse can serve as the link between the patient and family's presurgical assumptions and knowledge and postsurgical expectations.

Preoperative education should occur to some extent for every procedure performed. It is important for the basic information to be shared regarding the technical performance of the surgery and to discuss the intended results beyond the discussion that is required to meet informed consent standards. The best preoperative discussions occur with both the patient and the family. This allows for multiple individuals to participate in the education process and ask questions from multiple perspectives. For example, the patient may be most concerned about pain management while the family may be focused on potential discharge date. Interacting with the group will create more questions and answers and will improve the overall understanding of the surgical experience.

Other topics that can be discussed include where families wait during surgery, how soon the family can visit the patient, how often they can visit, what equipment will be visible, physical appearance of the patient, and anticipated recovery in nursing units such as critical care, progressive care, or medical surgical care. It is also important to discuss anticipated time frames for progress toward discharge and from which area in the hospital. The patient and family may also be concerned about pain control, nutrition (when can he or she eat regular food again), and how soon he or she can resume presurgical activity levels. These discussions extend beyond the routine explanation of the surgical procedure and address the emotional and intellectual expectations of the event.

Outcomes that are routinely measured postoperatively can be positively impacted by patient-centered preoperative education. It is widely accepted that patient outcomes such as reduced infection rates, patient and family satisfaction, treatment compliance, and length of stay are positively impacted by patients being well informed and aware of expectations regarding their care. St Jacques and colleagues (Hawes, 2006) report that patient education regarding surgical and anesthesia procedures, postoperative pain therapy, feeding, and logistic issues reduces delays, cancellations, and length of postoperative hospital stays.

Education and awareness are critical elements for error prevention and communication concerns. The nurse–patient relationship affords the opportunity to create a safe, open dialogue that will minimize fear and positively influence recovery.

SUGGESTED READINGS

Hawes D. Integrated Preoperative Patient Care. Prompte improving the convenience of quality care. 2006. Available at: http://www.prompte.com/integrated_preoperative_patient_care.pdf. Accessed August 6, 2008.

PREOPERATIVE USE OF HERBAL PREPARATIONS: IF YOU DO NOT ASK, THEY WILL NOT TELL

KATHERINE M. PENTURFF, RN, CAPA

WHAT TO DO: ASSESS

Most patients realize the importance of telling their physicians about their prescriptions and many carry detailed lists of the name, dose, and frequency of each prescription that they are taking. However, the same conscientious patients may consider herbal remedies and vitamins to be natural supplements rather than medicines. As many as 70% of patients who use herbal remedies or vitamins do not reveal the use of these preparations to their healthcare providers. There has been a recent increase in the use of herbal remedies in the United States for several reasons. The high cost of prescription medicines has driven many people to use what they may consider lower-cost alternatives. Increases in travel and exposure to other cultures have revived and expanded many ancient traditions. In a safety-conscious nation, advertising such products as "safe" and "all natural" has increased their appeal to the public. Herbs can be derived from flowers, shrubs, trees, algae, ferns, fungi, seaweeds, and grasses. They can be used fresh, dried, in alcohol (as tinctures), steeped as teas, simmered (decoctions), or may be extracted from vinegar, syrups, vegetable glycerin, or honey.

Echinacea, ephedra, garlic, ginkgo, ginseng, kava, St. John's wort, and valerian are some of the more commonly used herbal medications that may pose a concern during the perioperative period. A quick rule of thumb is that many herbals starting with the letter "G" may pose a perioperative hazard. Direct effects include bleeding from feverfew, garlic, ginger, ginkgo, and ginseng.

Cardiovascular instability can arise from ephedra, valerian, goldenseal, and licorice, increased sedative effects of anesthesia from kava, St. John's wort, and valerian, and hypoglycemia from ginseng.

Much inconsistency exists in the manufacture, potency, purity, and promotion of health claims regarding herbal preparations. They are not held to the same standards and regulations that the FDA maintains for the pharmaceutical industry. Although the Dietary Supplement Health and Education Act of 1994 placed the burden of product safety assurance on the manufacturer, the FDA has the responsibility to prove that the product is unsafe. Therefore, the product can only be removed from the market if the FDA has reason to suspect that it is unsafe.

Because of the potential risks associated with preoperative herbal use, the American Society of Anesthesiologists (ASA) suggests that all herbal medications should be discontinued 2 to 3 weeks prior to an elective surgical procedure. If a patient is unsure of what type of herbal preparation he is taking, he should be instructed to bring all bottles for evaluation. In the emergency setting, a thorough drug-intake history should be obtained from the patient or relative, including all herbal preparations and vitamins, so that proper precautions can be taken to prevent complications.

SUGGESTED READINGS

Ang-Lee MK, Moss J, Yuan C-S. Herbal medicines and perioperative care. *J Am Med Assoc.* 2001;286:208–216.

Herbal Medicines and Anesthesia. Available at: www.utsouthwestern.edu/utsw/cda/dept20768/files/78782.html. Accessed August 6, 2008.

Tsen LC, Segal S, Bader M, et al. Alternative medicine use in presurgical patients. *Anesthesiology.* 2000;93(1):148–151.

PREOPERATIVE USE OF DIET PILLS, ANOTHER "DO NOT ASK—WILL NOT TELL"

KATHERINE M. PENTURFF, RN, CAPA

WHAT TO DO: ASSESS

Obesity is a chronic condition that affects many people and the medications may be used to manage this condition. When patients who are on weight-reduction medications are facing surgery, precautions must be taken to avoid potentially dangerous interactions with certain anesthetic agents. Anesthesia providers recommend that weight-loss supplements be stopped 1 to 2 weeks prior to surgery. Two commonly prescribed appetite-suppressants that cause particular concern for the preoperative patient are sibutramine and phentermine. Some over-the-counter (OTC) weight-loss supplements are also contraindicated for these patients.

Sibutramine (Meridia®) is a controlled substance (Schedule IV) approved by the FDA for long-term use in weight management for people who need to lose more than 30 lb. Common side effects of sibutramine include increased blood pressure and pulse, since it acts on both the serotonin and catecholamine systems. Interaction with other medications, including some anesthetics, can result in Serotonin Syndrome, a potentially life-threatening condition characterized by confusion, myoclonus, hyper-reflexia, restlessness, ataxia, muscle rigidity, and nausea. While the symptoms are usually mild in most patients, it can progress quickly if left untreated. Because many of the early symptoms may be masked by or attributed to general anesthesia, identification and treatment may be delayed, leading to more serious outcomes. Mortality associated with Serotonin Syndrome is estimated to be approximately 11%. For these reasons, sibutramine should be stopped at least 2 weeks before elective procedures.

Phentermine hydrochloride (brand names Ionamin and Adipex-P) is a sympathomimetic amine similar to amphetamines, the prototype drugs of this class used in obesity. It is also a schedule IV controlled substance and acts as a central nervous system stimulant. Side effects include palpitations, tachycardia, hypertension, hypotension, and circulatory collapse. It is also typically discontinued 10 to 14 days prior to surgery.

Ephedra and ephedrine alkaloids are another class of medications that were previously used for OTC weight loss supplements. Derived from the Chinese botanical "Ma-huang," ephedra was banned by the FDA for sale in 2004 for weight loss and energy-enhancing products. Although less prevalent than before 2004, OTC derivatives of the botanical Ma-huang are available in the foreign market, and synthetic derivatives, ephedrine and pseudoephedrine, are available for medical use primarily as bronchodilators. Use and discontinuation of these preparations should be discussed with an anesthesia provider prior to surgery. While discontinuation of these medications preoperatively may be indicated, they should not be stopped suddenly without medical supervision.

Because of the lack of controlled studies regarding the safety and the inconsistency of the purity of herbal supplements, many anesthesia providers recommend stopping all herbal weight-loss supplements 2–3 weeks before undergoing an elective procedure. Thorough preoperative interviewing of patients will help identify those who are on medications or supplements that place them at risk of avoidable anesthetic complications.

SUGGESTED READINGS

Boyer EW, Shannon M. The serotonin syndrome. *N Engl J Med.* 2005;252(11):1112–1120.

Heyneman CA. Preoperative considerations: Which herbal products should be discontinued before surgery. *Crit Care Nurse.* 2003;23(2):116–124.

MERIDIA® (sibutramine HCl monohydrate) Capsules C-IV Use and Safety Information, MERIDIA_net. Available at: www.meridia.net/dsp_consumer_safety.html. Accessed August 6, 2008.

Nolan S, Bowld WJ, Scoggin A. Serotonin syndrome recognition and management. Available at: www.uspharmacist.com/oldformat.asp?url=newlook/files/feat/acf2fa6.htm.

Phentermine—Official FDA information, side effects and use. Available at: www.drugs.com/phentermine.html.

Tiner J, Miles R, Newland M. Recommendations and guidelines for preoperative evaluation of the surgical patient with emphasis on the cardiac patient for non-cardiac surgery. University of Nebraska Medical Center. 2006. Available at: webmedia.unmc.edu/anesthesia/Anesthesia%20Guide.pdf. Accessed August 6, 2008.

WIN Publication. Prescription medications for the treatment of obesity. Available at: win.niddk.nih.gov/publications/prescription.htm#meds. Accessed August 6, 2008.

DISCONTINUE MEDICATIONS BEFORE SURGERY

KATHERINE M. PENTURFF, RN, CAPA

When obtaining a patient's medical history, it is important to ask not only what medicines he is currently taking but also what medicines he has taken and discontinued in the last 2 to 3 weeks. Patients often do not realize the significance of "past" medications and may not reveal their recent use. When questioned about recent medication use, many patients will respond saying that they have not used a particular medicine in 2 to 3 days believing the medication to have lost any efficacy or side effects. Some medications continue to exert an influence on cardiac status and fluid and electrolyte balance for several weeks after their ingestion, such as corticosteroids, diuretics, monoamine oxidase inhibitors, and some weight reduction medications.

Corticosteroids are synthetic drugs that resemble cortisol, a hormone that is naturally produced by the adrenal glands, reducing inflammation and the activity of the immune system. When a patient has been on corticosteroids for more than 2 to 3 months, natural cortisol production by the adrenal glands is suppressed and may not be stimulated effectively if the patient is suddenly stressed, for example, by surgery. This acute adrenocortical insufficiency can precipitate hypotension and death; therefore, anesthesiologists must be informed when patients have taken 10 mg or more per day of corticosteroids within 3 months of surgery. This is necessary to continue maintenance doses for minor surgery or supplemental doses for moderate to major surgery.

If patients have taken diuretics, it is important for the healthcare provider to know why they were taken and why the patient stopped them. Inquire if the physician discontinued the medication due to a change in the patient's condition, or if the patient stopped it because of difficulty getting to the bathroom in time, a complaint heard frequently from orthopedic patients preparing for joint replacement. A patient who takes a diuretic for occasional dependent edema is not as likely to be affected by holding it preoperatively as a patient who takes one for congestive heart failure. Such a patient is more likely to become fluid overloaded during surgery with serious consequences, since diuretics have been shown to reduce the risk of death, delay heart deterioration, and improve exercise capacity in patients with congestive heart failure.

Monoamine oxidase inhibitors are a class of drugs used to treat depression in patients who do not respond to other, more commonly used drugs. Because of a potentially fatal reaction when these drugs are taken with other medications, especially some narcotics, it is important for an anesthesia provider to know if the patient has taken these within 2 to 3 weeks prior to surgery.

Meridia, an appetite suppressant, exhibits the common side effects of hypertension and tachycardia, and may have interactions with other medications, including some anesthetics. These interactions can result in Serotonin Syndrome—a potentially life-threatening condition characterized by a number of mental, autonomic, and neuromuscular changes.

SUGGESTED READINGS

Boyer EW, Shannon M. The serotonin syndrome. *N Engl J Med.* 2005;252(11):1112–1120.

Corticosteroids and corticosteroid replacement therapy. Available at: www.patient.co.uk/showdoc/40025317. Accessed August 6, 2008.

Monoamine oxidase inhibitors (MAOIs). Available at: www.mayoclinic.com/health/maois/MH00072. Accessed August 6, 2008.

Stevens LM. Diuretics reduce risk of death from congestive heart failure. Health Behavior News Service. Available at: todaysseniorsnetwork.com/diurectics_help.htm Accessed August 6, 2008.

What you need to know about corticosteroids. Available at: www.clevelandclinic.org/arthritis/treat/facts/steroids.htm. Accessed August 6, 2008.

MEDICATIONS FOR ERECTILE DYSFUNCTION AND THE PREOPERATIVE PATIENT

KATHERINE M. PENTURFF, RN, CAPA

WHAT TO DO: ASSESS

Erectile dysfunction (ED) is the inability to develop and maintain an erection for satisfactory sexual intercourse or activity in the absence of an ejaculatory disorder for at least 3 months. In the past, ED was often assumed to be either a psychologic problem or a normal part of the aging process, but ED is now known to be primarily organic, resulting from vascular, hormonal, or neurologic complications. In the United States, at least 10 to 20 million men less than18 years of age are affected. The prevalence of partial or complete ED is about 50% in men 40 to 70 years of age and increases with aging. Because of the sensitive nature of the disorder, many men who experience ED are reluctant to tell anyone, including their healthcare providers, that they are being treated for this condition.

Current treatment options include oral medications, surgical treatment, injections, and mechanical devices. Since the introduction of the first of the very effective oral phosphodiesterase type 5 inhibitors (PDE5 inhibitors) in 1998, other treatment options are being used less frequently. PDE5 inhibitors, marketed under the names of sildenafil (Viagra), vardenafil (Levitra), and tadalafil (Cialis), work by preventing the breakdown of phosphodiesterase type 5 in the corpus cavernosum during sexual arousal. All three drugs are contraindicated in patients who use nitroglycerin or nitrate-containing compounds, such as isosorbide mononitrate (Ismo, Monoket, Imdur), isosorbide dinitrate (Isordil, Sorbitrate), sublingual nitroglycerin tablets or spray (Nitro stat, Nitro lingual Spray), and transdermal nitroglycerin patches or paste (Minitran, Nitro-Dur, Transderm-Nitro). All PDE5 inhibitors cause direct coronary vasodilatation and potentiate the hypotensive effects of other nitrates, including those used to treat cardiovascular disease as well as recreational amyl nitrate, known as "poppers." For this reason, all nitrates are contraindicated for 24 h after the administration of any PDE5 inhibitor. These drugs can be of particular concern in the surgical setting if an anesthesia provider is unaware that the patient has had recent PDE5 inhibitors and prescribes nitrates for management of hypertension or reduced cardiac perfusion in the perioperative setting. It is vital that patients being treated with any PDE5 inhibitor be educated regarding the importance of disclosing this information to any healthcare provider. Nurses should be careful to obtain complete and accurate patient medical histories, including current and recent medication use, when admitting a patient to the hospital or when screening in a presurgical testing area for an upcoming surgery. Patients who have been identified prior to their surgery to be on a PDE5 inhibitor should be instructed to avoid its use for at least 24 h preoperatively.

SUGGESTED READINGS

Anawalt BD. Male sexual dysfunction. Last full review/revision June 2007. Available at: www.merck.com/mmpe/sec17/ch227/ch227c.html?qt=Vardenafil&alt=sh. Accessed August 6, 2008.

Lakin M. Erectile dysfunction. Available at: www.clevelandclinicmeded.com/medicalpubs/diseasemanagement/endocrinology/erectile/erectile.htm. Accessed August 6, 2008.

Make sure your preoperative patient is NPO

Katherine M. Penturff, RN, CAPA

Many patients understand preoperative diet instructions of NPO, from the Latin nulla per os, to be important to prevent nausea or vomiting post surgically. Few patients realize that the risk from having a full stomach when having general anesthesia, regional anesthesia, MAC (monitored anesthesia care), or even conscious sedation is much more serious than postoperative discomfort. Patients who are under the impression that NPO instructions are intended only to prevent postoperative nausea and vomiting and who have never had an issue with this in the past may be tempted toward noncompliance.

NPO after midnight on the day of surgery was initiated approximately 60 years ago as a practice that was intended to keep the stomach empty during surgery. Decreased gastric contents may prevent vomiting that could cause a patient to choke to death or aspiration of stomach contents into the lungs during surgery, which puts the patient at risk for aspiration pneumonia. In the past, NPO instructions for patients tended to be rigid and did not meet the needs of individual patients. Most facilities used "NPO past midnight" regardless of the patient's time of surgery, age, or the procedure to be done. This attempt to ensure an empty stomach caused hardships on some patient groups, especially infants and small children who could dehydrate quickly when deprived of oral intake for long periods of time.

Current recommendations by the American Society of Anesthesiologists (ASA) are more flexible and designed to meet the needs and comfort of the patient while maintaining his safety. The ASA Task Force on Preoperative Fasting now recommends that healthy patients of all ages should fast from solid food or nonhuman milk, including infant formula, at least six or more hours before elective procedures requiring general anesthesia, regional anesthesia, or sedation/analgesia, that is, MAC. If a meal is eaten ≥6h before surgery, it should be a light meal such as toast and clear liquids only, since fatty foods and proteins are subject to delayed gastric emptying. For neonates and infants who are breastfeeding, fasting is recommended for 4h. The Task Force also recommends fasting from intake of clear liquids for 2h before procedures requiring anesthesia or sedation. Clear liquids include, but are not limited to, water, fruit juices without pulp, carbonated beverages, clear tea, and black coffee. These recommendations apply to healthy patients who are undergoing elective procedures. They are not intended for women in labor or patients with other conditions that would affect gastric emptying or gastric volume such as pregnancy, obesity, diabetes, hiatal hernia, gastroesophageal reflux disease, ileus or bowel obstruction, emergency care, or enteral tube feeding.

These guidelines are not intended to override any instructions given by the patient's surgeon, who may have specific reasons for wanting a patient to be NPO longer than generally recommended. Educating patients on not only what they should do but also the rationale behind what they are asked to do may help improve their compliance and therefore improve the safety of having anesthesia with their procedures.

SUGGESTED READINGS

Margolis S. To fast or not to fast before surgery? *Yahoo Health News*. 2006. Available at: health.yahoo.com/experts/healthnews/123/to-fast-or-not-to-fast-before-surgery.

Practice guidelines for preoperative fasting and the use of pharmacologic agents to reduce the risk of pulmonary aspiration: Application to healthy patients undergoing elective procedures — A Report by the American Society of Anesthesiologists Task Force on Preoperative Fasting. Available at: www.asahq.org/publicationsAndServices/NPO.pdf.

REMOVE JEWELRY PREOPERATIVELY TO PREVENT SWELLING AND BURNS

JEANNIE SCRUGGS GARBER, DNP, RN

WHAT TO DO: IMPLEMENT

Healthcare facilities routinely have policies and procedures regarding the removal or taping of jewelry during surgical procedures. These policies are developed to minimize the risk of injury to the patient. If jewelry is not removed, there is an increased risk of swelling and burn at the jewelry site.

Swelling occurs during surgery due to tissue injury and fluid administration. Jewelry should be removed preoperatively to prevent additional swelling and to ensure that jewelry can be removed voluntarily and need not have to be cut off postoperatively due to swelling.

The risk of burns during surgery is a result of electrocauterization which may be used to stop bleeding. This instrument relies on an electrical current. If the patient is wearing metal jewelry that is in contact with his or her skin, an electrical burn may occur in the area of contact. A recent trend in body piercing has created further discussion of jewelry in the operating room. Body piercing is recognized as a common form of self-expression all over the world, yet there is little published literature regarding the specific care of these patients in the perianesthesia environment. It is recommended that all jewelry be removed, including body piercing, prior to an operative procedure.

The solution to this patient safety risk is fairly simple. Follow the healthcare organization policy and include removal of jewelry in the presurgical checklist process. The objective is to prevent patient injury and harm, and a simple, direct communication between patient and care giver can ensure the appropriate action. The human factors such as remembering to ask, providing the correct explanation, and the patients' acceptance of the request are the main factors to be considered in making this simple task occur for all operating room patients.

SUGGESTED READINGS

Jacobs VR, Morrison JE, Paepke S, et al. Body piercing affecting laparoscopy: Perioperative precautions. *J Am Assoc Gynecol Laparosc.* 2004;11(4):537–541.

Sheehan K. Communicating pre-operative instructions. *Can Oper Room Nurs J.* March 2005. Available at: http://findarticles.com/p/articles/mi_qa4130/is_200503/ai_n13639421. Accessed August 30, 2008.

ALLERGIES TO LATEX: HOW DO YOU KNOW?

JEANNIE SCRUGGS GARBER, DNP, RN

WHAT TO DO: ASSESS

Latex is everywhere in the healthcare environment. It can be found in gloves, tubing, tape, syringes, electrodes, ventilator equipment, etc. The incidence of allergic reactions to latex is increasing; therefore, identification and treatment is a priority for nurses. According to Behrman (2007), 1% to 5% of the population is latex to sensitive and patients with spina bifida, a history of numerous surgeries or healthcare events wherein they were exposed to latex are at a higher risk of experiencing latex allergy. Behrman (2007) also reports that some tropical fruits may also be linked to an increased risk of latex allergy. Agarwal and Gawkrodger (2002) report that the incidence is possibly 17% in healthcare workers and that prevention should be focused on the highest risk groups.

Nurses and other clinicians should be aware of the prevalence and risk of latex allergy in patients and providers. The nurse should include specific questions to patients regarding latex allergies when completing an assessment and addressing allergies in general. Patient assessment should also include an observation of any alert bracelets or jewelry. Skin should be assessed for integrity, color, as well as for the presence of rash or irritation.

In the event the patient has a known allergy to latex, latex-free gloves and equipment must be used to provide care. Patient education is the best course of prevention and treatment for latex allergy. Many healthcare organizations have latex-free standards for the operating room to prevent latex exposure to those who are at risk. Patients who have known allergies to latex should consider wearing Medi-Alert bracelets and/or have epinephrine available at all times. Latex allergy is a complex issue and needs further clinical research. Product development, manufacturing, and desensitization will be the work of the future.

SUGGESTED READINGS

Agarwal S, Gawkrodger D. Latex allergy: A health care problem of epidemic proportions. *Eur J Dermatol*. 2002;12(4):311–315.

Behrman A. Latex allergy. 2007. Available at: http://www.emedicine.com/emerg/topic814.htm#section~AuthorsandEditors. Accessed August 29, 2008.

INFORMED CONSENT: IS THE PATIENT REALLY INFORMED?

JEANNIE SCRUGGS GARBER, DNP, RN

WHAT TO DO: ASSESS

Informed consent is possibly one of the most important developments in the history of patients' rights. The concept was originally written in the 1947 Nuremberg Code for human experiments and now applies to medical and surgical treatment. This doctrine requires physicians to share certain information with patients before asking for their consent to treatment. Dictionary definitions of informed consent include: "a patient's consent to a medical or surgical procedure or to participation in a clinical study after being properly advised of the relevant medical facts and the risks involved, consent by a patient to a surgical or medical procedure or participation in a clinical study after achieving an understanding of the relevant medical facts and the risks involved or consent by a patient to undergo a medical or surgical treatment or to participate in an experiment after the patient understands the risks involved." (Informed consent, n.d.)

The clinician surely agrees with the above definitions and the intent of the laws surrounding informed consent; however, are patients really informed? For consent to be valid, "the patient must be competent, have adequate information to make a decision, and must not be under duress" (Department of Health, 2001 as cited in Anderson & Wearne, 2007). Making sure all of these criteria are met is difficult.

Nursing professionals are at the center of this dilemma: did the patient sign the consent and did he or she receive the information needed? Nurses, as patient advocates, are responsible for making sure that the patient is educated about the procedures and that the consent form is obtained, yet they may have little awareness of the actual process that occurs when the physician obtains the consent. It is within the nurses' role to assess whether or not the patient has a clear understanding of the impending procedure, what it is intended to accomplish, and whether or not the patient has an understanding about the risks, benefits, and alternatives. It is the physician's role to determine what and how information regarding the procedure is conducted. *The nurses should not obtain consent for a physician's procedures since they cannot sufficiently provide appropriate guidance to the patient for the risks, benefits, and alternatives.* Doing so jeopardizes the advocacy role the nurse has in the consent process.

The process of informed consent is an opportunity for physicians, nurses, and patients to work together to guide decision making and ultimately improve patient outcomes. The nurse is in an ideal position to follow up with patients after the informed consent is obtained to determine if the information shared was understood by asking open ended questions such as:

- Tell me about your discussion with your physician regarding your surgical consent.
- Tell me about the alternatives to surgery you discussed.
- What questions do you have for me about your surgery and your recovery?

These questions and discussion will clue the nurse into any areas that may need further explanation by the physician so that the patient can be fully informed. The clinician must avoid rushing through the informed consent process—time might be saved at the moment but at what cost?

SUGGESTED READINGS

Anderson O, Wearne M. Informed consent for elective surgery-what is best practice? *J R Soc Med*. 2007;100:97–100.

Informed consent. (n.d.). *The American Heritage® Dictionary of the English Language*. 4th Ed. Available at: http://dictionary.reference.com/browse/informed consent. Accessed August 6, 2008.

KNOW THE PROBLEMS ASSOCIATED WITH BOWEL PREPARATION PRIOR TO ENDOSCOPY

JEANNIE SCRUGGS GARBER, DNP, RN

WHAT TO DO: IMPLEMENT

On May 5, 2006, the U.S. Food and Drug Administrations (FDA) notified healthcare professionals and consumers of reports of acute phosphate nephropathy, a type of acute renal failure that is a rare, but serious adverse event associated with the use of oral sodium phosphates (OSP) for bowel cleansing. There is an increased risk of acute phosphate nephropathy for older individuals, individuals with kidney disease or decreased intravascular volume, and those using medicines that affect kidney function. When acute phosphate nephropathy occurs, renal impairment may be permanent and require chronic dialysis.

The FDA suggests that the following be considered when choosing a bowel cleanser for patients:

- Avoid use of OSP in patients with kidney disease, impaired renal function, perfusion, dehydration, or uncorrected electrolyte abnormalities.
- Avoid exceeding recommended OSP doses and concomitant use of laxatives containing sodium phosphate.
- Use OSP with caution in patients taking diuretics, ACE inhibitors, ARBs, and NSAIDs.
- Encourage patients to take the correct OSP dose and drink sufficient quantities of clear fluids during bowel cleansing.
- Obtain baseline and postprocedure labs (electrolytes, calcium, phosphate, BUN, and creatinine) in patients who may be at increased risk for acute phosphate nephropathy, including those with vomiting and/or signs of dehydration.
- Use hospitalization and intravenous hydration during bowel cleansing to support frail patients who may be unable to drink an appropriate volume of fluid or may be without assistance at home.

Healthcare providers must be aware of and monitor the risks associated with OSP therapy such as:

- Dehydration
- Abdominal pain or bloating
- Nausea
- Vomiting
- Headache
- Dizziness

Healthcare providers should assess the following as a part of patient preparation and education regarding bowel cleansing:

- Diet status
- Medications (especially diuretics, herbal supplements, etc.)
- Use of laxatives recently
- History of kidney problems
- Presence of other medical conditions

In order to prevent acute or chronic renal compromise as a complication of endoscopy procedure preparation, the healthcare provider must complete a thorough assessment of risks, monitor the patient condition closely, and educate the patient regarding options.

SUGGESTED READINGS

FDA (n.d.). Food and drug administration science background paper: Acute phosphate nephropathy and renal failure associated with the use of oral sodium phosphate bowel cleansing products. Available at: http://www.fda.gov/cder/drug/infopage/osp_solution/science_background.pdf. Accessed July 12, 2008.

FDA (n.d.). Patient information sheet: Oral sodium phosphate products for bowel cleansing. Available at: http://www.fda.gov/cder/drug/InfoSheets/patient/OSP_solutionPIS.pdf. Accessed August 6, 2008.

FDA. Information for healthcare professionals: Oral sodium phosphate products for bowel cleansing. 2006. Available at: http://www.fda.gov/cder/drug/InfoSheets/HCP/OSP_solutionHCP.pdf. Accessed August 6, 2008.

National Guideline Clearinghouse. (n.d.). Preparation of patients for GI endoscopy. Available at: http://www.guideline.gov/summary/summary.aspx?ss=15&doc_id=5680&nbr=3818. Accessed August 6, 2008.

PREPARE THE PATIENT FOR WHAT TO EXPECT DURING OPERATIVE CARE

JEANNIE SCRUGGS GARBER, DNP, RN

WHAT TO DO: PLAN

Preoperative education can be critical to the success of the postoperative recovery period. Patients must expect to receive education from the various healthcare providers that is informative, consistent, and understandable. The more informed the patient and family are, the more likely the patient will comply with the postoperative plan of care. As patients and families are more commonly internet savvy, many patients arrive to surgery knowing a great deal about the actual procedure, possible complications, and the postoperative course of treatment. It is the healthcare provider's responsibility to fully assess the patient's and family's level of understanding of anticipated care as well as to provide clarification and additional information as needed.

Patients should be encouraged to ask questions to their nurses, surgeons, anesthesiologists, respiratory therapists, physical therapists, etc. The informed consent process should include a review of the risks, benefits, and alternatives to surgery. A thorough medical history and assessment are necessary to provide information that may prevent complications postoperatively. Some healthcare issues can be life threatening during surgery if not identified preoperatively, such as latex allergy and medication allergies. Another important part of the preoperative assessment and education is the discussion regarding alcohol and tobacco use. Since these issues can compound potential operative complications, healthcare providers may alter the plan of care if excessive alcohol or tobacco use is identified. Patients should be encouraged to repeat themselves as much as they desire to provide constant reminders to the many providers that will participate in their care.

Preoperative patient education should provide an overview of what to expect before, during, and after surgery and include physical appearance, any equipment that may be present at the bedside, physical symptoms such as pain, tremors, cold chills, etc. Patients and families must also be involved in surgical site identification to minimize the risk of wrong site surgery.

Patients must also be educated about the potential complications of their procedure. They should be reminded of proper handwashing technique and measures that will be necessary to prevent wound infection. Patients should also be educated on the importance of deep breathing, use of pain management, and any other postoperative instructions.

Perhaps one of the most important reasons to provide preoperative education is to decrease anxiety related to this stressful event. According to Mitchell (as cited by Durling et al., 2007), patient's anxiety levels are decreased when preoperative education is provided. Patients and families become part of the postoperative care team when they are informed preoperatively, and that can only make for improved patient outcomes.

SUGGESTED READINGS

Durling M, Milne D, Huton N, et al. Decreasing patient's preoperative anxiety: A literature review. *Aust Nurs J.* 2007; 14(11):35.
[no authors listed] Patient education series: Tips for a safe operation. *Nursing.* 2007;37(8):43.

EDUCATE PATIENTS PRIOR TO CHEST TUBE REMOVAL TO AVOID BEING PUNCHED

JULIE MULLIGAN WATTS, RN, MN

WHAT TO DO: PLAN

Surprise is usually not a good thing during a medical procedure and the proper preparation of a patient can help avoid surprises. Hospitals across the country have developed preoperative assessment clinics, patient education areas, and written instructions for procedures. There are many reasons why these are good approaches to patient preparation. Education can be accomplished in a timely and efficient manner. Preoperative procedures in an outpatient area assist in completing pre-op paper work, admission processes, and help to streamline the admission. They also serve to reduce the patient's anxiety about inpatient procedures and the surgical procedure. Patients who are well prepared for procedures have less anxiety and are better able to participate in their care. Some studies have demonstrated shorter lengths of stay, less anxiety, less fear, better pain management, a more positive attitude, and identification of conditions that could contribute to postoperative complications.

Once a patient is in the hospital, he or she must rely on the staff to assist in preparing him or her for procedures. Patient preparation depends on individual nursing units, individual staff, patient expectations, and sometimes physician instructions.

The use of chest tubes is common in the hospital. Criteria for removal of tubes include decreased drainage, no air leaks, no respiratory distress, normal breath sounds or at the patient's baseline, the water-seal chamber does not fluctuate, and a chest X-ray shows lung re-expansion. When assisting with the removal of a chest tube, it is prudent to give prescribed pain medications 15 to 30 min prior to the procedure, depending on the medication and route of administration. Premedications are given to prevent pain and anxiety. A suture-removal kit, petrolatum gauze, regular gauze, and tape may be used. The procedure should be explained to the patient with instructions on how the patient may be required to participate. Usually patients are instructed to inhale and exhale during removal of a chest tube, with tube removal occurring during peak exhalation. By explaining the procedure and administering premeds, the patient will not be surprised by the swift removal of the tube, and this can avoid a painful surprise for both the patient and the physician.

SUGGESTED READINGS

Coughlin A, Parchinsky C. Go with the flow of chest tube therapy. *Nursing*. 2006;36(3):36–42.

McConnell E. Assisting with chest tube removal. *Nursing*. 1995;25(8):18.

Persaud D, Dawe U. Effects of a surgical pre-operative assessment clinic on patient care. *Hosp Top*. 1992;70(4):37–40.

Smeltzer S, Bare B. *Brunner & Suddarth's Textbook of Medical-Surgical Nursing*. 10th Ed. Philadelphia, PA: Lippincott Williams & Wilkins; 2004.

THE IMPORTANCE OF THE PREOPERATIVE PHONE CALL

ANTHONY D. SLONIM, MD, DrPH

WHAT TO DO: PLAN

As more and more surgery gets relegated to the ambulatory environment, there is less contact with patients prior to the procedure. Hence, new processes and procedures need to be in place to ensure that the patient's needs are able to be met when the patient shows up. If the procedure is going to be performed in the hospital, this issue does not pose a big problem. The patient has an operative course that is more difficult and then gets transferred to a bed in the intensive care unit. But, when the procedure is performed in an outpatient center, there may be little backup for the patient without transferring him or her urgently and by ambulance to a hospital. This is good neither for the patient nor for the staff in either location and may be partially improved with a preoperative phone call.

The preoperative phone call is performed in many perioperative areas to address patient needs prior to showing up on the morning of surgery and ensures the operating room staff that all preoperative work is complete. It serves as a reminder to not eat or drink and of what to bring, a validation of the procedure, and a check to ensure that all necessary preoperative testing is in hand. The patient can ask logistical questions about where to go, what time to be there, and who and what they should bring with them.

In the ambulatory surgery world, the outpatient phone call provides another important role to validate that the center can actually care for the patients their surgery, and their needs without the backup of the hospital. As a part of this, understanding the patient's medical and surgical history, prior anesthetic complications, new diagnoses, and medication lists is particularly important. The ambulatory surgery center and, often, the anesthesia team may have never met the patient before and need to ensure that while the surgeon feels comfortable, the remainder of the staff does too. The needs of the patient either by specific population or diagnosis have to be met by these centers. This includes the ability to ensure that processes are in place to protect the patient who may be an infant or child. In addition, the centers need to ensure that processes are in place so that patients with chronic, often asymptomatic, conditions like obstructive sleep apnea can be discharged to home safely.

Many ambulatory surgery centers are sophisticated places able to perform and support patients through many different types of procedures with very low complication rates. However, processes need to be in place to recognize when the needs of a particular patient may exceed the services that the center can provide. This is important since there is nothing worse than having a crisis develop during the intraoperative period or immediately postoperatively that cannot be managed by the center's staff.

A preoperative phone call will not identify all the potential problems or eliminate the need for urgent transfer, but it can assist with identification of some of the more common problems that may be better handled in a hospital surgery department.

SUGGESTED READINGS

Federated Ambulatory Surgery Association. Available at: http://www.ascassociation.org/about/press/june2.pdf. Accessed August 30, 2008.

Frequently asked questions about ambulatory surgery centers. Available at: http://www.ascassociation.org/faqs/faqaboutascs/. Accessed August 30, 2008.

Sleep apnea. Available at: https://www.ascassociation.org/resources/sleepapnea.pdf. Accessed August 30, 2008.

PREPARE THE PATIENT FOR SURGERY BOTH PHYSICALLY AND EMOTIONALLY

JEANNIE SCRUGGS GARBER, DNP, RN

WHAT TO DO: PLAN

As nurses prepare patients for the surgical experience, they are often focused on the technology, tasks, and procedures. Nurses must also remember the basic preparations that must be done so that the patient and family are prepared for the experience and not just the procedure.

All patients must be clean. It sounds simple, but is quite important. The skin must be cleansed to maximize comfort and to remove any drainage or secretions, which will prevent infection or irritation. A clean hospital gown is also important. Oral hygiene is a task that must not be overlooked for comfort, especially since the patient will have had nothing by mouth for a long period of time. Other simple things to remember include removing all hair accessories such as clips, headbands, and hair pieces to make head positioning easier and to prevent any electrocautery concerns. A disposable cap must also be placed on the patient prior to entering the operating room.

All makeup and nail polish should be removed so that a proper physical assessment can be performed to monitor oxygenation and circulation. It is also important to remove dentures, hearing aids, contact lenses, or other prosthesis. The nurse must be mindful of the patient's feelings and emotions related to removal of some of these items since body image and self-esteem may be of concern. Privacy and reassurance are necessary to help the patient be prepared for the surgery experience.

The patient's valuables must also be protected. Nurses must follow institutional policy and remember that the value of an object is in the eye of the patient, not the nurse. All items that the patient perceives as valuable are of value, so protect them accordingly.

All patients must also empty their bladder prior to entering the operating room and since patients may be very anxious, it is important to allow enough time for patients to have bathroom time that meets their needs.

The nurse must also collect vital signs and document how the patient was prepared. This documentation should address the task as well as the assessment and planning that occurred to get the patient to the operating room. Nurses must be aware of patient allergies and must be able to adapt the preoperative plan to meet individual patient and family needs. Patient education is also a critical component of patient preparation. Preoperative checklists are helpful, but the nurse is the individual who makes the plan for surgery successful.

SUGGESTED READINGS

Shallom L. Care of surgical clients. In: Potter P, Perry A, eds. *Fundamentals of Nursing*. Toronto, ON: Mosby-Elsevier; 2009, pp. 1387–1389.

ENSURE THAT THE PATIENTS UNDERGOING SURGERY MAINTAIN THEIR IDENTITY

JEANNIE SCRUGGS GARBER, DNP, RN

WHAT TO DO: PLAN

As patients are prepared for the surgical experience, we take off all their clothes, change their normal appearance by removing makeup, nail polish, body hair, and dentures, put a funny cap on their head, and dress them in a thin, unattractive hospital gown. After surgery, they look even more different than "normal" with swollen faces, swollen hands, drool, dry mouth, crusty eyes, drains, tubes, dressings that ooze body fluids, and sometimes with the inability to get out of bed to go to the bathroom. What an experience for those who are usually very independent.

The surgery experience can impact the body image short term or perhaps long term. If the patient is impacted long term, the nurse must be constantly aware of and assessing for the behaviors related to self-concept. Some indicators that patients may be struggling with their body image include not looking at themselves in the mirror, not looking at incisions, and refusing visitors. Another concern may be related to how well they will be able to go back to work, take care of their family, or participate in the activities they once enjoyed. The nurse must talk with the patient about these concerns and make the necessary referrals to social work and psychology.

The patient's family is critical in the assessment of the patient's self-concept. A preoperative assessment can also help the nurse keep in tune with any changes in self-concept that may occur as a result of the surgery.

Shalom suggests the following nursing actions to help patients with their self-concept:

- Maintain privacy
- Keep the patient clean
- Empty drains frequently
- Keep the patient environment clean and organized
- Talk with the patient about his or her concerns
- Talk with the family to support them as they help their family member

Regardless of how small or large a surgical procedure may be viewed by the healthcare provider, it may be a monumental, life-altering experience for the patient. The nurse is critical to this assessment and intervention and can make a difference in how the patient experiences the surgery, the perceptions of body image, and recovery.

SUGGESTED READINGS

Shallom L. Care of surgical clients. In: Potter P, Perry A, eds. *Fundamentals of Nursing*. Toronto, ON: Mosby-Elsevier; 2009, pp. 1405–1406.

301

OXYGEN-RICH ATMOSPHERE: USING A FACEMASK AND ELECTROCAUTERY DURING LOCAL ANESTHESIA

JEANNIE SCRUGGS GARBER, DNP, RN

WHAT TO DO: PLAN

Even though much progress has been made regarding operating room safety and the prevention of fires, there remains a risk of fire during surgical procedures. The use of electro-cauterization, which may be used to stop bleeding, and the oxygen-rich environment of the operating room are key potential causes of this safety concern. During local anesthesia procedures, the use of oxygen may be less contained when administered via face mask or cannula, resulting in more oxygen in the open air or outside the closed anesthesia system.

Batra et al. reported that operating room fires rarely occur; however, based on a study by the Emergency Care Research Institute, in approximately 72% of fires that do occur, "an oxygen-enriched atmosphere has been shown to have contributed to the fire and nearly 70% of these fires are related to the use of electro surgical equipment."

According to Podnos, the American College of Surgeons, Perioperative Committee suggests the following precautions to prevent fires in the operating room:

- Keep the electrocautery tip in the holster when it is not being used.
- Have power going to high-intensity light sources only when they are being used.
- Use only appropriately protected endotracheal tubes when operating near the trachea.
- Use air or air and oxygen mixtures in anesthetic gases.
- Avoid tenting of surgical drapes in a fashion that allows accumulation of oxygen or other flammable gases.
- Use water-soluble rather than oil-based substances to cover lanugo and other flammable parts on the body.
- Use fire-retardant surgical drapes.

Other suggestions include fire safety training for all employees and defined, clear roles and responsibilities of actions to be taken in the event of a fire.

Barker and Polson conducted a simulated operating room fire based on a reproduction of an actual event and speculated that the oxygen rich environment was a key contributor in this event. They made the following recommendations to improve fire safety in the operating room:

- Be certain that a fuel–oxidizer combination is not present in or near the surgical field
- When patient is not intubated and face mask or other oxygen administration is used, avoid large oxygen concentrations in the closed space within the surgical drapes
- If at all possible, flow air into the plastic mask rather than 100% oxygen
- If supplemental oxygen is required, use only the minimum amount needed to keep oxygen levels within acceptable range
- Be very cautious with flammable preparation solutions, especially when they are used on the head-neck region

The key messages for reducing operating room fires are education and awareness to promote prevention, skill in intervention when and if a fire occurs, and the need for continuing research to gain new knowledge that will ultimately improve the safety of the operating room environment.

SUGGESTED READINGS

Barker S, Polson J. Fire in the operating room: A case report and laboratory study. *Anesth Analg.* 2001;93:960–965. Available at: http://www.anesthesia-analgesia.org/cgi/content/full/93/4/960. Accessed August 6, 2008.

Batra S, Gupta R. Alcohol based surgical prep solution and the risk of fire in the operating room: A case report. *Patient Saf Surg.* 2008;(2):10. Available at: http://www.pssjournal.com/content/2/1/10. Accessed August 6, 2008.

Podnos Y, Williams R. Fires in the operating room [Electronic version]. *Bull Am Coll Surg.* 1997;82(8).

PREVENTING CORNEAL DAMAGE TO THE UNCONSCIOUS PATIENT

JEANNIE SCRUGGS GARBER, DNP, RN

WHAT TO DO: PLAN, IMPLEMENT, AND EVALUATE

Unconscious patients are in a compromised health status and are at increased risk for multisystem complications. Ocular care is often overlooked. Nursing care of the eyes is a simple task yet in the critically ill patient, research regarding best practices is lacking. According to a systematic literature review conducted by Joyce, the unconscious patient is at increased risk for eye injuries such as conjunctivitis, corneal ulceration, and long-term vision damage from ulceration and scarring. Keratitis, the inflammation and infection of cornea, is also a potential concern. Considering the potential complications and the unknown best practice in the unconscious patient, there has been very little research conducted in this area.

The patient, who experiences eye care with contaminated substances or has existing respiratory infections, is at increased risk for ophthalmic complications if he or she is unconscious for an extended period of time on the ventilator. Another possible issue in the ventilated patient is the diagnosis of "conjunctival chemosis" (edema) or "ventilator eye." Joyce reports that the drugs and pressures used in ventilated patients can cause an increase in intraocular pressure and fluid retention that results in swollen eyes and the potential for increased risk of drying and corneal abrasion.

How to best care for the eyes of the critical patient is debatable with many options are to be considered to prevent injury. Sivasankar et al. compared the use of ocular lubricants and tape to the use of goggles and sterile water gauze in comatose patients and determined that the latter was more effective in preventing corneal abrasions. The studies reviewed by Joyce indicate that covering the eye is better than instillations, yet either of these preventative measures is better than no treatment at all.

The nurse is in a position to assess and prevent eye injury in the critically ill or unconscious patient. Care should be taken to provide moisture or coverage to the eyes while the natural blink reflex is ineffective or nonexistent. The nurse should be aware of organizational policy and procedure and should inform and encourage other healthcare providers to pay attention to eye care in the unconscious patient. Although, according to Howell, corneal abrasions usually heal quickly with complete recovery of vision, by working together to create policy, practice, and research, eye injuries may be minimized in unconscious patient.

SUGGESTED READINGS

Howell R. Corneal abrasion. eMedicine. Article Last Updated: Jul 27, 2007. Available at: http://www.emedicine.com/emerg/TOPIC828.HTM. Accessed June 18, 2008.

Joyce N. Eye care for intensive care patients. A Systematic Review No. 21. *Adelaide: The Joanna Briggs Institute for Evidence Based Nursing and Midwifery*. 2002;6(1).

Sivasankar S, Jasper S, Simon S, et al. Eye care in ICU. *Ind J Crit Care Med*. 2006;10:11–14. Available at: http://www.ijccm.org/text.asp?2006/10/1/11/24683. Accessed August 6, 2008.

MARK THE CORRECT SURGICAL SITE

JEANNIE SCRUGGS GARBER, DNP, RN

In a review conducted by the Joint Commission (1998), the most common reasons for wrong-site surgeries were more than one surgeon, more than one procedure, time constraints, and unusual physical patient characteristics. Further review of the cases revealed that communication among healthcare providers was most often the key factor in the wrong-site surgery (Joint Commission, 1998).

The incidence of wrong-site, wrong-procedure, and wrong-person surgery can be prevented. The Joint Commission developed a universal protocol with the intent to eliminate this concern. The Joint Commission (2003) worked with diverse healthcare professionals to reach a common agreement on the following ideas or principles related to the topic as summarized in Table 303.1. The action steps that were developed based on the above principles are summarized in Table 303.2.

Unfortunately, "wrong-site, wrong-procedure and wrong-person surgeries are sentinel events that persist as a problem at the rate of 5 to 8 new cases each month and recently became the most frequently reported sentinel event in the Joint Commission's Sentinel Event database" (Joint Commission, n.d.). The protocol will need to be reviewed and revised over time to ensure that healthcare providers offer patients the best, up to date, evidence-based approach in solving this complex healthcare issue.

SUGGESTED READINGS

The Joint Commission (1998). Lessons learned: Wrong site surgery. Available at: http://www.jointcommission.org/SentinelEvents/SentinelEventAlert/sea_6.htm. Accessed August 6, 2008.

The Joint Commission (2003). Universal Protocol for Preventing Wrong Site, Wrong Procedure, Wrong Person Surgery™. Available at: http://www.jointcommission.org/PatientSafety/UniversalProtocol/. Accessed August 6, 2008.

The Joint Commission (n.d.). Facts about the Universal Protocol for Preventing Wrong Site, Wrong Procedure and Wrong Person Surgery™. Available at: http://www.jointcommission.org/PatientSafety/UniversalProtocol/up_facts.htm. Accessed August 6, 2008.

TABLE 303.1	JCAHO BASIC PRINCIPLES RELATED TO WRONG-SITE, WRONG-PROCEDURE, WRONG-PERSON SURGERIES—SUMMARIZED

The concern regarding wrong-site, wrong-procedure, and wrong-person surgery can and must be prevented.
Many strategies are needed to eliminate wrong-site, wrong-procedure, and wrong-person surgery.
Communication among all the members of the surgical team contributes to success.
The patient or designee should be part of the process.
The process must be standardized and protocol driven.
The protocol should allow for adaptation and interpretation to meet individualized patient needs.
Site marking should focus on those procedures of right and left or body parts with multiples.
The protocol should be applicable or adaptable to all operative and other invasive procedures regardless of setting.

Source: Joint Commission (2003).

TABLE 303.2	JCAHO UNIVERSAL PROTOCOL	
ACTION	**PURPOSE**	
Verify person, site, and surgery preoperatively	Ensure that all documents and studies are available and that they have been reviewed, consistent with each other and with the patient's expectations and with the team's understanding regarding the patient, procedure, site, and implants (if applicable). Any information that does not match must be reconciled prior to the procedure.	
Mark the operative site	To identify the incision site.	
Conduct a "Time out" immediately before the procedure	To create a final check to ensure right patient, procedure, and site.	

Source: Joint Commission (2003).

Training in Emergency Airway Placement Is Improved from Exposure in the OR

Francine B. Yates, RRT, RN, BSN

WHAT TO DO: PLAN

When a patient is in respiratory or cardiac distress or arrest, the first priority is to establish an airway. It is the task of all personnel involved—nurses, respiratory therapists, anesthetists, physicians, and residents—to ensure that this happens as quickly and safely as possible. When the staff does not perform adequately, the patient suffers with outcomes that could even be fatal.

If the intubation procedure is practiced first in the controlled setting of the operating room (OR) or simulation lab, patient outcomes may be improved. These instructions would include how to hold the laryngoscope, which side to put the tube in, and what type of patient monitoring needed to be performed. After participating in a class that gives verbal instruction and hands-on training with a simulator, a rotation in the operating room with an anesthesiologist would be very beneficial. This would assist the practitioner in learning the proper way to intubate and maintain an airway. The benefit of the operating room for this type of training is that it is a controlled environment.

Simulation centers have been established for the training of medical professionals. These centers use nonhuman simulators that can breathe, tell the provider what symptoms it is having, and exhale CO_2 to demonstrate appropriate tube placement. Machinery and medical equipment can be used on the mannequin, and cardiopulmonary resuscitation (CPR) can be performed without causing harm to a real patient. These centers also focus on training in communication and teamwork, and participants are trained in clinical procedures.

There are numerous mistakes that can happen when an inadequately prepared individual attempts to place an artificial airway. The most common error is placing the tube in the esophagus instead of the trachea, which will result in the stomach filling with air and becoming distended. This causes the patient to vomit and risks aspiration. Subsequent sequelae include aspiration pneumonia, extended ventilation periods, and nosocomial infections that prolong the patient's length of stay and compromise his condition.

A second, serious complication that can arise from lack of proper training on intubation is perforation of the trachea. When attempting to place an endotracheal tube (ETT), the practitioner must be able to identify the vocal cords, visualize them, and know where the ETT must be placed in reference to them. A blind and forceful intubation can result in tracheal perforation, resulting in the development of subcutaneous air throughout the chest, neck, and face. The patient cannot be properly ventilated, which results in other serious events, such as an emergency tracheostomy, anoxic brain injury, or death.

An inexperienced practitioner of any kind should not be allowed to intubate a patient without first having the appropriate training to learn the theory and to practice the proper technique of intubation. Part of this training should include a rotation in the OR with an anesthesiologist.

SUGGESTED READINGS

Carlson KK, Lynn-McHale, Weigand DJ. Endotracheal intubation (perform). In: *AACN Procedure Manual for Critical Care*. 5th Ed. Philadelphia: Elsevier; 2005;9–20.

Davis C. The perfect patient. *Nurs Stand*. 2005;19(20).

PATIENT SATISFACTION IN THE OPERATING ROOM

JEANNIE SCRUGGS GARBER, DNP, RN

WHAT TO DO: EVALUATE

Patient satisfaction in the operating room (OR) is generally measured preoperatively and postoperatively since patients are most often sedated during the procedure. However, with an increased use of local and regional anesthesia, the measurement of patient satisfaction during procedures can be done more readily than in the past. Patients may be awake, able to visualize the surgical procedure, to witness the interaction among the healthcare providers. Patient satisfaction is a quality measurement for the OR although there are few studies linking quality to patient satisfaction. Nurses and physicians strive to provide clinical care that is perceived as excellent by patients while providing ethical, competent, and technically proficient care. In the OR, equipment and technology can make the healthcare provider–patient interaction challenging. This challenge can negatively impact the patient's perception of caring, compassionate caregivers. The OR atmosphere is sterile, cold, and shiny—not warm, comfortable, and welcoming.

According to Hankela (1996), the following categories are potential concepts to use in measuring the patients' perceptions of their OR experience:

- Success of the surgery (was the desired outcome achieved?)
- Integrity
- Self-determination
- Environment
- Behavior of the OR nurses
- Actions by the OR nurses

Nurses are in a position to impact the patient's perception of each of these categories. Perhaps the most important category is how the nurse behaves and acts toward the patient. The patient needs to feel safe, secure, and supported throughout the OR experience. The nurse needs to listen and respond with kindness and compassion while continuing to execute the procedural processes within the OR.

There are abundant research opportunities within the OR related to the measurement of patient satisfaction. The information available is focused on the before and after perceptions of care—naturally the next step is to study and better understand how to best meet patient expectations intraoperatively.

SUGGESTED READINGS

Hankela S, Kiikkala I. Intraoperative nursing care as experienced by surgical patients. *AORN J.* 1996;63(2):435–442. Available at: http://findarticles.com/p/articles/mi_m0FSL/is_n2_v63/ai_19128844/pg_7?tag=artBody;col1. Accessed August 8, 2008.

RESIDENTS IN THE OPERATING ROOM: DO YOU KNOW THE ACGME'S COMPETENCIES?

JEANNIE SCRUGGS GARBER, DNP, RN

WHAT TO DO: EVALUATE

In 1999, the accreditation Council for Graduate Medical Education (ACGME) published six competencies that must be assessed as a part of the physician's resident education. Medical residents frequently rotate through the operating room, and surgical residents spend many waking hours in the surgical department. The operating room nurses are in a unique position to support and evaluate the development of the resident's competencies in the operating room. The ACGME competencies are listed and defined in Table 306.1.

These competencies must be taught and assessed throughout the residency program. Nurses serve as key resources for teaching, coaching, and evaluating as residents progress to higher levels of independence. A common statement made by residents is, "when you start your residency, find a nurse you can trust and develop a strong collegial relationship—he or she will be your best friend. If you do not develop this relationship, he or she may end up being your worst enemy." Unfortunately, there is some truth to this statement. New residents are

in an awkward position in that they are labeled as physicians yet have relatively no experience in independent decision making regarding patient care. Strong residents seek out resources and rely on interdependence to make patient decisions that will ultimately create more positive patient outcomes. Residents who are fearful of seeking advice or determined to be totally independent are unfortunately creating increased risk for negative patient outcomes or, for sure, making it much harder on themselves than necessary.

Operating room nurses have a great deal of face-to-face time with residents and are able to provide feedback to attending physicians regarding all the six competencies. Program directors and attending physicians can use the nurses' assessment to provide specific examples of strengths and opportunities for improvement and to facilitate a collaborative, interprofessional learning environment.

SUGGESTED READINGS

Greenberg JA, Irani JL, Greenberg CC, et al. The ACGME competencies in the operating room. *Surgery*. 2007;142(2): 180–184.

TABLE 306.1	ACCREDITATION COUNCIL FOR GRADUATE MEDICAL EDUCATION (ACGME) COMPETENCIES	
COMPETENCY	**DEFINITION**
Patient care	Able to provide appropriate clinical care to patients and families.
Medical knowledge	Able to demonstrate up-to-date awareness and use of scientific information to make diagnostic and treatment decisions.
Practice-based learning and improvement	Able to systematically evaluate patient care and analyze outcomes to improve practice.
Interpersonal and communication skills	Able to communicate effectively with patients, families, and other healthcare providers.
Systems-based practice	Able to practice with a global awareness of how their work fits within a larger system.

ANAPHYLAXIS IN THE OPERATING ROOM

JEANNIE SCRUGGS GARBER, DNP, RN

WHAT TO DO: ASSESS

Anaphylaxis is a severe allergic or unpredictable reaction to a medication. The situation is life-threatening and presents as:

- Sudden difficulty in breathing (constriction of bronchial muscles and swelling of the pharynx and larynx)
- Severe shortness of breath

Anaphylaxis is a crescendo process that can be fatal. Histamine is rapidly released into the system and impacts cardiovascular perfusion and oxygenation.

In the operating room, these symptoms may be less obvious due to anesthesia procedures supporting ventilation, the patient being covered by drapes, and the patient being unable to communicate any sensations that may indicate an allergic reaction. Determining the cause of the reaction can be difficult; however, the most common reasons for anaphylaxis in the operating room are

- Neuromuscular blocking agents
- Latex
- Antibiotics
- Various medications such as barbiturates, opioids, protamine, oxytocin, etc.

The treatment usually consists of the following: intravenous fluids, epinephrine, oxygen, or intubation. Early intervention and management of this situation will determine the success of treatment. This situation requires emergency intervention to prevent long-term implications or death. Patients who experience an anaphylactic reaction in the operating room must be informed postoperatively and educated on whether further allergy testing is needed and how to communicate the allergy to all healthcare providers in the future.

Some other diagnoses to be considered when determining whether an anaphylactic reaction has truly occurred are

- Asthma
- Arrhythmia
- Hemorrhage
- Myocardial infarction
- Medication overdose
- Sepsis

Anaphylaxis is not a common occurrence in the operating room; yet, when it does occur, the management is very complex. The patient is already in a compromised situation and is receiving numerous drugs that may be infused simultaneously. Surgeons, anesthesiologists, and nurses caring for the patient must work together to evaluate potential causes of the reaction and to provide the care needed to progress beyond the crisis.

SUGGESTED READINGS

Buckner S. Medication administration. In: Potter P, Perry A, eds. *Fundamentals of Nursing*. Toronto, ON: Mosby-Elsevier; 2009, pp. 691–692.

Reisacher WR. Anaphylaxis in the operating room. *Curr Opin Otolaryngol Head Neck Surg*. 2008;16(3):280–284.

PERIOPERATIVE NURSING: HOW DO YOU DEFINE IT?

JEANNIE SCRUGGS GARBER, DNP, RN

WHAT TO DO: PLAN

Perioperative nursing, like many forms of nursing, is undergoing constant change. How we assess quality, perform our daily work, and measure our success is different than in past. The operating room has always been dependent upon technology, but the increasing technology also creates additional challenges in using that equipment and caring for the patient.

Perioperative nurses have other, more traditional names such as OR nurses and Registered Nurses (RNs). The perioperative nurse works with a team of healthcare providers and the patients and their families to ensure quality surgical care for the patients. Various roles of the perioperative nurse may include

- Scrub Nurse
- Circulating Nurse
- RN First Assist
- OR Director, Manager, or Supervisor
- Consultant
- Educator
- Researcher
- Medical Sales Professional
- Nurse Anesthetist

The most likely environments where perioperative nurses work are hospitals, outpatient surgery facilities, and physician offices. As nurses carry out these roles, the balance between the patient's needs and the focus on the technology or equipment can be difficult to achieve.

Unfortunately, some people share the perception of OR nurses as less caring, less compassionate, and less of a "people person" than nurses who work in other specialties. Bull and Fitzgerald (2006) published an Australian RN's perception of OR nursing as "... theatre nurses are labeled like 'you're not a people nurse, you're not a people person, that's why you like theatre' and the nurses say they're not right, we have quite

intense contact with people, it's just very short and that's very true and you're also, even though our patients are asleep, they are still being cared for as if they are already awake and communicating. You care about patients, they're the most important factor in what you're doing... you can't be in the world where people are having a personal crisis as coming into an operating theatre. I mean, it must be the most, you know, tense time in people's lives almost, if they could say that, and a lot of our patients are awake throughout their surgery. I think that you have to marry them [technical and caring nursing]...."

Research questions to be explored related to OR nursing perceptions could include is there a relationship between a high level of focus on technology and patient safety? Are patient outcomes positively impacted when the intraoperative nurse is perceived as more caring or when she is perceived as more technical? Are the two categories separable and distinct? Most OR nursing research has focused on the preoperative and postoperative phases and not the intraoperative phase. Current intraoperative research is more likely related to staff perceptions, tasks, and nursing processes than it is about patient outcomes.

Perioperative or intraoperative nursing is evolving as all forms of nursing. The OR is a unique setting that requires a high standard for safety, competence, and compassion. As Bull and Fitzgerald (2006) suggest, nurses must be able to blend the traditional meaning of nursing care with the rapid infusion of technology in OR nursing to create safer patient environments.

SUGGESTED READINGS

Bull R, Fitzgerald M. Nursing in a technological environment: Nursing in the operating room. *Int J Nurs Pract*. 2006; (12): 3–7.

Hankela S, Kiikkala I. Intraoperative nursing care as experienced by surgical patients. *AORN J*. 1996;63(2):435–442. Available at: http://findarticles.com/p/articles/mi_m0FSL/is_n2_v63/ai_19128844/pg_7?tag=artBody;col1. Accessed August 8, 2008.

Intraoperative Blood Salvaging and Bloodless Surgery

Jeannie Scruggs Garber, DNP, RN

The process of recovering the blood lost during a surgical procedure is intraoperative blood salvage or autologous blood salvage. The recovered blood is reinfused into the patient. The prevalence of HIV, hepatitis, and other blood disorders has increased the concerns surrounding blood product administration, and autologous blood transfusion eliminates these problems. The blood salvaging procedure has most often been used in cardiothoracic and vascular surgery since blood loss during these operations is many times considered excessive.

There are different ways to collect and process the patient's blood during surgery, such as those that collect, wash, and save the blood cells, those that collect and directly reinfuse, and the process of ultrafiltration. There are numerous products available in use for these purposes and each surgeon and surgical team will decide which one is best for their patients. The benefits of using these forms of autologous transfusion include minimizing adverse transfusion reactions, decreasing the chance of human error in the process of transfusion, and overall conservation of blood bank donations. Human error, such as misidentification of patients, creates a much greater risk than the possibility of an adverse blood reaction.

Blood salvaging may also decrease costs if less blood-banked products are utilized. It is important to note that Jehovah's Witnesses may accept autologous blood while they will not accept other blood products or traditional transfusions. It does seem possible that the use of salvaged blood could minimize or prevent the need to use homologous blood transfusion; however, practice changes in the past several years have dramatically decreased the number of blood transfusions administered.

Other surgical options that minimize blood loss and the need for transfusion include minimally invasive surgical techniques, the use of erythropoietin preoperatively to produce red blood cells, volume expanders or blood substitutes, and self-donated or autologous blood use. Regardless of the choice the patient and healthcare provider make, to reinfuse the patient's own blood is an option to consider that may lessen the risk of blood-related complications and may improve the overall outcome of the surgical experience.

SUGGESTED READINGS

Freischlag JA. Intraoperative blood salvage in vascular surgery—worth the effort? *Crit Care.* 2004;8(S2):S53–S56. Available at: http://ccforum.com/content/8/S2/S53. Accessed August 10, 2008.

MEETING PHYSICIAN EXPECTATIONS: DO I EVER DO ANYTHING RIGHT?

JEANNIE SCRUGGS GARBER, DNP, RN

WHAT TO DO: EVALUATE

Physicians are knowledgeable, competent professionals who are taught how to be in charge, how to give directions, and how to evaluate situations. What they are not routinely taught in medical school is how to communicate effectively across disciplines and how teamwork can support and benefit their work and the patient's outcome. Have you ever heard these questions: Does anything meet his expectation? Or, if I (the nurse) behaved like that, I would be fired!

Most nurses can share stories of times when they carried out all the orders, provided the patient with appropriate nursing interventions, and the physician was not pleased with the nurse for some action or lack thereof. Similar scenarios are heard from nurses in administrative roles. The nurse carries out the task or project as discussed and planned, and the physician is still not pleased with the outcome and is very comfortable sharing his feelings in a demeaning or harsh manner.

Our expectations of physician behavior are formed throughout our lives as we observe from the patient's perspective. Whether the first memory of the physician is a time when he or she was looking in your ears to find a missing toy piece or a physician role being played on television, our idea of how physicians behave is determined at a young age. Once we enter into a healthcare professional role, our childhood image is either confirmed or tested. Is the image one of kindness, compassion, and comfort, or is it one of demands, superiority, and judgment?

As we practice our professional roles, physicians and nurses must work closely to provide leadership and patient care in many settings. The clinical roles are defined by license and tasks with the physician responsible for the medical diagnosis while the nurse is responsible for the nursing diagnosis and care. Collaboration among the professions is a critical element that impacts the quality of patient care and patient outcome. Recent health services research supports the value of collaboration in relation to patient outcomes and quality of work life for the providers.

As the nurse brings preconceived thoughts about the role of the physician and as the physicians bring self-image to their work, it is important to establish open communication that will create the best outcome for the patient. There is no room for ego or power struggles when a patient's outcome or an organizational process be can affected.

Nursing education has transitioned over the years to include instruction on topics such as assertiveness, effective verbal and written communications, and patient advocacy and physician relations. Some medical schools are starting to include these topics in their curriculum as well. Unfortunately, the traditional hierarchical hospital organization still exists today, and nurses may find themselves struggling to meet physician expectations.

Perhaps nurses must lead physicians to a new paradigm—a new way to work together. The best advice as you attempt to meet physician expectations: do what is right in a kind, compassionate way; be articulate; be respectful; and expect respect. We are all in this together with one purpose—to make a difference for the patient.

SUGGESTED READINGS

Baggs JG, Gedney J. Overview and summary. Partnerships and collaboration: What skills are needed? *Online J Issues Nurs.* 2005;10(1):56–59. Available at: http://web.ebscohost.com/ehost/detail?vid=3&hid=115&sid=399b8baa-0270–4e80–9a9a-ed7861bb1c4e%40sessionmgr102&bdata=JnNpdGU9ZWhvc3QtbGl2ZQ%3d%3d#db=byh&AN=16508342. Accessed August 8, 2008.

TEAMWORK IN THE OPERATING ROOM—HUDDLE AND DEBRIEF: IS THIS THE OR OR FOOTBALL?

JEANNIE SCRUGGS GARBER, DNP, RN

WHAT TO DO: IMPLEMENT

Patient safety, communication, and teamwork: how are they related in the operating room? Nurses and physicians carry out their work as individuals and as team members. In the operating room, a team exists when the individuals have a shared vision and expectation for the operative process and the patient outcome and mutual respect for each other. A simple technique labeled a huddle can serve as the point in time before a procedure begins to create that shared vision and create an environment that promotes teamwork. A debriefing can allow for a systematic review of the case including what went well, what could have been done differently, and what errors were avoided and to determine if outcome of the case met all of the original objectives for all involved. These same concepts are practiced routinely in football:

- Huddle—the team gathers pregame to discuss strategies and plans that will lead to winning the game.
- Debriefing—after the game, the team gathers to discuss how the game went and to evaluate the best plays and worst plays and to discuss how tomorrow will be different.

Healthcare teams can learn from this practice and make a difference in how healthcare is delivered tomorrow.

A huddle in the operating room may prevent medical error. The huddle is experienced when all members of the operating room team come together to discuss the plan for a case. The team is all inclusive, and the discussion can range from the physician sharing the specific technique to be used to students sharing their specific learning objectives for the day. This forum supports open communication and an opportunity for safety checks, safety discussions, equipment reviews, new technology summaries, and sharing of any unique characteristics for this patient and allows for questions and clarification.

Physician leadership is a key component to the success of the huddle. If the physician values communication and planning, the team will follow with the ultimate outcome being improved patient safety and teamwork. Potential problems can be identified, and solutions can be planned ahead during a huddle instead of waiting until a situation requires intervention. The practice of a huddle or debriefing has occurred informally in many organizations in many practice settings. Making communication an organized, formal process engrains the practice into the culture, promotes open communication and error identification, and creates a shared ownership for the patient outcome. Issues that arise are no longer "someone else's fault."

The debriefing in the operating room occurs at the end of the surgical procedure and provides an avenue for performance feedback, procedural review, and teamwork assessment. The sooner after the surgery, the better for the debriefing. Team members will have a real time account of the procedure, and all issues can be resolved to prevent similar error prone situations in future cases.

SUGGESTED READINGS

Edmondson A. Speaking up in the operating room: How team leaders promote learning in interdisciplinary action teams. *J Manag Stud*. 2003;40(6):1419–1452. Available at: http://www3.interscience.wiley.com/journal/118870438/abstract. Accessed August 11, 2008.

Medscape Today. Teamwork in the operating room. 2007. Available at: http://www.medscape.com/viewarticle/562998_2. Accessed August 11, 2008.

THINK CRITICALLY IN THE OPERATING ROOM

JEANNIE SCRUGGS GARBER, DNP, RN

The operating room is a complex microsystem within a complex organizational system. Human resources, patients, healthcare professionals, regulators, and processes are all interdependent in providing patient care. The operating room nurse must be able to think critically in diverse, complicated situations to create a safe environment for the surgical patient.

Nurses use the words critical thinking but what does it really mean? Good question, in that there is no consensus within the nursing profession regarding the definition of critical thinking. The concept of critical thinking is frequently connected to how nursing judgment occurs and how information is processed to make a decision that is intellectually sound and clinically appropriate for the situation.

Critical thinking, in general, is defined as a mental process of analysis and evaluation of information that creates a judgment. In order to be considered a critical thinker, one must collect information from multiple sources and make decisions based on an intellectual assessment of the findings. Critical thinking is judgment with a purpose to solve a problem or create a new situation. Logic is a component of critical thinking as well as experiences, prejudices, environment, and situation. Whether critical thinking can be taught or is an innate characteristic of individuals is debatable. Are individuals born with the cognitive ability and the behavioral attributes to support critical thinking or do individuals learn how to process information and then the behavior follows?

A critical thinker is always

- Asking why
- Asking for explanation
- Challenging the status quo
- Considering alternative options to problem solving
- Communicating how he or she thinks, what he or she thinks, and why

According to Reavis, Sandidge & Bauer (1998), the basic ideas behind systems theory support the idea that thinking patterns are complex and more than a simple processing of information. Nurses in the operating room demonstrate examples of critical thinking every day. They make decisions to prevent injury before, during, and after surgery; they provide patient education to address patient concerns, anxieties, and misconceptions; and they integrate practice standards with organizational expectations to mention just a few of the complex thought processes that occur.

Nurses are many times the link between the safe patient environment and the patient. Critical thinking and the ability to process multiple data sources and situations are key to maintaining the safety. The nurse must function somewhat like a computer—taking input from multiple sources, decoding it, and then making a decision to create an output that supports the patient's needs.

There has been little research regarding critical thinking and the possible links to patient safety in the operating room. The topic of patient safety is critical to nurses—how nurses think and solve problem might just be a key to improving patient safety.

SUGGESTED READINGS

Reavis C, Sandidge J, Bauer K. Critical thinking's role in perioperative patient safety outcomes. *AORN J*. 1998;68(5): 758–772.

ASSESSING THE PATIENT FOR RISK IN THE OPERATING ROOM

JEANNIE SCRUGGS GARBER, DNP, RN

WHAT TO DO: ASSESS

Experiencing a surgical procedure brings a certain degree of personal health risk. Patients with existing medical conditions are at greater risk for complications, and the nurse must complete a thorough preoperative assessment to help minimize the risk. Risk factors such as age, nutritional status, obesity, fluid and electrolyte balance, pregnancy, heart disease, diabetes, disease, medications, allergies, smoking and alcohol consumption habits, infection, etc. must also be discussed and assessed preoperatively to create the safest surgery experience possible.

The most important reason to complete the preoperative assessment is to establish baseline findings so that any variance from what is "normal" for that patient will be detected. In today's ambulatory and same day admission surgery setting, this can be quite challenging since the nurse may have limited time to conduct the preoperative assessment. It is becoming common practice for nurses to conduct the preoperative interview by telephone and then to conduct the physical assessment on admission. This practice calls for exceptional communication skills to gather the needed information and to allow a level of inquiry with the patient that determines risk or concerns related to the planned surgery.

Preoperative assessment for risks of surgery will allow the healthcare team in the operating room the opportunity to plan or anticipate possible complications. Patients at opposite ends of the age spectrum are the most vulnerable to surgical risk. The very young and the very old are compromised in some way already, and the surgery experience creates added stress and insult to the patient. The older patient's preoperative risk assessment should include a review of cardiovascular, integumentary, pulmonary, renal, neurologic, and metabolic systems. Any concerns identified within these systems should be communicated to the other operating room team members. If everyone is informed, everyone can be part of the ongoing assessment and perhaps be the team member that assesses the small change in patient condition that is an early indicator of a bigger concern to come. This awareness could be the key to preventing error, minimizing risk, and/or early intervention to increase patient safety.

It is also important to evaluate the patient's nutritional status or well-being. The malnourished patient should receive nutritional support and intervention prior to surgery unless it is an emergency. The obese patient is also at increased risk for complications such as hypertension, difficulty ambulating, increased oxygen consumption needs, and wound-healing concerns. The pulmonary assessment should include a routine physical exam as well as inquiry about any sleep disturbances, use of sleep apnea equipment, and smoking history. The knowledge about sleep concerns and smoking patterns will be helpful to the anesthesia providers as they plan sedation, intubation, and anesthesia.

Other significant information that is needed is the patient's medication history such as routine medications taken and reasons, history of drug abuse, usual daily alcohol intake, and any medication allergies or reactions experienced in the past. These findings can provide excellent guidance to the operating room team on which medications to administer and how to appropriately manage this patient through sedation and recovery.

Patients in the operating room are subjected to a procedure and environment that changes their "normal" status. The experience also subjects them to risk for intraoperative and postoperative complications that could be life threatening. The nurse's preoperative assessment of the patient is the key to minimizing risk and creating a safe environment so that the procedure can be successful.

SUGGESTED READINGS

Shallom L. Care of surgical clients. In: Potter P, Perry A, eds. *Fundamentals of Nursing*. Toronto, ON: Mosby-Elsevier; 2009, pp. 1368–1373.

KNOW HOW TO ASSESS AN IMPAIRED PROVIDER

ANTHONY D. SLONIM, MD, DrPH

WHAT TO DO: ASSESS

Patient safety is critically dependent upon the providers who deliver the care and the interactions that these providers have with one another. Providers want to do a good job for their patients but are sometimes unable to recognize when their performance can be compromised because of impairment. This impairment may be the result of medications, drugs, or alcohol but can also be related to sleep deprivation. The nurse needs to know how to identify these "at-risk" providers and what to do to ensure that patients are not harmed.

The impairment of providers by medications, drugs, and alcohol is not a new phenomenon. An estimated 10% to 15% of providers will experience a problem with addiction that compromises their ability to perform. These providers are at risk of hurting their patients, risking their livelihood, their families and their careers. Fortunately, most providers who receive treatment do well and recover. State medical board monitoring programs and a nonjudgmental approach toward these providers have been instrumental in securing success. The difficulty arises when the providers are not self-aware and do not believe that they have a problem.

Traditionally, the specialties with the highest risk for abuse and addiction have been anesthesiologists, emergency medicine providers, and psychiatrists. Two important characteristics distinguish this group including access to medications and stressful work conditions. There are a number of other medical disciplines including surgery and intensive care that may also be at risk given these criteria. Nonetheless, the nurse is in an important position to be able to identify these providers before they do harm to patients.

The warning signs of impaired providers are highly variable. There may be a change in appearance from the norm for that person. The provider may look tired, unshaven, and drowsy. A usually upbeat person will be "down." Their attention to detail may drift. Usually the fastidious provider may pay less attention and may be easily distracted. They may have behavioral outbursts. Some may show up to work with alcohol on their breath or be visibly under the influence.

The nurse has an immediate professional obligation to raise concerns when he or she perceives that something may be wrong. This includes the presentation of an impaired provider. When these circumstances arise, the nurse can attempt to speak with the providers to assess their current status. An approach of genuine concern is fine. "Hey, are you ok? You look more tired than usual" or "Rough night last night?" may provide the inroads to a useful conversation before the provider gets in the operating room. Do not be surprised if the provider becomes defensive. A follow-up question can continue to probe the situation. "Oh, well I was concerned because you don't look yourself today" may open the door to more direct conversations, but if it does not, the nurse needs to be prepared to follow appropriate hospital policy by discussing this with his or her director or nursing supervisor prior to allowing that provider to see the patient.

The issue of human factors or how humans interact with their environment, including the medical environment, has a profound impact on patient safety. Providers are humans and need to eat, sleep, and have bathroom breaks. Failure to allow these activities provides a distraction from patient care and can potentially jeopardize patient safety. Fatigue is one of the best examples of human factors, and there has been considerable attention to this topic in the last several years including one of the largest impact initiatives in recent medical history, the resident work hour restrictions. Nonetheless, there is concern on two levels with this initiative that nurses need to be aware of. First, just because the work hour restriction of 80 h is in place, 80 h is still a lot of time for a trainee with minimal experience performing highly technical procedures. Second, while the rule addresses resident trainees, other healthcare professionals, particularly attending physicians, are not subject to the rule and may have "grown up" in an era when you did what was expected for the patient. These are particularly important providers for the nurse to identify because they may not realize that their own performance is compromised.

In the operating room, mundane and monotonous tasks, particularly over long durations, may lead to problems. Anesthesiologists are particularly susceptible to the effects of fatigue over long cases. The nurses in the operating room, however, may find themselves in a difficult position, particularly for long cases when fatigue sets in during the operative course. Knowing how to appropriately escalate these situations so that the patient is protected is important for the nurse and the patient.

Healthcare providers are similar to professionals in other disciplines. They eat, drink, and sleep. Some will become addicted to drugs and alcohol; others will work themselves to exhaustion. The nurse needs to know how to recognize these impairments and what to do about them when they occur to protect the patient.

SUGGESTED READINGS

Baldisseri MR. Impaired healthcare professional. *Crit Care Med.* 2007;35(2 Suppl):S106–S116.

Biller CK, Antonacci AC, Pelletier S, et al. The 80-hour work guidelines and resident survey perceptions of quality. *J Surg Res.* 2006;135(2):275–281.

Boisaubin EV, Levine RE. Identifying and assisting the impaired physician. *Am J Med Sci.* 2001;322(1):31–36. Review.

Jagsi R, Weinstein DF, Shapiro J, et al. The Accreditation Council for Graduate Medical Education's limits on residents' work hours and patient safety. A study of resident experiences and perceptions before and after hours reductions. *Arch Intern Med.* 2008;168(5):493–500.

Luck S, Hedrick J. The alarming trend of substance abuse in anesthesia providers. *J Perianesth Nurs.* 2004;19(5):308–311.

DO NOT LET DISRUPTIVE BEHAVIOR IN THE OPERATING ROOM BE THE CAUSE OF HARM TO YOUR PATIENTS

ANTHONY D. SLONIM, MD, DRPH

WHAT TO DO: IMPLEMENT

For decades, the acknowledgment and tolerance of disruptive behavior in healthcare, particularly in the operating room, have been sensationalized in the popular press, the movies, and on television. Healthcare providers in these venues know all too well that these events have a negative impact on the function of the team and potentially the outcomes of the patients. As with most opportunities in healthcare, when providers are unable to uniformly address these challenges and problems, regulatory bodies step in to ensure that patients are safe. Recently, the Joint Commission released a sentinel event alert that highlights some of the problems related to disruptive behaviors, their impact on patients, and what institutions and providers need to do to ensure that improvements occur.

Healthcare environments where these behaviors tend to be demonstrated include high-stress environments with their own unique cultures. The behaviors may range from verbally abusive, which includes yelling, demeaning, and making fun of others, to physical outbursts, including throwing an object or pushing. Regardless of how they are manifested, all providers have a role in ensuring that these behaviors are not tolerated in healthcare.

Several important steps can help us to achieve this level of accountability. First, there needs to be a commitment to each other that we will not allow a colleague to be bullied by someone else. Stepping into the middle of an interaction and diffusing it demonstrates collegial support, when possible from the patient care area. If this cannot be done safely at that time, as it may harm the patient, a follow-up is important. Second, medical staff bodies have a code of conduct that addresses how physicians in particular need to behave in the hospital environment and participate as members of the team. Third, teamwork education is important for building and sustaining this work. Most physicians have not had any teamwork education or training and model behaviors that were passed down to them from their mentors and colleagues. Finally, a reporting system that tracks, trends, and offers support to the disruptive provider is an important step in eliminating these behaviors.

Disruptive behaviors in healthcare cannot be tolerated and often require nurses who are on the front line in the heat of the battle to advocate appropriately for their patients and other members of the team. Knowing your hospital's policies and procedures is important and can provide guidance, but only you can know when someone's behavior has "crossed the line." You feel it in the pit of your stomach. Do not allow that behavior to manifest itself as a bad outcome for the patient.

SUGGESTED READINGS

Rosenstein AH, O'Daniel M. Disruptive behavior and clinical outcomes: Perceptions of nurses and physicians. *Am J Nurs.* 2005;105(1):54–64. Available at: http://www.jointcommission.org/sentinelevents/sentineleventalert/sea_40.htm. Accessed August 29, 2008.

VHA Research Finds Disruptive Behavior Common in Operating Rooms; Behavior Linked to Adverse Events, Medical Errors, and Mortality. Available at: http://www.surgicenteronline.com/hotnews/67h613463885025.html. Accessed August 29, 2008.

316

OSTOMY EDUCATION IS ESSENTIAL FOR THE FRESH OSTOMY PATIENT

MELISSA H. CRIGGER, BSN, MHA, RN

WHAT TO DO: ASSESS AND IMPLEMENT

The care of an ostomy patient includes detailed information regarding site care, pouching, and diet. Ostomy is the surgical opening of a body cavity. The opening is called a stoma. Ostomy surgery can be performed due to surgery of the intestinal tract, trauma of the gastrointestinal tract, severe inflammation or infection, and cancer of the bowel or bladder. Fecal diversions are common forms of ostomies and include the ileostomy and colostomy. An ileostomy (an ileal opening) is created in cases when the entire colon is removed as with cancer whereas the colostomy (opening of the colon), depending on its location, is used to allow fecal material to be eliminated.

When caring for the ostomy patient, it is important that the nurse educates the patient on proper assessment of the stoma. The nurse should always inspect the stoma for a beefy red color. An ostomy that is pale, bluish, or black is indicative of poor circulation. The patient and the nurse should report any abnormal color immediately to the physician. The nurse should also educate the patient that initially the stoma will be edematous due to the surgery, but as the stoma heals, the site may be a rose-red color and will shrink within 6 to 8 weeks of surgery. The patient should be aware that initial drainage from the ostoma might contain the presence of some blood or mucus. The patient should be observant of the drainage and be aware that fecal drainage can take up to 48 h to occur in the ileostomy patient.

Proper pouching is another topic that must always be discussed in the patient with an ostomy. The patient should be aware that to change the pouch, the patient must have a pouch with an attached or separate skin barrier, paste, pouch closure device, and adhesive remover.

The nurse should educate the patient that the appliance should be removed and reapplied at regular intervals (as frequently as every 3 days and as infrequently as every 14 days). If the pouch leaks, the appliance should be changed to prevent skin breakdown from fecal material. The stoma should be measured, and the appliance should be measured and cut based on the stoma measurement, especially during the first 6 to 8 weeks when the stoma is more edematous. Once edema subsides, the measurement of the stoma should remain the same. The patient should be aware of the importance of emptying the pouch when it is ½ to ⅓ full. If the pouch is allowed to fill more than this level, the seal of the barrier could be compromised. For the patient with complaints of pouch odor, the nurse should instruct the patient on the use of deodorant sprays such as Banish to control odor. Another technique is to add a couple of drops of mouthwash to a piece of toilet tissue.

With ostomies, dietary management is another aspect of ostomy education. Patients are usually encouraged to eat soft diets initially, which progresses to a more regular consistency. However, the patient must be aware that high fiber foods should be avoided in the initial postoperative phase. This includes food such as:

- Celery
- Coconut
- Corn
- Cabbage
- Coleslaw
- Citrus fruits
- Peas
- Popcorn
- Spinach
- Dried fruit
- Nuts
- Sauerkraut
- Seeds
- Skin of fruits and vegetables

The patient should be encouraged to eat at regular time periods, to chew food well, and to drink adequate fluids. The patient should avoid foods that cause gas and avoid gaining excessive amounts of weight.

Regardless if the patient has an ileostomy or colostomy, nurses must remember that skin assessment, pouching education, and diet education are of the utmost importance. Remember that the stoma should be beefy red; if not, notify the physician. Also the educated patients will better manage their stoma.

SUGGESTED READINGS

Linton AD. The patient with an ostomy. In: *Introduction to Medical-Surgical Nursing*. 4th Ed. St. Louis, MO: Saunders-Elsevier; 2007, pp. 396–401.

Williams LS, Hopper PD. Nursing care of patients with lower gastrointestinal disorders. In: *Understanding Medical Surgical Nursing*. 2nd Ed. Philadelphia, PA: F.A. Davis Company; 2003; pp. 525–529.

IMPORTANCE OF DANGLING BEFORE ACTIVITY IN THE POSTOPERATIVE PATIENT

MELISSA H. CRIGGER, BSN, MHA, RN

WHAT TO DO: IMPLEMENT

Remember that activity should be increased slowly with dangling performed prior to ambulation due to the risk of orthostatic hypotension. The postoperative patient requires thorough nursing care. One area of concern for the patient who has had an invasive surgical procedure is the potential for impaired physical mobility. As with all postoperative patients, the nurse must remember to implement the proper level of activity based on the physician's order. For the patient with activity orders for ambulation, the nurse must always remember to assist the patient to a dangling position prior to actually mobilizing the patient.

Orthostatic hypotension occurs when the patient's systolic blood pressure drops suddenly with a change in posture. In order to qualify as orthostatic hypotension, the systolic blood pressure must drop 20 mm Hg during the change of position from lying to standing position or from sitting to standing position. Those patients that suffer from orthostatic hypotension may complain of light-headedness and dizziness.

The nurse caring for the postoperative patient with activity orders must remember the importance of progressing slowly when getting the patient out of bed for the first time. Prior to getting the patient out of bed, the nurse should remember to first raise the head of the bed slowly to allow the patient to adjust to the position change. If the patient complains of dizziness or light-headedness with raising the head of the bed, the position should be lowered with the nurse obtaining vital signs and allowing the patient to rest for up to 1 h. Once the patient has rested, the nurse should attempt to raise the head of the bed again.

Once the patient has achieved the sitting position without complaints of dizziness and light-headedness, the nurse should then attempt to dangle the patient on the side of the bed. Dangling should occur for at least 1 to 2 min prior to the nurse attempting to ambulate the patient. Once the patient has been able to tolerate dangling, the nurse can attempt ambulation. Upon rising, the patient should have eyes facing forward and should rise slowly. The nurse should remember that depending on the surgical procedure and the patient's strength, the patient may require the assistance of two healthcare workers for ambulation. The patient might also benefit from the use of a gait belt.

The nurse should be aware of signs of orthostatic hypotension, which include complaints of dizziness, light-headedness, feeling faint, and skin pallor. The patient who verbalizes any of these symptoms should be allowed to return to the sitting position and then back to the lying position. The nurse should also obtain vital signs upon first attempt of ambulation postoperatively. These vital signs should be performed while sitting as well as standing. The nurse should also return the patient to bed if orthostatic hypotension occurs (e.g., patient's sitting blood pressure was 120/80 and upon standing, the patient's blood pressure dropped to 80/40).

Should a patient become faint, the nurse must remember that safety is of utmost importance. If this occurs during ambulation with the assistance of one nurse, the nurse should assist the patient either to bed or to a chair. If neither is available, the nurse should control lowering the patient to the floor to prevent injury. For the patient with two healthcare workers assisting in ambulation, the second healthcare provider can walk behind the ambulatory patient with a wheelchair. If the patient becomes dizzy or faint, the wheelchair is easily accessible to provide a safe sitting position. Obtain vital signs and notify the physician immediately if syncope occurs.

Remember to check the activity order. Dangling is important to provide adjustment for the cardiovascular system after prolonged bed rest or surgery. Dangling should always be performed to assist with the prevention of orthostatic hypotension.

SUGGESTED READINGS

Linton AD. Surgical care. In: *Introduction to Medical-Surgical Nursing*. 4th Ed. St. Louis, MO: Saunders-Elsevier; 2007, pp. 274–276.

Williams LS, Hopper PD. Nursing care of patients having surgery. In: *Understanding Medical Surgical Nursing*. 2nd Ed. Philadelphia, PA: F.A. Davis Company; 2003, pp. 170–171.

PREVENT WOUND DISRUPTION IN OBESE PATIENTS

MONTY D. GROSS, PhD, RN, CNE

WHAT TO DO: IMPLEMENT

Obese patients are at higher risk of experiencing wound disruptions in the postoperative period. Despite a seemingly unremarkable recovery, with minimal pain and moderate discharge, some patients can experience difficulty with skin closure in the postoperative period. Most wound sutures or staples holding the skin together stay in place for 7 to 10 days. Earlier removal may jeopardize the integrity of the site since the patient's obesity causes increased stress on the incision. These patients include patients with obesity and poor nutrition and those taking medications such as steroids that impede wound healing. When an activity order to get the patient out of bed is given, the patient should be assisted to the bedside chair, provided with an abdominal binder, and provided with a call bell to ask for assistance when completed.

Disruption of abdominal wounds in obese patients is a source of morbidity and mortality. Infection is one of the more common causes of wound disruption. Obesity is an independent risk factor for wound complications. Healing is delayed and infection is more likely because of poor subcutaneous vascular supply.

Vacuum-assisted wound closure devices can decrease wound edema, closure time, and wound bacterial colony counts. Wound vacuums provide negative pressure and enclose the wound area to promote healing. Due to the fact that dressing changes are less frequent, new tissue growth is disrupted and pain reduced.

Obese patients need extra consideration with abdominal wounds. Sutures should not be removed prematurely. Abdominal binders may be used to provide extra support while the wound heals. This is especially important as the patient's activity level increases. Vacuum-assisted closure devices are a proven method to heal complicated wounds.

SUGGESTED READINGS

Heller L, Levin S, Butler C. Management of abdominal wound dehiscence using vacuum assisted closure in patients with compromised healing. *Am J Surg*. 2006;191(2):165–172.

Kore S, Vyavaharkar M, Akolekar R, et al. Comparison of closure of subcutaneous tissue versus non-closure in relation to wound disruption after abdominal hysterectomy in obese patients. *J Postgrad Med*. 2000;46(1):26–28.

MALIGNANT HYPERTHERMIA IN THE PACU

JEANNIE SCRUGGS GARBER, DNP, RN

Malignant hyperthermia (MH) is a hereditary condition of uncontrolled heat production that results from the administration of anesthetic agents and can occur during or after anesthesia. The first hour postsurgery is a particularly critical time for this life-threatening complication.

The diagnosis of MH should be suspected when an elevated level of carbon dioxide is noticed, which is an early sign, and may occur during induction of anesthesia or postoperatively. Other signs and symptoms include tachypnea, premature ventricular contractions, labile blood pressure, cyanosis, mottling, and muscular rigidity. Regardless of when it occurs, immediate diagnosis and treatment are necessary. Diagnosis is complex and must be made early to prevent a life-threatening situation.

The treatment for MH is largely supportive, but there is specific therapy available. The drug of choice is dantrolene sodium. Its use and the avoidance of future anesthesia for at-risk patients have greatly reduced the mortality from MH. Other treatments may include cooling blankets and ice packs, blood pressure medications, or other drugs specific to symptoms.

The best way to prevent MH is through the detection of those at risk prior to surgery. A family history of death during general anesthesia or having a high body temperature during or after general anesthesia is the most likely indicator that a person may be susceptible to MH. The nurse can play a vital role in prevention of this situation by collecting an accurate patient and family history preoperatively. Patients may also wear a medical alert bracelet to communicate this in case of an emergency. A resource for patients or professionals about MH is the Malignant Hyperthermia Association of the United States at www.mhaus.org or the 24 h hotline at 800–644–9737.

This anesthetic complication remains incompletely understood and ongoing research may provide hope for saving lives of postoperative patients in the future.

SUGGESTED READINGS

Litman R, Rosenberg H. Malignant hyperthermia: Update on susceptibility testing. *J Am Med Assoc.* 2005;293(23): 2918–2924.

Malignant Hyperthermia Association of the United States (MHAUS) (n.d.). Available at: www.mhaus.org.

FREQUENT POSTOPERATIVE MONITORING

JEANNIE SCRUGGS GARBER, DNP, RN

WHAT TO DO: EVALUATE

The postoperative patient requires close observation and evaluation for early detection of complications or detrimental changes in condition that could result in negative outcomes. Patients who have undergone a surgical procedure and had anesthesia are at increased risk for airway, circulatory, and neurologic complications, and postanesthesia nurses are the most likely clinicians to anticipate and identify life-threatening situations.

Postoperative care is a complex, sometimes rapidly changing, scenario. In order for compromised patients to be identified, the nurse must maintain close observation and monitoring of all the major organ systems of the patients' postanesthesia. The nurse should begin with an assessment of the patients' airway. The tongue is the most common cause of airway obstruction postoperatively, so it is imperative that nurses support the patients in keeping an appropriate position to maintain an open airway. Once the airway is ensured, attention can be turned to the breathing. The respiratory rate, breathing patterns, lung sounds, and oxygen saturation should be monitored for each patient. The level of consciousness and color change should also be noted. The circulatory system is also at risk following surgical intervention. Circulatory parameters to be monitored include heart rate, cardiac rhythm, blood pressure, capillary refill, pulses at multiple points, and extremity color. Another circulatory complication is hemorrhage either internally or at the surgical site. The nurse must pay close attention to the patients' blood pressure, changes in heart rate and respiratory rate, pulse strength, skin assessment including change in temperature, moisture, or color, and sudden onset of restlessness. Once the As, Bs, and Cs are ensured, attention can be turned to other important elements of the evaluation.

The patients' temperature should be monitored to determine hypothermia, potential infection, or the possibility of malignant hyperthermia. Fluid and electrolyte balance must be assessed immediately postoperatively and is best evaluated with lab values, skin turgor, cardiac and neurologic assessments, and by measuring fluid intake and output. The skin should be assessed for rashes and color changes that could signal hemodynamic concerns and for evidence of pressure or positioning changes during surgery. The gastrointestinal and genitourinary tracts should also be part of the assessment process to check bowel sounds, intake, and output and rule out abdominal distention. Pain should also be assessed and treated immediately during the postoperative recovery phase.

The postoperative recovery phase demands close monitoring and frequent nursing evaluation to quickly identify and prevent postoperative complications and negative patient outcomes.

SUGGESTED READINGS

Schallom L. Care of surgical clients. In: Potter PA, Perry AG, eds. *Fundamentals of Nursing*. Toronto, ON: Mosby-Elsevier; 2009, pp. 1393–1399.

PNEUMONECTOMY PATIENTS WITH CHEST TUBES SHOULD NOT BE PLACED ON WALL SUCTION

FRANCINE B. YATES, RRT, RN, BSN

WHAT TO DO: IMPLEMENT

The incidence of pulmonary surgery is increasing as a result of smoking and chronic obstructive pulmonary disease, empyema, tumors, or masses. Postoperative care should be provided by the thoracic surgeon and multidisciplinary teams that are trained in the care of thoracic patients. Multiple complications such as respiratory failure, tachyarrhythmias, and renal failure need to be recognized and managed quickly and efficiently to reduce the risk of catastrophic events. It is important that staff members that care for these patients are familiar with the different types of surgeries, the anatomy of the procedure, what systems are initially affected, and the use of chest tubes and fluid replacement.

Pneumonectomies are not as common as thoracic procedures such as wedge resections, lobectomies, or thoracoscopies, and they are somewhat more difficult to manage postoperatively. Fluid replacement and blood pressure are two areas of management that make this procedure a nursing challenge. Pneumonectomy patients are kept dry in the operating room to reduce the risk of postpneumonectomy edema. The onset of this complication is rapid with increasing shortness of breath and infiltrates, suggesting pulmonary edema in the opposing lung. Pneumonectomy patients are often hypotensive after surgery and it is preferable to use inotropic agents to increase the blood pressure rather than fluid administration. If edema develops, it can be managed with fluid restrictions and diuretics.

An additional challenge with a pneumonectomy patient is chest tube management. Should a chest tube be required postoperatively, it is imperative that the anatomy and physiology of the pneumonectomy is understood. Pneumonectomy patients experience a type of postoperative rotation and mediastinal shift toward the surgical side since the lung tissue has been removed and air exits from the pleural space. The retention of air added to accumulating fluid can cause deviation of the mediastinum toward the remaining lung. Several adverse conditions can occur if the air accumulation occurs too rapidly after thoracotomy closure, such as arrhythmias, hypotension, and postpneumonectomy edema. A large shift toward the remaining lung can impair venous return or compromise lung function on the "good" side. Chest tubes, when required for bleeding or pleural drainage, should be attached to water seal at all times. If the chest tube is placed on wall suction, this mediastinal shift may occur too rapidly. With each cough, air is expelled, increasing the shift. In turn, this can cause over-distention of the remaining lung, which increases the risk for pulmonary edema. Placing the chest tubes on suction may also initiate cardiac herniation if the pericardium was entered or result in sudden death due to bronchopleural fistula.

Competencies and education should be required of all nursing staff for chest tube management in thoracic surgery. Each type of pulmonary surgery may require a chest tube at some point. Chest tube set up, management, and troubleshooting skills as well as attention to details are needed to ensure patient safety and recovery.

SUGGESTED READINGS

Deslauriers J, Mehran R. *Handbook of Perioperative Care in General Thoracic Surgery*. St. Louis, MO: Mosby; 2005, pp. 241–242, 264–267, 318–319.

Lynn-McHale Weigand DJ, Carlson KK. Closed chest drainage system. In: *AACN Procedure Manual for Critical Care*. 5th Ed. Philadelphia: Elsevier; 2005, pp. 151–169.

ACTIVITY LEVELS FOR THE TOTAL HIP ARTHROPLASTY

MELISSA H. CRIGGER, BSN, MHA, RN

WHAT TO DO: IMPLEMENT

Remember that joint mobility is reduced in the total hip arthroplasty patient. Total hip arthroplasty involves the insertion of a two-piece device (an acetabular cup and a femoral component) into the pelvic acetabulum and femur. The most common complication of this surgery is subluxation or total dislocation of the hip and requires that the patient as well as the nursing staff be aware of correct positioning.

There are many nursing interventions to ensure correct positioning of the total hip arthroplasty. Postoperatively, the use of an abduction pillow or placing pillows between the patient's legs can ensure correct positioning. The primary purpose for the use of pillows or the abductor pillow is to prevent adduction of the hip. Whenever the patient is turned, pillows should be placed between the patient's legs to prevent internal rotation or adduction. The nurse should also remember to turn the hip and legs concurrently to prevent dislocation. A key goal for the nurse is to prevent adduction after surgery.

Other concerns of positioning include preventing hyperflexion (flexing the joint more than 90°) and internal rotation. The patient should be educated not to flex the hip more than 90°. Some physicians initially order the patient not to sit at an angle more than 60°. This requires the use of a reclining chair. As the patient progresses, the physician will allow positioning to increase up to 90°. The patient needs to avoid bending at the waist to pick up objects. Bending at the waist could lead to hyperflexion, which could lead to subluxation of the prosthesis. Another potential cause of subluxation is when the patient attempts to don his or her own socks, shoes, or stockings. It is recommended that the patient does not put on his or her own socks or shoes for at least 6 weeks to 2 months. Should the patient need to pick up items, the patient should receive an assistive device from occupational therapy, such as a grabber. This reduces the need to bend at the waist, which could lead to hyperflexion.

The patient also has to be aware of the need for a raised toilet seat if he or she is to be discharged. The use of a raised toilet seat allows toileting without causing hip flexion of more than 90°. The nurse must always educate the patient not to cross his or her legs due to the potential of internal rotation and adduction. The nurse must also educate the patient to recognize symptoms of subluxation and total dislocation. This includes pain in the affected joint, any loss of function, and deformity of the affected extremity or shortening of the affected limb.

Immobility is another concern for the total hip arthroplasty patient. Physicians usually encourage early ambulation, that is, within the first day postoperatively. Due to immobility, the patient is at risk for joint stiffening, skin breakdown, and pulmonary issues. The nurse must remember to reposition the patient as ordered by physician at least every 2 h and inspect for pressure points or skin breakdown. Cough and deep breathing exercises and the use of incentive spirometer, which should be an expected order postoperatively, should be instructed to the patient. The nurse must always assess lung sounds through auscultation. Abnormal lung sounds are indicative of retained secretions and atelectasis.

Education is extremely important for the total hip arthroplasty patient. Positioning and breathing exercises can make the difference in whether or not a patient ends up with postoperative complications such as subluxation, total hip displacement, possible atelectasis, and skin breakdown.

SUGGESTED READINGS

Linton AD. Connective tissue disorders. In: *Introduction to Medical-Surgical Nursing*. 4th Ed. St. Louis, MO: Saunders-Elsevier; 2007, pp. 893–899.

Williams LS, Hopper PD. Nursing care of patients with musculoskeletal and connective tissue disorders. In: *Understanding Medical-Surgical Nursing*. 2nd Ed. Philadelphia, PA: F.A. Davis Company; 2003, pp. 774–777.

COMMON MEASURES FOR SAFE CAST CARE

MELISSA H. CRIGGER, BSN, MHA, RN

WHAT TO DO: EVALUATE

Remember that cast care requires observation and education. Casts are used to hold the fractured bones in alignment. The goal of cast application is to secure the position of the fractured bone, thus allowing early mobility and a reduction in pain. The cast can also be used to correct deformities and support weak joints. There are different types of material used for casting. Plaster of Paris and fiberglass are durable materials that are used. Plaster of Paris casts are hot when applied for about half an hour due to the chemical reaction that occurs when the plaster is wet. It requires 24 to 72 h drying time. During this drying time, the plaster of Paris cast must be handled gently to prevent indentations that can cause pressure points. When the cast is dry, it is hard, with a shiny white coat. Fiberglass casts require less drying time. They harden within 10 to 15 min and often allow weight bearing within 30 min of application. The patient who has received a plaster of Paris cast must receive education on cast care, which includes not getting it wet. The patient with a fiberglass cast may get the cast wet. Other possible materials that can be used for cast application include thermolabile plastic and thermoplastic resins.

Post procedure care of a cast requires observation of the casted limb. The nurse must remember to assess edema of the extremity and complete neurovascular checks in areas distal to the fracture and compare these assessments to the unaffected extremity. These assessments should be performed every 1 to 2 h for the first 24 h, and every 4 h afterward. This assessment includes

- Pulse checks of the affected extremity
- Assessment of skin color
- Capillary refill time
- Sensation

The nurse should remember that edema is often present with a fracture. The casted limb should be elevated for the first 24 to 48 h. Ice can also be applied to the casted limb. The nurse must also remember to assess for cast tightness, which could lead to compartment syndrome. Cast tightness must be relayed to the physician immediately so that an order for bivalving (cutting the cast down two sides) can be ordered to reduce pressure. The nurse must also observe any drainage or odors coming from inside the cast. Both are signs of infection. In case the cast was applied over the wound, the physician may decide to cut a window into the cast to allow for observation of the wound and to allow for the provision of wound care. Any window should always be taped in place to prevent exposure of skin.

Due to the roughness of the cast, it is necessary for the nurse to maintain skin integrity. The skin around the cast should be assessed for redness and irritation. If the cast edges are causing irritation, then they should be trimmed or petaled (application of moleskin or adhesive strips over the edges to prevent irritation). The patient must receive education not to insert foreign objects into the cast and not to apply lotion or powder on the skin around the cast. This could lead to injury of the tissue as well as provide a medium for microorganism growth. The patient should always be educated on the signs of infection, which include drainage, odor of the cast, and elevated temperature.

SUGGESTED READINGS

Linton AD. Fractures. In: *Introduction to Medical-Surgical Nursing*. 4th Ed. St. Louis, MO: Saunders-Elsevier; 2007, pp. 914–922.

Williams LS, Hopper PD. Nursing care of patients with musculoskeletal and connective tissue disorders. In: *Understanding Medical-Surgical Nursing*. 2nd Ed. Philadelphia, PA: F.A. Davis Company; 2003, pp. 782–786.

REMEMBER THAT TRACTION CARE REQUIRES OBSERVATION OF THE PULLEY SYSTEM AND LINE OF PULL

MELISSA H. CRIGGER, BSN, MHA, RN

WHAT TO DO: EVALUATE

Traction is recognized as a system that exerts a pulling force to create proper alignment of a fractured bone. Traction can be applied to the skin or attached directly to the bone through metal pins or wires. Skin traction, also known as Buck traction, involves the application of a boot with Velcro or a sling, which is then attached to the skin. This type of traction is often used for pain control due to muscle spasms that can occur with bone fractures. Skin traction is applied most often preoperatively to hip fractures. Weight of less than 5 to 10 lb is usually applied during skin traction to prevent injury to the surrounding tissue. Skeletal traction allows heavier weights to be applied (15 to 30 lb). Skeletal traction involves the use of pins, screws, wires, or tongs that are surgically implanted into the bone.

When applying traction, the nurse should remember that complications could occur due to its use. These complications include impaired circulation, breakdown of skin, soft tissue injury, and improper fracture alignment. The nurse should also be aware that pin site infection as well as osteomyelitis could occur in those patients that receive skeletal traction. Due to the potential for complications, the nurse must always monitor neurovascular checks (pulse checks of affected extremity in conjunction with unaffected extremity, assessment of skin color, capillary refill time, and presence of sensation). Traction must always be maintained for fractures and include the following assessment and interventions:

- Knots, pulleys, ropes, and weights are inspected at least once per shift to keep them intact
- The weight system must remain free of obstructions and should never be sitting on the floor
- Weights should never be removed and lifted while in use
- The patient should be properly aligned in bed with feet not touching the footboard
- When repositioning the patient, the nurse should always obtain assistance from other staff members due to the potential for injury in lifting the patient with weight system in place
- For patients with skeletal traction, the pin sites should always be observed for redness, drainage, and odor, which are indicative of infection
- For patients receiving Buck traction (skin traction), the nurse should always inspect the skin for signs of skin breakdown as well as pressure points and irritation of the skin due to equipment

The use of skeletal traction can be linked to pin site infection and osteomyelitis. The nurse must always monitor vital signs and report any elevated temperature to the physician. The nurse must remember that the elderly client has an increased risk for developing skin ulcers, especially on the heels. The importance of skin assessment cannot be stressed enough. Another concern with traction is that it causes increased immobility. The patient must receive education regarding the importance of cough and deep breathing to prevent stasis of lung secretions.

SUGGESTED READINGS

Linton AD. Fractures. In: *Introduction to Medical-Surgical Nursing.* 4th Ed. St. Louis, MO: Saunders-Elsevier; 2007, pp. 914–923.

Williams LS, Hopper PD. Nursing care of patients with musculoskeletal and connective tissue disorders. *Understanding Medical-Surgical Nursing.* 2nd Ed. Philadelphia, PA: F.A. Davis Company; 2003, pp. 782–786.

ENSURE CORRECT NASOGASTRIC TUBE PLACEMENT

MONTY D. GROSS, PHD, RN, CNE

WHAT TO DO: EVALUATE

Nasogastric tubes provide a route for patients to receive nutritional support and medications or, in some cases, have stomach contents removed. However, improper insertion or maintenance can cause serious injury.

Large-bore tubes such as the single-lumen Levin tube or double-lumen gastric (Salem) sump tube with a blue pigtail and antireflux valve allow for administration of products and the extraction of gastric contents. These tubes are especially helpful to remove poisons, toxins, or drugs ingested by the client. This is often accomplished by connecting the tube to intermittent or constant low-pressure suction. It is important to keep the blue pigtail clear of stomach contents or fluid to prevent excess vacuum pressure from developing within the stomach. If the blue pigtail becomes blocked, it can be cleared with 20 mL of air. When removing contents, the blue pigtail end of the tube must be kept above the patient's stomach to prevent a siphoning effect. The blue end of the reflux valve is inserted into the blue pigtail to assist with this function.

Small-bore feeding tubes are more flexible and less irritating to the patient. Because small-bore tubes are more flexible, extracting contents from the stomach is often impossible as the tube may collapse when suction is applied. A guide wire filling the inner lumen of the tube is often used to facilitate passage of the tube through the oral pharyngeal anatomy and into the stomach or small intestine. To prevent injury to the patient, inspect the tube for a guide wire protruding through the tube wall prior to attempting to insert the tube. The guide wire is carefully removed after the placement of the tube is confirmed.

It is critical to determine that the tube is correctly positioned prior to administering food or medications. The inadvertent instillation of food or medications into the lungs can be lethal and results from inadvertent confirmation of tube placement. Be sure to check your hospital's policy regarding the method confirming placement. Historically, auscultating for the injection of an air bolus of 20 to 30 mL into the stomach was used to determine tube placement. Unfortunately, auscultating for tube placement is unreliable. There are more reliable ways to assess for tube placement.

Gastric pH testing is one method to help determine tube placement. The pH of gastric contents should be <5. However, after about 24 h, tubes often migrate into the small intestine. The pH in the small intestine is normally between 6 and 8. Using a 50 mL syringe, aspirate 5 to 10 mL of secretions. Gastric secretions are normally green to tan in color. Respiratory secretions are usually light yellow with mucus and a pH of >6. Testing for gastric pH should occur at least 1 h after administering medication or food to avoid the pH altering effect of medications and food. However, this method is not feasible when the patient is on continuous tube feeding. Tube feeding formulas will raise the pH of the gastric contents. After the initial placement of the feeding tube and when in doubt of the tube's position, an X-ray should be obtained.

Remember to be sure that the tube is in the correct location before administering any medication or substance into the patient. New tube feeding design variations will be available. Appropriate training and guidelines for their use need to be adopted by hospitals to ensure appropriate use.

SUGGESTED READINGS

Smith S, Duell D, Martin B. *Clinical Nursing Skills: Basic to Advanced Skills.* Upper Saddle River, NJ: Pearson; 2008.

PREVENTION OF INFECTION IN ORTHOPEDIC SURGERY PATIENTS IS EVERYONE'S JOB

JULIE MULLIGAN WATTS, RN, MN

WHAT TO DO: PLAN

Preventing infections in hospitals takes everyone's effort and should not be an option. Hospitals cannot afford to ignore recommendations and standards that will improve infection prevention. Hospital-acquired infections cost hospitals more than $30 billion a year, resulting from the 2 million infections that occur. The average cost to manage an infection is $15,000. Preventing infection in orthopedic surgery patients is imperative due to the risk of oseteomyelitis, a serious infection that is difficult to treat.

Prophylactic antibiotics and other infection control processes are used to minimize the risk of infection in this population. Osteomyelitis is a bone infection that requires long courses of antibiotics for treatment. Often, the surgical site must be re-explored and bone, prosthesis, and internal fixation devices removed.

Many healthcare and regulatory organizations have proposed recommendations and set standards to improve hospital acquired infections. Some include the Joint Commission for the Accreditation of Healthcare Organizations (JCAHO), The Surgical Care Improvement Project (SCIP), the World Health Organization (WHO), and various others. The SCIP is a national partnership of organizations working to reduce surgical complications. The goal of SCIP is to reduce the incidence of surgical complications nationally by 25% by 2010.

The SCIP recommends prophylactic antibiotics one hour prior to surgery, proper hair removal without the use of razors, and maintaining normothermia in colorectal surgery patients immediately after the operation. Postoperative wound infections are to be diagnosed during the indexed hospitalization. While most individuals with direct patient care responsibilities are focused on handwashing, sterile technique, and isolation procedures, those working in other hospital departments need to realize their role in preventing infection and work as a team with caregivers.

Some hospitals have transitioned to patient-centered care or other strategies that promote teamwork by focusing efforts on the patient. The aim is to provide excellent care that is closer to the patient and makes staff and patient interactions less complicated. Good communication, staff development, and collaboration are characteristic of an effective team approach. Cross training of staff or development of new roles could help to improve the environment of care when it comes to preventing infection. Orthopedic staff, including caregivers, dietary staff, and environmental services staff, should all work together to keep the patient area clean to avoid wound infections in the orthopedic patients.

SUGGESTED READINGS

Hagenstad R, Weis C, Brophy K. Strike a balance with decentralized housekeeping. *Nurs Manage*. 2001;31(6):39–43.

McGaughey B. Saving lives and the bottom line. Hospitals must answer growing pressure to act on homegrown infections. *Mod Healthc*. 2006;36(5).

Medicare quality improvement community. Surgical Care Improvement Project: A national quality partnership. Available at: http://www.medqic.org. Accessed May 10, 2008.

Smeltzer S, Bare B. *Brunner & Suddarth's Textbook of Medical-Surgical Nursing*. 10th Ed. Philadelphia, PA: Lippincott Williams & Wilkins; 2004.

KNOW HOW TO PREVENT INFECTION IN YOUR BURN PATIENTS

JEANNIE SCRUGGS GARBER, DNP, RN

WHAT TO DO: IMPLEMENT

According to Murray, "approximately 500,000 persons seek medical treatment for burns every year in the United States. Of these, approximately 40,000 are hospitalized for burn injuries. Typically, 4,000 people die from fire and burns every year; nearly 75% die at the scene of the incident or during initial transport. Of those who reach medical care, infection is a major cause of morbidity and mortality." The skin is one of the largest organs of the human body and serves as a physical shield for the body against infection. Burn wounds interrupt this barrier and allow microorganisms' direct access to internal organs. This direct access creates a fertile ground for infection. Typical symptoms of a burn wound infection include change in wound color, redness, warmth, increased tenderness, elevated temperature, increased heart rate, shortness of breath, and elevated blood sugar.

Murray lists the following as risk factors for potential burn wound infections:

- Extremes of age, both young and old
- Comorbidities such as obesity and diabetes
- Immunosuppression
- Invasive devices
- Burns involving more than 30% of total body surface area
- Full-thickness burns
- Failure to cover burns or failed skin graft resulting in prolonged open burn wounds
- Improper early burn care

Medical and nursing care of the burn patient should focus on preventing infection. If wound infection occurs, debridement may be done and topical antimicrobials used. Church et al. suggest that "topical antibiotic agents should first be applied directly to the patient's dressings before application to the burn wound to prevent contamination of the agent's container by burn wound flora." While topical antimicrobials are considered state of the art, prophylactic systemic antibiotics are not indicated. In fact, definitive narrow spectrum antibacterial agents should be used based upon the results of burn tissue cultures. Nurses often become concerned because of fever, tachycardia, and other elements of systemic inflammation, which are representative of the body's response to burns and do not require antimicrobial therapy. Other considerations in caring for the burn wound patient include making appropriate consultative decisions about infectious disease management, plastic surgery, dietician services, physical therapy, and occupational therapy to assist in guiding therapy.

Since infection is a critical concern for burn wound patients, healthcare providers must focus on preventing nosocomial infections by being attentive to handwashing, patient room assignments, and proper isolation techniques. Infection control practitioners are key members of the healthcare team in monitoring, educating, preventing, and researching burn wound care.

SUGGESTED READINGS

Church D, Elsayed S, Reid O, et al. Burn wound infections. *Clin Microb Rev.* 2006;19(2):403–434.
Murray C. Burn wound infections. eMedicine from WebMD. 2008. Available at: http://www.emedicine.com/med/topic258.htm. Accessed July 9, 2008.

KNOW THAT HYPERBARIC OXYGEN MAY HELP IN COMPLEX WOUND CARE

JEANNIE SCRUGGS GARBER, DNP, RN

WHAT TO DO: IMPLEMENT

Hyperbaric oxygen therapy (HBO) is the delivery of 100% oxygen at increased atmospheric pressure. In studies of chronic wound management, HBO therapy has been found to enhance wound healing. During HBO, cells become saturated with oxygen to promote the healing process.

Hyperoxia and increased nitric oxide production are the key components related to the effectiveness of HBO. Oxygen is necessary for the healing process to occur and nitric oxide regulates microcirculation and endothelial cells through vasodilation. HBO is useful for treating chronic wounds resulting from peripheral vascular disease, diabetes, radiation necrosis, mixed soft-tissue infections, refractory osteomyelitis, and some traumatic wounds. Patients with pneumothorax, recent sinus surgery, chemotherapy, seizures, claustrophobia, and fever are not eligible for HBO.

HBO treatments range from 1 to 2 h and may be scheduled for up to 20 sessions; however, frequency and duration are dependent upon the diagnosis and patient condition. Patients are monitored at all times during the procedure, but the nurse requires specific understanding of the physics of pressure and the delivery of care in isolated surroundings.

Nursing care of the hyperbaric patient requires a focus on patient education, monitoring, and ongoing assessment of the wound healing process. The nurse must work with the interdisciplinary team of physicians, dieticians, and technicians and with the patient and significant others to determine educational needs and interventions.

SUGGESTED READINGS

Boykin J. Hyperbaric oxygen therapy helps heal chronic wounds. *Nursing.* 2002. Available at: http://findarticles.com/p/articles/mi_qa3689/is_200206/ai_n9128200. Accessed August 7, 2008.

Hyperbaric oxygen therapy. Available at: http://altmed.creighton.edu/o2tx/hbot.htm. Accessed August 7, 2008.

FAILED BACK SURGERY SYNDROME

JEANNIE SCRUGGS GARBER, DNP, RN

WHAT TO DO: EVALUATE

Failed back surgery syndrome (FBSS) is the term used to describe the results of unsuccessful back or spine surgery. There are no other failed surgery syndromes, making the FBSS unique and complex for the patient and healthcare providers to understand.

Back or spine surgery alters anatomy but, unfortunately, may not eliminate back pain. The most typical reason that pain is not relieved is that it is being caused by something other than the back anatomy. According to Talbot and Asher, the debate over the causes of FBSS continues; however, some potential causes of a failed surgery or continued pain after surgery include

- Failure to fuse and/or implant failure, or a transfer lesion to another level after a spine fusion
- Recurrent stenosis or disc herniation, inadequate decompression of a nerve root, preoperative nerve damage that does not heal after a decompressive surgery, or nerve damage that occurs during the surgery
- Scar tissue considerations (interrupts normal neurologic functioning)
- Postoperative rehabilitation (continued pain from a secondary pain generator)
- Technical aspects of the operation were not successful
- The surgery was not performed at the site that causes the pain
- The surgery performed was not actually necessary
- The patient was a poor fit for a successful surgery (improper selection of patient)
- The diagnosis was incorrect
- Complications of surgery arose

FBSS can create chronic disability and pain and has fallen into a no-man's land between surgery and medicine for treatment. It is widely recognized that many patients with FBSS also have psychosocial or work related issues associated with the chronic pain and discomfort. Selecting the best treatment for FBSS requires a complete assessment with imaging technologies, review of the patient's medical and surgical history, and physical examination. Usually, treatment is conservative and uses rehabilitation (exercise, physical therapy, and stimulators) or implantable pain management pumps before considering follow up surgery.

Patient selection plays a key role and the decision to proceed with an initial surgery should be shared by the patient and provider. The patient history and timing of symptoms are the most critical findings when considering FBSS as a diagnosis. The most common complaint of patients with FBSS is their difficulty or inability to perform routine activities without experiencing pain. Sometimes the only treatment is narcotics and use of these drugs can be as difficult to live with as the pain itself.

Other than repeating surgery or a lifetime of narcotics, spinal cord stimulation (SCS) or intraspinal drug infusion therapy may be considered. Neurostimulation creates a change in sensation from pain to tingling. Colella (2003) suggests that clinicians need to be mindful that patients with FBSS have very few treatment options and may be willing to try SCS to decrease symptoms. The intraspinal drug option is more invasive, yet, it allows for less systemic side effects.

Possible issues with the intraspinal drug therapy are catheter movement, mechanical issues with the pump, and infection. Patients with FBSS should be encouraged to maintain physical activity and be reminded of proper body mechanics for routine body positions. Since this is a chronic illness, it is not uncommon for the healthcare provider to identify anxiety and/or depression as an additional diagnosis. Patients with this syndrome need ongoing education, reassurance, and reassessment regarding the best individualized treatment options.

SUGGESTED READINGS

Asher A. What is failed back surgery syndrome? About.com: Back and neck pain. 2006. Available at: http://backandneck.about.com/od/faqs/f/failedbackfbss.htm. Accessed August 7, 2008.

Colella C. Understanding failed back surgery syndrome. *Nurse Pract.* 2003;28(9):31–43. Available at: http://www.tnpj.com/pt/re/nursepract/fulltext.00006205–200309000–00005.htm; jsessionid=L7vNws24ynGJ9nbj7pTVGxzsJ0XjpFxhy4cz31gSG9J2J1QsD4ZY!536197444!181195628!8091!-1. Accessed August 7, 2008.

Talbot L. Failed back surgery syndrome. *Br Med J.* 2003;327:985–986. Available at: http://bmj.bmjjournals.com/cgi/content/full/327/7421/985. Accessed August 7, 2008.

Ulrich P. Failed back surgery syndrome: What is it and how to avoid it. Spine-health. 2003. Available at: http://www.spine-health.com/treatment/back-surgery/failed-back-surgery-syndrome-what-it-and-how-avoid-it. Accessed August 7, 2008.

POST-OP ALCOHOL WITHDRAWAL SYNDROME

JEANNIE SCRUGGS GARBER, DNP, RN

WHAT TO DO: ASSESS AND EVALUATE

It is difficult for healthcare providers to identify individuals with alcohol use disorders because either the patients do not self report or the provider simply does not ask the right questions. The consequences of not knowing this information may be life threatening in the postoperative period.

Alcohol is the most abused drug worldwide and causes death and life altering illness. History taking and screening for alcoholism are critical to minimizing patient risk when undergoing a surgical procedure. The history of alcohol use includes quantity per day, past alcohol use, and a thorough assessment of behavioral changes related to alcohol consumption. The provider must also inquire about high risk behaviors such as drinking and driving, social drinking, and any previous attempts to decrease alcohol consumption.

Screening tools have been developed to support healthcare providers in determining the level of alcohol dependence of an individual. One tool is the CAGE questionnaire with four questions:

- Have you ever felt the need to cut down on your use of alcohol?
- Has anyone annoyed you by criticizing your use of alcohol?
- Have you ever felt guilty because of something you've done while drinking?
- Have you ever taken a drink to steady your nerves or get over a hangover?

The interpretation of this screening relies on the finding that if two or more of the CAGE questions are answered "Yes," then the specificity is 89+% and implies a high likelihood that the patient is alcoholic.

Another common term for alcohol withdrawal syndrome, used in the past, is delirium tremens or DTs. The signs and symptoms associated with alcohol withdrawal are:

- Fever (often low-grade)
- Sweating
- Tachycardia
- Tremor

- Disorientation, hallucinations, and sleep disturbance
- Agitation and anxiety
- Seizures

Seizures may occur within hours after stopping drinking; however, the syndrome related to alcohol withdrawal may not occur for several days.

It is important for the healthcare provider to be aware of other diagnoses that can be confused with alcohol withdrawal syndrome such as:

- Sleep withdrawal, sensory deprivation, and an unfamiliar environment
- Drugs (polypharmacy: steroids, sedative-hypnotics, narcotics, atropine, cimetidine, digoxin, etc.)
- Infection (chest, operative site, and urinary tract)
- Fluid and electrolyte disturbances
- Neurologic diagnosis
- Hypotension
- Major organ dysfunction
- Endocrine diseases

Healthcare providers should also be aware of the comorbid conditions that can compound the course of alcohol withdrawal syndrome. Issues such as malnutrition, vitamin deficiencies, cardiac disease, liver disease, and gastrointestinal symptoms can make the diagnosis and treatment of alcohol withdrawal syndrome complex. The use of sedation in itself can lead to respiratory depression, intubation, and increased risk of infection. Patient assessment is the key to preventing unanticipated alcohol withdrawal syndrome. Healthcare providers must be educated on appropriate screening and treatment options for alcohol withdrawal syndrome to possibly prevent post-op complications.

SUGGESTED READINGS

Alcohol and Other Drugs: A Handbook for Health Professionals (n.d.). Chapter 16: Surgery and substance abuse. National Centre for Education and Training on Addiction (NCETA) Consortium. Australian Government Department of Health and Ageing. 2004. Available at: http://www.aodgp.gov.au/internet/aodgp/publishing.nsf/Content/handbook/$FILE/chap16.pdf. Accessed August 7, 2008.

Hopley & Schalkwyk. Alcohol withdrawal syndrome. Anesthesist.com. 2006. Available at: http://www.anaesthetist.com/icu/manage/drugs/ethanol/aws/Findex.htm#index.htm. Accessed August 7, 2008.

Postoperative cognitive decline (delirium) is a real problem for patients and demands early identification by nurses

Jeannie Scruggs Garber, DNP, RN

WHAT TO DO: ASSESS AND EVALUATE

Delirium is an acute state of confusion that may be reversible. The onset of symptoms is sudden, and the severity of symptoms may be different at various times during the day. Delirium can last briefly as in hours or can become an ongoing lifelong health concern. Most patients with delirium are disoriented to their surroundings and have short-term memory loss. Delirium is also evident through disorganized thinking and speech difficulties. According to Monk, 10% to 15% of elderly patients will experience delirium postoperatively. The immediate and ongoing post operative assessment is critical to identify cognitive decline or delirium.

Possible physiologic causes of delirium include electrolyte imbalance, cerebral anoxia, hypoglycemia, medications, tumors, subdural hematomas, cerebrovascular infection, infarction, and hemorrhage. Elderly adults in the acute-care setting are at increased risk for delirium. Patient assessment preoperatively and postoperatively and early intervention are critical to the success of the treatment of delirium.

The short-term concerns related to cognitive decline are patient safety and determination of the underlying cause of the delirium. The long-term concerns related to cognitive decline are more focused on the psychosocial aspects of independence and one's ability to achieve the previous level of physical activity.

Monk suggests that cardiothoracic and orthopedic surgery create the greatest risk for developing postoperative delirium. Healthcare providers who have worked with patients with major surgery experiences have many stories on how cognitive function was temporarily or permanently different after the surgery experience. In the past 10 years, more and more clinical studies have investigated postoperative cognitive decline.

Cognitive decline postoperatively is not just limited to the elderly; however, cognitive impairment post-op is fairly common after major surgical procedures in the oldest age groups. Despite these findings, healthcare providers are not always aware of or attentive to the risk of postoperative cognitive decline.

Future research needs to focus on the mechanisms of postoperative cognitive decline, the long-term effects that postoperative cognitive decline have on cognitive function, and how the risks of anesthesia related to postoperative cognitive decline can be impacted with anesthesia practice changes. The most valuable information the healthcare provider can have preoperatively is a baseline cognitive assessment so that any postoperative changes can be identified and treated early in an attempt to minimize the long-term effect and to improve patient outcome.

SUGGESTED READINGS

Ballard C, Clack H, Green D. Postoperative cognitive decline, dementia and anesthesia. *Br J Hospital Med*. 2007;68(11): 576–577.

Lueckenotte A. Older adult. In: Potter P, Perry A, eds. *Fundamentals of Nursing*. Toronto, ON: Mosby-Elsevier; 2009, pp. 201–202.

Monk T. (2003). Postoperative cognitive dysfunction: The next challenge in geriatric anesthesia. Emery A. Rovenstine Memorial Lecture. Available at: http://10085.hostinglogin. com/saga1/Rovenstine2.ppt#1.

POSTOPERATIVE PAIN MANAGEMENT IN THE ELDERLY: THERE ARE IMPORTANT THINGS TO REMEMBER

JEANNIE SCRUGGS GARBER, DNP, RN

WHAT TO DO: ASSESS AND EVALUATE

Elderly patients require special consideration when assessing and managing their postoperative pain. Many times, they already have several medical conditions, take multiple medications, and may experience some level of pain routinely that they believe as part of the normal aging process. The elderly patient may also have sensory changes such as reduced hearing or vision that will impact communication and the ability to conduct the pain assessment. Another concern in assessing the elderly patient is the possibility of impaired cognitive ability.

The elderly postoperative patient requires frequent assessment for pain and ongoing evaluation of treatment effectiveness. The cumulative effects of pain medications are important in the elderly, and routine pain medication orders may need to be altered to better meet the aging patient's needs.

It is important for the nurse to know that elderly patients may use different words to express discomfort. They may not use the word "pain" but might instead use words such as ache, hurt, or tender. As with all patients, the first component of a pain assessment is to ask the patients to describe what they are feeling in their own words or by using a predetermined tool or scale. The patient's family or caregivers may also be instrumental in assessing postoperative pain. They may have insight into behaviors that will serve as indicators of pain. It is also important for nurses to describe the treatment for pain as "pain medicine" instead of using the word "drug."

The fear of becoming dependent on pain medications may be of concern to the elderly patient and families just as it is to younger populations. Although there are additional concerns with the elderly and pain medication such as sensitivity to dose or duration of effect, it is the nurse's responsibility to provide education and information that will support short-term pain relief and facilitate recovery. As with all patients, it is important for the pain to be controlled so that the patient can fully participate in ambulation, repositioning, coughing, deep breathing exercises, etc. to facilitate healing and minimize postoperative complications. Minimizing the pain that the patient experiences is key to the recovery process.

Another factor in working with the elderly postoperative patients is their perception of the healthcare provider's role in "taking care of them." If they believe that the doctors and nurses are doing everything they can to help them, they may not be aware of the need to actively participate in managing their care and controlling their pain. Preoperative assessment and education are crucial to make sure that the patients are aware of and understand their role in asking for pain therapy and in helping to manage the experience of pain. The preoperative discussion also helps to reduce anxiety for the patient and family and establish expected outcomes. If possible, provide preoperative education in a quiet, uninterrupted area with low noise levels. Since many elderly patients have sensory changes, the less the distraction, the more likely communication will be effective. Other reminders in communicating with the elderly are to speak clearly, not too fast, and to assess for understanding after each key point. It is also important to remember that it may take longer for the elderly to process the information; so allow the patient time to respond before advancing to the next topic of discussion.

One of the most common concerns postoperatively related to pain medication is the adverse effect of respiratory depression. In the elderly patients, this is of concern due to their increased sensitivity to the medications prescribed and as a result of the anesthetic agents taking longer to metabolize than in younger patients. The nurse must monitor respiratory rate and pattern as well as signs of adequate oxygenation and communicate with the physician if medication dosages need to be altered.

Caring for the postoperative elderly patients can be challenging. Managing their pain is complex and requires strong assessment skills. It has been well documented that surgical outcomes are much better when pain is managed appropriately.

SUGGESTED READINGS

Buckner S. Medication administration. In: Potter P, Perry A, eds. *Fundamentals of Nursing*. Toronto, ON: Mosby-Elsevier; 2009, p.1386.

Lauzon C, Laurie M. An ethnography of pain assessment and the role of social context on two postoperative units. *J Adv Nurs*. 2008;61(5):531–539.

McDonald DD. *Postoperative Pain Management for the Aging Patient Geriatrics Aging*. 2006;9(6):395–398. Available at: http://www.medscape.com/viewarticle/537057_3.

Pasero C, McCaffery M. Pain in the elderly. *Am J Nurs*. 1996;96(10):38–45.

MAKE THE SPONGE COUNT COUNT

JEANNIE SCRUGGS GARBER, DNP, RN

WHAT TO DO: EVALUATE

Patient safety in the operating room is a topic of great concern. One major element of concern is the retention of foreign bodies during surgery. Retained foreign bodies and supplies such as sponges, needles, and instruments being left in the patient during surgery is rare but does happen. Gwande and colleagues have reported that sponges are the most common foreign bodies retained during an operative procedure and that the current reporting is probably low since there is no mandatory hospital reporting requirement for foreign body retention rates.

The reasons for foreign bodies being retained during surgery can be categorized into surgical factors, patient factors, and human factors. These categories include situations such as emergency surgery when the process is out of the ordinary, patient obesity or comorbid conditions that need unanticipated attention during surgery, or simple distractions or failure to follow policy or procedure.

It is well documented that the most common negative outcomes of retained foreign bodies after surgery are sepsis, wound infection, repeat surgery, increased length of stay, readmission to the hospital, and possibly death. Nurses and physicians in the operating room are constantly striving to prevent the retention of foreign bodies by implementing policies, procedures, and changing processes. Unfortunately, foreign bodies continue to be left in surgical sites leading to higher healthcare costs and legal concerns. The typical safety procedure used in hospitals is focused on the human counting and documenting of sponges, needles, equipment, etc. Most hospital policies promote the following action steps when a sponge count is incorrect:

- The surgical site closing is stopped.
- A follow-up sponge count is done.
- The patient remains under anesthesia during process.
- The surgical site may be temporarily closed while x-rays are taken.

- The x-rays are read by a radiologist.
- If the sponge is found, the patient returns to the operating room for sponge removal.
- If the sponge is not found, the process is documented, and the patient is monitored for possible complications of foreign body retention.

The simple solution and direction are to just follow the policy and procedure to minimize risk. Following protocol with great precision and detail can be the first line of prevention regarding foreign body retention, but relying on this to prevent all errors is unreasonable due to the human factors involved in the process.

In the past few years, there have been many technologic attempts to help solve this risk issue; however, healthcare providers continue to struggle with use of the technology. Clinical research in this area is desperately needed to improve patient safety.

Some of the outcome measures that could be used to help address this safety concern include:

- An evaluation of the time per operating room staff member (circulating nurse and scrub technician) spent on sponge and instrument counts.
- Focus on the processes related to the act of counting such as initial counts, ongoing counts, final counts, etc.
- Measuring the time spent in searching for a missing sponge or how the counts are most frequently resolved.
- Documentation of other activities going on in the operating room during the time of the discrepancy.
- Evaluation of teamwork and communication as factors in resolving the count concern.

SUGGESTED READINGS

Pelter MM, Stephens KE, Loranger D. An evaluation of a numbered surgical sponge product. *AORN J*. 2007;85(5): 931–936,938–940.

Sugicount Medical (n.d.). Surgical sponge counting techniques: Fast facts. Available at: http://www.surgicountmedical.com/fastfacts.cfm. Accessed August 7, 2008.

USE INCENTIVE SPIROMETRY IN YOUR POSTOPERATIVE SURGERY PATIENT TO PREVENT PULMONARY COMPLICATIONS

JEANNIE SCRUGGS GARBER, DNP, RN

WHAT TO DO: IMPLEMENT

Pulmonary complications are not uncommon in the postoperative patient. The fact that there is an incision in either the chest or abdomen that creates discomfort directly impacts the ability to take deep breaths and is a major contributor to the most common postoperative respiratory complication—atelectasis. This occurs as a result of splinting, shallow breathing, a deactivation of surfactant, and alterations in chest wall function and physiology postoperatively. The objective of postoperative incentive spirometry is to maximize lung volume and keep the alveoli open for optimal air exchange.

Incentive spirometry also facilitates the movement of secretions to minimize the risk of infection. Incentive spirometry education should occur preoperatively. The healthcare provider should be aware of preoperative lung volume to assess progress postoperatively. A thorough pain assessment is one component of the respiratory assessment. Pain medications can be given prior to incentive spirometry to maximize lung volume with these exercises.

Pullen offers the following guidelines for healthcare providers as they support the patient while using incentive spirometry:

- Explain the reason for incentive spirometry while helping them inflate their lungs.
- Explain that deeper breaths make the indicator move more, and the higher the indicator the better for their lungs.
- Provide pain assessment and medications to maximize respiratory function.
- Position the patient as upright as possible.
- Instruct the patient on proper technique in using the spirometer.
- Encourage the use of spirometer as much as possible, and suggest every hour, if awake, with five or more deep breaths and coughs.
- Initiate spirometry immediately after extubation.
- Teach proper incisional splinting to minimize discomfort.

Incentive spirometry is a simple, effective exercise that can prevent major respiratory postoperative complications in surgery patients. Healthcare providers must not underestimate the implications of incentive spirometry in improving patient outcomes postoperatively.

SUGGESTED READINGS

Harton S, Grap M, Savage L, et al. Frequency and predicators of return to incentive spirometry volume baseline after cardiac surgery. *Progr Cardiovasc Nurs.* 2007;22(1):7–12.

Pelus S, Kaplan D. What the new guidelines offer for preoperative risk reduction. *Patient Care.* 2006;40(10):18–25.

Pullen R. Teaching bedside incentive spirometry. *Nursing* 2003;33(8):24.

Westwood K, Griffin M, Roberts K. Incentive spirometry decreases respiratory complications following major abdominal surgery. Available at: http://www.thesurgeon.net/site/CMD=ORA/ArticleID=24b618a6-b33f-4ae1-9558-9371ad26ab7d/0/default.aspx. Accessed August 18, 2008.

POSTOPERATIVE CARDIOTHORACIC SURGERY: MOBILIZATION

JEANNIE SCRUGGS GARBER, DNP, RN

WHAT TO DO: IMPLEMENT

Cardiothoracic techniques have advanced significantly over the past 10 years. Until recently, patients remained intubated till postoperative day (POD) 1 and sometimes longer depending on hemodynamic stability. Current practice goals are for extubation to occur within the first 4 to 6 h after surgery if possible. This practice minimizes pulmonary complications and promotes earlier respiratory and hemodynamic stability. Same day extubation supports self-regulated turning, coughing, and deep breathing, which are critical to the recovery process. On-time or early extubation also encourages mobility.

Most cardiothoracic patients, extubated postoperatively, are and walking in their room on POD 1. By POD 2, they are walking in the hall with oxygen as needed and with a progressive reduction in assistance. Some patients may not meet this expectation and that is usually due to requiring mechanical ventilation for longer than the anticipated durations, a past medical history that delays or complicates recovery, such as chronic obstructive pulmonary disease, stroke, or obesity.

If the primary reason for delayed mobilization is related to a respiratory complication, the treatment may include prolonged ventilation, respiratory treatments, pulmonary toilet and additional medications, and suctioning. Pneumonia is the biggest concern when mobilization is delayed. If extubated, the incentive spirometer can be a valuable mechanism to promote deep breathing and coughing.

Many patients who experience delayed mobilization come to the operating room with pre-existing conditions that complicate the postoperative recovery process. Some of the more common conditions include chronic obstructive pulmonary disease, skin breakdown, arthritis, independence, and balance or mobility concerns.

Another issue to be considered that impacts mobilization is pain management. Depending on the surgery, pain management may be the single most important factor in the success of early mobilization. Healthcare providers must provide adequate pain assessment and intervention to support the patient in early ambulation.

Mobilization of the postoperative cardiothoracic patient is a collaborative effort among nursing, medicine, respiratory, and other therapies as needed. Protocols, standard orders, and practice guidelines can be instrumental in facilitating the patient's progress with mobilization. Early mobilization speeds up recovery, decreases the possibility of postoperative complications, and minimizes the length of stay.

SUGGESTED READINGS

Bojar R. *Manual of Perioperative Care in Adult Cardiac Surgery*. 4th Ed. Boston, MA: Blackwell; 2005.

Postoperative Cardiac Surgery: Low Cardiac Output Syndrome

Jeannie Scruggs Garber, DNP, RN

WHAT TO DO: ASSESS AND EVALUATE

Since cardiac surgery is rarely the first line of coronary artery disease intervention, it is now common for patients who come to the operating room for cardiac surgery to have already experienced many interventional procedures over the course of time to treat their disease. The patient therefore arrives to the operating room with a potentially compromised heart muscle that has recovered time and time again to insult or intervention. This situation creates the possibility for postoperative complications. One of the most common complications is low cardiac output syndrome (LCOS).

LCOS is a complex syndrome when perfusion is suboptimal and the cardiac index is less than $2.0 L/min/m^2$. A low cardiac output increases the risk of life-threatening complications such as renal failure, neurologic insult, and respiratory failure. Healthcare providers must provide timely diagnosis and intervention to improve the patient outcome. Patients with LCOS present with hemodynamic changes that represent poor perfusion, such as hypotension, tachycardia, cool, clammy skin, restlessness, change in mental status, and tachypnea. The treatment for these patients is identified through good multidisciplinary critical care and may include the use of pressors, inotropic agents, and mechanical support such as intra-aortic balloon pumps.

Patients to be observed closely for this possible complication are those who have experienced multiple myocardial infarctions (MIs), stents, angioplasties, and have a compromised ejection fraction. However, the situation of LCOS is not as prevalent as in the past. There are a number of potential reasons for this including

- More surgeries are being performed off pump
- Patients receive earlier ambulation
- Operating room time is less
- For cases in which pump is used, the pump time is less
- Cardioplegia solutions are warmed and not administered cold

Most facilities have standard orders, protocols, and guidelines to support the provider's decision making regarding assessment and intervention postoperatively. The nurse at the bedside is the primary consistent patient-care provider and may be the first to identify hemodynamic changes that indicate LCOS. Healthcare providers must be educated on the signs, symptoms, and assessment skills needed to make this diagnosis in order for treatment to be expedient and for further complications to be prevented.

SUGGESTED READINGS

Bojar R. *Manual of Perioperative Care in Adult Cardiac Surgery.* 4th Ed. Boston, MA: Blackwell; 2005.

Kučukalić F, Kulić M, Pandur S, et al. Management of low cardiac output syndrome. HealthBosnia.com. 2001. Available at: http://www.healthbosnia.com/cvsa/abstracts/131.htm. Accessed August 7, 2008.

Postoperative cardiac surgery: bleeding

Jeannie Scruggs Garber, DNP, RN

WHAT TO DO: ASSESS

One of the possible postoperative cardiac surgery complications is bleeding or coagulopathy. The preoperative assessment is critical in assessing the potential for bleeding, and the postoperative assessment is critical to early intervention if bleeding occurs. Patients on aspirin or anticoagulant therapy are at increased risk for postoperative bleeding. Depending on the type of surgery performed, there are usually multiple sites of cannulation and anastomosis as well as graph sites and tube insertion sites that create potential bleeding sites.

Other possible causes for bleeding include pump time, hypothermia, and the intraoperative use of heparin (C.D. Jennings, personal communication, July 24, 2008). Heparin can be maintained in adipose tissue for up to 4 h and may have an impact on bleeding; so it is important to monitor for this effect hours after the drug is administered.

Nursing care of the patient postoperatively requires constant monitoring and assessment for signs of bleeding such as hypotension, tachycardia, oozing from chest tube insertion sites, bleeding at incision, and blood in the urine. Lab values should also be assessed frequently to support early detection of internal bleeding. Treatment options vary by practitioner and institution and may include protamine sulfate, antifibrinolytic agents, or fresh frozen plasma.

If bleeding occurs and it is difficult to control, there is potential for further complication of cardiac tamponade. Healthcare providers must be aware of the signs and symptoms of tamponade to provide timely intervention. The symptoms of cardiac tamponade are decreased or absence of chest tube drainage, hypotension, narrowed pulse pressure, tachycardia, jugular venous distention, increased central venous pressure, and muffled heart sounds (Urden L et al., 2002 as cited by Martin and Turkelson, 2006).

Hemodynamic assessment is ongoing and includes cardiac output and index measurements, blood gases, coagulation studies, and physical assessment. In the event when bleeding is not controlled through treatment efforts, return to the operating room for emergency surgery may be necessary.

SUGGESTED READINGS

Bojar R. *Manual of Perioperative Care in Adult Cardiac Surgery.* 4th Ed. Boston, MA: Blackwell; 2005.

Martin C, Turkelson S. Nursing care of the patient undergoing coronary artery bypass grafting. *J Cardiovasc Nurs.* 2006; 21(2):109–117.

A POSTOPERATIVE ARTERIAL BLOOD GAS IS ONLY ONE PARAMETER TO ASSESS POSTOPERATIVE RESPIRATORY FUNCTION

JEANNIE SCRUGGS GARBER, DNP, RN

WHAT TO DO: ASSESS AND EVALUATE

Surgery insults the normal exchange of air and oxygen at the "macro" level between the atmosphere and the lungs. However, the "micro" respiratory system is also compromised and represents alterations in the transfer of oxygen from the alveoli to hemoglobin across the alveolar-capillary membrane. With these changes, the possibility of postoperative respiratory complications such as atelectasis, respiratory failure, sputum retention, and pneumonia are increased. Some subsets of postoperative patients, such as those after cardiac surgery, are particularly vulnerable to the complications that surgery presents. Up to 30% to 60% of these patients may experience hypoxemia. As with other possible complications postoperatively, the patient's preoperative history is the key to detecting, preventing, and managing the patient's care.

Significant pulmonary factors to be assessed preoperatively include

- Smoking history
- Other medical conditions that may impact respiratory health (heart failure, gastrointestinal disease, etc.)
- History of chronic obstructive pulmonary disease
- Use of steroid medications
- Nutritional status
- Review of medications that might impact respiratory function (i.e., Amiodarone)
- History of environmental irritants (i.e., asbestos, coal, etc.)

Patients arrive in the postoperative recovery area in a variety of respiratory conditions. Some may be intubated and mechanically ventilated while others are on low concentrations of oxygen.

Respiratory function is monitored closely while intubated, with early extubation being a desired outcome. The longer the patient remains intubated, the more concern there is for respiratory complications. Many institutions are attempting to extubate patients on the day of surgery, which allows the patient to ambulate earlier and ultimately impacts the patient's length of stay in the hospital. To achieve the desired early extubation, healthcare providers must monitor and maintain stability of oxygenation and neurologic and hemodynamic status. It is important that the other body

systems are working as effectively as the respiratory system prior to extubation. The patient should not be extubated based purely on an arterial blood gas alone.

The preoperative and postoperative phases are critical to maintaining oxygenation; however, there are also intraoperative factors that impact respiratory function and the potential for complications. These factors include

- Length of surgery
- Amount of anesthetic medications used during surgery
- Amount of fluid infused during surgery
- Patient positioning during surgery

Typical postoperative management of the surgery of the patient's respiratory status includes

- Frequent physical assessment
- Arterial blood gas analysis
- Pulse oximetry
- Endotracheal tube suctioning
- Turn, cough, and deep breathing
- Incentive spirometry after extubation
- Early mobilization
- Pain medication
- Maintenance of body temperature
- Postoperative chest X-ray for tube and line placement verification

Timely extubation is very important for minimizing respiratory complications. The sooner the patient can be extubated, the sooner the patient can mobilize and can begin to turn, cough, and deep breathe and incentive spirometry. The universally accepted criteria for readiness for extubation include

- Easy to awaken
- Able to respond to commands
- Hemodynamically stable
- Breathing at a normal respiratory rate per minute without mechanical assistance

Caring for the postoperative surgery patient can be complex and challenging. It is critical that healthcare providers understand the importance and significance of respiratory stability in relation to the overall patient recovery postoperatively. Moving the patient from surgery through extubation and return to normal respiratory function as quickly as possible will minimize complications and ultimately decrease hospital length of stay.

SUGGESTED READINGS

Bojar R. *Manual of Perioperative Care in Adult Cardiac Surgery*. 4th Ed. Boston, MA: Blackwell;2005.

Martin C, Turkelson S. Nursing care of the patient undergoing coronary artery bypass grafting. *J Cardiovasc Nurs*. 2006;21(2): 109–117.

Teba L, Omert LA. Postoperative respiratory insufficiency. American Family Physician. Available at: http://findarticles.com/p/articles/mi_m3225/is_n6_v51/ai_16874737. Accessed August 18, 2008.

Perioperative cardiac ischemia is one worth paying attention to

Jeannie Scruggs Garber, DNP, RN

WHAT TO DO: ASSESS AND EVALUATE

Since coronary artery disease (CAD) is a leading cause of disease and mortality in adults, patients arriving in the operating room may have already experienced other treatment options for their CAD, such as angioplasties, stents, and multiple medications. While the range of incidence for perioperative ischemia and infarction varies widely between 20% and 60%, there is often difficulty in identifying a cause. It is known that the impact or clinical significance of a myocardial infarction (MI) postoperatively can range from minimal to catastrophic. As with MIs that are not associated with surgery, the more hemodynamically unstable the patient, the more likely long-term survival will be impacted. The preoperative assessment is critical in identifying patients at increased risk for perioperative ischemia and MI.

The factors to consider include:

- site of CADs (left main, or three vessel disease)
- history of MI
- prevalence of ischemia
- left ventricular function
- history of cardiac surgery
- history of carotid artery concerns
- length of surgery and time on bypass

During surgery it is important for the nurse and other providers to be aware of the preoperative risk factors and to monitor conditions such as changes in blood pressure, tachycardia, and alterations in tissue perfusion and oxygenation. These become particularly important during critical times of the procedure, including when anesthesia is induced and during extubation. There is also the possibility of a reperfusion MI as the patient is coming off cardiopulmonary bypass. These physiologic changes are in addition to the more routine issues of clots, alterations in pre-existing grafts, or vasospasm that may accompany the stress of the surgery.

Immediately postoperative, the patient is unable to communicate the presence of pain; therefore, the ischemia or MI is usually diagnosed through new electrocardiogram (EKG) changes or hemodynamic instability. Treatment for a suspected MI in this population is generally the same as for patients who have not had cardiac surgery. Acute ischemia with hemodynamic changes may result in transportation to the cardiac cath lab or a return to the operating room if a graft is the reason.

Myocardial ischemia and infarction are two of the most concerning conditions in the postoperative period and most likely to impact the long-term survival of the patient. The nurse needs to appropriately assess patients in the postoperative period, be alert for ischemic changes on electrocardiogram, control pain, temperature, and anemia, and ensure the administration of prescribed β-blockers for treatment of the underlying CAD.

SUGGESTED READINGS

Bojar R. *Manual of Perioperative Care in Adult Cardiac Surgery*. 4th Ed. Boston, MA: Blackwell; 2005.
Priebe HJ. Triggers of perioperative myocardial ischemia and infarction. *Br J Anaesth*. 2004;93(1):9–20. Available at: http://bja.oxfordjournals.org/cgi/content/full/93/1/9. Accessed August 18, 2008.

POSTOPERATIVE STROKE IN THE CARDIAC SURGERY PATIENT

JEANNIE SCRUGGS GARBER, DNP, RN

WHAT TO DO: ASSESS AND EVALUATE

Patients who experience cardiac surgery are at risk for neurologic complications. The most common reasons for stroke associated with cardiac surgery are reduced perfusion or emboli that can occur either during surgery or postoperatively. The risk factors for stroke in this patient population include:

- history of vascular disease
- anticoagulation therapy preoperatively
- manipulation of the aorta during surgery
- age
- history of previous stroke
- carotid bruit
- hypertension
- history of transient ischemic attacks

If any of the above is present, it may be necessary for further diagnostic testing to be conducted prior to cardiac surgery to fully understand the origin of the symptoms and to minimize postoperative complications.

Neurologic assessment skills are critical for the postoperative nurse. The preoperative assessment provides a baseline perspective for the patient's normal neurologic assessment. It is important to consider other disease processes or causes of any neurologic change. Some conditions to consider are:

- alcohol use and the potential for alcohol withdrawal syndrome
- dementia
- psychosis
- hypoglycemia
- hypoxia

After surgery, the patient will be unable to speak due to intubation and sedation; therefore, the nurse must be able to conduct a neurologic assessment beyond orientation to person, place, and time. As the patient begins to awaken, pupil size and light reaction should be assessed. The nurse must know that normal pupillary reaction will return over time as anesthetic and paralytic agents are metabolized.

The neurologic assessment also serves as a key indicator for readiness for extubation. The patient should progress to follow simple instructions such as squeezing hands, nodding head, and moving feet. The nurse should assess for equal strength on each side. The nurse must also talk with the family members to inform them of the normal neurologic progression postoperatively.

SUGGESTED READINGS

Bojar R. *Manual of Perioperative Care in Adult Cardiac Surgery.* 4th Ed. Boston, MA: Blackwell; 2005.

Martin C, Turkelson S. Nursing care of the patient undergoing coronary artery bypass grafting. *J Cardiovasc Nurs.* 2006;21(2): 109–117.

POSTOPERATIVE CARDIAC SURGERY DYSRHYTHMIAS

JEANNIE SCRUGGS GARBER, DNP, RN

WHAT TO DO: ASSESS AND EVALUATE

Postoperative monitoring of the cardiac surgery patient includes paying close attention to cardiac rhythm and rate as they are key indicators of hemodynamic stability and successful recovery. Changes in heart rhythm are not uncommon after surgery; therefore, constant assessment is necessary.

The most common overall dysrhythmia post-op cardiac surgery is atrial fibrillation. The most common dysrhythmias early in the postoperative recovery are ventricular and later in recovery are supraventricular dysrhythmias.

The common factors associated with dysrhythmias post-op cardiac surgery include:

- hypothermia
- anesthetic agents
- fluid and electrolyte imbalances
- metabolic stability
- physical manipulation of the heart muscle
- myocardial ischemia
- pain
- anxiety
- sedation

Treatment for dysrhythmias depends on the clinical symptoms of the patient. The nurse must assess the patient's condition beyond the monitor to aid in determining the correct treatment. Perhaps the most critical indicators to evaluate are the hemodynamic stability indicators such as blood pressure, cardiac output, and neurologic perfusion.

In some institutions, epicardial pacing wires are inserted during procedure closure that allow for temporary pacing in the event a dysrhythmia occurs. Placement of pacing wires is more common in patients who undergo valve surgery as heart block is of concern. Pharmacologic treatment is the primary means of treating most dysrhythmias and each surgeon or institution makes the decisions regarding which agents to use routinely.

Most organizations utilize standard protocols in caring for the postoperative cardiac surgery patient and the nurse is responsible for implementing the protocol as needed.

SUGGESTED READINGS

Bojar R. *Manual of Perioperative Care in Adult Cardiac Surgery.* 4th Ed. Boston, MA: Blackwell; 2005.

Martin C, Turkelson S. Nursing care of the patient undergoing coronary artery bypass grafting. *J Cardiovasc Nurs.* 2006;21(2):109–117.

IS IT POSSIBLE THAT POSTOPERATIVE ADHESIONS ARE THE CAUSE OF YOUR PATIENT'S ABDOMINAL PAIN?

JEANNIE SCRUGGS GARBER, DNP, RN

WHAT TO DO: ASSESS

An adhesion is a band of scar tissue that binds two parts of tissue together. It may be thin or thick and may or may not create problems for the patient. Adhesions develop when the body's normal healing process reacts to surgery, infection, trauma, or radiation and are most common in the stomach, pelvis, and heart. The most common sites of adhesions and their types are presented in Table 342.1.

Unfortunately, there is no systematic way to prevent adhesions. Attention to good operative and postoperative practices is usually highlighted as a mechanism for preventing the development of adhesions. Adhesions can present as pain, obstruction, and problems with pregnancy. Patients and healthcare providers need to consider that adhesions may be the culprit of abdominal pain in the patient with prior laparoscopic or open surgical interventions.

SUGGESTED READINGS

Ellis H, Moran BJ, Thompson JN, et al. Adhesion related hospital readmission after abdominal and pelvic surgery: A retrospective cohort study. *Lancet.* 1999;353:1476–1480.

Johns A. Evidence based prevention of post-operative adhesions. *Hum Reprod Update.* 2001;7(6):577–579. Available at: http://humupd.oxfordjournals.org/cgi/reprint/7/6/577. Accessed August 18, 2008.

Post-operative adhesions. SyntheMed, Inc. Available at: http://www.synthemed.com/post-op_adhesion.htm. Accessed August 16, 2008.

TABLE 342.1	ADHESIONS—MOST COMMON SITES AND THEIR TYPES
ABDOMINAL	**USUALLY A SURGERY COMPLICATION**
Adhesions	Usually painless Complication of adhesions is small bowel obstruction or pelvic pain Symptoms occur, may be, months or years later Surgical treatment is not necessary unless an obstruction is present Further treatment may be needed if patient experiences severe abdominal pain, fever, nausea, and vomiting, or infrequent bowel movements can be a recurring problem (since surgery is the cause and the cure)
Pelvic adhesions	Usually a surgery complication Can be related to any organ in the pelvis (uterus, bladder, ovaries, etc.) May be related to pelvic inflammatory disease
Heart adhesions	Scar tissue that forms in the pericardial sac May be a result of surgery, rheumatic fever, or infection May lead to reduced heart function

Postoperative paralytic ileus: Do not let it slow your patient down

Jeannie Scruggs Garber, DNP, RN

WHAT TO DO: ASSESS

Paralytic ileus is intestinal paralysis that prohibits the passage of food through the intestine and leads to intestinal blockage. Paralytic ileus is usually a complication of surgery but can be a result of certain medications, injuries, or illnesses.

The primary symptoms of paralytic ileus are absent bowel sounds, constipation, and bloating. Ileus or paralytic ileus occurs because peristalsis stops. Peristalsis is the rhythmic contraction that creates movement through the bowel. Infection can also cause an ileus and is one of the most common causes of bowel obstruction in infants and children.

Another possible cause of ileus is a reduction in the blood supply to the abdomen. The way the bowel is manipulated during surgery can cause normal bowel peristalsis to stop. Usually this condition only lasts for several days postoperatively and normal bowel function returns with no further complications.

The most common symptoms of paralytic ileus are

- Abdominal pain
- Bloating
- Nausea
- Vomiting
- Constipation
- Lack of abdominal gas
- Lack of peristalsis
- Lack of bowel sounds

Diagnosing paralytic ileus requires physical assessment of the abdomen, including a bowel sound check with a stethoscope, abdominal X-ray, and/or abdominal ultrasound. Depending on the severity of symptoms, treatment may include nasogastric suction (to alleviate vomiting and distention), intravenous fluids, maintaining nothing by mouth except for sips of water or ice chips, and labs to evaluate fluid and electrolyte balance. Continuing treatment depends on responsiveness to the nonsurgical treatments offered. Further evaluation may include colonoscopy, or exploratory surgery.

Missing this diagnosis could lead to life threatening complications. Healthcare providers must be aware of the signs and symptoms of paralytic ileus and provide ongoing abdominal assessment to allow for early diagnosis and treatment.

SUGGESTED READINGS

Medicine.Net (n.d.). Definition of ileus: paralytic. Available at: http://www.medterms.com/script/main/art.asp?articlekey=7208. Accessed August 7, 2008.

WD. Misdiagnosis of paralytic ileus. 2008. Available at: http://www.wrongdiagnosis.com/p/paralytic_ileus/misdiag.htm. Accessed August 7, 2008.

POSTOPERATIVE URINARY COMPLICATIONS

JEANNIE SCRUGGS GARBER, DNP, RN

WHAT TO DO: EVALUATE

The most frequent postoperative urinary problem after general surgery is urinary retention; however, more severe complications such as anuria, blockage, infection, or renal failure may also occur. These complications increased the length of stay and hospital costs. As healthcare organizations continue to focus on improving patient outcomes while attempting to reduce costs, attention must be paid to postoperative urinary complications.

Urinary retention is usually due to the surgery-induced temporary disruption in the nervous system that regulates the elimination process. General surgeries that last more than a few hours may result in the placement of a urinary catheter to prevent bladder distention postoperatively. The possibility of infection must also be investigated as a possible contributing factor to urinary retention. Depending on the surgery, the patients' ability to regain voluntary control over urination may take 6 to 8 h after anesthesia. If epidural or spinal anesthesia is used, the sensation of bladder fullness is also disrupted. Healthcare providers must conduct an assessment that includes palpation and percussion of the bladder as well as an assessment for discomfort or tenderness. If a urinary catheter is in place, the assessment should include checking urine flow as well as urine color and odor.

Another possible postoperative complication is anuria. This is most likely due to situations such as postoperative shock, chemical injury to the kidneys, or a blocked urinary tract. Anuria must be quickly evaluated and treated and fluid input monitored closely as diagnosis and treatment are initiated.

Postoperative urinary tract infection is another common, postoperative complication, especially in women. Causes may include urinary catheterization, decreased urinary output, and incomplete bladder emptying. If the patient has symptoms, they are usually urinary frequency and pain with urination. Early diagnosis and treatment are usually effective and symptoms resolve quickly.

A blockage in the urinary tract may result from the surgical procedure or from stricture or long-term catheterization (especially in male patients). The symptoms are generally painful urination and a decrease in urine output and flow.

Acute renal failure can also be a complication post-operatively and can be classified as prerenal, renal, and postrenal failures. Prerenal failure is the most common reason for acute renal failure and is a direct result of low fluid volume, while the renal category is caused by pre-existing diseases such as hypertension or drugs and the postrenal category results from obstruction.

SUGGESTED READINGS

Belt E. Acute urinary tract complications following general surgical procedures. *West J Med*. 1949;71(2):126–129.

Merchant R, Sui K, Ismail N, et al. The relationship between postoperative complications and outcomes after hip fracture surgery. *Annals Acad Med*. 2005;34:163–168.

BE ALERT FOR SURGICAL SITE INFECTIONS IN POSTOPERATIVE PATIENTS AND REMEMBER THAT WHEN THE UNFORTUNATE OCCURRENCE OF A WRONG SITE/SIDE PROCEDURE OCCURS, BOTH SURGICAL SITES ARE AT RISK FOR INFECTION

BETSY HARGREAVES ALLBEE, BSN, CIC

WHAT TO DO: ASSESS AND EVALUATE

Wrong site procedures are the most frequently reported sentinel events. Wrong site surgery is a broad term used to describe errors such as the wrong patient, wrong body part, or wrong side of the body. In 2005, there were 88 wrong site cases reported in the United States. Policies and protocols outlining methods to avoid wrong site procedures are available through the Association for Operating Room Nurses and The Joint Commission.

The unexpected occurrence of a wrong site surgery is a serious issue that causes physical and psychologic injury to the patient. To compound this traumatic event, the patient often still requires surgery on the intended site. It would be prudent, following a wrong site surgical error, to be meticulous in all aspects of care during the postoperative period. The incidence of a surgical site infection, especially on a healthy individual seeking elective surgery, is low. It is estimated that of the 40 million operations performed annually in the United States, approximately 2% to 5% of patients will develop a surgical site infection. These statistics suggest that a patient with a wrong site infection is not predisposed to infection.

Surgery causes physical disruption of the skin, interfering with the body's first line of defense against infection. Surgical site infections are the third most frequently reported hospital associated infection (nosocomial) identified in the United States. Surgical site infections increase mortality, readmission rates, length of stay, and costs for the patients who incur them. A surgical site infection results in 7.3 additional postoperative hospital days. Clinically, a surgical site can be considered infected when purulent drainage is present at the incision site. This may be associated with local swelling, erythema, tenderness, wound dehiscence, or abscess formation. Local signs and symptoms may not always be present, nor are they necessarily due to infection. As a result, a widely adopted definition of a surgical site infection is a surgical site draining a purulent exudate.

The centers for disease control and prevention (CDCP) developed surgical wound definitions that are widely used throughout the world. There are three general categories of surgical site infections. These are based on the location of the operative site and include (1) superficial incisional, (2) deep, and (3) organ/space. A superficial incisional surgical site infection involves only the skin or subcutaneous tissue of the incision. A deep surgical site infection involves deep soft tissue (e.g., fascial and muscle layers) of the incision. An organ/space surgical site infection involves any part of the anatomy (e.g., organs or spaces), other than the incision, which was opened or manipulated during an operation. Generally, infections related to the operative procedure are classified as surgical site infections if they occur within 30 days of the incision. One caveat to this rule involves the placement of an implantable device. If an implant is inserted and an infection, that appears to be related to the operative procedure, develops within 12 months of the procedure, it is considered hospital associated. An implant is defined as a nonhuman derived implanted foreign object (e.g., prosthetic heart valve, nonhuman vascular graft, mechanical heart, hip prosthesis, etc.) that is permanently placed in a patient during the operative procedure.

Host factors such as age, obesity, nutritional status, and the presence of underlying disease such as diabetes, malignancy, peripheral vascular disease, and pre-existing infection contribute to the risk of developing a surgical site infection. A prolonged preoperative stay also has adverse effects, including the proliferation of endogenous microorganisms, which can more heavily contaminate the surgical site, procedural interventions that allow microorganisms to gain access into the body (such as mechanical ventilation and central venous catheter use), and the use of antibiotics that can alter the host's normal flora and promote the acquisition of hospital-acquired multidrug-resistant pathogens. The length of the surgical procedure is an important risk factor for the development of a surgical site infection. Lengthy procedures have been associated with an increase in the contamination of the wound and an increase in tissue damage from drying, prolonged retraction, and manipulation.

Recommendations for the prevention of a surgical site infection include:

- Appropriate use of antibiotics
- Appropriate hair removal (clippers)
- Thorough cleaning around the incision site
- Maintenance of postoperative glucose control
- Maintenance of postoperative normothermia

- Treating all infections remote to the surgical site before performing the elective procedure and postponing elective operations on patients with remote infections until the infection has resolved
- Keeping the preoperative hospital stay as short as possible
- Appropriate hand hygiene of healthcare workers

Other recommendations specific to the postoperative period include:

- Protecting the incision with a sterile dressing for 24 to 48 h postoperatively
- Washing hands before and after dressing changes and before any contact with the surgical site (when there is more than one surgical site/incision, hands should be washed between sites)
- Using sterile technique during incision dressing changes
- Educating the patient and family regarding proper incision care, symptoms of a surgical site infection, and the need to report such symptoms

Adverse event are more frequent occurences in the healthcare environment than should be tolerated. Steps should be taken to prevent the occurrence of two adverse events in one patient. Events such as wrong site surgery and surgical site infection are preventable. Active involvement of the healthcare team and adherence to established evidence-based guidelines will promote patient safety.

SUGGESTED READINGS

Mangram AJ, Horan TC, Pearson ML, et al. Guideline for prevention of surgical site infection. *Am J Infect Control.* 1999;27:97–134.

Martone WJ, Jarvis WR, Cluver DH, et al. Incidence and nature of endemic and epidemic nosocomial infections. In: Bennett JV, Brachman PS, eds. *Hospital Infections.* 3rd Ed. Philadelphia, PA: Lippincott-Raven; 1992, pp. 577–592.

The Joint Commission. Universal protocol: Facts about the universal protocol for preventing wrong site, wrong procedure and wrong person surgery. 2003. Available at: http://www.jointcommission.org/PatientSafety/UniversalProtocol/.

POSTOPERATIVE PAIN MANAGEMENT

JEANNIE SCRUGGS GARBER, DNP, RN

WHAT TO DO: IMPLEMENT

The postoperative patient will most likely experience pain. Depending on the type of surgery performed, the pain can range from a minor ache to severe or excruciating pain. The nurse must establish a pattern of pain assessment and intervention to help the patient maintain comfort, reduce oxygen consumption, and prevent complications.

Patients must also receive preoperative education and information regarding what type of pain and sensations they will experience postoperatively and be taught how they will be managed. The patients need to be prepared and knowledgeable about the protocol for pain management and how they can participate in their pain management to make it the most effective possible. They need to know what types of pain medications are available, how they will be administered, and how to maximize pain relief. Preoperative education should also be shared with the patient's significant others who will be supporting the patient after surgery. They can be the eyes and ears for assessment and for communication with healthcare providers during the times when the patient may be unable to communicate.

The fear of becoming dependent on pain medications may be of concern to the patient and families. The nurse can be a source of accurate information regarding the importance of short term pain relief that will aid the recovery process. It is important for the pain to be controlled so that the patient can fully participate in ambulation, repositioning, coughing, deep breathing exercises, etc. To facilitate healing and minimize postoperative complications. Minimizing the pain that the patient experiences is the key to the recovery process.

The nurses' pain assessment must include:

- Attainment of the patients' description of pain in their words or according to a pain assessment tool (such as on a scale of 1–10, with 10 being the worst pain you have ever experienced)
- Assessment of patient behavior that indicates pain (grimacing, movement, crying, laughing, etc.)
- Observation of how the pain impacts the patient's ability to ambulate, verbalize, breathe, etc.
- Discussion regarding how interventions are working or not working and how this compares to the patient's previous experiences in dealing with pain
- Establishing the patient's expectation of pain relief and making a plan to reach that goal collaboratively

It is also important for the nurse to remember that the effects of medication on pain relief can be augmented by additional interventions such as relaxation, music therapy, imagery, and/or the application of heat or cold. Pain management is critical for the postoperative patients and directly impacts their recovery time and their overall perception of the surgical experience. Nurses are key players in educating, assessing, diagnosing, and intervening this patient population to make a difference in outcome.

SUGGESTED READINGS

Buckner S. Medication administration. In: Potter P, Perry A, eds. *Fundamentals of Nursing*. Toronto, ON: Mosby-Elsevier; 2009, p.1386.

Lauzon C, Laurie M. An ethnography of pain assessment and the role of social context on two postoperative units. *J Adv Nurs.* 2008;61(5):531–539.

Ensure Postoperative Deep Breathing and Incentive Spirometry Where Appropriate, but Chest Physiotherapy Adds Relatively Little Value in Reducing Postoperative Pulmonary Complications

Anthony D. Slonim, MD, DrPH

WHAT TO DO: IMPLEMENT

The postoperative patients require attention to a number of details to ensure that their organ systems return to a normal state of functioning. These are often inconvenient for the nurse and may be uncomfortable or painful for the patient, but a failure to carry out these postanesthesia activities will create complications for patients. One of the more frequent complications is atelectasis. Atelectasis, or collapse of the alveoli, occurs often and presents as postoperative fever, tachypnea, or increased work of breathing. Importantly, this can occur from being postoperative, but can also be a complication of immobility in the postoperative course.

Patients who receive general anesthesia during surgery are intubated and mechanically ventilated. Their lungs accommodate, for the duration of the surgery, positive pressure breathing, which allows the ventilator to push air into their lungs. This is in contrast to the routine, negative pressure breathing that the nonventilated patients perform with their respiratory muscles. This mode of breathing and the anesthetic gases can lead to atelectasis in the postoperative phase of care.

One of the most important mechanisms available for the postoperative patient is the use of deep breathing exercises and incentive spirometry. The ability of the patient to perform these activities is often limited by incisional pain, fatigue, and general postoperative deconditioning. Nurses need to be careful that they do not fall into the trap of enabling the patients in their ability to ignore these activities. Pain medications can be offered, mobilization of the patient can take place, and education on splinting of the surgical wound can be offered, but incentive spirometry and deep breathing must occur.

In addition, the nurse is often busy providing care to other patients who require attention. While suctioning is often well attended to, deep breathing exercises may be prioritized to a lower level because the needs of other patients require the nurse's attention. Using other members of the team, like respiratory therapy professionals, may be helpful in allowing the nurse to meet the needs of all patients and pay particular attention to pulmonary toilet to prevent postoperative respiratory complications.

While deep breathing and incentive spirometry are both important adjuncts to the rehabilitation of the postoperative patient's respiratory status, it is also important for the nurse to know what does not add value. Chest physiotherapy may add considerable distress to the postoperative patient, but does little to reduce postoperative pulmonary infections. Nurses who prioritize their activities to interventions that make a difference may be doing themselves and their patients a better service.

SUGGESTED READINGS

Pasquina P, Tramèr MR, Walder B. Prophylactic respiratory physiotherapy after cardiac surgery: Systematic review. *Br Med J.* 2003;327:1379.

Shea RA, Brooks JA, Dayhoff NE, et al. Pain intensity and postoperative pulmonary complications among the elderly after abdominal surgery. *Heart Lung.* 2002;31(6):440–449.

Stiller K, Montarello J, Wallace M, et al. Efficacy of breathing and coughing exercises in the prevention of pulmonary complications after coronary artery surgery. *Chest.* 1994;105: 741–747.

Westerdahl E, Lindmark B, Eriksson T, et al. Deep-breathing exercises reduce atelectasis and improve pulmonary function after coronary artery bypass surgery. *Chest.* 2005;128: 3482–3488.

LISTEN TO YOUR PATIENT'S LUNGS POSTOPERATIVELY TO ASSESS FOR EARLY COMPLICATIONS AND PROVIDE A BASELINE

EDWARD HUMERICKHOUSE, MS, MD

WHAT TO DO: ASSESS

If you remember your "ABC's" of basic life support, you know that without an adequate airway, all is lost. Nurses must know what their patients' lungs sound like and follow them routinely with appropriate documentation. There is no more important time to make the initial assessment than when the patient returns to the ward postoperatively. This will provide the baseline upon which other nurses will detect changes and be able to communicate those changes to the surgeon.

To listen to the lungs appropriately in the postoperative setting, the patient needs to be sitting upright or rolled to one side with the mouth open. Please do not hyperventilate the patient. It is ok to take a few seconds between each series of breaths. With a warmed stethoscope diaphragm firmly applied to bare skin, start at the apices (trapezius from behind and right above clavicles in front) and work your way down, comparing each side to the other before going lower. In other words, listen to each apex and compare before moving down. On the back side, listen to the space between the spine and scapula instead of on the scapula. Do not forget to listen laterally as well. On the front of the patient, do the same, listening lateral to the sternum and around the lateral bases. In female patients, the breast may need to be lifted. In postoperative thoracic patients, the dressing or chest tube may be in the way, complicating portions of the examination. Note that in your assessment.

Hopefully, the main sound that you hear is "vesicular." This is normal air movement into and out of the alveoli. Note that the inspiratory phase is longer and louder than the expiratory phase. Absence or local reduction of lung sounds in a field may be a normal postoperative finding depending upon how deeply the patient is breathing and what surgery was performed. These findings should be documented and compared to the physician's physical exam. These findings may also be abnormal if effusions or a pneumothorax has started to develop, so serial postoperative assessments are important.

Another commonly heard sound is "tracheal" or "bronchial" breath sounds. This is normal if you are listening over the trachea. Both phases are clearly audible, though again, inspiration takes longer than expiration. It is essentially unfiltered white noise. Hearing tracheal breath sounds in the periphery is abnormal.

This suggests that the "filter" created by our alveoli has been bypassed. This happens most frequently when the alveoli are compressed or filled with fluid such as with atelectasis, tumors, pneumonia, or heart failure.

Wheezes are high pitched "musical" sounds that indicate airway obstruction. They are most commonly heard on expiration with the general consensus that inspiratory wheezes are more advanced a disease than wheezes that occur only at the end of expiration. Wheezes are most commonly associated with asthma and emphysema, but can also be heard with pneumonia and CHF. Wheezes in the postoperative setting may represent an exacerbation of one of these diseases as a response to surgery. A wheeze that is loudest in one particular spot and seems to diminish as you get further away should make you wonder about aspiration of a solid material. The real importance of wheezes is following their changes.

Stridor is similar to wheezing, except that it is quite loud and you hear it best over the trachea. Stridor is caused by upper airway obstruction. Expiratory stridor is generally associated with lesions in the lower trachea or main bronchi. Inspiratory stridor is closer to the palate. Postoperative stridor may represent important postoperative airway complications that need to be addressed.

Crackles, rales, and crepitations are all about the same thing. They are associated with lower airway and alveolar pathology and sound like the name "crackle." They are common in pneumonia and CHF, but can also be heard in chronic lung diseases such as idiopathic pulmonary fibrosis. Crackles that clear with a solid cough or deep breath are usually benign and indicate temporary closure of alveoli (such as temporary patches of atelectasis first thing in the morning). Other crackles need to have documentation of their size and location.

The nurse needs to know what the common lung sounds are postoperatively so that appropriate assessments regarding their changes can be made, causes identified, and the surgical team notified when therapy needs to begin.

SUGGESTED READINGS

Odom-Forren J. Postoperative patient care and pain management. In: Rothrick JC, ed. *Care of the Patient in Surgery*. 13th Ed. St. Louis, MO: Mosby; 2007, 246–270.

Orient J. *Sapira's Art & Science of Bedside Diagnosis*. 3rd Ed. Baltimore, MD: Lippincott Williams & Wilkins; 2005, pp. 307–317.

REMEMBER THE UNIQUE NEEDS TO ENSURE SAFETY OF THE POSTOPERATIVE PEDIATRIC PATIENT

ANTHONY D. SLONIM, MD, DrPH

WHAT TO DO: IMPLEMENT

The postoperative care for special patient populations requires attention by the nurse. Among the many groups with special needs are pediatric patients. Pediatric patients come in a variety of sizes and shapes. Aside from ensuring that postoperative nurses undergo age specific competency training, the pediatric patient experiencing surgery may also have a number of chronic conditions that are important to address.

Premature babies experience problems related to the immaturity of their organ systems. Further, this immaturity and the problems related to organ dysfunction persist past the newborn period and manifest themselves as sensitivity to anesthetics and narcotics of the respiratory systems of these patients.

Children may also have a number of congenital abnormalities including cyanotic heart disease, airway anomalies, and developmental delays that require expertise by the postoperative care staff. The monitoring of oxygen saturation in the postoperative arena is commonplace; for the child with cyanotic disease, the nurse needs to know the acceptable saturation for the child, which may be as low as 70% to 80%. Patients with congenital airway problems as a part of a congenital syndrome require special monitoring that includes ventilation and the child's ability to maintain the airway.

Another major challenge in dealing with children in the postoperative period is development. Children by their nature have different levels of ability, but the stress of surgery will often cause children to regress to prior developmental levels and act out. The family may become anxious by this and needs to be supported.

Finally, the most challenging piece of dealing postoperatively with a child is the recognition that the nurse is actually dealing with three patients when the parents are added into the postoperative arena. This is important since the parents' and child's needs have to be met. This begins with explaining to the parents what to expect preoperatively, assuring attention to the child's pain postoperatively, and answering questions and concerns objectively and with a caring tone.

The care of the child and family postoperatively is both rewarding and challenging. Postoperative nursing care can make a difference in the child's and family's ability to successfully overcome this stressful period.

SUGGESTED READINGS

Stow J. Pediatric surgery. In: Rothrick JC, ed. *Alexander's Care of the Patient in Surgery*. 13th Ed. St. Louis, MO: Mosby; 2007, pp.1066–1142.

REMEMBER THE SPECIAL NEEDS OF YOUR POSTOPERATIVE ELDERLY PATIENTS

ANTHONY D. SLONIM, MD, DRPH

The geriatric patient has a number of concerns that contribute to problems in the postoperative period, including aging physiologic systems, ability to tolerate medications, and sensory and motor dysfunctions. The elderly patient is also more likely to experience a complication related to other organ systems, such as postoperative myocardial infarction or stroke, than younger patients.

The aging of the elderly patients' physiologic systems affects their ability to recover from anesthesia, heal wounds, and manage medications in the perioperative period. They have a slower metabolism and require longer periods of time to excrete medications. Further, dosage adjustment and drug selection become important for the elderly to minimize complications related to interactions.

Elderly patients experience visual and hearing deficits that limit their ability to remain oriented to their environment. Patients experience difficulties related to the effects of medications and being without their usual supportive aids like eyeglasses and hearing aids. Postoperative electrolyte abnormalities can contribute to delirium and lead to further problems with orientation. These patients become agitated and disoriented. They try to get out of bed, may be restrained or administered with medications to calm them down, which only worsens their ability to function independently. The nurse can assist through reorienting the patient, providing appropriate aids for hearing and vision, providing a protective environment, and minimizing the use of sedative medications. Patients with these difficulties often experience gait abnormalities related to both the administered medication and the disorientation. Supervised ambulation and bedrails when the patient is bedbound are essential in preventing falls and injuries postoperatively.

Finally, because of the aging physiologic systems, the elderly patient needs to be monitored for decompensation related to any number of organ systems. The stress of surgery increases the need for the patient's organs to perform. This is manifested most commonly as alterations in the cardiovascular system with perioperative ischemic disease, congestive heart failure, and stroke. However, other organ systems may decompensate and develop new problems related to the surgery or medications, including the kidneys, lungs, and liver. Patients formerly in control of their diabetes or hypertension may now require the addition of medications to achieve baseline status.

The geriatric patient is an important population that is in need of perioperative care. They have unique needs and problems that make them a challenging group to care for, but one that is rewarding for the nurse.

SUGGESTED READINGS

Allen SL. Geriatric surgery. In: Rothrick JC, ed. *Alexander's Care of the Patient in Surgery*. 13th Ed. St. Louis, MO: Mosby; 2007, pp. 1143–1164.

351

KNOW WHEN AND HOW TO USE A BLOOD AND FLUID WARMING DEVICE

DORIS S. DUFF, BS, RN IV, CEN

WHAT TO DO: IMPLEMENT

Homeostasis is the body's method of maintaining a constant internal environment, including body temperature, pH, blood glucose levels, and osmotic pressure of the blood, so that the cells, tissues, and organs of the body function appropriately. Alterations in thermoregulation, a major homeostatic mechanism, can result from trauma and other critical illnesses. Hypothermia is a common life-threatening problem, particularly in the resuscitative phases of trauma and shock, since it affects the blood's ability to clot. The first step in the treatment of hypothermia begins with the prevention of further heat loss. This can be accomplished by warming the patient through the use of overhead lamps, room thermostats, warming blankets, and warming assistive devices.

Prewarmed fluids should be administered to patients who that require emergent transfusion or large-volume resuscitative care. These fluids should be warmed for routine administration and can also be warmed as an active intervention to increase body temperature. Blood and fluid warming devices are used in the emergency department (ED) and in the intensive care unit for the purpose of warming blood and intravenous solutions so that homeostasis can be maintained. The use of blood and fluid warming devices, such as a Level 1 fluid warmer or a Thermo 900®, should only be used by those who are knowledgeable in the device's use. Manufacturer guidelines and hospital policy should be adhered to while using these devices. Further, since these devices may be used relatively infrequently, nurses should review their use and be tested on their knowledge and ability to use these machines effectively through annual competencies. The device's safety features are intended to prevent patient and user injury. Nursing actions to circumvent these safety features may result in a hazardous condition and injury to the patient or staff.

Many of the newer fluid warmers and infusers are electrical, having extended intravenous (IV) poles, and allow for the delivery of large volumes of warmed fluids. These devices represent one more piece of patient care equipment around a busy bedspace where the extended IV poles and electrical cords present potential hazards to staff working in a fast-paced environment. The accidental spillage of blood and electrolyte-containing fluids around these devices can create electrical and fall hazards and loss of valuable resources for acutely ill patients. For the patient, excessive heating of the blood can injure blood cells and destroy his or her oxygen carrying capacity. The excessive heating of IV fluids can also lead to patient burns. Finally, the nurse's assessment skills are critical for large-volume infusers to ensure that the patient does not become fluid overloaded.

SUGGESTED READINGS

Environmental emergencies: Hypothermia. In: Jenkins J, Braen GR, eds. *Manual of Emergency Medicine*. 5th Ed. Philadelphia, PA: Lippincott Williams & Wilkins; 2004, p. 488.

Soreide E, Smith C. Hypothermia in trauma victims–Friend or Foe? *Int. Trauma Crit Care Symp*. 2005;18–20. Available at: http://www.itaccs.com/traumacare/archive/05_01_Winter_2005/friendorfoe.pdf. Accessed August 8, 2008.

ENSURE THAT EPIGLOTTITIS IS CONSIDERED IN PATIENTS WITH RESPIRATORY DISTRESS CAUSED BY AN UPPER AIRWAY ETIOLOGY SINCE APPROPRIATE SAFETY MECHANISMS NEED TO BE PUT IN PLACE

DORIS S. DUFF, BS, RN IV, CEN

WHAT TO DO: ASSESS

Epiglottitis is a life-threatening condition defined as swelling of the epiglottis and the periepiglottic folds. The most common cause of epiglottitis is infection, although trauma and chemicals are also major contributors. Children of 3 to 7 years of age are the most vulnerable to epiglottitis where, traditionally, most cases involved infections with *H. influenza* Type B. These infections have dramatically decreased due to the improved use of vaccination against this organism. In adults, patients of 20 to 40 years of age are the most commonly affected age group. Since 1973, adult deaths have decreased from 32% to 7% due to earlier recognition, improved treatment, and current vaccination programs. Thermal epiglottitis is another type of epiglottitis in adults caused by drinking hot liquid or solid foods or from using illicit drugs by inhaling metal pieces from crack cocaine pipes or the tips of marijuana cigarettes. Nonetheless, when it presents in adults, epiglottitis is often misdiagnosed as strep throat. The nurse needs to maintain a high index of suspicion for this more serious disorder.

In epiglottitis, symptoms of severe sore throat and fever develop very rapidly and progress to the signs of drooling, inability to swallow liquids, and unexplained tachycardia. A child will often assume a "tripod" or "sniffing" position. Care must be taken to keep the child calm and as quiet as possible and allow the parent or caregiver to hold and stay with the child. Emergency airway equipment should be readily available in the room with the patient, regardless of age, in the event those symptoms worsen or progress or if laryngospasm develops. Complete airway obstruction can occur in as few as 6 h of onset. Active interventions, including examination of the airway using tongue blades, the establishment of intravenous access, or obtaining throat cultures, should be avoided. An immediate lateral neck X-ray is the most important diagnostic aid for the physician. The patient should remain under very close observation with the administration of humidified oxygen unless it causes agitation. Anesthesia and otolaryngology consults should be requested emergently, and an artificial airway should be provided, preferably in the operating room. Once complete airway obstruction and respiratory arrest have occurred, bag valve mask-assisted respirations should be followed with laryngoscope-guided oral intubation or cricothyrotomy by the most experienced member of the team.

Remember, epiglottitis is a life-threatening condition. Although the incidence has subsided, if not identified and treated early, it can be deadly. Emergency airway management equipment should be kept readily available and the patient intubated as needed. Aside from airway management, an X-ray of the neck for accurate diagnosis takes priority over other procedures.

SUGGESTED READINGS

Epiglottitis. eMedicineHealth: Practical Guide to Health. Available at: http://www.emedicinehealth.com/epiglottitis/article_em.htm. Accessed May 5, 2008.
Jordan K, ed. *Emergency Nursing Core Curriculum*. 5th Ed. Philadelphia, PA: WB Saunders; 2000, pp. 568–569.

OUT OF SIGHT SHOULD NOT BE OUT OF MIND

DORIS S. DUFF, BS, RN IV, CEN

WHAT TO DO: ASSESS

One of the ultimate challenges in emergency nursing is to be a good triage nurse. It requires a skilled, astute, compassionate, and culturally competent healthcare professional with a great deal of common sense and intuition. Some patients present to the emergency department (ED) with very unique complaints and may report using unique home remedies that can be outside the clinical expertise of the triage nurse. Nonetheless, these patients need to be assessed and treated appropriately. Their management starts with the assessment skills in triage.

Complication from a pessary is not a common ED complaint, but do not be caught off guard. A pessary is used as a nonsurgical approach to the treatment of pelvic organ prolapse. Pessaries are removable devices placed in the vagina to support pelvic organs or other gynecologic conditions such as a malpositioned uterus. A pessary can help to manage and slow down the progression of prolapse by adding support to the vagina and increasing tissue and muscle tightness. Symptoms improve and may be completely eliminated in women using a pessary. Potential risks include bleeding, open sores on the vaginal wall, and vaginal tears. The manufactured varieties of pessaries are made of rubber, plastic, or silicone materials with the most common types being inflatable, doughnut, and Gillhorn. They come in a variety of sizes and should be fitted carefully by the physician to hold the pelvic organs in position without causing pain. Once fitted, the pessary should not cause any pain and should be removed on a regular schedule for cleaning. Cleaning schedules are determined by the type of pelvic organ prolapse and the specific brand.

On occasion, the patients elect to try remedies that are handed down from generation to generation or are cultural in their origin. The use of foreign materials in body cavities are not new experiences for the ED triage nurse but are important to keep in mind. Even homemade pessary has been tried. Items such as potatoes and sponges have been used. The patients are simply attempting to get relief from a physical situation, like uterine prolapse, but may be too embarrassed to seek medical care. Hence, they might consider the insertion of an untraditional device, such as a pessary, into the vagina to help with their problem. Once inserted, patients may actually forget or may be embarrassed to admit that they have placed the object there when they present to the ED for treatment.

Patients do not understand the complexities of medical treatments or devices. They may use a home remedy to manage their health issue and develop additional complications. Sometimes they may forget that they have a foreign material in place, particularly if it is out of sight. A thorough assessment that begins with cultural sensitivity, a history of complaints, a thorough physical assessment, and a caring and thoughtful approach can assist a patient who may be experiencing complications from a home remedy, resulting in unintended consequences.

SUGGESTED READINGS

Grossman VGA. *Quick Reference to Triage*. 2nd Ed. Philadelphia, PA: Lippincott Williams & Wilkins; 2003, p. 5.

Vaginal Pessaries, Incontinence & Overactive Bladder Health Center. WebMD. Available at: http://www.webmd.com/urinary-incontinence-oab/vaginal-pessaries. Accessed May 5, 2008.

BE SURE TO HAVE PATIENTS UNDRESS COMPLETELY

DORIS S. DUFF, BS, RN IV, CEN

WHAT TO DO: ASSESS

"Triage" is a French word which means "to sort." It is a major component of the emergency medical system and an expectation of emergency nursing practice. Emergency department (ED) nurses require experience, professionalism, sensitivity, and concern. The primary goals of triage are to quickly identify patients that have emergent, life-threatening conditions and regulate the flow of patients through the ED. To facilitate these goals, the triage nurse establishes rapport and communicates with the patient and family to gather information so that appropriate interventions can begin. After a thorough assessment, conditions are prioritized and appropriately expedited depending upon the classification of the acuity.

The triage environment often prevents a complete assessment of the patient's complaint, which is often more thoroughly completed by the primary nurse once the patient is placed in a treatment room. However, it is essential to perform a primary assessment to determine the effectiveness of a patient's As, Bs, and Cs: Airway, Breathing, and Circulation. Assessment is performed rapidly, and if a problem is identified, immediate interventions can be performed. A head-to-toe approach is common. Start by examining the head and upper body, as well as extremities. Do not forget the subjective information from the patient. Ask about sensations such as vision or hearing changes, numbness or tingling, shortness of breath, and pain. Assess oxygenation and perfusion by checking oxygen saturations and

peripheral pulses. Ideally, the entire body should be examined to allow for a complete assessment.

Focused assessments on the patient's specific complaint are also beneficial. When a patient is in distress, focusing on that particular system assessment may be necessary. For example, if a patient presents with a bleeding chest wound, a focused thoracic assessment gets priority. However, always follow up with a complete head-to-toe approach.

When gathering information from the patient, maintain patient privacy. A thorough assessment includes looking at the patient and looking under the patient's clothing for signs of hidden injury or illness. It also means asking very personal questions that may cause embarrassment, especially if friends or family members are present. Assessing a patient, even in a busy ED, can and should be done in a respectful and considerate manner.

Triage in the ED can be done quickly, effectively, and with respect to the patient's privacy. Remember to respectfully remove the patient's clothing to enable a thorough assessment, including visualization, gathering subjective information, and providing quick treatment for injuries. Gathering this information quickly and accurately in a professional manner will help improve the flow of patients and their satisfaction in the ED.

SUGGESTED READINGS

ENA orientation to emergency nursing. *Assessment and Priority Setting Module*. Des Plaines, IL: Emergency Nurses Association; 2000.

Grossman VGA. *Quick Reference to Triage*. 2nd Ed. Philadelphia, PA: Lippincott Williams & Wilkins; 2003, pp. 3–7.

THE NURSE NEEDS TO BE AWARE OF UNCOMMON MEDICAL CONDITIONS THAT PRESENT AS COMMON PROBLEMS: NECROTIZING FASCIITIS IS ONE SUCH CONDITION

DORIS S. DUFF, BS, RN IV, CEN

WHAT TO DO: EVALUATE

A patient arrives to the triage desk complaining of flu like symptoms for several days and pain in his arm. He relates that he injured his arm while changing a tire in the rain a few days prior to presentation. The patient is noted to have a high fever and is placed in a treatment room. The physician writes orders for blood cultures looking for a source of infection and treating the patient. Several hours into the emergency department (ED) stay, the patient has not improved despite intravenous fluids and analgesics. While waiting for the remaining laboratory results, it is noted that the patient now has redness that has become apparent on his arm. Upon returning to the patient's room with the physician, the nurse notes that the redness has increased on the patient's skin and now has a shiny appearance. The ED physician orders antibiotics, blood skin cultures, and a surgery consultation. The patient is kept informed of his condition, but an urgent approach is definitely in order. The redness progresses rapidly and requires close, frequent monitoring.

Necrotizing fasciitis (NF) is pronounced *neck-row-tize-ing fash-e-i-tis* and often called "the flesh eating bacteria." It is an infection of the soft tissue that spreads very rapidly along the fascia and can lead to death if not treated quickly. The bacteria most commonly associated with this infection is Group A streptococcus. It can develop from a local injury with either superficial or deep infections or can result in the postoperative period. Clinical symptoms include fever, tachycardia, darkening of the tissue underneath the skin, and severe pain that is out of proportion to the local infection or injury. Late signs are a foul odor and drainage. Marking the lines of demarcation is helpful in evaluating the rapid progression of this infection.

The patient requires isolation and frequent monitoring of his or her vital signs. Admission to an intensive care unit is essential. Often, therapy consists of broad spectrum antibiotics and repeated surgical debridement. Complications of NF include gangrene requiring amputation, loss of tissue and function, and death. Remember that NF often presents with pain out of proportion to the injury, spreads extremely quickly, and must be treated aggressively with antibiotics and surgery.

SUGGESTED READINGS

Necrotizing Fasciitis. In: Nettina SS, ed. *Lippincott Manual of Nursing Practice*. 8th Ed. Philadelphia, PA: Lippincott Williams & Wilkins; 2006, p. 1103.

Necrotizing Soft Tissue Infection, Medline Plus Medical Encyclopedia. Available at: http://www.nlm.nih.gov/medlineplus/ency/article/001443.htm. Accessed August 3, 2008.

TOXIC SHOCK: WHEN A FOREIGN BODY CAN GET YOU

DORIS S. DUFF, BS, RN IV, CEN

WHAT TO DO: ASSESS AND EVALUATE

Toxic shock is a syndrome caused by a toxin. The toxin is usually produced by Staphylococcus bacteria but can also be produced by other bacteria, such as *Clostridium sordellii*, which has been associated with fatalities due to medical abortions. Toxic shock syndrome (TSS) is a form of septic shock. TSS can occur in children, women using tampons during their menses, and postmenopausal women as well as men. Risk factors include foreign bodies, such as nasal packing and tampons, menstruation, use of barrier contraceptives, childbirth, surgical wounds that are packed with gauze, and current *S. aureus*-bacterial infection.

The body's inflammatory response to this syndrome is characterized by a high fever, nausea, vomiting, diarrhea, and a widespread rash that looks like sunburn. In 1 to 2 weeks, the skin begins to peel including the palms of the hands and soles of the feet. The patient can have confusion, headaches, muscle aches, hypotension, and seizures. The kidneys and liver demonstrate signs of failure, but any organ can deteriorate as its perfusion is compromised. The treatment depends upon identification and removal of any foreign material such as tampons or nasal packing. Surgical wounds should be drained. Supportive treatments include intravenous fluids, vasopressors to maintain blood pressure, organ supportive therapies like dialysis, and antibiotics to treat the infection.

As a preventive measure, female patients should be instructed to avoid highly absorbent tampons and to change tampons frequently. Remember that toxic shock is a bacterial infection often related to a foreign object in a body cavity; identifying and removing this object is the first step to dealing with the syndrome.

SUGGESTED READINGS

Harvath, CA. *Emergency Nurse Core Curriculum*. Lippincott Williams & Wilkins, Philadelphia; 2006.

Medical Encyclopedia. Toxic shock syndrome. Available at: http://vsearch.nlm.nih.gov/vivisimo/cgi-bin/query-eta?v%3Aproject=medlineplus&query=toxic+shock+syndrome&x=44&y=5. Accessed August 3, 2008.

KNOW THAT COMMON PRESENTING COMPLAINTS MAY BE SIDE EFFECTS OF THE PATIENT'S MEDICATIONS LIKE ORAL CONTRACEPTIVES

DORIS S. DUFF, BS, RN IV, CEN

WHAT TO DO: ASSESS

Assessing the use of oral contraceptives (OCs) by women in the emergency department (ED) is important. OCs increase the risk factors for certain conditions. Identifying their use by patients may help identify the cause of the patient's presenting complaint. For example, the use of estrogen-containing oral contraceptives can cause headaches.

OCs have been associated with a variety of complications. While taking OCs, women who have hypertension have a 1.5 times greater risk for stroke. Higher estrogen doses in the OCs predispose women to a greater risk of stroke. Women below 35 years of age, who do not smoke and have a normotensive blood pressure, have less of a risk of ischemic stroke related to OC, but this risk increases with age.

A common serious event in women who use OC pills is venous thromboembolism. A venous thrombosis occurs when the fibrin, red blood cells, platelets, and leukocytes form a mass in the cardiovascular system. This risk is highest in the first year of OC pill use and is not related to the estrogen content of currently available OCs. Although the risk of venous thromboembolism increases with age, obesity, and recent surgeries, women who take OCs are at higher risk of venous thromboembolism than women who do not. Pulmonary embolism and deep vein thrombosis (DVT) are different manifestations of venous thromboembolism. Patients with a venous thromboembolism are also at greater risk for cerebral vascular accidents.

The dose and type of progestin may influence the effect of the OC on the metabolism of lipids and on the coagulation and fibrinolytic markers. OC pills that contain desogestral and gestodene are usually associated with a higher risk of venous thromboembolism than other OCs.

OCs have serious side effects. It is important to assess your patients to identify if they are using OCs and what type they are using. Otherwise your patients' risk for headaches, stroke, or DVT may be underestimated.

SUGGESTED READINGS

Aegidius K, Zwart J-A, Hagen K, et al. Oral contraceptives and increased headache prevalence. *Neurology*. 2006;66:349–353.

Cerel-Suhl SL, Yeager BF. Update on Oral Contraceptive Pills American Family Physician 11/1/99; 1–14. http://www.aafp.org/afp/991101ap/2073.html. Accessed on August 2, 2008.

Snyder JA. *Emergency Nurse Core Curriculum*. Lippincott Williams & Wilkins, Philadelphia; 2006.

ESOPHAGEAL VARICES ALWAYS NEED TO BE CONSIDERED IN THE PATIENT PRESENTING WITH AN UPPER GASTROINTESTINAL BLEEDING

DORIS S. DUFF, BS, RN IV, CEN

WHAT TO DO: PLAN

Esophageal varices are veins that are located in the lower esophagus and result from portal hypertension. They can extend into the upper esophagus and stomach. Portal hypertension is most often caused by cirrhosis from alcoholism. When these vessels rupture, it can be a life-threatening emergency. The rupture of esophageal varices is responsible for approximately 10% of upper gastrointestinal (UGI) bleeding and occurs more frequently in men. Diligence on the part of the nurse to identify patients with potential esophageal varices is critical to effectively planning the patient's care. Failure of the nurse to recognize the risks that varices pose is a potentially serious mistake with serious consequences. The insertion of a nasogastric tube in these patients increases the risk of rupturing these vessels and causing subsequent hemorrhage.

The symptoms of esophageal varices include hematemesis, hypotension, and tachycardia. These patients have a reduced hematocrit. Diagnosis is made based on the patient's history and decreased platelet count. Patients may complain of a feeling of blood filling up in their mouth, but they do not often vomit forcefully. Preparations should be made to insert a Minnesota or Sengstaken–Blakemore tube to temporarily stop the bleeding. This should only be performed by a physician experienced in the procedure. However, bleeding can be better controlled by endoscopic sclerotherapy, which is successful in 90% of cases. Gastric lavage has been a practice of emergency department nurses in the past for the control of UGI bleeding; however, this may not be the best practice to manage esophageal varices since it can impede normal coagulation mechanisms or disrupt clots that are beginning to form. Communication with the physician is important so that the nurse can help prepare the patient for the selected treatment. Treatment is focused at keeping the patient hemodynamically stable. Oxygen, ECG monitoring, and the insertion of large bore intravenous catheters are standard practices. Administration of normal saline and blood products is necessary to restore intravascular volume in the acutely bleeding patient. Octreotide is the drug of choice to manage variceal bleeding. It helps reduce the portal pressure by increasing clotting and hemostasis by decreasing splanchnic blood flow.

Patient behaviors such as straining, lifting heavy objects, sneezing, and gagging generally increase the pressure in the portal veins, and the patient should be instructed to avoid these types of behaviors to reduce the chances of spontaneous rupture and bleeding. Patients should also be encouraged to stop drinking alcohol and smoking. Remember to always assess a patient for esophageal varices prior to inserting an orogastric or nasogastric tube.

SUGGESTED READINGS

Cumming SP and Cummings PH. Abdominal Emergencies. In: Sanders Jordon K. *Emergency Nurse Core Curriculum.* Lippincott Williams & Wilkins, Philadelphia; 2006.

A LITTLE HONEY CAN CAUSE A LOT OF HARM

DORIS S. DUFF, BS, RN IV, CEN

WHAT TO DO: PLAN

Botulism is caused by a neurotoxic spore. It is found in the soil in the form of a bacterium (*Clostridium botulinum*) and when ingested can lead to blurred vision, slurred speech, difficulty swallowing, and descending muscle weakness. It can be transmitted to humans through air, open wounds, or food. Improper home canning and undercooked food are common sources of ingestion. It can also be found in maple syrup, corn syrups, and honey. Honey, in particular, has many supposed benefits that include the reduction of allergy symptoms. It also has known antibiotic properties and has traditionally been used for upset stomach. New evidence suggests that honey can also help prevent the growth of *Helicobacter pylori* and may alter the effects of cancer-producing carcinogens. There are also descriptions of honey being applied topically for gangrene and burns.

However, as mentioned previously, botulism can be found in honey. Infants have immature gastrointestinal tracts that allow botulism spores, when ingested, to germinate and produce botulism toxin. Very small amounts can lead to paralysis of the respiratory muscles, respiratory failure, and if untreated, death. Infants less than 12 months should not be given honey. Infantile botulism begins with constipation that appears 3 to 30 days after ingestion of the honey. The baby becomes listless and has a weak cry and poor feeding. As the disease progresses, the infant begins drooling. The gagging and sucking reflexes diminish next. Infants with prior head control often lose this ability, which is an important clinical sign. Respiratory arrest can occur gradually or suddenly. Infants who become sick enough for admission often require mechanical ventilation in a pediatric intensive care unit and have very long admissions averaging a month or more with several more weeks on the general pediatric floor. Infants receiving a correct diagnosis and appropriate supportive care often have a good recovery. The Center for Disease Control is usually contacted when a case is suspected. The patient is managed with oxygen and ventilation. Fortunately, fatalities remain low, but the most important part is to remember that this can be prevented by not giving honey to an infant less than 12 months because of the risk of neonatal botulism.

SUGGESTED READINGS

Honey and infant botulism. Available at: http://www.drgreene.org/body.cfm?id=21&action=detail&ref=825. Accessed May 9, 2008.

Act quick, time can be muscle with a compartment syndrome

Doris S. Duff, BS, RN IV, CEN

WHAT TO DO: ASSESS AND EVALUATE

A patient presents to triage with a forearm injury. He winces as the triage nurse barely touches his arm to obtain his pulse. Fascia is a tough, nonelastic membrane that envelopes the muscles, nerves, and blood vessels that form the multiple compartments of the extremities. When the compartment pressures increase from an outside force such as a cast or from an internal force such as injection of a foreign body, such as from a paint gun, the vascular and neurologic structures can become compromised. The microcirculation is initially obstructed, leading to edema, which also increases the pressure. The arteries remain patent until the pressure exceeds the systolic blood pressure. The forearms and lower legs are the most commonly affected sites, although the hands, digits, and feet can also be involved.

Symptoms include pain that is out of proportion to the injury, paresthesia, pallor, paralysis, and pulse, which are the "five P's" of assessment for vascular insufficiency and compartment syndrome. Pain is intense and is increased with palpation over the compartment. A pulse is usually present, and there is hyposthesia along the nerve that crosses the affected compartment. Pallor is related to the obstructed microcirculation and weakness that results from ischemia of the motor fibers in the affected nerves. A compartment pressure and laboratory values should be obtained. The nurse measures compartment syndrome pressures with a manometer. Pressures less than 10 mm Hg are considered normal. Lab studies and a urinalysis for myoglobinuria and an orthopedic's consult will likely be ordered. The patient should be monitored closely and the findings documented so that repeated evaluations can be performed as needed. The treatment includes an emergent fasciotomy. All forms of external compression should be removed, and any interventions that may impede circulation should be avoided. Ice should not be applied since this will continue to promote vasoconstriction. The extremity should not be elevated excessively since arterial flow may become impaired. Pain should be assessed and analgesics administered. Evaluation of the ongoing pain is an important part of the care.

SUGGESTED READINGS

Semonin–Holleran R. Environmental Emergencies. In: Sanders Jordan K. *Emergency Nurse Core Curriculum.* Lippincott Williams & Wilkins, Philadelphia; 2006.

Walker J. Specific Life Threatening Complications Associated with Orthopedic Injuries. In: Sanders Jordon K. *Emergency Nurse Core Curriculum.* Lippincott Williams & Wilkins, Philadelphia; 2006.

REMEMBER NOT ALL PATIENTS THAT ACT CRAZY ARE IN FACT, CRAZY. THERE MAY BE IMPORTANT CLINICAL CONDITIONS RESPONSIBLE FOR THEIR CONDITION THAT CAN BE TREATED. WERNICKE ENCEPHALOPATHY IS ONE SUCH CONDITION

DORIS S. DUFF, BS, RN IV, CEN

WHAT TO DO: PLAN

Wernicke–Korsakoff syndrome is a brain disorder that is caused by thiamine deficiency. It involves the loss of specific brain functions. Wernicke encephalopathy can damage nerves in both the central and peripheral nervous systems. Alcoholics with poor nutrition, including a lack of thiamine (otherwise known as Vitamin B1), are at risk. Alcohol interferes with the breakdown of thiamine in the body, which is necessary for the body to use glucose. Deficiencies of thiamine result in a reduction in cerebral glucose utilization, but the symptoms involve specific areas of damage. Lesions in the brainstem lead to ocular motor signs. The patient may exhibit diploplia, abnormal eye movements, and drooping eyelids. Ataxia is also a sign of damage to the cerebellum and leads to gait and stance abnormalities. The gait is often unsteady and uncoordinated. A wide-based short-stepped abnormality exists and may prevent the patient from standing or walking without assistance. Because the nerve cells are not destroyed, some improvement in the patient's symptoms occurs with the administration of thiamine.

The Korsakoff syndrome is a psychosis that tends to develop after the Wernicke symptoms resolve. Areas of the brain involving memory are damaged. The patients can tell detailed stories about their experiences or situations in an attempt to hide their memory loss (confabulation). The patients believe these stories to be true and make a compelling case to their providers. Causes of this condition also include patients with persistent emesis (such as hyperemesis gravidum, gastric malignancy, intestinal obstruction, and bariatric surgery), systemic diseases (such as malignancy, tuberculosis, AIDS, and uremia), starvation (such as anorexia or prisoners of war), and iatrogenic conditions (such as chronic hemodialysis, refeeding after starvation, and intravenous hyperalimentation). The goals of the treatment include the control of symptoms and the prevention of progression of the syndrome. Patients who are unconscious, lethargic, or comatose are monitored carefully. The administration of thiamine intravenously is the most common treatment. Symptoms of confusion, delirium, and vision can improve with thiamine administration; however, it will not improve the memory loss from the Korsakoff psychosis.

SUGGESTED READINGS

Wernicke-Korsakoff syndrome. Medline Plus. Available at: http://www.nlm.nih.gov/medlineplus/ency/article/000771.htm. Accessed August 3, 2008.

KNOW HOW AND WHEN TO INSERT A NASOGASTRIC TUBE AND WHEN TO AVOID IT

DORIS S. DUFF, BS, RN IV, CEN

WHAT TO DO: PLAN

The general purpose for inserting a nasogastric tube (NGT) into a patient in the emergency department (ED) is to decompress the stomach by removing air and gastric contents. The tube is inserted through either the mouth or a nare into the stomach. Gastric lavage can also be performed with the NGT to remove clots and blood from patients with gastrointestinal bleeding. In trauma patients, the NGT is inserted to assist in the prevention of vomiting and aspiration. Gastric contents can be analyzed to assist in clinical diagnosis. Other uses are to remove toxic substances, prevent gastric dilatation and aspiration, and administer radiopaque-contrast media. The size and type of the tube are dependent on the reason for placement. The smallest tube, appropriate for the intervention, should be used to prevent stress to the esophageal sphincter. Placement is usually verified by aspiration of gastric contents, use of CO_2 detectors, auscultation of air over the epigastrium when air is instilled via a cath-tip syringe, or chest X-ray.

Caution must be taken while inserting the NGT. Patients who have a potential cervical spine injury should be manually immobilized for the procedure, and caution should be taken during insertion to prevent movement of the cervical spine. Patients who have massive facial trauma, head injury, or skull fractures should have the tube inserted by the orogastric route to prevent potential insertion into the brain via the cribiform plate or ethmoid bone. Patients with esophageal varices are at risk for rupture and hemorrhage when a tube is inserted. Inserting NGTs in patients who have ingested a caustic substance can further damage the esophagus. Inserting an orogastric tube alongside of the cuffed endotracheal tube can be deceiving, and placement should be confirmed by the above methods prior to use. In the pediatric patient, NGTs are inserted for gastric decompression. Children swallow large amounts of air when they are in distress, and this causes gastric distention that can affect ventilation. Infants should have orogastric tubes inserted as opposed to NGTs since they are obligate nose breathers. Care should be taken when inserting NGTs in children because the diameter of their air passages is smaller, and their tongues are proportionately larger for their oral cavity.

SUGGESTED READINGS

Rossoll L. Insertion of orogastric and nasogastric tubes. In: Proehl JA. *Emergency Nursing Procedures*. 4th Ed. Philadelphia: Saunders, 2009.

KNOW WHAT TO DO WHEN YOUR PATIENT IS ASSAULTED BY A SNAKE IN THE GRASS

DORIS S. DUFF, BS, RN IV, CEN

WHAT TO DO: ASSESS, IMPLEMENT, AND EVALUATE

Patients bitten by snakes commonly bring the snake into the emergency department (ED) with them, which is often intriguing to staff and other patients. Many EDs allow the patient to bring in a dead snake to assist in the identification of poisonous versus nonpoisonous snakes and to see the size of the snake to approximate the amount of venom that was potentially injected.

The bites of venomous snakes result in one- to two-puncture wounds whereas nonvenomous snakes have up to four rows of top teeth and two rows of bottom teeth and may not always leave a mark on the skin. Snake saliva contains an anticoagulant that increases bleeding for several hours at the site of the bite. Home remedies, including pouring kerosene or alcohol on these bites, should be discouraged. Patients will often arrive with "tourniquets" applied above the site of the bite to reduce blood flow and stop the venom from getting into the heart. Tourniquets should also be discouraged. However, bands placed close to the bite that allow the insertion of two fingers between the band and the body are usually suggested if the bitten patient has a long travel time to reach the ED. These bands can generally stay in place for 1 to 1½ h. Suction devices are also not recommended; nor do they incise the wound in the prehospital arena, which can lead to damaged nerves, tendons, and vessels and an increased risk of infection.

Plan on keeping the patient calm, keeping the wound as immobile as possible, and getting to the ED quickly. Increased activity, fear, and intake of fluids and food speed up the circulation and cause the venom to act quicker. Avoid ice to the area as this leads to tissue destruction and amputation. The treatment consists of tetanus prophylaxis, intravenous access, blood work, and antivenom, as indicated. Copperhead bites generally do not require antivenom. The patient's age, clinical history, and the number of bites are all important in planning the treatment. Patients can be observed in the ED for several hours prior to being transferred or discharged.

SUGGESTED READINGS

Snakes—the good, the bad and the beautiful. Mother Earth News. Available at: http://www.motherearthnews.com/Nature-Community/2006–06–01/Snakes-The-Good-the-Bad-and-the-Beautiful.aspx. Accessed August 3, 2008.

COMA OCCURS FROM A NUMBER OF DIFFERENT CONDITIONS. IN ORDER TO APPROPRIATELY CARE FOR THE PATIENT, THESE CONDITIONS NEED TO BE ADDRESSED QUICKLY AND SPECIFICALLY

DORIS S. DUFF, BS, RN IV, CEN

WHAT TO DO: PLAN

Coma is a generic term that refers to an altered state of consciousness. It can result from a number of different clinical conditions, including acute trauma, diabetic ketoacidosis (DKA), stroke, alcohol abuse, or hypoglycemia. Of importance, the airway, breathing, and circulation need to be maintained while the causative problem is identified and rectified quickly in the emergency department (ED).

DKA is defined as a deficiency of insulin that results in metabolic acidosis, hyperglycemia, and ketosis. It can occur with Type II diabetes mellitus but is most frequently associated with Type I diabetes mellitus. The insulin deficiency leads to several physiologic changes, including decreased glucose intake at the cellular level, free fatty acid release, and an increase in gluconeogenesis by the liver. Hyperglycemia leads to osmotic diuresis with dehydration, hyperosmolality, and electrolyte depletion. The stress hormones have anti-insulin effects and stimulate the release of free fatty acids. The free fatty acids are converted to ketones that release hydrogen ions, leading to metabolic ketoacidosis. Acidosis affects myocardial contractility and cerebral function. Stressful events and infection, missing insulin doses, and the new onset of diabetes are some of the more common precipitating events for DKA. The symptoms of DKA include fatigue, nausea, vomiting, polyuria, and polydipsia. When untreated, these can progress to stupor and coma. After assurance of the airway, breathing, and circulation, these patients require volume expansion with isotonic fluids and insulin to treat their hyperglycemia and metabolic derangements.

Coma can occur from a number of other causes that are not associated with diabetes, such as cerebrovascular accidents (CVAs). CVAs are neurologic deficits that arise from a defect affecting the vasculature of the brain. Adequate cerebral blood flow can be compromised by a clot, narrowing of a vessel, or a rupture of a weakened blood vessel. The clinical picture is related to the vessel involved, the extent of the damage, and collateral flow that is available to the injured area. Patients at highest risk for a CVA include diabetics, those with hypertension, and those with a history of smoking and drug use. These patients can have weakness on unilateral extremities, slurred speech, or an inability to speak. For patients presenting acutely with ischemic stroke as a cause for their coma, the use of thrombolytic medications can be considered. Mostly, the care for stroke patients is supportive.

Alcohol is one of the most commonly abused drugs in the United States. Alcoholism is a chronic illness characterized by an impaired control over drinking. Alcohol is metabolized in the liver. Patients can be belligerent, demanding, difficult, and dangerous, making care of these patients challenging. The symptoms of intoxication and withdrawal may mimic or mask other potentially life-threatening illnesses. Patients who have had an increase in alcohol ingestion can exhibit slurred speech, confusion, and ataxia. Many of these patients can benefit from hydration and the assurance that they do not have thiamine deficiency.

Hypoglycemia is a reduction in the serum glucose level less than 50 mg/dL and is one of the most common endocrine emergencies. Once glucose levels are below 35 mg/dL, brain damage can begin. Hypoglycemia occurs for many reasons, but diabetes and alcohol ingestion are two of the biggest reasons. These patients can exhibit symptoms similar to CVAs—unilateral weakness of extremities, slurred speech, or inability to speak; therefore, patients exhibiting altered levels of consciousness should be urgently tested for hypoglycemia.

Regardless of the cause of coma, it becomes important for the nurse to be prepared to assess the blood sugar upon the patient's arrival. Hypoglycemia and hypoglycemia related to alcohol toxicity are the two readily treated emergencies that can prevent brain damage. Patients with CVA are often diabetic, and hyperglycemia will often accompany their body's stress response from the CVA and worsen their outcome. Therefore, it should be treated aggressively. Finally DKA will present with hyperglycemia, and the diagnosis may then become apparent. The testing of a glucose level for the patient who arrives in the ED in coma is the first order of business after assurance of the As, Bs, and Cs and well within the practice of nursing.

SUGGESTED READINGS

Jordan KS, ed. *Emergency Nursing Core Curriculum*. 5th Ed. Philadelphia, PA: Saunders; 2000, pp. 263–265, 409–411, 625–627.

THE SKIN IS THE WINDOW TO THE BODY, AND RASHES MAY REPRESENT IMPORTANT SYSTEMIC DISEASES

DORIS S. DUFF, BS, RN IV, CEN

WHAT TO DO: ASSESS

Skin rashes are a common complaint, and patients often present to the emergency department (ED) for treatment because they are frightened. Many rashes are benign and are treated with antihistamines or steroids, resolving quickly in a few days. However, it is important to know when the rash represents a more important problem with the patient. Forgetting to attend to a skin rash that is serious may mean that you will miss an important infection or organ failure. Petechiae are tiny pinpoint red lesions found on the skin that form when blood vessels break. Petechiae do not blanch when pressure is applied to the skin. This allows them to be differentiated from other rashes that may be more benign. Purpura is a collection of blood under large flat areas of the body that do not blanch with pressure. Petechiae and purpura can present together as signs of more severe disease and when accompanied by fever, may represent a medical emergency such as overwhelming sepsis or meningitis. The cause of the sepsis or meningitis can be a number of different organisms, including *H. Influenza, Neisseria meningititis*, or *S. pneumoniae*. Regardless of the causative organism, the patient's body will exhibit similar symptoms that often begin with petechiae and progress to purpura as the other manifestations become apparent.

Because these diseases progress rapidly and death occurs within only a few hours, patients with fever should be assessed carefully after removing all their clothes to ensure that they do not have dermatologic signs of more severe disease. The treatment for one of these bacterial conditions should be started as early as possible after blood cultures and spinal fluid are obtained. In these cases, healthcare workers should wear protective masks to prevent the spread of these suspected pathogens.

SUGGESTED READINGS

Pierce-Peabody S. Meningitis. In: Sanders Jordon K. *Emergency Nurse Core Curriculum*. Lippincott Williams & Wilkins, Philadelphia; 2006.

Thoroughly Search the Acutely Ill Psychiatric Patient Being Cared for in the Emergency Department

Elizabeth A. Gilbert, ADN, BA-CS

WHAT TO DO: PLAN

As behavioral health resources dwindle in the community, emergency departments (EDs) are caring for increased numbers of acutely ill psychiatric patients presenting for treatment. The psychiatric patient population has different needs than patients presenting with medical problems. The routine equipment and tools of our trade necessary to care for a majority of the patients that present to the ED can be hazardous to psychiatric patients or staff if a violent or self-destructive patient is cared for without attention to what can cause harm.

In the absence of a secured psychiatric area, ED staff members need to remember to remove any items that pose a threat to either the staff or the patient. For example, cardiac monitor cables are commonly found at the bedside in the ED. A psychiatric patient can use them to hang himself/herself or strangle a staff member. Other commonly used items that need to be always checked include sharp instruments such as scissors, scalpels and needles, and medications.

Remember to check specific facility policies and guidelines for searching psychiatric patients. It is frequently a common practice to have psychiatric patients change into paper scrubs or a hospital gown, and their belongings searched and removed from them while they are in the ED. Searching their belongings will allow staff to remove any hazardous items, such as weapons, drugs, matches, and lighters that were brought in with the patients.

The ED environment itself needs to be designed to eliminate potential hiding places where the patients can hide items that can be used to hurt themselves and others. Psychiatric patients frequently demonstrate poor impulse control, and may take items left around the ED while they are unattended. Other items that ED staff members need to be aware of that can be hazardous to the psychiatric patients are belts, shoelaces, silverware from meal trays, soda cans, or items commonly worn around the necks of employees, such as a stethoscope or badge lanyard. These items can be used to assault staff members or to attempt suicide. Toiletry items such as mouthwash and razors, emergency call bell light cords, and shower curtain hooks can also be hazardous.

Finally, it is important for the nurse to develop an understanding of common psychiatric diagnoses to provide appropriate treatment modalities and a safe environment. For example, the nurse must remember that it is during the manic phase of bipolar disorder that the patient is particularly susceptible to poor judgment and is unable to control impulses. Patients with schizophrenia frequently experience auditory and visual hallucinations that they interpret as instructing them to harm themselves or others. Collaborating with the ED physician and the psychiatry service to stabilize the patient on medication is critical to patient and staff protection. Maintaining situational awareness also facilitates a safe environment and allows the patients to be cared for with attention to their needs.

SUGGESTED READINGS

Manton A. Psychiatric patients in the ED—How can the system respond? *ENA Connection Online*. April 2004; 28(3).

Challenges to conscious sedation in the emergency department

Elizabeth A. Gilbert, ADN, BA-CS

WHAT TO DO: PLAN

Conscious sedation is a procedure that is frequently performed in the emergency department (ED) during painful procedures, such as fracture reductions, in both adult and pediatric populations. The nurse must be trained in airway management, be knowledgeable of sedation medications and their side effects, and be able to identify risk factors that patients may present with, which can lead to adverse outcomes. Conscious sedation can be defined as the administration of medications to produce a state of amnesia while the patient maintains his or her own protective airway reflexes. The patient maintains an ability to follow simple commands but is unable to recollect the procedure.

The nurse must remember to explain the procedure to both the patient and family, who may be at the bedside during the procedure, especially the parents of pediatric patients. The patient may cry out loud while the procedure is being performed. This may be interpreted by family as ineffectiveness of the medication. Reassuring the family is important. The nurse must also remember to explain the effects of the different medications used since many of the effects can be alarming. For example, ketamine commonly causes nystagmus or postprocedure nightmares that can be of concern to families. The nurse must be familiar with the facility policy regarding conscious sedation. It is critical to always ensure that the room is stocked with appropriately sized emergency equipment such as a bag valve mask, oxygen source, and suction set-up. They should be tested and available should an emergent need arise. All materials, including the medications, reversal agents, and paperwork, should be brought to the bedside so that the nurse can maintain a presence with the patient until the procedure is complete and the patient has adequately recovered from the sedation.

It is important to obtain a medical history that includes any chronic illnesses, an accurate list of current medications, smoking, alcohol, and drug history, when the patient last drank or ate anything, and allergies and adverse responses to anesthesia. It is also important that the nurse remember to perform a complete baseline physical assessment, particularly of the airway, pulmonary, and cardiovascular systems, and a complete set of vital signs, including a temperature and pulse oximetry reading. Placing the patient on a cardiac monitor and continuous pulse oximetry will assist in managing the patient's cardiopulmonary and oxygenation status and monitoring for side effects of the medication, such as slowed breathing, hypotension, or desaturation. The nurse may have to support the patient's airway with positioning, with supplemental oxygen, and by encouraging the patient to breathe deeply. The nurse must avoid giving an excessive amount of medication that can decrease the patient's ability to support his or her own airway.

Continuous monitoring until the patient is fully awake, able to tolerate fluids by mouth without nausea or vomiting, and vital signs remain stable, including a normal temperature, is an essential discharge criterion. The patient and family should verbalize understanding of discharge instructions, including contact information for the ED, should they have any concerns regarding the procedure or the sedation.

SUGGESTED READINGS

Pascarelli P. The role of the nurse during intravenous conscious sedation. *Orthop Nurs.* 1996;15(6):23–25.

KNOW HOW TO SOLICIT EMBARRASSING INFORMATION DURING THE TRIAGE HISTORY

ELIZABETH A. GILBERT, ADN, BA-CS

WHAT TO DO: ASSESS

All patients presenting to the emergency department (ED) for treatment go through a triage process, which allows ED staff to obtain information and determine the priority of treatment. The nurse needs to be skilled in soliciting accurate information through a chief complaint and a brief and targeted medical history, performing a rapid physical exam, and determining the severity of the illness. While it is important and self-evident to the nurse that patients should be forthcoming with medical information, including an accurate list of current medications to facilitate appropriate treatment, some patients may be apprehensive about being completely honest about their medical history or current medications because of embarrassment.

An example of one such medication is Viagra. Viagra is a phosphodiesterase inhibitor that is prescribed for erectile dysfunction, which may result from several diseases, including heart disease, diabetes, psychologic distress, obesity, low testosterone levels, or lifestyle choices such as alcohol, smoking, or drug use. Cialis and Levitra are other examples of drugs in this class of medications.

Patients presenting to the ED with chest pain should be questioned and encouraged to provide an accurate listing of medications, especially those taken within the past 24 to 36 h. Phosphodiesterase inhibitors are contraindicated with nitrates due to the risk of severe hypotension and altered perfusion; therefore, the treatment of the patient's chest pain will have to be modified. Of note, α-blocker(s), such as Hytrin, Flomax, and Cardura, are also contraindicated with phosphodiesterase inhibitors due to the risk of severe hypotension. Patients on combination drug therapy are at higher risk for side effects and should be monitored more closely.

Several things can be done by the ED nurse to facilitate a thorough history. First, ensure that the patient has privacy to share this information; usually a curtain in the triage room is inadequate to ensure a patient's confidentiality with these intrusive questions. Second, ensure that you make the patient comfortable prior to diving into the sensitive areas of the history. A casual conversation about his or her job or family may break the ice and allow the professional relationship to be built prior to asking more difficult questions. Third, tell the patient how important it is for him or her to share this information with specifics about his or her case. For example, "I am really glad you came in with this chest pain, it is always better to get these things checked out. It is important for us to know if you are taking any medications that can interfere with your treatment here. We are finding that many patients are now on medications like Viagra to help them with sexual activity. Are you taking any of these medications?" Fourth, be calm. The triage area in a busy ED can often be busy and chaotic. Allowing the patient to know that your focus is on him or her for this interval of time can be helpful. Our patients do not want to be a burden, and although we may not say it, a harried look on a busy night can send nonverbal cues. Finally, be matter-of-fact. If the patient sees that asking the question is making you uncomfortable, he or she will be uncomfortable responding.

SUGGESTED READINGS

Erectile dysfunction. MayoClinic.com. Available at: http://www.mayoclinic.com/health/erectiledysfunction/DS00162/DSECTION=treatments%2Dand%2Ddrugs. Accessed August 3, 2008.

Do not forget to inquire about home remedies

Elizabeth A. Gilbert, ADN, BA-CS

WHAT TO DO: ASSESS

Complimentary and alternative medicine has been used for centuries. One reason for the popularity of these therapies is the common belief that they are natural and therefore safe. This is a common misbelief that often leads to self medication with supplements that have unknown components and dosing practices. Many of the currently available supplements have not been tested on pregnant women or children and interact with prescription medications. In the United States, herbal supplements are regulated as foods, not drugs. This means that they do not have to meet the same standardization for safety and manufacturing processes that is required of medications. This lack of standardization leads to inconsistent effectiveness and organ damage, particularly the liver. The nurse needs to be diligent in learning about some of the more common therapies that patients self-administer, their side effects and interactions with prescription medications, and provide appropriate education to the patients.

Aloe is one of the more common herbal remedies. It is generally known as a topical agent for burns, which produces analgesia and anti-inflammatory effects at the burn site. It is also used orally as a laxative. The long-term use of aloe as a laxative should be avoided. Aloe is contraindicated in pregnancy and in children. It interacts with antiarrhythmics, cardiac glycosides, loop diuretics, thiazides, and steroids by increasing their effects. It should not be used as a laxative if the patient is experiencing abdominal pain of unknown origin, Crohn disease, ulcerative colitis, or suspected intestinal obstruction.

Black Cohosh is another common herbal therapy that is used by women to treat symptoms of menopause and premenstrual syndrome (PMS). It is also used in combination with St John's wort to treat mood disorders and depressive symptoms. Black Cohosh should not be used during pregnancy or in children. It can interact with antihypertensive medications by increasing their effects and causing severe hypotension. In high doses, Black Cohosh can cause vomiting, headache, dizziness, and extremity pain. While it can help ease PMS and menopausal symptoms, Black Cohosh should not be used for longer than 6 months. Black Cohosh should not be confused with Blue Cohosh, which is used as an anticonvulsant and antispasmodic. Blue Cohosh increases menstrual flow and frequently has gastrointestinal and cardiac side effects.

St John's wort has been in some limited clinical studies. It has been approved for use in anxiety and depressive moods. It has significant interactions with prescription medications. It should not be used with monoamine oxidase inhibitors because of the danger of precipitating hypertensive crisis. The use with immunosuppressants can result in decreased serum levels of the prescription drug. It should also be avoided with certain SRI medications since this can also increase the effects and result in serotonin syndrome.

Echinacea is another common herbal therapy used to alleviate cold symptoms and acute and chronic respiratory infections. Echinacea is contraindicated in immunosuppressed patients and those with autoimmune disorders since it alters the effects of immunosuppressant medications. Echinacea should be used for a limited time, recommended no longer than 8 weeks. Chronic use can lead to hepatotoxicity. While there are many more therapies that could be listed, these common ones and their effects are used most often. The nurse needs to remember to ask the patients about all medications they are taking, including over-the-counter and herbal therapies. If the nurse does not inquire specifically about these medications, the patients are not likely to offer the information since they generally do not consider these remedies as a part of their medication regimen.

SUGGESTED READINGS

Decker GM, Myers J. Commonly used herbs: Implications for clinical practice. *Clin J Oncol Nurs*. 2001;5(2):13.

National Center for Complementary and Alternative Medicine. Herbal supplements: Consider safety, too. Available at: http://nccam.nih.gov/health/supplement-safety/. Accessed August 3, 2008.

ALWAYS HAVE A PROCESS TO ENSURE THAT YOU HAVE THE RIGHT PATIENT SINCE IT IS THE FIRST STEP TOWARD ESTABLISHING A CULTURE OF SAFETY IN THE EMERGENCY DEPARTMENT

ELIZABETH A. GILBERT, ADN, BA-CS

WHAT TO DO: PLAN

Developing a consistent practice in patient identification is imperative for avoiding mistakes that could lead to mistreatment or adverse outcomes for the patient. In today's busy emergency department (ED), it is highly probable that there will be two or more patients with the same or similar names or other demographic information. Because there are frequently multiple caregivers for any patient, the nurse must remember to verify the patient's identity prior to performing a procedure or administering a medication or therapy such as transfusion.

Two essential components of good nursing practice in the ED are to ensure that there is clear communication between caregivers and to develop and accept a culture of safety. Clear communication between caregivers is imperative. The nurse must remember to allow time for questions and clarify as needed whether the information is between two nurses as in shift report or between two disciplines like the pharmacist and the nurse. Questioning things that do not seem right is also essential. For instance, if the nurse were to review lab results on a patient that seemed to be inconsistent with what was expected, she should take the time to verify that they were, in fact, correctly collected and resulted. Taking the time to verify results can ensure that the patient is treated correctly.

A culture of safety is important for the patient and nurse's relationship and the relationship between the nurse and the hospital. The nurse needs to make a personal commitment to patient safety by following appropriate processes such as patient identification. However, it goes further than this in terms of interacting with the patient and family, keeping them informed of their treatment status, and allowing them to ask questions. The nurse needs to avoid feeling "challenged" when patients ask questions. Nurses also need to feel comfortable to question or "stop" an action or treatment that does not seem appropriate. Many organizations are working with a program called TeamSTEPPS to facilitate effective communications and teamwork among healthcare providers. These efforts pay large dividends in terms of helping nurses to be understood and recognized for their expertise and the skills they bring to patient care.

Finally, having a reporting process in the organization to evaluate poor outcomes is also very important. Event reports and root cause analysis can be used to evaluate existing processes and identify opportunities to change processes that have lead to incidents. Continually evaluating training processes and ensuring that nursing staff is competent and informed of existing policies are also important. Encouraging staff to share information and concerns about issues is essential. Nursing staff members need to feel that the organization is willing to listen to their concerns.

Developing a culture of safety begins with nurses and their ability to ensure that their own clinical processes are hardwired and evidence based. It continues through the nurse's interaction with others including other providers and the hospital. When we all work together, the result will be a more optimal patient-care experience for our patients.

SUGGESTED READINGS

Making Healthcare Safer. *A Critical Analysis of Patient Safety Practices Promoting a Culture of Safety*. Available at: http://www.ahrq.gov/clinic/ptsafety/. Accessed August 3, 2008.

TeamSTEPPS: National Implementation. About the National Implementation Plan. Available at: http://teamstepps.ahrq.gov/aboutnationalIP.htm. Accessed March 8, 2008.

FOLEY CATHETER USE IN POST-TURP PATIENTS—LEAVE IT IN...PLEASE!

ELIZABETH A. GILBERT, ADN, BA-CS

WHAT TO DO: IMPLEMENT

The emergency department (ED) nurse needs to have an appreciation for postoperative care, especially with same day surgical procedures where the patient may present to the ED emergently due to a complication of the procedure. A transurethral resection of the prostate (TURP) is performed in men for a variety of reasons including prostate cancer, benign prostatic hyperplasia, recurrent urinary tract infections from an enlarged prostate, bladder stones, weakened or damaged bladder, or the inability to empty the bladder leading to kidney damage. The use of a Foley catheter post-TURP is standard practice for postsurgery irrigation and to prevent urinary retention. Continuous bladder irrigation is used for the first 24 h to prevent urinary retention from blood clots. Once the irrigation is stopped, the urine will form small clots that will generally pass through the catheter without difficulty. Occasionally, the catheter will become clogged, and urinary retention will result, particularly if the patient is not maintaining an adequate fluid intake.

Patients with urinary retention will present to the ED with complaints of decreased urine output and lower abdominal pain. On physical examination, the nurse will note a distended bladder and an obviously uncomfortable patient. The nurse must have an understanding of this particular post-op procedure and resist the temptation to remove or replace the catheter. By removing the catheter, the nurse runs the risk of not being able to replace the catheter or causing increased bleeding. The nurse must always remember to consult with the treating physician about the treatment plan for the patient. The standard approach for the treatment of a clogged urinary catheter would be to irrigate by hand with sterile normal saline and attempt to remove the clots. This may take 10 to 15 min but is often successful in unclogging the catheter and allowing the bladder to empty. Once patent, the nurse should avoid allowing large amounts of urine to escape quickly from the bladder, which can result in painful bladder spasms. The nurse needs to remember to record the amount of urine emptied from the bladder. Once patency is ensured, the catheter needs to be connected back to a leg bag, and urine flow monitored. The nurse should remember to educate the patient on maintaining an adequate fluid intake to avoid clotting of the catheter. Verify physician follow up with the patient.

SUGGESTED READINGS

Transurethral resection of the prostate. Available at: http://www.swedish.org/body.cfm?id=7. Accessed August 3, 2008.

KNOW THAT DIFFERENT DOSING PATTERNS EXIST FOR DROPERIDOL DEPENDING UPON THE INDICATION

ELIZABETH A. GILBERT, ADN, BA-CS

WHAT TO DO: IMPLEMENT

Medications have different uses, intervals, and dosages depending upon the indications for use, and it is important to ensure that you have the correct dose for the indication. Droperidol is a medication that is most frequently used as an antiemetic for postoperative nausea in lower doses and as an antipsychotic medication in higher doses. A low dose is 0.625 to 1.25 mg. A higher dose is 5 to 10 mg. Droperidol is in the class of drugs referred to as a dopamine receptor antagonist, but it also has some histamine and serotonin antagonist properties. Droperidol received a "Black Box Warning" in 2001 because of concerns that it caused QT prolongation and Torsades de Pointes. With the emergence of other antiemetics, such as ondansetron, which has better efficacy in children and equal efficacy in adults for relieving nausea, droperidol has been used less frequently in the emergency department (ED) setting.

However, with this reduced use, it becomes even more important for the nurse who will be administering droperidol to inquire about any cardiac history and any related medications. Patients with a history of coronary artery disease, high blood pressure, congestive heart failure, electrolyte imbalances, or heart rhythm disorders should not receive droperidol. Droperidol may interact with a number of cardiac medications. If the physician is aware of the patient's history and would still like to have droperidol administered, the nurse needs to remember to place the patient on a cardiac monitor and administer a low dose. The nurse will need to remember to tell the patient receiving droperidol to report any side effects such as a faint feeling, a fast or pounding heartbeat, or fluttering in the chest. The patient will need to be monitored for extrapyramidal side effects such as dystonia and neuroleptic malignant syndrome. If these side effects should occur, the nurse needs to treat them promptly. In appropriate individuals, and with proper evaluation, Droperidol can be used safely in the ED setting, but it is important for the nurse to know the different dosing strategies with this drug, particularly with its less frequent use.

SUGGESTED READINGS

Domino K, Anderson E, Polissar N, et al. Comparative efficacy and safety of metoclopramide for preventing postoperative nausea and vomiting: A meta-analysis. *Anesth Analg.* 1999; 88:1370.

Droperidol. Available at: http://www.providence.org/health-library/contentViewer.aspx?hwid=d00219a1&serviceArea=generic. Accessed May 8, 2008.

PATHOLOGIC WATER INTOXICATION IN THE EMERGENCY DEPARTMENT

ELIZABETH A. GILBERT, ADN, BA-CS

WHAT TO DO: ASSESS

Water intoxication can be seen in patients who present to the emergency department (ED) and often in those who present with hyponatremia. Water intoxication is most frequently associated with athletes who engage in high intensity sports, such as endurance events. Their prolonged and profuse sweating places the athletes at risk of upsetting the balance of blood sodium. By drinking only water, a relatively hypotonic fluid, during the event, they are not replenishing the sodium lost in their sweat. These patients most often present with nausea, muscle cramps, and confusion, and if left untreated, the hyponatremia can lead to seizures, coma, and death.

Nurses in EDs may see another presentation of water intoxication that has a pathologic origin. Psychiatric patients with schizophrenia are also at risk for water intoxication; however, this presentation often goes unnoticed until the late signs occur. Schizophrenic patients have abnormally high levels of antidiuretic hormone (ADH). The combination of high levels of ADH and excessive water intake, which occurs frequently with schizophrenia, can cause a patient to gain 20 to 30 lb of water weight! Nurses need to remember that these patients are at risk and monitor their fluid intake while they are in the ED. Placing the patient in a water-free environment is difficult, so the nurse may have to come up with creative ways for maintaining fluid restriction. The nurse will also need to remember to be cognizant of subtle signs of hyponatremia, such as muscle cramps, nausea, and increased confusion, and intervene appropriately. While scientists and researchers do not clearly understand the mechanism of pathologic water intoxication, efforts to identify medications that may be effective for these patients and improve their lives continue. ED nurses need to maintain awareness for the risk factor that water can create for patients and an understanding of when they are becoming symptomatic and what dangers can occur if they remain untreated.

SUGGESTED READINGS

Goldman M. UIC researchers to study new drug for schizophrenic patients. University of Illinois Psychiatric Clinic, Department of Psychiatry. Available at: http://www.psych.uic.edu/news/new_schizophrenia_drug.htm. Accessed August 3, 2008.

Goldman MB, Luchins DJ. Prevention of episodic water intoxication with target weight procedure. *Am J Psychiat.* 1987;144:365–366.

Goldman MB, Robertson GL, Luchins DJ, et al. The influence of polydipsia on water excretion in hyponatremic polydipsic schizophrenic patients. *J Clin Endocr Metab.* 1996;81:1465–1470.

THE ELECTRONIC MEDICAL RECORD...JOB SECURITY FOR NURSES

ELIZABETH A. GILBERT, ADN, BA-CS

WHAT TO DO: PLAN

Many hospitals are moving to electronic medical records (EMRs) to document and store patient's health information and to improve the safety and integration of the healthcare experience for patients. EMRs have several advantages that facilitate optimal patient care. Caregiver notes are legible and time stamped. They cannot be changed by another caregiver. Physician orders are legible and are frequently designed to comply with regulatory requirements. All caregivers are able to document the patient record, and the documentation is simultaneously accessible to all, facilitating communication between disciplines. Many EMRs have built-in safety features and decision support, such as interaction checking during provider order entry when the provider is warned that two drugs of the same class are being prescribed. This has the potential to greatly reduce medication errors.

While the EMR has many advantages, there are also some disadvantages that also need to be considered when nurses begin to use these applications. First, confidentiality issues remain a concern. The nurse needs to gain access only to those records that they have a professional reason to read. Simple curiosity is not only unprofessional but also it may result in a harsh penalty for breach of confidentiality. The penalty may be more severe if the patient is a psychiatric patient. Passwords become even more important to ensure confidentiality and screens need be logged off when not in use. Second, another disadvantage an EMR is the use of templates in charting. While the template may save time and focus the nurse on a line of pertinent questions as it pertains to the patient's chief complaint, it should not substitute for clinical judgment and inquiring about information that is not in the template. Third, the nurses must avoid becoming so preoccupied with completing the EMR that they overlook the patient. Patients deserve the attention that only a professional nurse can provide. Finally, the nurses have to be careful that they do not become overreliant on the computer so that the failure to receive a prompt about a dosage or medication is considered okay. Computers are designed and implemented by people and sometimes the programming is incorrect and should be challenged. While an EMR is a valuable tool and can enhance the quality of care for the patient, the nurse must remember to continue to document nursing assessments, actions, and observations so that the patient can continue to receive high quality care.

SUGGESTED READINGS

Likourezos A, Chalfin DB, Murphy DG, et al. Physician and nurse satisfaction with an electronic medical record system. *J Emerg Med*. 2004;27(4):419-424.

KNOW HOW TO CARE FOR THE PATIENT WITH JIMSON WEED AND OTHER HALLUCINOGENIC POISONINGS

ELIZABETH A. GILBERT, ADN, BA-CS

WHAT TO DO: IMPLEMENT

Emergency departments (EDs) experience the presentation of patients who have ingested substances for their hallucinogenic effects. Typically, the patient is brought in by friends or relatives because of bizarre behavior, agitation, or hallucinations. Some patients will be able to tell the ED staff members what they have ingested, and some will not. The management of these patients begins with a primary survey, starting with the ABCs of resuscitation. Hallucinogenics can be ingested through a variety of routes such as inhaling, smoking, snorting, or ingesting.

Jimson weed is a common poisoning that has been used for centuries. It is a member of the belladonna family and has strong anticholinergic properties. It grows freely alongside roads and in pastures. Although farmers and gardeners may sustain an unintentional exposure, it is more commonly used by teenagers who intentionally misuse it for its hallucinogenic and euphoric effects. The nurse must try to get an accurate account from the patient or friends of what he or she may have ingested. The nurse must also recognize the presenting symptoms of atropine poisoning—dilated pupils, flushed, warm dry skin, dry mouth, tachycardia, hypertension or hypotension, delirium with hallucinations, jerky myoclonic movements, and hyperthermia. Frequently the mneumonic "blind as a bat, mad as a hatter, red as a beet, hot as a hare, dry as a bone, the bowel and bladder lose their tone, and the heart runs alone" is used to describe the symptoms. Management of Jimson weed poisoning will be supportive. The nurse needs to remember to provide for the patient's safety by providing a nonstimulating environment to assist with hallucinations and agitation and administer sedatives as needed. Frequent monitoring of vital signs is important, including temperature. Manage hyperthermia with cooling blankets if needed. Depending on the dosage ingested, the symptoms will usually resolve in 24 to 48 h. It is important for the nurse to educate the patient and family on the hazards of Jimson weed and other hallucinogenics.

SUGGESTED READINGS

Chan K. Jimson weed poisoning: A case report. *Permanente J.* 2002;6(4):28–30.

Jimson Weed Fast Facts. Available at: http://www.doitnow.org/pages/525.html. Accessed August 3, 2008.

KNOW YOUR INSULIN TYPES

ELIZABETH A. GILBERT, ADN, BA-CS

WHAT TO DO: IMPLEMENT

Insulin is a life-saving medication that is a daily essential for many patients with diabetes. There are many types of insulin stocked in the emergency department (ED). Each insulin preparation has a different onset and peak effectiveness, which makes the administration of insulin a risky business that mandates that nurses review these medications and their effects regularly. Patients that present to the ED with problems related to diabetes management typically have hyperglycemia, diabetic ketoacidosis, or hypoglycemia. Hypoglycemia in the ED is easily managed. Hyperglycemia is managed with a regimen that includes insulin.

Insulin types typically stocked in the ED are regular insulin, NPH insulin, and Lantus. EDs usually do not stock long-acting insulin because patients are not kept and managed in the ED for extended periods of time. Regular insulin is short-acting insulin, with an onset of 30 to 60 min. It peaks in 1 to 5 h and lasts 6 to 10 h. Frequently in the ED, regular insulin is administered intravenously for hyperglycemia and may be mixed in an infusion to be administered to the patient with diabetic ketoacidosis. Regular insulin is approved for subcutaneous, intramuscular, or intravenous administration. NPH insulin has a duration of 16 to 24 h. NPH insulin is approved for subcutaneous administration only. Lantus insulin would be considered long-acting insulin with an onset of 1 h, no peak, and duration of 24 h. This insulin is not used frequently in the ED. Subcutaneous is the preferred administration route for insulin because the absorption through fatty tissue is more efficient. The abdomen is the desired administration site.

The nurses must pay attention to the reason that the insulin is being ordered so that they can achieve the desired outcome. The nurse should always draw insulin up in the appropriate syringe, remember to verify the type of insulin that is being given, and do verification that the dose is correct before administering it to the patient.

SUGGESTED READINGS

Hodgson BB, Kizior R. *Saunders Nursing Drug Handbook*. Philadelphia, PA: W.B. Saunders; 2008, pp. 618–620.
Insulin preparations. *FDA Consum Mag*. 2002. Available at: http://www.fda.gov/fdac/features/2002/chrt_insulin.html. Accessed August 3, 2008.

BE CAREFUL WHEN ADMINISTERING MEDICATIONS TO KIDS IN THE EMERGENCY DEPARTMENT

ELIZABETH A. GILBERT, ADN, BA-CS

WHAT TO DO: IMPLEMENT

Children have a number of reasons that make them more at risk for medication errors than adults. These include differences in size, weight, developmental status, and drug distribution. Errors can occur at many points in the medication delivery process, including prescribing, dispensing, and administering, and in documenting the medication given. The most common source of medication errors in children is dosage calculations. Consistently instituting checks and balances into one's practice will reduce the risk for error in the emergency department (ED).

The nurse must always remember that children's medications are dosed by weight. The child should be weighed for accuracy and assurance that the right units (lb vs. kgs) have been used. If possible, the nurse should avoid taking the parents' word for how much their child weighs. The nurse should have the knowledge of the medication that will be given and minimize distractions while calculating dosages and preparing and administering the medication. "High risk" drugs calculations, such as insulin, sedation medications, and heparin doses, should be double-checked by another nurse. The nurse must always question illegible orders or orders that do not seem to make sense. Following protocols and facility policies will contribute to safety. Having readily available drug information sources is also important as is utilizing the appropriate equipment for properly preparing and administering medications. Oral medication syringes should only be used for oral liquid to avoid inadvertent intravenous administration. Intravenous medications may also require small doses and need to be drawn up using the appropriate syringes. Using a tuberculin syringe will allow more accurate dosing than using a 1 mL syringe due to the increments in tenths. The nurse should always draw up insulin in an insulin syringe because the dosage of units is demarcated on the syringe.

Medication administration for children in the ED is important, and the nurse should avoid overriding safety features on medication administration equipment such as intravenous infusion pumps, should remain updated on medications through educational offerings, and should develop sound clinical practices that are important for protecting these vulnerable patients.

SUGGESTED READINGS

Hughes R, Edgerton E. Children's health: Nurses can take steps to prevent pediatric medications errors associated with dosing and administration. Agency for Healthcare Research and Quality. Available at: http://www.ahrq.gov/research/jun05/0605RA17.htm. Accessed August 3, 2008.

The Joint Commission. Sentinel event alert, Issue 39. Available at:http://www.jointcommission.org/SentinelEvents/SentinelEventAlert/sea_39.htm. Accessed August 8, 2008.

GET THE MOST USE OUT OF THE EQUIPMENT YOU USE FOR PATIENT CARE

ELIZABETH A. GILBERT, ADN, BA-CS

WHAT TO DO: PLAN

Emergency department (ED) nurses utilize many pieces of equipment on a daily basis. It is important for the ED nurse and support staff to understand the proper use of the equipment and to be able to use it to its full potential to enhance patient care. It is the responsibility of the organization to provide the necessary information and training for all staff members who will be using the equipment, and it is the responsibility of the nurse and staff to learn to use the equipment properly and ask appropriate questions if they do not understand its functions.

Patient safety must remain a priority at all times. One monitoring device that is common to the ED is the cardiac monitor. This device will provide continuous monitoring for cardiac rhythms, blood pressures, respiratory rates, and pulse oximetry. The monitor has many more functions available to the nurse, including arterial pressure monitoring and ST segment monitoring; cardiac outputs and central venous pressures monitoring are possibilities if a pulmonary artery catheter is in place. However, the nurse needs to be careful not to use components in the ED that should be performed in another setting. Using specialty equipment infrequently and with inadequate knowledge can be a setup for a major safety event.

It is certainly appropriate for nurses in the ED to be able to set specific alarm parameters and they can split a screen to view other assigned patients should they be delayed in another room for an extended period of time. The cardiac monitor can also calculate drug doses for intravenous infusions. Nurses must remember to enter all the appropriate patient information such as name, weight, and medication they wish to administer. The monitor will calculate and printout a titration table. The monitor will store information and show trends and history when requested.

The functionality of the monitoring equipment will be dependent upon the specific equipment that is purchased for the department. The availability of medical monitoring equipment in the ED can assist the nurse in providing optimal patient care as long as the device is used consistently with the care provided in the setting. The nurse should avoid feeling apprehensive about the use of technology and seek to learn as much of the functionality of the equipment as is useful while remembering that the equipment can often do more than the setting in which it is being used.

SUGGESTED READINGS

Drew BJ, Califf RM, Funk M, et al. AHA scientific statement: Practice standards for electrocardiographic monitoring in hospital settings: An American Heart Association Scientific Statement from the Councils on Cardiovascular Nursing, Clinical Cardiology, and Cardiovascular Disease in the young: Endorsed by the International Society of Computerized Electrocardiology and the American Association of Critical-Care Nurses. *J Cardiovasc Nurs*. 2005;20(2):76–106.

IT's AN ED, NOT AN ICU

ELIZABETH A. GILBERT, ADN, BA-CS

WHAT TO DO: EVALUATE

As emergency departments (EDs) become increasingly overcrowded, they experience multiple challenges in providing patient care. Besides long wait times, longer turn around and throughput times, and decreased patient satisfaction, there are challenges that arise for ED nurses trying to care for inpatients being housed in the ED. Providing intensive care unit (ICU) level of care in the ED is particularly challenging. There are a number of reasons why the critically ill patient should be transferred as soon as possible to the ICU.

First, one of the factors that contribute to the challenge of providing ICU level of care in the ED is nurse-to-patient ratios. The typical nurse-to-patient ratio in the ED is 1:4, although it may be higher in a rapid care area. Patients in any one assignment often have a mixed acuity. The delivery of critical care to patients who are critically ill demands that the typical staffing ratio in the ICU be 1:1 or 1:2, depending on acuity. Critically ill patients who are receiving care from a nurse with a higher ratio will fail to get the care justified by their severity.

Second, another factor contributing to the challenge of caring for an ICU patient in the ED is the unpredictable volumes that occur in the ED. At any one time, the volume of patients arriving to the ED can shift causing staff to be inconsistent in the care they provide to the critically ill patient who demands intensive monitoring. The constant reprioritization and workload reassignment create multiple handoffs and problems for the ICU patient who requires consistency in care.

Third, processes for obtaining medications and other treatment requirements for inpatients that are being housed in the ED are also challenging. Inefficiencies in acquiring equipment and performing inpatient functions only serve to distract the ED nurse from his or her ED work.

Fourth, ED nurses have neither the familiarity with the equipment nor the core competencies in critical illness that the ICU patient will require. Hence, the ED nurse needs to collaborate with the treatment teams to ensure the patient receives optimal care. Overcrowding and inpatient holds are becoming standard procedures for EDs. The nurse needs to identify care needs and seek out educational opportunities to correct them. The goal needs to be to decrease the length of stay for inpatient holds in the ED, particularly for the vulnerable ICU patient who deserves the specialized care that his or her condition demands.

SUGGESTED READINGS

Morgan R. Turning around the turn-arounds: Improving ED throughput processes. *J Emerg Nurs*. 2007;33(6):530–536.

METHODS FOR ACHIEVING HEMOSTASIS IN THE TRAUMATIC TONGUE LACERATION

RICK MCCRAW, RN, MBA, CMTE

WHAT TO DO: PLAN

Patients who present with injuries where the bleeding is uncontrollable pose a unique challenge in the emergency department (ED) environment. Thankfully for most of these patients, the emergency care provider has a continuum of options for achieving hemostasis that range from noninvasive and simple to complex. The usual strategies for bleeding control range from simple things, such as direct pressure to the wound or pressure on the arterial supply proximal to the injury, to direct cautery or ligature of the bleeding vessel itself. When the area that is bleeding is confined within a small space or is noncompressible, several new challenges are created. One example of such a situation is when the injury is to the tongue.

The tongue is a large single muscle that is quite vascular. It is also contained within the oral cavity. The good news is that many lacerations to the tongue heal very quickly and often do not require treatment beyond supportive management.

However, there are certain tongue injuries that do require repair, and it is those that we will discuss, including those that are more than 1 cm, those that are multi-layered, and those where the bleeding cannot be controlled by other means. Since the tongue is so vascular, bleeding can be profuse. To make things even more dangerous, the patient's airway can quickly become compromised by blood that is aspirated, making airway protection the number one priority with any injury to the mouth or face. Some simple techniques for hemostasis are effective in tongue lacerations but are also difficult to achieve. Direct pressure is an example of such a technique. Since the tongue can be difficult to get a good grip on, the use of a gauze pad to pull the tongue out and then apply pressure both above and below with the wound in between may be a successful method to control the bleeding till normal clotting occurs.

If suturing is selected as an option to control the bleeding, then appropriate measures must be taken to ensure that an emergency airway can be achieved if the patient's normal airway is compromised. The use of conscious sedation may also be considered due to the extremely uncomfortable and panic-inducing nature of procedures such as these. Having good patient cooperation will certainly boost the potential to have a good outcome for the procedure and will make for a better experience for the patient overall.

Injuries of this type are certainly difficult for the nurse to handle in the ED setting. Being prepared and remaining calm (you and your patient) are two essential steps in being able to prevent the tough case from becoming a nightmare. Anticipating the things that can go wrong and having a plan in place and equipment ready for those eventualities are the hallmarks of the really good emergency provider.

SUGGESTED READINGS

Control bleeding. Available at: http://www.ic.sunysb.edu/Stu/wilee/e-zine-controlbleeding.html. Accessed July 15, 2008.

Infection Control is Critical for the Modern Day Emergency Department

Rick McCraw, RN, MBA, CMTE

WHAT TO DO: PLAN

The emergency department (ED) is neither a sterile environment nor does it need to be. With more and more cases of resistant infections presenting for treatment, cross-contamination is a danger to everyone in this setting, including patients, staff, and visitors. This issue is further complicated by the volume of patients that flows through the traditional ED. Depending on the size of the ED, several hundred patients per day may be seen. When an additional two to five family members per patient are added in, the containment of germs becomes essential for preventing the spread of disease and is becoming more and more an almost overwhelming task. There are several strategies that can assist the ED in becoming a safer environment from an infection control perspective.

As important as infection control is, frequently the worst offenders have been hospital employees themselves. The national patient safety goal of "wash in and wash out" has been instrumental in raising awareness of the importance of handwashing within healthcare, but providers are still having difficulty achieving appropriately high levels of compliance for our patients. Hence, we subject patients who present to the ED with cross-contamination from other patients we may have already treated. While there is a great value in the use of clean latex gloves for the prevention of the spread of infection, gloves alone are not enough and may be porous; therefore, washing after degloving is also of prime importance. At the turn of the century, hospitals, like many expensive buildings, had silver doorknobs. As hospitals became more mainstream and opulence in construction was curtailed, the silver doorknobs were replaced by other less precious metals. What was not known was that silver was also bacteriostatic. When silver was no longer used, the transmission of microbes

from hand to doorknob climbed dramatically, resulting in many more hospital infections. This continued until handwashing became an accepted practice to curtail the transmission of disease. Besides the providers, the equipment in the ED can be a source of contamination. Fomites can often spread disease. It becomes increasingly apparent that we need to consider the transmission of microbes on our stethoscopes and other patient-care equipment including otoscopes, blood pressure cuffs, stretchers, counter tops, and mattresses. Decontaminating these surfaces on a regular basis when contaminated can assist in preventing the spread of infectious diseases to patients.

Finally, for patients who are in the ED to have a wound repaired or receive an invasive procedure like a central venous catheter, the importance of decontaminating the wound and ensuring that appropriate care is delivered through antisepsis during and after the procedure is critical. Applying appropriate dressings and maintaining their sterility are important even in a busy ED.

While the ED will never be on par with the operating suite in terms of its sterility, there are fundamental practices, including good cleaning technique, that can make a difference between the spread of infection to patients and the transmission of microbes to our staff and families. Good nursing care supported by the use of appropriate barriers, gloving, and handwashing can assist us in making the difference.

SUGGESTED READINGS

CMS seeks to add 9 hospital-acquired conditions to no-pay list. Availableat:http://www.ama-assn.org/amednews/2008/05/12/gvsb0512.htm.

DeMarco P. Your life is in hospital workers' (clean) hands. *Toxic Alert*. Available at: http://www.toxicslink.org/art-view.php?id=60. Accessed on July 8, 2008.

Slavin H. Ionic silver—The powerful defense against viruses and other microbes. National Health Federation, September 2006. Available at: http://www.thenhf.com/articles_360.htm.

CONSIDERATIONS MADE IN THE SEDATION OF THOSE WITH IMPENDING NEUROLOGIC OR NEUROSURGICAL EVALUATION

RICK MCCRAW, RN, MBA, CMTE

WHAT TO DO: IMPLEMENT

Frequently, patients who present with neurologic insults are difficult to assess due to the symptoms of their injury or illness. Many brain injuries can cause cognitive impairment, the result of which can be an inability of the patient to cooperate with the simplest of commands. In brain or neurologic injury, the patients may also experience coma, agitation, seizures, delusions, hallucinations, or any combination of these symptoms that also alter their consciousness.

Despite the difficulties in management of these patients, it is essential for the neurosurgeon or neurologist to be able to observe and assess this behavior first hand. The nursing challenge is to be able to differentiate between the ominous signs of a deteriorating underlying clinical condition and a behavioral manifestation of the patient. As an emergency nurse, the goal is not to control the behavior of these patients who may pull their IV out, take their cervical collar off, or generally be uncooperative with attempts at treatment. While the routine use of sedation for convenience is never indicated, there are important times when the patients' behavior has become a danger to themselves, and chemical or physical intervention is required to prevent injury. For example, the stroke patient who is hallucinating and trying to crawl out of the bed, despite being unable to walk, may require additional restraint or sedation.

The objective in these situations is always to use the least amount of restraint or medication with the shortest duration that achieves effective control of symptoms. For controlled sedation, drugs such as propofol may be a good choice, since it has a very short half life and can be titrated as needed to achieve the desired level of sedation. Alternative agents include benzodiazepines.

Often simple nursing measures such as reassurance and 1:1 care can be enough to get a patient who is confused but not combative through until his or her neurologic evaluation can be completed. If the nurse takes time, the patient may benefit by getting a good and thorough neurologic evaluation early in the course of his or her hospital stay.

SUGGESTED READINGS

Galvin AA. Sedation. In: Proehl JA, *Emergency Nursing Procedures*. 4th Ed. Philadelphia: Saunders; 2009, pp. 842–846.

Murphy's Law as it Pertains to the Checking for Allergies!

Rick McCraw, RN, MBA, CMTE

WHAT TO DO: ASSESS

Most of us are familiar with Murphy's basic law that states that anything that can go wrong will go wrong. I would assume there is a Murphy's Law for medication allergies that would say "If you do not ask about a patient's allergy status prior to the administration of a medication, your patient will in fact be allergic to that medication." For all nurses who have given medications, an assurance of the five Rights for medication safety is something learned from the very start of nursing school:

• Right Patient
• Right Drug
• Right Route
• Right Time
• Right Dose

While not included in these five Rights, it is also imperative to check a patient's allergy history, especially when the medication is being given for the first time or in an emergency setting. There is also increasing difficulty in understanding the cross reactivity between drugs of different drug classes. The use of interaction checking and allergy checking in many electronic sources and formularies provides important and useful information at the point of care when the medication is ordered.

Of course, these tools do not relieve the burden of simply communicating with our patients and inquiring with them or their family about medication allergies.

For example, the patient who, when asked about allergies, says that he or she took the medication once and it made him or her itch will need to be interrogated in greater detail to see if he or she had a local rash (indicating a minor local reaction) or urticaria (possibly suggesting a much more serious systemic allergic response). Good nursing practice is a bit like detective work. The patient may not know what is important and what is not and omit details that are significant. The nurse will need to ask probing questions and piece information together to achieve the best course of action.

Since a patient's condition is dynamic, all information is subject to change and must constantly be updated and compared. Allergic history is one example of a potentially changing set of data elements that the caregivers must never allow themselves to become complacent about.

Changes in the patient's sensitivity can turn a medication that a patient has taken many times from friend into foe. The medication nurse's diligent observations may be the patient's last defense against a bad reaction. Remember to assess for allergies to medications!

SUGGESTED READINGS

Allergic reaction: Topic overview. WebMD. Available at: http://www.webmd.com/allergies/tc/allergic-reaction-topic-overview. Accessed July 8, 2008.

Murphy's Law site. Available at: http://www.murphys-laws.com/. Accessed July 8, 2008

The Five Rights of Medication Administration. Available at: http://www.dora.state.co.us/NURSING/news/TheFiveRights.pdf. Accessed July 8, 2008.

NOT ALL STATUS EPILEPTICUS IS ASSOCIATED WITH CONVULSIONS

RICK MCCRAW, RN, MBA, CMTE

WHAT TO DO: IMPLEMENT

Most emergency providers treat recurrent seizures as a self-limiting situation where the treatment really focuses on protection of the patient's airway and body during the "convulsive" phase of the seizure. Once the acute phase has passed, the reasons for the patient's seizure are then explored through diagnostic testing like anticonvulsant blood levels, alcohol or drug withdrawal, CT scanning for intracranial pathology, or trauma.

There are some cases, though, where the ability to detect a discrete beginning and end to the seizures is difficult. Nonconvulsive status epilepticus consists of electrical seizure activity that persists even when the associated movements are fragmentary or absent. Since the physical manifestations are no longer present, providers lose their more typical overt signs of the seizure and are unable to detect if the patient is still experiencing status or not. In these patients, seizure activity remains on electroencephalogram (EEG). When confronted with this difficult situation, some important differences in care need to be addressed.

In the patient with nonconvulsive status epilepticus, the assessment always begins with the basics, airway protection, ensuring adequate oxygenation, ventilation, and circulation. The nasopharyngeal airway placement is sufficient to maintain the airway for some patients, particularly if the seizures have stopped and the patient is awakening or may be postictal. For other patients, endotracheal intubation is necessary. In this setting, if neuromuscular paralysis is required, rapid sequence induction may be necessary to stop the seizures long enough to secure the airway. The use of short-acting paralytic agents can facilitate airway control, yet ensure that the ongoing seizure activity is not masked. If a longer-acting neuromuscular blocker is used, the placement of EEG monitoring is indicated to ensure that the patient does not have continued status epilepticus with a masking of the physical manifestations. Further, succinylcholine, a very useful agent for rapid sequence intubation, may be relatively contraindicated since many patients with status epilepticus experience hyperkalemia and acidosis and this drug raises the potassium level.

After securing the airway, patients with nonconvulsive status epilepticus can have their breathing and circulation assessed and managed like other status epilepticus patients before turning the attention to some of the underlying causes. Since ongoing seizure activity consumes large quantities of blood sugar, rapid glucose determination and correction should be performed. The establishment of intravenous access, ideally in a large vein, is the preferred route for anticonvulsant administration because it allows therapeutic tissue levels to be attained more rapidly.

Careful monitoring and aggressive treatment of status epilepticus are essential in the emergency department setting since failure to diagnose and treat adequately could contribute to permanent brain damage and a much worse outcome that might otherwise be seen. Remember that not all status epilepticus is represented by convulsions.

SUGGESTED READINGS

Huff JS. Status epilepticus. eMedicine from WebMD. Available at: http://www.emedicine.com/emerg/fulltopic/topic554.htm#sectioñIntroduction. Accessed July 8, 2008.

Kaplan PW, Fisher RS. *Initiators of Epilepsy*. 2nd Ed. Available at: http://www.ncbi.nlm.nih.gov/books/bv.fcgi?indexed=google&rid=imitepil.section.1476. Accessed July 8, 2008.

Allergies: Rash versus hives, local versus systemic

Jennifer Bath, RN, BSN, FNE, SANE-A

WHAT TO DO: EVALUATE

Allergic reactions can be as minor as a rash or as life threatening as anaphylactic shock. Most allergic reactions seen in the emergency department (ED) are minor and can be treated with a few medications. However, some allergic reactions will be fatal to the patient. Allergies can be caused by many things such as environmental sources (e.g., dust, pollen, insects, and animal dander) or common items found around the house, including foods or medications (e.g., eggs, peanuts, etc.).

Rashes are an inflammation of the skin and can range from an irritation, such as a diaper rash, to chronic problems, such as psoriasis. Rashes are common manifestations of allergic reactions but vary in their character. Hives are a buildup of fluid under the top layer of your skin. Hives occur when histamine is released into the blood causing the vessels to stretch and intravascular fluid to leak. This fluid then accumulates and forms lesions called wheals that cause intense pruritus. The physical manifestations of hives will usually disappear within 24 h. A local allergic reaction usually involves pain, swelling, redness, itching, and hives. Most local allergic reactions are not life threatening; however, even when local, the airway can sometimes be involved. The most common local reactions are from insects like bees.

A systemic allergic reaction is called anaphylaxis. Anaphylaxis is a rapid multiorgan systemic reaction that occurs within seconds to minutes of exposure to an allergen. This can be fatal if not treated promptly. The most common allergen in anaphylaxis is medications. However, anaphylaxis can be caused by a number of other products like bees or peanuts. Other symptoms associated with anaphylaxis include hives, flushing, shortness of breath, congestion, wheezing, stridor, respiratory distress, hypotension, weak and irregular pulses, chest tightness, cardiac irritability, and diaphoresis. Often the patients' skin will appear warm and dry, but as the reaction progresses, it will become pale and cool. This is a sign that the cardiovascular collapse accompanying their shock is getting worse. Patients with anaphylaxis will often communicate an impending sense of doom, uneasiness, and apprehension.

It is important to recognize the difference between a local and a systemic reaction. Local reactions usually only involve the area affected, where the patient was exposed or stung. A systemic reaction will involve multiple body systems like the skin, airway, lungs, and heart and require immediate recognition and treatment. The treatment often involves subcutaneous epinephrine (1:1,000 concentration), antihistamines, isotonic fluids for shock, and supportive care of the airway, breathing, and circulation.

SUGGESTED READINGS

Allergic reaction: Topic overview. Available at: http://www.webmd.com/allergies/tc/allergic-reaction-topic-overview. Accessed July 8, 2008.

Beach S. How allergies work. Available at: http://www.health.howstuffworks.com/allergy2.html. Accessed July 8, 2008.

TRIAGE IS NOT OVER WHEN THE VITAL SIGNS ARE TAKEN

JENNIFER BATH, RN, BSN, FNE, SANE-A

WHAT TO DO: EVALUATE

Triage plays an important role in every emergency department (ED). Triage is the process of gathering information from patients as they present in the ED to assign a priority score. Those with the most life-threatening or potentially life-threatening problems go before those with problems that are less severe. Effective triage is even more important now with the problem of overcrowding and longer waiting times before being seen by a physician. The three most serious consequences of triage include those patients who sit too long in the ED waiting room and decompensate because of a failure to be reassessed, those patients who are so tired of waiting that they leave the ED without being seen and experience a deterioration of their condition, and those patients who are undertriaged from their presentation to the ED and experience adverse events while waiting. All three of these highlight the need for triage to be a very active and dynamic process.

There are several methods of ensuring effective triage and addressing these problems. First, because of longer wait times, patients should be reassessed every 2 h while waiting. A repeat set of vital signs should be taken, and the patient should be asked if his or her condition has worsened while waiting. The patient's triage level may change if his or her reassessment demonstrates that his or her condition has worsened. Second, undertriage occurs when a lower acuity is assigned to the patient than is actually warranted by the patient's risk factors and physical signs and symptoms. A patient who is undertriaged has an increased chance for an adverse outcome because of a longer waiting time than his or her condition warrants. Ensuring the accuracy of triage and testing the ED nurses' capabilities at providing triage services are important. Third, understanding why patients leave without being seen and evaluating their outcomes are an important approach to better understand how triage works in the ED. Finally, another way to help reduce errors in triage is to ensure that the nurse assigned to triage is properly trained. The Emergency Nurses Association (ENA) recommends that a nurse have at least 6 months of ED experience before being assigned to triage. The triage nurse must have good assessment skills, be organized, know how to prioritize, be a good interviewer, have a good knowledge of diseases, and be able to pick up on subtle clues to perform accurate triage. The ability to implement standing orders while the patient is waiting to be seen by the physician can also help improve patient outcomes. For instance, ordering an X-ray for an extremity injury or collecting a urinalysis for a complaint of abdominal pain can speed up patient flow through the ED. Initiating diagnostic tests early will decrease the amount of time the patient is in the ED.

The triage process has been evaluated over the past several years. New systems for triage are being developed and many use a five-level system. The ENA and the American College of Emergency Physicians (ACEP) advocate for standardized triage process and support the five-level triage system. Two commonly used acuity systems, the ENA's Emergency Severity Index (ESI) and the Canadian Triage and Acuity Scale (CTAS), utilize the five-level process. The five-level system considers the patient's vital signs and presentation and accounts for the number of resources the patient will need while in the ED. This helps ensure that all patients are triaged appropriately. Algorithms have been developed that help assign a triage level to the patient. These can be posted in the triage room for reference. Skillful triage provides for prompt assessment and treatment in a busy ED. Assessing for critical information helps establish appropriate patient priorities. This improves outcomes, efficiency, and patient satisfaction.

SUGGESTED READINGS

Derlet R. Triage and ED overcrowding: Two cases of unexpected outcome. *West J Emerg Med.* 2002;3(1):8–9.

Funderburke P. Exploring best practice for triage. *J Emerg Nurs.* 2008;34(2):180–182.

Twedell DM. Priorities of care: Triage Models. In: Sanders Jordon K. *Emergency Nurse Core Curriculum.* Philadelphia: Lippincott Williams & Wilkins; 2006, pp. 24–27.

KNOW THE CONDITIONS THAT MIMIC ABUSE

JENNIFER BATH, RN, BSN, FNE, SANE-A

WHAT TO DO: ASSESS

Healthcare providers come in contact with children who have been abused and need to appropriately refer these children to social service agencies when the provider is suspicious. It is important when abuse is suspected that a thorough medical and family history is completed and a thorough examination is performed to rule out a medical cause for the injury or illness.

There are many diseases and cultural practices that may mimic abuse because of the physical changes they cause. A few of the more commonly seen conditions will be described here. Mongolian spots are a congenital defect that is present from birth and usually disappears by the age of five. They are blue, brown, or blue–black patches of skin found primarily over the lower back and buttocks. Mongolian spots are more common in people with pigmented skin, primarily from the African-American population. These spots are generally mistaken for bruises.

Osteogenesis imperfecta (OI) is a condition in which the bones are brittle and break easily, sometimes for no apparent reason. It is caused by a defect in collagen synthesis. The signs and symptoms include easy bruising, blue, gray, or purple sclera, hearing impairment, laxity of joints, and spinal curvature. It is very common for practitioners to care for these children and misdiagnose them as being abused. However, it is also important to realize that just because a patient has OI, it does not mean that he or she also cannot be abused.

Coining, cupping, and spooning are Southeast Asian cultural practices for healing that involves putting warmed oil on the chest, back, and rib cage and rubbing a coin, spoon, or cup repeatedly over the areas until petechia or purpura develops. Patients will often have patterned bruises and welts in a linear fashion from coining and spooning and circular bruises from cupping. The context of the therapy must be analyzed in these cases before accusing the family of abuse.

Staphylococcal scalded skin syndrome (SSS) is an infection caused by the *Staphylococcus aureus* bacteria. SSS mimics a burn and has a scalded appearance due to epidermal erythema, peeling, and necrosis. It has a generalized appearance, whereas most burns related to abuse are local. It usually involves the inguinal and perigenital areas but can also be seen elsewhere. It primarily affects infants aged 1 to 3 months but can be seen in older children. To diagnose SSS, a culture of the lesions is collected to isolate the Staph infection.

Hair tourniquets involve wrapping a thread or piece of hair around an infant's penis, finger, or toes. The patient develops swelling and erythema in the area distal to the thread or hair. The affected digit or penis becomes edematous, discolored, and painful.

Lichen sclerosus is a chronic benign inflammatory skin disorder that involves the vulvar and perianal areas. The hymen is not involved. It is often misdiagnosed as sexual abuse because the genitalia will have a bruised appearance and may be bleeding. The lesion has a figure of eight or hourglass pattern with skin that becomes thin and will tear very easily causing bleeding. Chicken pox and impetigo are frequently misdiagnosed as cigarette burns due to their appearance. Other diseases like idiopathic thrombocytopenia purpura, Henoch-Schonlein purpura, hemophilia, and leukemia can also be mistaken for bruising from physical abuse.

It is important to obtain an accurate patient and family history and complete physical examination. Protecting children who are being abused is very important. However, it is just as important to rule out medical reasons before falsely accusing someone of being an abuser, which has adverse consequences of its own.

SUGGESTED READINGS

Broduer AE, Monteleone JA. *Child Maltreatment: A Clinical Guide and Reference*. Philadelphia, PA: G. W. Publishing, Inc; 1994.

Hammer R, Moynihan B, Pagliaro E. *Forensic Nursing: A Handbook for Practice*. Boston, MA: Jones and Bartlett; 2006, p. 654.

Lynch V. *Forensic Nursing*. St. Louis, MD: Elsevier Mosby; 2005, pp. 82–84.

CPR: Get it right!

Jennifer Bath, RN, BSN, FNE, SANE-A

Cardiopulmonary resuscitation (CPR) provides life-sustaining care in the setting of an acute cardiopulmonary arrest. Despite the fact that so many healthcare providers are familiar with CPR and have been trained, CPR is often performed incorrectly; even by doctors and nurses. The two major errors that occur when performing CPR include overventilation and chest compressions that are neither deep nor fast enough. Studies performed on in-hospital cardiac arrest demonstrate that 48% of the time compressions were inadequate. Many providers will share that the reason for these errors is a concern of hurting the patient. Unfortunately, the failure to provide effective compressions can often lead to a patient's death since it is the compressions that are needed to substitute for the heart's pumping action and push the blood through the body. When CPR is performed well, the survival for out-of-hospital cardiac arrest doubles.

Recently, bystander CPR has been revised to hands-only CPR. This is mainly for those who have not had CPR training or those who are unsure of their ability to perform CPR correctly. Hands-only CPR is used only on witnessed, adult cardiac arrests. Any cardiac arrest in an infant or child, an unwitnessed cardiac arrest, or an arrest due to respiratory problems should still be treated with conventional CPR. Hands-only CPR improves survival if started immediately and not stopped until emergency medical services arrive. There appears to be no negative impacts on patient outcomes when hands-only CPR is performed.

One solution to the problems with ineffective CPR may lie in improved training since CPR skills deteriorate after only a few months if not practiced routinely. At the very least, the two messages of adequate but not overventilation and of hard and fast compressions should be reinforced for all healthcare providers. Hard and fast compressions increase the patient's chance of survival. Computer guided CPR is a hope for the future. Computer guided CPR is a process in which a computer alerts the providers if the compressions are too slow or shallow or if ventilations are too fast.

SUGGESTED READINGS

Berg R, Cave D, Page R, et al. *Hands-only CPR Simplifies Saving Lives for Bystanders.* 2008. Available at: http://www.american heart.org/presenter.jhtml?identifier=3057167. Accessed July 27, 2008.

CPR: Are we doing it wrong? *The Harvard Medical School Family Health Guide.* June 2005. Available at: http://www.health.harvard. edu/fhg/updates/update0605c.shtml. Accessed July 27, 2008.

A TEAM APPROACH IS NEEDED IN CODE SITUATIONS IN THE EMERGENCY DEPARTMENT

Jennifer Bath, RN, BSN, FNE, SANE-A

WHAT TO DO: IMPLEMENT

Anyone who has ever worked a cardiac arrest knows it can be a high-stress situation. A life hangs in the balance and the team is there to do what it can to save that life. Many hospitals have code teams, consisting of staff members who respond to the codes. One advantage of having a code team is that there are established roles for each member of the team. In the emergency department (ED), there usually is no code team response since the ED staff are expected to handle cardiac arrests often enough and as a part of their daily work and competencies.

However, unless the members of the ED practice and rehearse their responses as a team, they may be unprepared to act in synergy when the patient needs them most. If you have more than one person doing the same task, certain tasks or procedures may either be duplicated or not performed at all. For example, when there is a lack of clarity around task assignment, two people may both end up giving medications and no one would record the events that occur during the code. This can lead to problems for the patient since the documentation helps to keep the team organized on task and expectant of the next interventions.

Code teams usually have designated roles for each member, such as the first responder, team lead, defibrillator operator, recorder, intubator, intravenous (IV) nurse, med nurse, floor nurse, and crowd controller. Roles will differ from team to team depending on the staff availability. The first responder is the person who finds the patient. Their job is to call for help, assess the airway, breathing, and circulation, and initiate basic life support. In the past, nurses would call for help and clear the room to make space for the code team rather than starting CPR and attending to the patient. Mock codes have assisted the nursing staff in becoming more confident in these emergent situations and have resulted in earlier activation of resuscitation. Having "Mock Code Drills" on a routine basis can help to keep the staff prepared for the real event.

The first responder will also make sure the crash cart is at the bedside and the patient's chart is available. The team leader, usually an ED physician, will lead the resuscitation efforts. The defibrillator operator is responsible for monitoring the patient's rhythm, calling out any rhythm changes, delivering shocks, and printing strips for the record. The recorder is the person who logs all events and interventions during the code. This is an essential role, since they will be keeping track of times that medications were given so that they can notify the team when the next dose is due. The team leader is often responsible for intubation, but some hospitals have anesthesist respond to the code and handle this procedure. The IV nurse makes sure the patient has at least one, if not two, working IV site and regulates the flow of fluids. The role of the medication nurse can be completed by two nurses, one standing at the cart and preparing the medications and the other administering the medications. The floor nurse is responsible for notifying the family and the patient's primary doctor of what is happening. Crowd control can be performed by nonclinical personnel to keep the area free of all unnecessary personnel and bystanders.

Beyond the personnel, it is important during a code to ensure that the clinical processes are also performed appropriately. When giving medications during a code, ensuring that the name of the drug and dosage are called out loud verified with the order and again upon administration will help to prevent any errors. In the ED, like in other locations of the hospital, it is critical to ensure that everyone knows his or her role on the team when a critical incident or code arises. Role assignment is usually the job of the team leader, but if the leader is ineffective at this task, the role of the team members is to assist him or her and ensure that they are attending to their duties, the most important of which is role assignment. Be an advocate for your patient. Establish roles early on as to prevent confusion while actually caring for the patient experiencing a cardiac arrest.

SUGGESTED READINGS

Ehrhardt B, Glankler D. Your role in a code blue. *Nursing*. January 1996. Available at: http://findarticles.com/p/articles/mi_qa3689/is_199601/ai_n8744476.

Walker A, Shaffner D, Miller M, et al. Mock CPR "codes" expose weakness in hospital emergency response for children. John Hopkins Medical Institutions. February 2008. Available at: http://www.hopkinschildrens.org/pages/news/pressdetails.cfm?newsid=105.

KNOW WHEN ABDOMINAL PAIN MAY INDICATE AN ECTOPIC PREGNANCY

JENNIFER BATH, RN, BSN, FNE, SANE-A

WHAT TO DO: ASSESS

Abdominal pain is one of the most common complaints that patients present with in the emergency department (ED). Causes of abdominal pain are diverse because of the many structures and organs in the abdominal cavity. Abdominal pain in the female is of great concern, especially if they are pregnant. Ectopic pregnancy is always a concern in the pregnant female who presents with abdominal pain. If not recognized and treated in a timely manner, a ruptured ectopic pregnancy can be fatal.

Ectopic pregnancies occur when a fertilized egg is implanted outside the uterine cavity. The most common site is the fallopian tubes, and 98% of all ectopic pregnancies are tubal in nature while the other 2% occur in the cervix, abdomen, or ovaries. As the egg develops into a fetus, it causes the tube to tear and eventually rupture. Signs and symptoms of an ectopic pregnancy include severe and sudden onset of unilateral pelvic pain, abdominal tenderness and guarding, positive pregnancy test, late or missed period, syncope, shoulder pain, and vaginal bleeding. Often patients state that they would feel better if only they could just move their bowels. If rupture has occurred, then the patient may be exhibiting signs of shock such as hypotension, tachycardia, light-headedness, dizziness, have a decreased level of consciousness with cold, clammy skin, and decreased capillary refill. Only 50% of the patients will present with a typical presentation, while the other half will present with generic complaints such as nausea, fatigue, abdominal cramping, shoulder pain, and breast fullness. The first warning signs the patient will see are light vaginal bleeding and unilateral lower abdominal or pelvic pain.

There are many reasons an ectopic pregnancy can occur. Some of the causes are scarred tubes, damaged or misshapen tubes, and sometimes the cause is unknown. Risk factors for an ectopic pregnancy include a T-shaped uterus, previous ectopic pregnancy, inflammation or infections such as pelvic inflammatory disease or gonorrhea, fertility drugs, smoking, previous abdominal surgeries such as a tubal ligation, and women between the ages of 35 and 44 years. Use of birth control pill is also a risk factor. If a woman becomes pregnant on birth control, she is more likely to have an ectopic pregnancy.

Normal pregnancies are possible once a woman has had an ectopic pregnancy. The patient will need to be closely monitored for the first 5 to 6 weeks after conception to make sure another ectopic pregnancy has not occurred. Treatment is usually an injection of methotrexate if the pregnancy is found early enough. Methotrexate stops the cell growth and dissolves the existing cells. Typically, only one administration is needed, but if the patient has no response after the first administration, a second administration may be given. Surgery is required if the patient fails to respond to methotrexate or if there is a rupture. Sometimes it is possible to remove the ectopic tissue, but if there is significant damage, then the entire tube must be removed. Emergency surgery is done if heavy bleeding, signs of shock, or tube rupture occurs.

While there is no way to prevent an ectopic pregnancy, the risk can be reduced by limiting the number of sex partners, using condoms, and not smoking. Because ectopic pregnancies occur in 2% of all pregnancies and are the leading cause of pregnancy-related death in the first trimester, it is important to recognize patients with the potential for an ectopic pregnancy so that treatment can be initiated quickly.

SUGGESTED READINGS

Mayo Clinic Staff. *Ectopic Pregnancy*. 2007. Available at: http://www.mayoclinic.com/health/ectopic-pregnancy/DS00622. Accessed July 27, 2008.

DRAWING BLOOD FROM THE IV LINE: TIME SAVERS OR NOT?

JENNIFER BATH, RN, BSN, FNE, SANE-A AND JEANNIE SCRUGGS GARBER, DNP, RN

WHAT TO DO: EVALUATE

Drawing blood from intravenous (IV) sites is a common practice. The question posed is—does this technique save time as compared to direct phlebotomy? According to Ernst and Ernst (2003), "phlebotomy is the most underestimated procedure in healthcare." The process of determining the best venous access and accurately performing the skill appears to be a simple task. However, the clinician must be aware of "anatomy, physiology, and of the consequences that poor judgment can have on the specimen as well as the potential for injury to the patient." The clinician must weigh the factor of time against the potential consequences when determining whether to use the IV site for blood draws.

The most common concern regarding IV site blood drawing is sample hemolysis. In a 2003 study by Grant, emergency department (ED) samples were evaluated for hemolysis in relation to the blood drawing technique used. The findings revealed that samples obtained using IV sites had "significantly more hemolysis than drawing blood with straight needles." Other potential risks associated with IV access blood draws include contamination of blood cultures, contamination by IV fluids, air embolism, and infection. A benchmark by the American Society of Clinical Pathologists (ASCP) for the ED suggests a rate of less than 2% for hemolysis of specimens. Most EDs fail to meet this benchmark. The ASCP recommended that the best practice is to perform a venipuncture on all patients. One solution is to have a dedicated phlebotomist in the ED. However, staff shortages and costs make this difficult for most institutions. Opportunities to decrease the frequency of hemolyzed samples may be impacted by education and quality improvement activities. Educating staff on phlebotomy practices, reinforcing policies related to blood draws, and working in the lab to monitor samples to see if certain nurses have higher incidences of hemolysis are a few helpful strategies. That way, individual education can be done with those staff members.

Emergency Medical Services (EMS) agencies have also started to draw blood through IV sites when they initiate them. This is done to help save time in obtaining labs in critical patients. As with blood drawn through IVs in the ED, the blood EMS draws has a higher incidence of hemolysis because it is being drawn through the IV site. A blood specimen drawn too quickly can also cause hemolysis. This leads to the patient having to be restuck once he or she is in the ED. So, is it really better to draw blood through the IV site? Not really, when you evaluate the literature. It can actually add time to treatment of your patient and lead to delays in getting lab results, which in turn leads to longer ED stays in an already overcrowded ED.

As healthcare providers, we want to minimize pain to our patients, which is why drawing blood through the IV is a widely used practice. However, in the long run, it seems more important to get the lab tests in a timely manner by sticking the patients a second time than trying to prevent the pain of two sticks, which they may get in the end anyway.

SUGGESTED READINGS

Dugan L, Leech L, et al. Factors affecting the hemolysis rates in blood samples drawn from newly placed IV sites in the ED. *J Emerg Nurs.* 2005;31(4):338.

Ernst D, Ernst C. Phlebotomy tools of the trade: Part 3: Alternative sites for drawing blood. *Home Healthc Nurs.* 2003;21(3):156–158.

Grant M. The effect of blood drawing techniques and equipment on the hemolysis of ED laboratory blood samples. *J Emerg Nurs.* 2003;29(2):116–121.

Lowe G, Stike R, Pollack M, et al. Nursing blood specimen collection techniques and hemolysis rates in an ED: Analysis of venipuncture versus intravenous catheter collection techniques. *J Emerg Nurs.* 2008;34(1):26–32.

IV MEDS—HOW FAST IS TOO FAST?

JENNIFER BATH, RN, BSN, FNE, SANE-A

WHAT TO DO: EVALUATE

A majority of medication errors occur with intravenous (IV) medications. A study done in the United Kingdom found that 49% of all medication errors were related to IV meds and that a majority of those were medications that were given too fast. Errors with IV meds are a problem because once the drug is given, there is nothing to stop it from entering the patient's circulatory system. The errors can be minor, with little to no adverse effects. But they can also be major. For instance, giving Vancomycin too fast can cause hypotension and Red man syndrome, a flushing of the upper body. Every IV medication has a specific rate of infusion. Some medications can be given quickly, but others need to be given more slowly. Sometimes medications need to be given slowly to monitor the effect of the drug on the patient. Others will lead to cardiac arrest if given too quickly. Many nurses may not be familiar with the drug being administered and the rates at which it needs to be administered.

There are ways to safe guard against rapid administration of medications. One is to be familiar with the drugs most commonly used by your unit. If it is a drug you are unfamiliar with, use your resources and get clarity. You could ask a coworker, but better yet is to call the pharmacy or look it up in a medication handbook. Never give a drug you are not familiar with; it can lead to serious problems. Another way to help safeguard patients is by providing alerts to the staff on high-risk medications. Include the maximum rate in milligram per minute in the alert. If medication administration records (MARs) are used, having notes and other decision support tools under the medication about administration times can be helpful. Lists of high-risk drugs and how fast they can be given can be posted in medication rooms. If the medication has to be obtained from the pharmacy, the pharmacy staff can place brightly colored label warning that the drug has to be administered over a certain amount of time.

Dilution is another way to avoid rapid administration. If it is a medication that needs to be given over more than a minute, you can dilute it and use a syringe pump or give it as an IV piggyback. If a medication is packaged as 5 mg/1 mL and 1 mg/1 mL, use the 1 mg/mL package as it is a less concentrated dose and therefore less room for error. Just remember, if you need to monitor the patient for effects of the drug, you need to remain at the bedside to do so. You cannot just hang the med and leave.

Be aware that the most common form of medication error is in the form of an IV medication and that it is usually because the med is given too fast. So be familiar with the medications you are giving, the adverse effects, and the rate of infusion. Knowledge is the key to reducing the number of errors with IV med administration.

SUGGESTED READINGS

Nichols PK, Agius CR. Toward safer IV medication administration: The narrow safety margins of many IV medications make this route particularly dangerous. *Am J Nurs*. 2005;105(3):25–30.

The Institute for Safe Medication Practices (online). Horsham, PA. Available at: http://www.ismp.org/newsletters/acutecare/articles/20030515.asp. Accessed May 15, 2005.

LOCARD'S PRINCIPLE AND ITS APPLICATION TO THE VICTIM OF VIOLENCE

JENNIFER BATH, RN, BSN, FNE, SANE-A

WHAT TO DO: ASSESS

Locard's principle states that when two objects come into contact, traces from those objects will transfer from one to the other in both directions. Every contact you have, you leave a part of you behind. This is important to remember when dealing with victims of crime. When these patients present to the emergency department (ED), managing threats to life is always first and foremost, but preserving evidence is also important. In many crimes, including rape, the only evidence to the crime may be on the victim. The patient is the crime scene.

Evidence is something we need to be aware of with any patient who is the victim of a crime. Some hospitals have nurses called Sexual Assault Nurse Examiners (SANE) who deal with victims of sexual assault or Forensic Nurse Examiners (FNE) who deal with all manners of victims of violent crimes. If your hospital employs these types of nurses, utilize them.

There are many key points to remember in evidence collection. Chain of custody is one of the most important points. Chain of custody identifies those individuals who have control and are responsible for any evidence. It includes the proper collection, documentation, transportation, and storage of evidence. Chain of custody is achieved by keeping a written record of who has possession or control over the evidence. You must document the name of the person releasing the evidence, the person receiving it, and the date and time of transfer. Every time evidence changes hands, this data must be documented. This protects against the allegations of tampering with or loss of evidence. The goal is to keep handling of the evidence to a minimum.

Photography is one of the main forms of evidence collection done on almost all cases. Along with photographs, a written record of injuries should be kept. It is important to document size, shape, color, location, and any patterns of injury in the record. The use of body diagrams is also recommended. With any piece of evidence, there are some general rules to follow. Items need to be bagged, placed in a container or envelope separately, sealed with a tape, and labeled with your name, date, time, patients name, medical record number, what item is in the container, bag, or envelope, and, if appropriate, where it came from. With clothing, remember to never cut through a hole, stain, or defect in patient's clothes as it will alter the evidence. If clothing needs to be cut, cut at least 6 inches away from any hole, stain, or defect if possible. Clothing needs to be bagged separately in paper bags, never plastic or recycled bags. Never place clothing directly on the floor since this will contaminate the evidence. When undressing a patient, place two sheets on the floor, one on top of the other. Have the patients stand in the middle and undress, bagging each item of clothing as they remove it. After the patient has removed all clothing, fold and collect the top sheet. This collects any debris or trace evidence that may fall off the patient as he or she is changing. Bag this sheet as evidence also. If the patient cannot stand, make sure to collect the sheet under him or her on the stretcher or ambulance cot since there may be evidence transferred there as well. Bullets should be handled carefully so as not to destroy any evidence on the bullet itself. It is best to wrap the bullet in gauze and place it in an envelope or specimen container with only one bullet per container. Seal and label as described earlier. For victims of sexual assault or rape, there are preassembled evidence kits that come with most of what you will need for the rape exam. It is important to note that once you break the seal on a kit, it must never leave your possession until it is turned over to the police. Wherever you go, it goes.

Some patients who may require evidence collection are children or the abused elderly and special attention needs to be given when dealing with these patient populations' needs. For additional information on evidence collection, ask your local police or SANE/FNE to review the finer points of evidence collection with you. Remember to treat the patient; first preserve and collect evidence because the victim is the crime scene.

SUGGESTED READINGS

Crowley S. *Sexual Assault: The Medical-Legal Exam.* Stamford, CT: Appleton and Lange; 1999, pp. 104–113.

Hammer R, Moynihan B, Pagliaro E. *Forensic Nursing: A Handbook for Practice.* Boston, MA: Jones and Bartlett; 2006, p. 654.

MUNCHAUSEN SYNDROME

JENNIFER BATH RN, BSN, FNE, SANE-A AND JEANNIE SCRUGGS GARBER, DNP, RN

WHAT TO DO: ASSESS

Munchausen syndrome (MS) is a condition that all healthcare workers in the emergency department (ED) need to be familiar with. We have all seen the frequent flyer who presents 15 times in 2 weeks for the same back pain that just will not go away. MS is the most severe condition in a class of disorders known as factitious disorders named after Baron von Munchausen who was known for embellishing stories about his life and travels. Patients with this condition present with physical or mental illness, although physical symptoms predominate. MS is characterized by the intentional creation of physical symptoms. Patients present to the healthcare setting with a self-inflicted or fictitious illness. They will lie about or fake their symptoms, alter diagnostic tests (e.g., by putting blood in their urine to fake a kidney stone), or engage in self-injurious behaviors. Some patients will repetitively complain of certain symptoms such as back pain while others will actually inflict injury or pain on themselves so they will actually be ill.

Patients with this condition have an inner need to be seen as ill or injured. These patients often contrive stories about their history and make up signs and symptoms. Often they present with hypoglycemia, hemoptysis, rashes, abscesses, fever, hematuria, or seizures. The DSM–IV states "All organ systems are potential targets and the symptoms presented are limited only by the person's medical knowledge, sophistication, and imagination" (APA, 1994). Factitious disorders such as MS are consciously motivated, carefully and intelligently crafted, and quite believable until diagnostic tests prove otherwise. MS is different from the diagnosis of hypochondria. Those with MS know that they are making up their symptoms and those with hypochondria are convinced that a real illness exists.

The actual cause of MS is unknown. But there are a number of predisposing factors that are true physical disorders that involved several or extensive hospitalizations during their childhood, a history of abuse or neglect, employment in healthcare, and significant or traumatic prior relationships with a doctor.

The symptoms most commonly seen in MS include

- Dramatic but inconsistent medical history
- Unclear symptoms that become more severe or change once treatment has begun

- Predictable relapses following improvement in the condition
- Extensive knowledge of hospitals or medical terminology and textbook descriptions of illnesses
- Presence of multiple surgical scars
- Appearance of new or additional symptoms following negative test results
- Presence of symptoms only when the patient is alone or not being observed
- Willingness or eagerness to have medical tests, operations, or other procedures
- History of seeking treatment at numerous hospitals, clinics, and doctors' offices, possibly even in different cities
- Reluctance by the patient to allow healthcare professionals to meet with or talk to family, friends, or prior healthcare providers
- Problems with identity and self-esteem

The diagnosis is very difficult considering the dishonesty that underlies the syndrome. The possibility of physical and mental illnesses must be evaluated before considering the diagnosis of MS. Given the diagnosis is so difficult, there are no reliable statistics on MS but it is considered rare in the United States. MS is also very difficult to treat. Most individuals who are diagnosed deny the diagnosis and treatment. Treatment, once they are identified, includes changing their thinking and behavior along with psychotherapy. To date, there are no medications available to treat the disease, but medications can be used to treat the related disorders like depression or anxiety. So when you have a patient who comes to the ED for repeated complaints, he or she may not be drug seeking; he or she could be suffering from MS.

SUGGESTED READINGS

Cleveland Clinic Center for Consumer Health Information. Available at: www.clevelandclinic.org/healthcare-info.
Cutter D, Hsich G. (n.d.). Munchausen syndrome. Available at: http://my.clevelandclinic.org/disorders/factitious_disorders/hic_munchausen_syndrome.aspx. Accessed June 14, 2008.
Hammer R, Moynihan B, Pagliaro E. *Forensic Nursing: A Handbook for Practice*. Boston, MA: Jones and Bartlett; 2006, p. 654.
Lynch V. *Forensic Nursing*. St. Louis, MD: Elsevier-Mosby; 2006, pp. 82–84.

THE BAITED TRAP: OVERRIDING SAFETY FEATURES OF CLINICAL ALARMS

JENNIFER BATH, RN, BSN, FNE, SANE-A AND JEANNIE SCRUGGS GARBER, DNP, RN

WHAT TO DO: EVALUATE

Clinical equipment is developed with extensive safety and alarm features intended to prevent harm to patients. Clinicians are educated about the safety features and aware of their purpose; however, overriding these features is common practice. Healthcare equipment alarms and their effectiveness have been the focus of many research studies. The issue is of such interest and significance that in 2004, the American College of Clinical Engineering Healthcare Technology Foundation (AHTF) started a project to evaluate the literature and analyze adverse event reporting regarding the clinical alarm system. It is widely noted that alarms, auditory and visual, are frequently viewed as inaccurate intrusions to practice. How do we balance the understanding of the desire for accurate, useful equipment safety features and the reality of what technology can offer with the need to keep the patient safe?

Why do nurses and other clinicians override safety features? According to Hyman and Johnson (2008), alarms may not be effective, may not be received, may be set up incorrectly, may be ignored, or the work environment may simply be too busy to allow response. Nurses are working in a sensory filled environment, using numerous pieces of equipment simultaneously while setting up and responding to the patient requests, alarms, and the communication of many healthcare professionals. The AHTF (2007) study findings suggest that in critical environments, there are so many alarms that it "challenges human limits for recognition and action." Edworthy and Hellier (2005) reported a similar finding stating that practitioners are overusing their sense of hearing and experiencing high false alarm rates. Other considerations for why safety features and alarms are overridden include alarms may be from the general environment and may not be always related to patients, the alarm process is a systems concern and cannot be solved by individuals, and excessive false alarms have desensitized practitioners to their usefulness. Figure 395.1 demonstrates the complexity of alarms in the clinical setting (Philips and Barnsteiner, 2005).

There have been a number of technologic advances in healthcare in the past decade and many of these are used frequently in the emergency department (ED). There are devices and equipment to monitor the heart, breathing, blood pressure, and support organs when

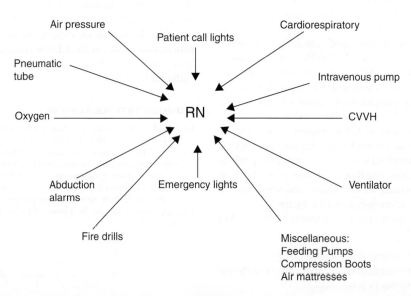

FIGURE 395.1. Clinical alarm complexity. (From Phillips. *Crit Care Nurs Quart.* 2005;28(4):317-323.)

they fail. There are intravenous pumps that calculate and administer medications and fluids and warn if the dose is too high. But as important as all these advances are, the technology is only as good as the providers using them. All of the monitors, pumps, and devices have alarms that let the user know when something is wrong. Whether it is because the blood pressure is too low or the medication dosage too high, there are alarms and safeguards in place to protect the patient. Unfortunately, these safety features require the nurse to be actively engaged with the device to ensure the appropriate delivery of care. Clinical judgment needs to be used to set appropriate alarm limits and ensure that they are realistic for the patient's condition. For example, if you have a patient on a nitroglycerin drip and set the blood pressure limits to a systolic low of 50, ineffective patient monitoring will result. The patient must be admitted to the monitor before it is used, and every time a safety feature is overridden, the nurse should take a second look. The newer medication pumps have drug libraries programmed into them, which store information on numerous drugs. They have set low and high limits for the drugs and even provide warning messages for certain drugs that may need closer monitoring. Heparin, for example, will warn the programmer to watch for bleeding, a common side effect of this medication.

Many times, providers will override alarms or turn them off altogether. It is no secret that in a busy ED, the number of alarms is often overwhelming. In addition, the number of false alarms due to leads being off a patient or a patient moving excessively desensitizes the staff to the meaning of the alarm and creates rework. The safety features exist to assist the nurse in monitoring the patient while the nurse is performing other duties. Ensuring that staff members are educated on new equipment and tested on their competencies so that patients can benefit from the full capabilities of the equipment is essential. Teach them how to use it effectively. Safeguard your patients and yourself by using the safety features that were designed to help them.

Clinical equipment safety features are a limited, yet important tool that supports patient assessment and intervention (AHTF, 2007). It is imperative that new

equipment purchases be evaluated regarding alarm sound (so as not to duplicate an existing alarm sound), false alarm potential, and usability by the clinician. The complexity of the setup for the safety features should also be a consideration. Clinicians must also become an integrated part of equipment development and evaluation.

Phillips and Barnsteiner (2005) reports that The Joint Commission on Accreditation of Healthcare Organizations (JCAHO) National Patient Safety Goal No. 6 addresses the safety of clinical alarms by requiring the testing of alarms, appropriate alarm set up, and the use by the clinician. These requirements are understandable, yet insight is lacking in how to accomplish the goal, considering the complexity of the healthcare environment. Chambrin, Ravaux, Calvelo-Aros, Jaborska, Chopin, and Boniface (as cited in Phillips and Barnsteiner, 2005) observed over 3,000 alarms in a critical care environment with only 5.7% of alarms determined to be significant. This finding further supports the ongoing dilemma regarding alarms and overrides. Does the nurse respond to every alarm? Research indicates that the answer to this is "no." Should the nurse respond to every alarm? Research findings related to this question create more questions than answers. If the patient is you or your family member, my guess is that your answer to both the questions is "yes."

SUGGESTED READINGS

Clinical Alarms Task Force. Impact of clinical alarms on patient safety: A report from the American College of Clinical Engineering Healthcare Technology Foundation. *J Clin Eng.* 2007;32(1):22–33.

Dulak S. Technology today: Smart IV pumps. RN Web. 2005. Available at: http://rn.modernmedicine.com/rnweb.

Edworthy J, Hellier E. Fewer but better auditory alarms will improve patient safety. *Qual Saf Healthc.* 2005;14(3):212–215.

Hyman W, Johnson E. Fault tree analysis of clinical alarms. *J Clin Eng.* 2008;33(2):85–94.

McConnell E, Nissen J. The use of medical equipment by Australian registered nurses. *J Clin Nurs.* 1993;2(6):341–348.

Phillips J, Barnsteiner J. Clinical alarms: Improving efficiency and effectiveness. *Crit Care Nurs Quart.* 2005;28(4):317–323.

PA-PSRS Patient Safety Advisory. Smart infusion pump technology: Don't bypass the safety catches from the Pennsylvania Patient Safety Authority. 2007;4(4). Available at: http://www.psa.state.pa.us/psa/lib/psa/advisories/.

KNOW HOW TO TELL THAT THE DEFIBRILLATOR IS REALLY SYNCHRONIZED

NANCY F. ALTICE, RN, MSN, CCNS, CNS-BC

WHAT TO DO: IMPLEMENT

Both ventricular and supraventricular dysrhythmias can be cardioverted by delivering a direct current shock. When a ventricular rhythm is chaotic in appearance or the patient is hemodynamically unstable, the shock can be delivered with a standard defibrillator, which will discharge the electrical shock as soon as the discharger or "deliver shock" button is pushed. But in the case of a more organized rhythm in a patient who is not in a severe crisis, the electrical shock needs to be timed with the patient's cardiac cycle so that a shock is not delivered during ventricular repolarization. Delivering a shock during the T wave could result in ventricular fibrillation. To prevent this, the defibrillator has a setting that allows for the synchronization with the patient's QRS complex. By simply pushing the synchronization button, the defibrillator will mark the QRS complex as the place where the defibrillator will deliver the shock. The defibrillator equipment becomes more sophisticated with each model that is released. But the basic premise of synchronization timing is that the machine is looking for the tallest wave on the EKG and interpreting this tall wave to be the R wave. A prudent nurse will always double-check when the synchronization button is on to see where the synchronization indicator is marking the EKG. It should be on the R wave. Occasionally thought, the EKG may have some abnormalities due to the patient's underlying condition. In some leads, the tallest wave may be the T wave. If the synchronization marker is designating the T wave as the place where it will fire, the nurse should immediately look for another EKG lead in which the QRS is indeed the tallest wave. Always determine where the synchronization marker is located before cardioverting the patient.

SUGGESTED READINGS

2005 American Heart Association. Guidelines for cardiopulmonary resuscitation and emergency cardiovascular care, Part 5: Electrical therapies. *Circulation*. 2005;112:IV-34–IV-46. Available at: http://circ.ahajournals.org/cgi/content/full112/24_suppl/IV-35.

Conover MB. *Understanding Electrocardiography*. 8th Ed. St.Louis, Mo: Mosby; 2002.

ENSURE THAT THERE IS REALLY A PULSE WITH THE RHYTHM ON THE MONITOR

NANCY F. ALTICE, RN, MSN, CCNS, CNS-BC

WHAT TO DO: EVALUATE

Technology sometimes draws our attention away from the basics of clinical assessment. Numerous monitors contribute to our assessment of the patient's clinical status. It is easy to keep our eyes fixed on the monitors and assume that the data we see are providing sufficient information. There are times, however, when the data give false assurances. In the case of EKG monitors, the rhythm seen on the monitor is only one piece of the necessary information. It is essential to know whether the rhythm is accompanied by a pulse. Pulseless electrical activity (PEA) will quickly deteriorate into a lethal arrhythmia due to lack of myocardial oxygenation but there could be a delay of several minutes before this change is noted. The sooner resuscitation begins, the higher the chance of successful recovery. The key in PEA is to find a treatable underlying cause. The causes of PEA are referred to in Advanced Cardiac Life Support as the 5 Hs and 5 Ts. These are outlined in Table 397.1.

TABLE 397.1	ADVANCE CARDIAC LIFE SUPPORT'S 5 Hs AND Ts
THE 5 Hs	**THE 5 Ts**
Hypoxia	Tension pneumothorax
Hypovolemia	Tamponate (cardiac)
Hypothermia	Thrombosis (cardiac)
Hypokalemia or hyperkalemia	Thrombosis (pulmonary)
Hydrogen ions (acidosis)	Tablets (overdose)

Always remember to assess for a pulse when a different EKG rhythm is noted on the monitor.

Other sources of misleading data include transcutaneous pacing artifacts. Because the transcutaneous pacing method delivers electrical shock through the chest wall, skeletal muscle contraction can be expected. This muscle movement sometimes leaves a motion artifact on the EKG that can occasionally mimic an actual QRS complex. Always check for a pulse when initiating any form of artificial pacing.

Mechanical ventilation can cause changes in intrathoracic pressure, which can cause changes in arterial waveforms seen in patients who have arterial lines placed in the femoral artery or aorta. These pressure changes would not be high enough to mimic a real BP but could serve as a source of confusion when trying to establish cardiac death.

In a patient who was previously alert, progression to PEA would be very obvious. But in a busy ICU, a patient who is sedated and mechanically ventilated could be pulseless for a few minutes without an obvious change in appearance. Do not assume that a pulse is present just because an electrical rhythm appears on the monitor screen. Assess the pulse and other signs of adequate perfusion such as skin color. Remember to treat the patient, not the monitor!

SUGGESTED READINGS

American Heart Association. Guidelines for cardiopulmonary resuscitation and emergency cardiovascular care, Part 5: Electrical therapies. *Circulation*. 2005;112:IV-34–IV-46. Available at: http://circ.ahajournals.org/cgi/content/full112/24_suppl/IV-35.

Pulseless electrical activity. Available at: http://www.fpnotebook.com/CV42.htm.

DURING TRANSFERS, ALWAYS ENSURE THAT YOU HAVE BEEN GIVEN THE RIGHT PATIENT AND REPORT AND ARE SENDING THE RIGHT PATIENT AND REPORT FOR MORE DEFINITIVE CARE OR PROCEDURES

ANTHONY D. SLONIM, MD, DRPH

WHAT TO DO: EVALUATE

In the emergency department (ED), patients are often coming and going at rapid speeds and it is not unusual for an individual provider to be involved with the care of hundreds of patients in an individual shift. Therefore, it becomes important to ensure that healthcare providers appropriately track the identity and whereabouts of patients they are caring for. Patient identification and geographic locators in the ED have assisted with these tasks, but it is essential that the nurse ensures that the care is directed to the right patient at the right time.

On the receiving end, it is not uncommon for the emergency medical services (EMS) to deliver several patients at any given time either from the scene of a motor vehicle accident or multicasualty event. Many patients will not be identified, may have alterations to their mental status, and may not be carrying identification, which all adds to the confusion and the potential for medical errors in the ED. Ensuring a positive identification and labeling of patients from their entrance to the ED is imperative, particularly if multiple EMS crews are delivering patients simultaneously. ED clinicians have compensated by identifying the "48 year old

with the acute MI" or the "kid hit by a car," but when the ED quickly fills up with multiple victims from a single accident, this approach falls apart quickly.

When working quickly, the immediacy of these decisions becomes apparent. Often there is a need for diagnostic testing, either laboratory or radiologic, and on occasion, the need for emergent surgery or admission to intensive care. When this occurs, the nurse in the ED, who has failed to identify the patient, may compound the problem by then transferring the patient to another location and perhaps getting procedures on the wrong patient. For these reasons, ensuring that the correct patient being sent out of the ED is clearly labeled and the receiving department is ready to assume the care of the correct patient is imperative. When transporting to radiology or the ICU, the identification at transfer should be the first step of the handoff. Failure to do so may lead to confusion and incorrect procedures, particularly when the patient is unable to cooperate.

SUGGESTED READINGS

Stehr S, Simpson D. Victim identification and management following the collapse of the World Trade Center towers. Available at: http://www.colorado.edu/hazards/research/qr/qr148/qr148.html. Accessed August 3, 2008.

THE EMERGENCY DEPARTMENT (ED) DOES NOT NEED TO PROVIDE ALL THE CARE A PATIENT NEEDS, BUT ALWAYS NEEDS TO ENSURE THAT THERE IS A PLAN FOR FOLLOW-UP AND THE PATIENT UNDERSTANDS WHAT TO DO

ANTHONY D. SLONIM, MD, DrPH

WHAT TO DO: EVALUATE

The emergency department (ED) exists to provide a number of functions for the community. The ED is available 24×7 when the patient's primary care physician may not be available. The ED exists to allay anxiety for patients who are worried about a particular condition and are too nervous to wait for an appointment. The ED exists because patients who cannot afford healthcare need a place to go and know that they will be turned away. While these examples are clear to the ED nurse, they help to point out several important deficiencies with the healthcare system in the United States. Nonetheless, they exist and are part of the work that EDs perform every day.

To adequately fulfill the obligation to patients, EDs need to ensure that they are not only identifying through the triage process those patients who are in need of urgent assistance and treatment but also doing what needs to be done to ensure that the emergent therapy is provided to the patient. There is another important obligation that is often unnoticed but is just as important for the care of the ED patient, and that has to do with follow-up. The follow-up falls discretely into two separate categories—patient follow-up and diagnostic follow-up.

All patients being discharged from the ED require a follow-up appointment either with their primary care provider or with an on-call specialist. Hospitals usually maintain lists of these providers who are available for unassigned patients to ensure that the community receives the care that it needs. The patients also need appropriate direction on what to do if their condition deteriorates either before reaching that referral or in the short term. For many, that means returning to the ED for re-evaluation. ED providers often become legitimately concerned about the patient who re-presents to the ED within a 24 or 48h time frame with the same complaint or symptoms. These patients require attention to their concerns and appropriate testing to ensure that their condition has not deteriorated and can still be managed as an outpatient.

Once patients are discharged from the ED, the ED also has the burden to ensure that for the diagnostic testing performed as a part of the ED visit, those diagnostic test results are being followed up and shared with the patients and their care provider. Often, laboratory results may only be processed in batches or radiology results may be over-read by radiologists in the morning. In these circumstances, the ED has an obligation for providing an appropriate follow-up of this testing to the patients.

The ED is an important resource for many patients and often provides life-saving interventions. For those patients who are discharged, appropriate follow-up of the patients and their ED course needs to be ensured.

SUGGESTED READINGS

Emergency room visits: How to follow up. Revolution Health. Available at: http://www.revolutionhealth.com/conditions/first-aid-safety/emergency/after-emergency/. Accessed August 8, 2008.

Kyriacou DN, Handel D, Stein AC, et al. Factors affecting outpatient follow-up compliance of emergency department patients. *J Gen Intern Med.* 2005;20(10):938–942.

ENSURE THAT THE PATIENTS BEING DISCHARGED FROM THE EMERGENCY DEPARTMENT (ED) KNOW WHAT TO DO TO IMPROVE THEIR CARE INCLUDING MEDICATIONS, DIET, AND FOLLOW-UP

ANTHONY D. SLONIM, MD, DrPH

WHAT TO DO: IMPLEMENT

The care of the patient in the emergency department (ED) is a complex proposition. Patients spend their lives doing pretty well with only episodic visits to the ED when they feel they are in crisis. Two important things result from these crises-like interventions that may affect a patient's safety. First, the patient and his or her family are in crisis and as a result, they do not think clearly, nor do they articulate the problems they are having. Second, the ED personnel need to perform, often based on inadequate information, across multiple specialty problems to appropriately position the patient's complaint within a broader context of care. This is not easy for the providers, but it is also very difficult for the patients upon ED discharge when they need clarity about what has occurred and how to address their medication, diet, and activity regimen after discharge.

Medication reconciliation is an important process for understanding what medications a patient is taking and how they may interact with the presenting problem in the ED. Often, the healthcare provider gets a pretty clear understanding about the patient's problems (often better than the patients themselves) by reviewing the medication list. Patients, unfortunately, may not know why they are taking medications or what they are being treated for. After discharge from the ED, the providers need to make a decision and provide guidance to the patients about whether they should continue or discontinue medications after discharge. The problem is that with the vast array of new specialty medications available, often the ED is making these decisions in concert with a primary care doctor or, alternatively, from a deficit of knowledge about the underlying conditions and their treatment. This is compounded often by a lack of integrated medical records that fail to provide clarity to the ED to solve these issues.

Nonetheless, after the acute management is over, the ED owes it to the patients to provide a plan for the medications of discharge and what the patients should do with their home medications if they are affected. Further, directions regarding diet, activity, and follow-up need to be provided upon ED discharge to the patient and family. These directions should be articulated back to the nurse with a demonstration of understanding so that the patient receives appropriate postdischarge care.

SUGGESTED READINGS

Engel KG, Heisler M, Smith DM, et al. Patient comprehension of emergency department care and instructions: Are patients aware of when they do not understand? *Ann Emerg Med.* 2008; 53(4):454–461.e15. Epub 2008 Jul 10.

Moss JE, Flower CL, Houghton LM, et al. A multidisciplinary care coordination team improves emergency department discharge planning practice. *Med J Aust.* 2002;117(8): 435–439.

401

PRIOR TO METHOTREXATE ADMINISTRATION FOR ECTOPIC PREGNANCY, THE NURSE MUST CHECK THE LABS AND VERIFY THE DOSE

MARY S. WARD, RN, BS, OCN

WHAT TO DO: PLAN

Ectopic pregnancy is defined as any pregnancy that occurs outside of the uterus. It is the most common first trimester pregnancy complication and the one that carries the highest mortality for first trimester pregnancies. Women with ectopic pregnancy, sometimes referred to as "tubal pregnancy" because the most frequent presentation is in the fallopian tubes, often present to the emergency department with complaints of abdominal pain with or without vaginal bleeding. The woman may not even know that she is pregnant. Pregnancy is confirmed by elevated β human chorionic gonadotrophic (HCG) levels and an ultrasound that confirms the pregnancy has implanted the embryo outside of the uterus. At this point, the physician has two options to offer the patient: surgery to remove the pregnancy and tube or medication. Medication will preserve the tube and usually will preserve fertility. It is a good option if the pregnancy is not too advanced, there is a confirmed fetal cardiac heartbeat, and the woman is assessed to be able to comply with follow-up visits. The last requirement is critical. If the patient is unable or unwilling to follow up with an obstetrician in 4 to 7 days, medication is not a good option. Follow-up lab values are the only way to confirm the effectiveness of this treatment.

The most common and most efficacious medical treatment to date is the use of methotrexate, a chemotherapeutic agent that is a member of the class of antimetabolite agents. When given as a single dose, it has up to 94% effectiveness. Side effects are minimal and include mild nausea, vomiting, mouth sores, alopecia, and immunosuppression. The standard dosage of methotrexate is $50 \, \text{mg}/\text{m}^2$. Accurate dosing of this drug requires that a patient's current height and weight be obtained. Because methotrexate is an antineoplastic agent, guidelines for administration are the same as those for administration in an oncology setting.

Chemotherapeutic agents have the highest reported risk for medication errors of all drug classes and when they occur, they are the most serious. This is due in large part to the fact that they are dosed individually. The administration of methotrexate for ectopic pregnancy is no different. Protocols for administering the drug in this setting require that labs be performed and evaluated prior to the mixing of the drug. These labs should include a complete blood count with a differential, a chemistry profile, a β-HCG level, and a type and screen. If any of the lab values are abnormal, the physician should be notified and the treatment options re-evaluated. If the patient is immunocompromised, is human immunodeficiency virus positive, or has renal or liver compromise, administration of the drug is contraindicated. The type and screen are necessary to determine the patient's blood type and screen for the possibility of Rh seroconversion and the need for anti-D immunoglobulin.

It is also the administering nurse's responsibility to understand how to calculate the body surface area and verify the dose being given to the patient. It should be understood that the physician writing the order has already done this. The body surface area can be easily calculated by taking the square root of height in inches multiplied by the weight in pounds and divided by 3,131 or taking the square root of height in centimeters multiplied by the weight in kilograms and divided by 3,600.

The total BSA is then multiplied by the dose ($50 \, \text{mg}/\text{m}^2$) and is administered to the patient. The drug is given intramuscularly and may be administered in more than one injection. It is the administering nurse's responsibility to be aware of any complications that might be a contraindication for administration. It is also the nurse's responsibility, as the one administering the drug, to know the dose and the side effect potential of the drug. The risks for overdosing or underdosing the drug and for toxicities are as real for this administration of methotrexate as they are for administering it to a cancer patient.

SUGGESTED READINGS

ACEP Clinical Policies Committee and Clinical Policies Subcommittee on Early Pregnancy. American College of Emergency Physicians. Critical issues in the initial evaluation and management of patient presenting to the emergency department in early pregnancy. *Ann Emerg Med*. 2003;41:123–133.

Kelly H, Harvey D, Moll S. A cautionary tale: Fatal outcome of methotrexate therapy given for management of ectopic pregnancy. *Obstet Gynecol.* 2006;107(2):439–441.

Lipscomb GH, McCord ML, Stovall T, et al. Predictors of success of methotrexate treatment in women with tubal ectopic pregnancies. *New Engl J Med.* 1999;341(26): 1974–1978.

Miller JH, Griffin E. Methotrexate for ectopic pregnancy in the emergency department—one hospital's protocol competencies. *J Emerg Nurs.* 2003;29(3):240–244.

Polovich M, White JM, Kelleher LO. *Chemotherapy and Biotherapy Guidelines and Recommendations for Practice.* 2nd Ed. Pittsburgh, PA: Oncology Nursing Society; 2005.

Uzelac PS, Garmel SH. *Early Pregnancy Risks, Current Diagnosis and Treatment Obstetrics and Gynecology,* 10th Ed. New York, NY: Lange Medical Books/McGraw-Hill Medical Publishing Division; 2007.

TERM BIRTH IS NOT A CRISIS

LYNDA COOK SAWYER, RNC, BSN, MBA

WHAT TO DO: EVALUATE

Labor starts slowly, naturally, after 39 weeks of a wonderfully healthy pregnancy. The mother spends the next 4 to 5 h accomplishing tasks that she knew she had time to do. Contractions are mild and pleasantly manageable, just enough tightening to cause a slightly alerted mindset of "this is probably the real thing." Her childbirth classes have prepared her for the early phases of labor and she is not scared. The baby, normally quiet in the morning, stretches and turns every now and then.

A healthy labor that starts naturally will gradually progress through the early phase to the active phase. As the contractions become stronger, longer, and closer together, the mother will seek more physical support and knowledgeable company. For some, it is a midwife who comes to her home or meets her in a birthing center or hospital; while for others, it is the nurses and doctors in a hospital's labor and delivery department. Regardless of the location of the laboring mother or the credentials of her chosen attendants, there is no need for hurried, harried, and excitable overtones. There is no emergency unless and until an emergency presents itself; term, active labor is not an emergency. And if you are working in a birthing center or hospital labor and delivery unit, term, active labor should not be a surprise either. Be prepared for the actively laboring family.

For a term labor and an ambulatory, conscious mother, focus on the variable factor that will determine an emergency, the fetus. Obtain fetal heart tones. Between contractions, let the mother know calmly what you need to do. For example, "Mrs. Jones, I need to listen to the baby." She will respond—she may not speak to you, but she will position herself for you to monitor the baby. Your movements should be purposeful, yet calm and unrushed. Your words need to be encouraging and be offered in normal to quiet volumes. Be respectful of her work. If the fetal heart tones are within normal limits, let her know that. If the fetal heart tones are nonreassuring, let her know that too. Tell her that you need to listen to the baby during a contraction and then you move to accommodate that auscultation. Do not expect the mother to "lie still."

Thwarting the mother's labor progress at this stage because you need to gather data unrelated to her stage of labor ("Do you live in a house or an apartment?") is distracting and unhelpful. Knowing that the fetal heart tones are strong and reactive allows you to move to the next order of business—the presenting part. To gather this information, begin with the status of her membranes—ruptured or intact? Ask her about any vaginal bleeding. While some bloody show and mucus are expected, active bright red bleeding is not. Whether her membranes are ruptured or not, perform a vaginal exam for a full-term, actively laboring woman. Do not perform a digital vaginal exam in the presence of bright red bleeding.

Let the mother know that you need to check her cervix and that you will wait on her. "Mrs. Jones, I need to check your cervix." Again, she may not answer you depending on her stage of labor, but she will move to allow you to check her cervix…between contractions, usually. Actively laboring women do not want to be checked during a contraction—while you know this is ok to do, it is distracting, uncomfortable, and possibly frightening for her.

With strong fetal heart tones and a vertex fetus, there is no emergency. All other intake information and data and routine admission processes can be conducted methodically and calmly between contractions until the birth is imminent. Your gentle and respectful support will reflect positively on the mother's reactions to her own labor—if you do not act like birth is a medical emergency, she will not either.

SUGGESTED READINGS

Korte D, Scaer RM. *A Good Birth, A Safe Birth*. 3rd Ed. Boston, MA: Harvard Common Press; 1992.

McCutcheon-Rosegg S. *Natural Childbirth the Bradley Way*. Revised Ed. New York, NY: Penguin-Plume Corporation; 1996.

THE MOST IMPORTANT PERSON IN THE LABOR OR BIRTHING ROOM IS NOT A HEALTHCARE PROVIDER

LYNDA COOK SAWYER, RNC, BSN, MBA

WHAT TO DO: EVALUATE

When in labor, women love to be surrounded by beautiful things, calming smells, and knowledgeable, supportive attendants. It is not uncommon these days to have the baby's father present for prenatal exams, labor, and birth. Indeed, it is not uncommon to have three or more support people arrive and attend the mother while she is laboring. Some women invite the baby's to-be siblings to share in the excitement of birth. Add to the group the mother's birth attendant(s) including midwife, doctor, doula, and labor nurse and you quickly have an entire crowd!

As healthcare providers in hospital and birthing center venues, we have become accustomed to this phenomenon that is wholly American in its nature. This is alright. Our labor spaces in the hospital setting are larger, now, as the mothers most often expect to give birth where they labor and we have not decreased our need for birthing equipment (bowls, gloves, gowns, drapes, instruments, syringes, medications, etc.). Labor, Delivery, Recovery Rooms (LDRs) and Labor, Delivery, Recovery, and Postpartum Rooms (LDRPs) are the norm, now, in many hospital obstetrical settings while all-in-one-room care is the norm for all birthing centers. It still might be crowded and yes, we still may ask all but the essential support person(s) to step out, but there is still space to attend the mother as she gives birth vaginally.

Let us prepare for the childbirth in this LDR. There is the mother (of course), the father (good), the mother's mother (Gram to-be) and the mother's sister (Aunty to-be), the mother's chosen doula (great), the labor nurse (employed by the facility), and the midwife or physician. That is seven people... with an eighth to emerge momentarily. The facility's baby nurses are called to the room as the fetal head begins to crown. That will make nine human beings in the room awaiting the birth of the tenth.

It is very easy for each and every one of us to focus on the fetus as birth is imminent. Each of us is doing a little something to assist the fetus to come faster— holding the mother's legs in the "right position" if she is in the generally-used semi-recumbent position for pushing, coaching, and counting aggressively as another contraction appears on the fetal monitor, cheering loudly with each millimeter of descent, reading the fetal monitor and interpreting the fetal heart tones aloud for all to hear, managing the mother's intravenous fluids and the lines that provide them, laying out the birth stuff, preparing the warmer for receipt of the newborn, and the physician or midwife, gowned and gloved, usually perched on a stool between the mother's legs. We busy ourselves with the importance of our work according to our assigned role in this labor and birth.

Notice, however, that the most important person in the room, the mother, is getting the least attention from eight of the nine adults present—sometimes herself included, which would make that nine of the nine adults. Our stuff, our things, her legs, the fetal presenting part, the monitor, the mother's ability to hold her breath and push without making noise, the introitus and perineum, and the infant warmer are not important to the birth of a term baby. The mothers who have been trained in traditional childbirth classes believe this activity to be essential, so despite their own internal directions, they acquiesce to the activities and direction of the "professionals."

The arrival and presence of the trained birth attendants and healthcare personnel is not a cause for a shift in the focus. The attention to the arrival and busyness of healthcare professionals in the room is a diversion of attention from the laboring mother. The attention generated by their arrival also diverts the attention of the mother's support people. They begin to watch in fascination, the busyness of the healthcare professionals; they wait in expectation of a role assignment from the healthcare professionals.

Actively redirect that attention to the mother. When she and everyone in the room are focused on her needs, she will be more actively in tune with the descent of the fetus and choose the best position for her to push—allowing her to push more effectively with contractions and rest more deeply between contractions. Focus on her will initiate the psychologic process in her that she will be the parent–guardian, fully responsible for the care and protection of her infant, not the healthcare professionals and extended family. The entire busyness necessary for the safe environment of birth needs to fade into the background and be unnoticed. For while all the stuff, all the processes, all the support people, and all the expertise of birthing professionals are complimentary to the birthing process, the mother is the most important person in the room.

SUGGESTED READINGS

Brodsky PL. *Control of Childbirth: Mothers Versus Medicine through the Ages*. Jefferson, NC: McFarland; 2008.
McCutcheon-Rosegg S. *Natural Childbirth the Bradley Way* Revised Ed. New York, NY: Penguin-Plume; 1996.

The perineum and introitus were built to pass a term fetus. In the absence of extreme congenital needs of the fetus, the perineum does not need help, preparation, or "more room"

Lynda Cook Sawyer, RNC, BSN, MBA

WHAT TO DO: IMPLEMENT

There used to be a time when every mother in a hospital's postpartum unit had stitches in her bottom if she had birthed vaginally. Whole industries of medical supplies mushroomed to meet the comfort demands of these healing women: sitz baths—at first, hard-plumbed into rooms centrally built down the hall for "q shift" episiotomy-care, and then, more cheaply built (but individual and private) plastic sitz baths that could be used over the mother's own commode in her room and taken home with her upon discharge. There were roll-around/bedside or built-in heat lamps for use as the mother reclined on the bed, knees up and spread wide while the light and heat from the bulb warmed the fresh episiotomy repair and the skin of her perineum. Ice packs—first in latex gloves—are now built-in to the peri-pads and dermoplast spray is used to cause a freezing sensation, and then topical numbness, directly at the site.

Episiotomies are still the most common, routine surgical procedure performed in hospital obstetrics today. However, today, there are many mothers requesting not to be cut during the vaginal birth of their child. "But they will tear!" you gasp. Possibly. Research published in 1989 found that women were five times more likely to suffer a severe laceration through the anus and rectal sphincter (a "fourth degree perineal laceration") requiring restorative surgery if they had received an episiotomy (a "second degree perineal incision") first (Enkin et al.,1989). In other words, the episiotomy to enlarge the vaginal outlet may actually be linked to the major tears they are purported to prevent.

The introitus (opening leading to the vagina) and the perineum (the skin between the introitus and the anus) are pliable. With increasing, but gentle, pressure, it will stretch to accommodate the emerging fetal head or buttocks. Some birthing practitioners are uneducated to the birthing techniques that allow this normal stretching. Also, birthing positions that encourage uniformity in the application of the fetal presenting part on the introitus is a major contributor to perineal lacerations and the false belief that perineums need an episiotomy to release the fetus at birth.

First, assist the laboring mother into upright or side-lying positions—these positions enable the uterus with the fetus to line up directly over the cervix, the pelvic outlet, the vagina, and the introitus. Equalizing the pressure during descent of the fetal presenting part assists with the application of uniform pressure on the introitus, thus allowing for maximum stretching of the perineum. The lithotomy or supine position will cause the presenting part to lie along the void space of the rectum, thus "bulging outward" at the perineum with the introitus superiorly located at the time of birth. The pressure is not uniform around the circumference of the introitus and damage to the perineum, rectum, and anus is probable with vaginal birth.

Second, do not massage or "hold open" the vagina. It was thought at one time that these measures would assist in easing the perineum into a full thinning and stretch. Now, we know that these types of maneuvers are more likely to cause friction that triggers the body's response to rush fluids to the region. A swollen perineal area does not effectively stretch.

Third, in the absence of fetal distress, allow birth to occur. Rushing the fetal descent mechanically (with forceps or vacuum) or emotionally (loud cheering/coaching) can cause the mother to artificially expel her baby by force before the perineum and introitus are ready—this leads to lacerations and tears that would have otherwise been unnecessary.

What can you do? Apply clean wet washcloths, wrung out in hot water, to the mother's perineum as it is stretching. The mother's grateful moan of relief will let you know that the moist heat and the pressure it takes to hold it in place at the introitus as her baby is beginning to crown is the best thing you have done all day.

SUGGESTED READINGS

Block J. *Pushed*. Cambridge, MA: Da Capo Press; 2007.
Enkin M, Kierse M, Chalmers I. *Effective Care in Pregnancy and Childbirth*. Oxford, England: Oxford University Press; 1989.
Korte D, Scaer RM. *A Good Birth, A Safe Birth*. 3rd Ed. Boston, MA: Harvard Common Press; 1992.

LABORING WOMEN BELIEVE WHAT HEALTHCARE PROFESSIONALS TELL THEM. TELL THEM SOMETHING NICE ABOUT THEMSELVES

LYNDA COOK SAWYER, RNC, BSN, MBA

WHAT TO DO: IMPLEMENT

I have heard birth stories for the length of my career in nursing. Mothers of all ages, 14 to 90, remember what was said to them and about them during their labors. Something about the energy of birth, the concentration during contractions, and the relief between contractions burns certain statements into the mothers' minds forever. In the midst of all doubts and fears, a laboring mother will believe what she hears.

A fully pregnant woman's body is nothing that she could have ever imagined. Granted, she has had 9 months to get used to the constantly changing form, but the exponential growth of her abdomen, the fat deposits laid on her buttocks, hips, and thighs, the over-roundness of her breasts, and the likely swelling of her face, neck, hands, and feet have distorted her perception of self regardless of her actual size or weight gain. Now, in labor and probably naked under a flimsy hospital gown amidst virtual strangers she just met an hour or so ago, it does nothing for her positive body image.

Then the doubts of "good mothering" wash over this woman's every laboring thought. Will I be able to labor right? Will I birth right? Will I poop while I'm pushing? Can I breastfeed? Will my body work? Will I embarrass myself? Will I scream? Will I cuss…yell at my husband…kick the doctor?....

Those of us in the business of childbirth see women like this everyday. We are used to the shapes, the inability to mobilize on a dime, the guarded awareness of nudity, and the apprehension of "doing it right." It would be very easy for us to shrug-off our "next patient's" emotional concerns, but we shouldn't. We may work with these body types, birth processes, and extreme maternal doubts every day, but we do not work with "her" everyday.

The physical act of an unmedicated labor draws the woman's attention inward, demanding her full focus during every contraction. However, between contractions, she is fully cognizant of what is happening and what is being said to her and around her. And with that awareness comes all the apprehensions and misperceptions of her own body image and future mothering abilities. A medicated mother may be drowsy or aware but without sensations of labor. Regardless of this, laboring women who are not involved in the throes of contractions believe and remember what they hear during labor. Tell them something nice.

Here are some nice things said by healthcare professionals in the environment of labor and birth, which are cherished by mothers years after the births of their children:

"Awwwwww, you're the perfect size for having a baby! Look at that beautiful tummy…"

"You just do what you have to do (during contractions); it's my job to work around you, not the other way."

"The nurse kept telling me, 'You are doing great.' …and she meant it."

"You're a beautiful person. I can only imagine the mother you'll be."

SUGGESTED READINGS

Kelleher J. *Nurturing the Family: The Guide for Postpartum Doulas.* Philadelphia, PA: Xlibris Corporation; 2002.

Simkin P. *The Birth Partner: A Complete Guide to Childbirth for Dads, Doulas, and All Other Labor Companions.* 3rd Ed. Boston, MA: Harvard Common Press; 2007.

MOTHERING IS LEARNED BY WATCHING

LYNDA COOK SAWYER, RNC, BSN, MBA

WHAT TO DO: EVALUATE

The basic tenet of being a mother—raising a baby, a child, or a teenager—is associated with simply having the guardianship of a baby, a child, or a teenager. The complete acceptance of this little person through caring and protection is parenting while the demonstration of caring through complete selfless nurturance is mothering.

The activities of mothering run from the changing of diapers to the provision of basic healthcare. Feeding a child can be awfully tricky too whereas calming an overly tired newborn can seem impossible. Bathing a wiggly infant, wrestling a toddler into clothing, providing loving discipline and boundaries to a preteen, and saying just the right thing to a teen's broken heart are all examples of mothering.

Folding clothes, cleaning a house, and preparing a meal are all examples of adult, like responsibilities; adding a child to the mix reduces the previously practiced adult childlike again. Learning to fold baby clothes, cleaning a house around a preschooler bent on destroying a house, and preparing a meal that a child will eat are entirely different processes altogether. This is mothering.

Today's mother most likely grew up in a family with one or no siblings. Emphasis for learning and free time was directed at academic and social achievements and extracurricular activities as opposed to caring for younger siblings and babysitting. They were more likely to graduate high school and most of them went on to participate in some college. As a result, the number of first-time mothers in the 30+ age range has increased. It is completely likely, therefore, to have a 30-something mother with a college degree and a professional career having her first baby but knowing nothing about diapering, infant feeding, infant swaddling, and normal infant behaviors—sounds, temperature, sleep patterns, etc. Regardless of her education or intelligence level, a new mother is often hesitant to verbalize, "I do not know how to care for my baby. Can you teach me?"...this is the last thing she wants anyone to know or suspect.

Therefore, in today's birthing facilities, it could be entirely possible that the nurse caring for the mother's newborn in a birthing center or hospital setting is this mother's first opportunity to observe newborn care. Removing the infant to a separate and closed nursery to change diapers, rock and settle a crying baby, or feed the baby interferes with the mother's ability to watch you provide this care. Do not stand over her and try to talk the mother through a task with your words—this would be same as her reading a book. She needs to watch you perform the activities of daily care. Allow the mother to see the process in action and then encourage her to practice it whenever she would like. Move slowly and with purpose. Speak to the baby with kind and gentle words. Yes, we all know that you can wrap a blanket tighter and faster than this and you probably do not need to speak to the newborn either, but remember...the mother is learning. Model the action in the same way as a mother would do it herself. Gently.

Your role as a postpartum nurse professional is to prepare this new family for discharge. For observing the coordination you use to fold the blanket, hold the baby, place the baby on the blanket, and fold the corners for a nice, tight swaddle is intimately more beneficial to this mother's education in newborn care than anything you could ever tell her with words or give her to read.

SUGGESTED READINGS

Kelleher J. *Nurturing the Family: The Guide for Postpartum Doulas.* Philadelphia, PA: Xlibris Corporation; 2002.

Simkin P. *The Birth Partner: A Complete Guide to Childbirth for Dads, Doulas, and All Other Labor Companions.* 3rd Ed. Boston, MA: Harvard Common Press; 2007.

IT WAS CALLED "THE URGE TO PUSH" BEFORE IT WAS CALLED "LABORING DOWN"

LYNDA COOK SAWYER, RNC, BSN, MBA

WHAT TO DO: IMPLEMENT

A fully dilated cervix is not an indication for the mother to be coached to "Push!" A fully dilated cervix is an indication that the uterus has completed its work of contracting from the fundus to its base, the lower uterine segment. The fundus pushes downward while the uterus as a whole pulls upward, stretching the cervix up and over the fetal presenting part. The intact fetal membrane acts as a smooth, cylindrical surface to wedge and hold the cervix open. If the membranes have been ruptured, the presenting part—be it the fetal head, the fetal buttocks, or a foot or two—is left to provide the surface over which the cervix must be pulled.

As the largest part of the baby's head (the circumference around his eyebrows and ear-tips) passes through the fully dilated cervix, it will bulge into the vaginal cavity. While the tissues of the vaginal floor are made to receive the passing of the entire term fetus, it gains its space by compressing the mother's rectum. When this final step occurs, the mother will alert you to her strong "urge to push" either verbally by stating "the baby is coming!" or involuntarily by pushing.

Often, a laboring mother will be "fully dilated" upon digital examination of her cervix, but has no urge to push. In the absence of emergent criteria—hemorrhage, nonreassuring fetal heart tones, etc.—this space between transition and the urge to begin pushing should be received as normal and even necessary. The time may span 15 to 30 min or more as the fetus completes any necessary internal rotations for passage through the maternal pelvis. Contractions may space from 1–2 min (as was needed for transition) to 4–5 min. The uterus will fully relax between contractions allowing optimal blood perfusion to the placenta and hence, to the fetus; the mother will have a moment to relax before beginning the next phase of labor.

Waiting for the uterus and fetus to join in the efforts of birth can significantly decrease the amount of time needed for this stage of labor. The uterine muscle coupled with the urge to push creates a more focused type of pushing than when the mother is simply pushing without this involvement. Maternal abdominal muscles pressing externally to the uterus are not what expel the fetus. The fundus pushing the fetus directly from above provides the direct impetus for birth. The overwhelming urge to push supplied by the physical compression of the rectum directs the mother's efforts and focuses her muscle usage to those muscles that are most useful for birth—lower abdominal and rectal. In addition, she will relax the perineal muscles through which the fetus needs to pass. (It is simply not an easy maneuver to push with the total involvement of the lower abdominal and rectal muscles while contracting the perineal muscles—think Kegal exercise.)

Today, with 90% epidural rates in some medical birthing facilities, the indication for the mother to begin pushing is a fully dilated cervix. Her cervix is checked often in anticipation of reaching this stage of labor. Disconnected from most sensations in the pelvic region of her body, the belief is that the mother will not be able to tell her care providers that she feels pressure. Pushing, if begun at the time when a fully dilated cervix is discovered, can drag out 30–60 additional minutes without the full involvement of the uterine and rectal muscles. This tires the mother physically and deflates her emotionally—"the baby is not coming." With the full involvement of the uterus, however, the uterus will do much of the work and the mother's pushing efforts will become complimentary. The size of the fetus, the type of the presenting part, and the flexibility of the mother's bony structures determine exactly how long this third stage of labor will be, but utilizing the musculature in its intended manner can only help the process, not delay it.

With all of this in mind, if your laboring mother is term, without an epidural, the fetal heart tones are reassuring, and the contractions begin to space remarkably during her transition phase of labor, suspect the end of the transition phase and complete dilatation; perform a digital exam if you must. Encourage her to rest. Explain the physiology if she or the support persons are curious. When the fetal presenting part completes its internal machinations, proceeds through the pelvis, and the vaginal vault expands to receive the fetus, the mother will most definitely alert you that she has an urge to push.

If the laboring mother has chosen to use an epidural, this phase will all happen in the same order if allowed. Her contractions will space, the fetal heart tones will be reassuring, and when the fetal presenting part proceeds through the pelvis and the vaginal vault expands to receive the fetus, the mother will most definitely alert you that she feels some type of pressure. The difference between this and what was previously taught as proper management of labor is that healthcare personnel did not wait for this "pressure." Via digital exams, we would announce for the pushing to begin! Now, waiting for the mother to indicate that she is "feeling pressure" is called "laboring down."

Knowledgeable birth attendants, however, will tell you that this is not a new phenomenon created by intuitive doctors for the ultimate in birth management when utilizing epidural anesthesia in labor; it is a physiologic normality—the urge to push—lost to the bedside practice for a long time in our sea of epidural anesthesia.

SUGGESTED READINGS

Roberts JE. The "push" for evidence: Management of the second stage. *J Midwifery Wom Health*. 2002;47(1):2–15.

Simpson KR, James DC. Effects of immediate versus delayed pushing during second-stage labor on fetal well-being; a randomized clinical trial. *Nurs Res*. 2005;54(3):149–157.

THE NURSE SHOULD GIVE DEPO-PROVERA (MEDROXYPROGESTERONE ACETATE) USING THE Z-TRACK INTRAMUSCULAR INJECTION METHOD

CATHERINE A. CHILDRESS, RN, MSN

WHAT TO DO: IMPLEMENT

Depo-Provera should be given deep into the muscle. The Z-track method is recommended for intramuscular (IM) injections. Potter and Perry (2005) described the Z-track method as involving (1) changing to a new needle before injection, (2) moving the skin down before injection, and (3) waiting 10 s after injecting the medication. A new needle is applied so that no medication remains on the outside of the needle. Moving the skin down creates a zigzag path through the tissue that seals the needle track to avoid tracking of medication. Waiting 10 s allows time for the medication to absorb. Avoid massaging the site after the injection of Depo-Provera because massage accelerates absorption and decreases the period of effectiveness.

The preferred site for a Z-track method is the ventrogluteal muscle that is situated deep and away from major nerves and blood vessels. Injuries such as fibrosis, nerve damage, abscess, tissue necrosis, muscle contraction, gangrene, and pain have all been associated with the common IM sites except for the ventrogluteal site. To locate the ventrogluteal site, place the palm of the hand with thumb toward the groin on the patient's greater trochanter and then extend the index finger to the anterior iliac spine making a V with the middle finger. The injection is given in the center of the V.

IM injections can cause pain. A major deterrent to Depo-Provera is the painful injection that discourages many patients from its use. Fletcher conducted a randomized, controlled trial to see if pinching a fold of skin in the gluteal region before the injection of Depo-Provera would reduce the pain. A total of 78 patients participated in the study. Depo-Provera was administered in the gluteal region, with 39 receiving the pinch before and during the injection while the other 39 just received the injection. The participants were asked if their pain was severe. Six in the pinch group were severe compared to 15 in the injection-only group. The pinch method appears to be useful in decreasing the pain of injection. Fletcher notes that other studies have described similar methods that have also decreased the pain of injections.

The nurse should administer Depo-Provera using the Z-track method and the ventrogluteal site, pinching a fold of the skin, and avoiding massaging after the injection. The nurse should use a 21–23 gauge, "½–3" needle to penetrate deep into the muscle, which depends on the patient's weight and adipose tissue.

SUGGESTED READINGS

Family planning. In: Murray SS, McKinney ES, eds. *Foundations of Maternal-Newborn Nursing*. 4th Ed. St. Louis, MO: Saunders; 2006, pp. 832–855.

Fletcher H. Painless Depo-medroxyprogesterone acetate (DMPA) injection using the "pinch technique." *J Obstet Gynecol*. 2004;24(5):562–563.

Hunter J. Intramuscular injection technique. *Nurs Stand*. 2008;22(24):35–40.

Medication administration. In: Potter PA, Perry AG, eds. *Fundamentals of Nursing*. 6th Ed. St. Louis: Mosby; 2005, pp. 822–909.

THE NURSE SHOULD ENCOURAGE OPEN-GLOTTIS BREATHING DURING STAGE 2 OF LABOR AND DELIVERY

CATHERINE A. CHILDRESS, RN, MSN

WHAT TO DO: IMPLEMENT

A usual practice in the United States is to have women in the second stage of labor use coached, closed-glottis pushing that institutes the Valsalva maneuver. The Valsalva maneuver increases intrathoracic pressure and eventually reduces blood pressure, which results in decrease in blood flow to the placenta. Closed-glottis pushing reduces blood flow to the placenta, which causes fetal hypoxia. Fetal hypoxia will lead to fetal distress during labor. It can be detected on an electronic fetal monitor. Severe fetal distress can result in neonatal complications and the need for intrapartum operative deliveries.

Simpson and James (2005) conducted a randomized clinical trial (RCT) on 45 eligible women who were assigned to either the immediate pushing group or the delayed pushing group. The immediate pushing group was coached to use closed-glottis pushing for about three to four times during each contraction. The women in the delayed pushing group were assisted to a left lateral position at 10 cm dilatation until they felt the urge to push. They were encouraged by the nurse to bear down with contractions without holding their breath (open-glottis). Fetal oxygen desaturation was significantly greater in the immediate pushing group. There were significant differences between groups in the number of variable decelerations. This study suggested that pushing with the open-glottis technique in nulliparous women with epidural anesthesia was more favorable for fetal well-being than the traditional provider-coached, closed-glottis pushing. The authors noted that these results were consistent with the older RCTs cited in the review of literature of this study.

The laboring patient should rely on her natural urge to push. The woman should bear down with the contraction without holding her breath. Begin each contraction by taking a cleansing breath, then take a breath and exhale while pushing 4 to 6s at a time. Women can be encouraged to grunt or vocalize along with pushing. This method will avoid the Valsalva maneuver and promote fetal well-being. The nurse should always monitor for variable decelerations during the second stage of labor. Severe variable decelerations with nonreassuring fetal heart rate should be reported to the physician immediately. The laboring woman should be encouraged to use the left lateral position whenever possible.

SUGGESTED READINGS

Murray SS, McKinney ES. Nursing care during labor and birth and intrapartum fetal surveillance. In: *Foundations of Maternal-Newborn Nursing*. 4th Ed. St. Louis, MO: Saunders; 2006, pp. 266–334.

Simpson KR, James DC. Effects of immediate versus delayed pushing during second-stage labor on fetal well-being. *Nurs Res.* 2005;54(3):149–157.

ASSESS THE BLOOD PRESSURE OF A WOMAN IN LABOR IN BETWEEN THE CONTRACTIONS

CATHERINE A. CHILDRESS, RN, MSN

WHAT TO DO: EVALUATE

The laboring woman will experience uterine contractions that increase in frequency, intensity, and duration during the labor process. These contractions cause the blood flow to the placenta to gradually decrease, shunting its blood to the woman's circulatory system, which will increase her blood pressure. The increase in maternal blood pressure will reduce placental blood flow, which can lead to fetal hypoxia and distress.

Other causes of an increased blood pressure also need to be considered. Anxiety will cause a slightly elevated blood pressure when the woman is admitted to the labor and delivery unit. The increasing contractions during labor will cause pain that will stimulate the sympathetic nervous system to release catecholamines. These will stimulate the α-receptors, causing vasoconstriction, which will also raise the woman's blood pressure.

The nurse should attempt to reduce the laboring woman's anxiety on admission and throughout the labor process. Nonpharmacologic and pharmacologic methods should be implemented to minimize the discomforts of labor. Teach the woman relaxation and breathing techniques. The laboring woman's blood pressure should be assessed when she is not having a contraction.

SUGGESTED READINGS

Murray SS, McKinney ES. Nursing care during labor and birth. In: *Foundations of Maternal-Newborn Nursing*. 4th Ed. St. Louis, MO: Saunders; 2006, pp. 266–305.

ASSESS THE BLOOD PRESSURE OF A PREGNANT WOMAN IN THE LATERAL POSITION

CATHERINE A. CHILDRESS, RN, MSN

WHAT TO DO: EVALUATE

A woman lying in supine position will experience a reduction in blood pressure due to her enlarging uterus, particularly in the second and third trimester of pregnancy. The increasing size of the uterus impedes the blood return from the lower extremities, reducing the return of the blood to the heart. Placental blood flow can also decrease if she remains in a supine position, which can lead to fetal hypoxia and distress. The side-lying position relieves the pressure, allowing the blood to return to the heart.

Other factors that could cause a reduction in blood pressure during pregnancy need to be considered. These causes may result from conditions that are associated with pregnancy itself or unrelated but coincidental. For example, a woman who is experiencing severe nausea and vomiting can develop dehydration that, if severe, may lead to hypotension. Similarly, a symptom of pregnancy induced anemia or cardiomyopathy may adversely affect the patient's blood pressure. Alternatively, systemic infections or trauma, while they can present during pregnancy, is also a common cause of hypotension in the nonpregnant patient.

The nurse should carefully assess a pregnant woman's blood pressure in the lateral recumbent position. The woman should be taught to avoid lying in the supine position for extended periods of time. The nurse should determine if other factors are contributing to the woman's blood pressure reading, teach measures to prevent anemia, and treat nausea and vomiting early in the course of their presentation.

SUGGESTED READINGS

Murray SS, McKinney ES. Physiologic adaptations to pregnancy. In: *Foundations of Maternal-Newborn Nursing*. 4th Ed. St. Louis, MO: Saunders; 2006, pp. 109–149.

TAKE PRENATAL VITAMINS WITH BEVERAGES THAT DO NOT CONTAIN CAFFEINE AND NOT COFFEE OR MILK

CATHERINE A. CHILDRESS, RN, MSN

WHAT TO DO: IMPLEMENT

Pregnancy is a time when the nutritional needs of a woman are increased. Most diets are inadequate to meet the increased needs of some vitamins and minerals such as vitamins B_6, D, and E, folic acid, iron, calcium, zinc, and magnesium. The nurse has a major role in the prenatal nutrition education of the mother in preparing her for the delivery of a healthy newborn. Obstetricians prescribe prenatal vitamins for their patients to meet this increased demand. The absorption of some of these vitamins and minerals is affected by how the prenatal vitamin is taken (Table 412.1).

A prenatal vitamin should be taken with a meal. The fat-soluble vitamins require the ingestion of fats for absorption. The nurse should assess what time of the day is best for the pregnant woman to take her prenatal vitamins. Teaching her to take the prenatal vitamin with water or orange juice may be the best. Women should be cautioned not to take more than the

TABLE 412.1	THE AFFECT OF DIETARY PRODUCTS ON THE ABSORPTION OF DIETARY MINERALS	
MINERAL	DECREASES ABSORPTION	INCREASES ABSORPTION
Iron	Calcium	Ascorbic acid
	Phosphorus in milk	Meat
	Tannin in tea	Fish
	Coffee	Poultry
Calcium		Vitamin D

recommended dose of prenatal vitamins and to keep their vitamins out of the reach of children.

SUGGESTED READINGS

AAP & ACOG. Specialized counseling. In: *Guidelines for Perinatal Care*. 6th Ed. Washington, DC: ACOG; 2007, pp. 89–93.

Murray SS, McKinney ES. Nutrition for childbearing. In: *Foundations of Maternal-Newborn Nursing*. 4th Ed. St. Louis, MO: Saunders; 2006, pp. 173–201.

A PREGNANT WOMAN SHOULD PERFORM SHOULDER RELAXATION AND PELVIC TILT EXERCISES FOR BACK PAIN

CATHERINE A. CHILDRESS, RN, MSN

WHAT TO DO: IMPLEMENT

The enlarging uterus during the third trimester of pregnancy creates a progressive lordosis. This strains the muscles and ligaments of the back, often causing back pain. Back pain can interfere with activities of daily living and increase the blood pressure. Hypertension in pregnancy can decrease placental perfusion leading to possible fetal hypoxia and intrauterine growth restriction.

Morkved et al. (2007) conducted a randomized clinical trial (RCT) to assess if a 12-week training program during pregnancy could prevent or treat lumbopelvic pain. Included in the study were 301 healthy nulliparous women at 20 weeks gestation. The women were randomly assigned to the training group or control group.

Interventions in the training group included daily pelvic floor muscle exercises, low impact aerobics, and light stretching, breathing, and relaxation exercises. The control group received the routine information given by the healthcare providers. At 36 weeks of gestation, the training group reported significantly less lumbopelvic pain (44%) versus the control group (56%). The women in the training group also had significantly higher scores on functional status. The authors reported that there were two previous studies using muscle training systems with similar results.

The nurse should assess the pregnant woman's exercise routine. Pregnancy is not the time to begin a new exercise routine; however, the nurse should teach the woman to perform exercises to relax the shoulders and thighs to prevent backaches. Shoulder exercises involve shoulder circling. Tailored sitting and the pelvic tilt will relax the thighs. Advise the woman that exercising supine is not safe because of the adverse effects it may have on venous return and circulation to the placenta.

SUGGESTED READINGS

Morkved S, Salvesen K, Schei B, et al. Does group training during pregnancy prevent lumbopelvic pain? A randomized clinical trial. *Acta Obstetrica et Gynecol*. 2007;86(3):276–282.

Murray SS, McKinney ES. Physiologic adaptations to pregnancy and complications of pregnancy. In: *Foundations of Maternal-Newborn Nursing*. 4th Ed. St. Louis, MO: Saunders; 2006, pp. 640–643.

CUP ONE HAND AGAINST THE UTERUS AT THE SYMPHYSIS PUBIS WHEN MASSAGING AN ATONIC UTERUS

CATHERINE A. CHILDRESS, RN, MSN

WHAT TO DO: IMPLEMENT

The uterine muscles contract in the postpartum period to return the uterus to its nonpregnant size and control bleeding. Should the uterus fail to contract and become "boggy," the patient can experience postpartum hemorrhage. Severe bleeding is the leading cause of maternal death and uterine atony is the cause in 80% of the primary postpartum hemorrhages. Postpartum women with risk factors for uterine atony should be identified to facilitate early detection of postpartum hemorrhage. Risk factors for uterine atony are presented in Table 414.1.

TABLE 414.1	RISK FACTORS FOR UTERINE ATONY
Prolonged labor	
Augmented labor	
Rapid labor	
History of postpartum hemorrhage	
Overdistended uterus	
Operative delivery	
Chorioamnionitis	
Urinary retention	

An atonic uterus should be massaged to restore the muscle tone. The nondominant hand should be cupped against the uterus at the symphysis pubis to prevent trauma while the dominant hand massages the uterus.

On admission, the postpartum nurse should identify the patients at a risk for uterine atony. A fundal assessment should be performed frequently to identify the early signs of uterine atony. Should the uterus be not firmly contracted, the nurse should use the appropriate technique to massage the fundus. The woman should be taught about the purpose of the uterine contractions, the normal blood flow, and how to massage her uterus.

SUGGESTED READINGS

American College of Obstetrics and Gynecology. ACOG Practice Bulletin: Clinical management guidelines for obstetricians-gynecologists Number 76, October 2006: Postpartum hemorrhage. *Obstet Gynecol.* 2006;108(4):1039–1047.

Murray SS, McKinney ES. Physiologic adaptations to pregnancy. In: *Foundations of Maternal-Newborn Nursing.* 4th Ed. St. Louis, MO: Saunders; 2006a, pp. 109–149.

Murray SS, McKinney ES. Complications of pregnancy. In: *Foundations of Maternal-Newborn Nursing.* 4th Ed. St. Louis, MO: Saunders; 2006b, pp. 640–643.

To express clots from a uterus after massaging for an atonic uterus for postpartum hemorrhage provides pressure over the lower uterine segment

Catherine A. Childress, RN, MSN

WHAT TO DO: IMPLEMENT

An atonic uterus must be massaged during a postpartum hemorrhage to prevent further blood loss. Severe bleeding is the leading cause of maternal death. Uterine atony is one of the most common causes of early postpartum hemorrhages. An atonic uterus needs to be massaged using the nondominant hand cupping the lower uterine segment while massaging with the dominant hand. The clots must be expelled once the uterus is firm to allow the uterus to contract properly. The nondominant hand should be kept firmly just above the symphysis pubis while the dominant hand presses firmly on the uterus to expel the clots. The pressure applied over the lower uterine segment with the non-dominant hand prevents uterine inversion.

While attempting to perform massage and express clots for the atonic uterus, it is important for the nurse to remain cognizant of the whole patient. This requires an attention to the As, Bs, and Cs of care airway, breathing, and circulation and appropriate volume resuscitation with isotonic fluids or packed red blood cells as appropriate for hemorrhagic shock. In addition, the uterus that fails to respond to stimulation may be benefited by oxytocic medications. The patient often becomes anxious during these episodes because of both the circumstances and the acute bleeding. This requires calm yet deliberate and methodical interventions to allay fear, ensure hemodynamic stability, and address the cause of the uterine atony.

SUGGESTED READINGS

American College of Obstetrics and Gynecology. ACOG Practice Bulletin: Clinical management guidelines for obstetricians-gynecologists Number 76, October 2006. Postpartum hemorrhage. *Obstet Gynecol.* 2006;108(4):1039–1047.

Cashion K. Nursing care of the postpartum woman. In: Lowdermilk DL, Perry SE, eds. *Maternity and Women's Health Care.* 8th Ed. Philadelphia, PA: Mosby; 2004;173–183.

Murray SS, McKinney ES. Physiologic adaptations to pregnancy. In: *Foundations of Maternal-Newborn Nursing.* 4th Ed. St. Louis, MO: Saunders; 2006, pp. 109–149.

ADMINISTER VITAMIN K AND HEPATITIS B VACCINES TO THE NEWBORNS

CATHERINE A. CHILDRESS, RN, MSN

WHAT TO DO: IMPLEMENT

The neonates lack vitamin K, which puts them at risk for clotting deficiencies and hemorrhagic diseases of the newborn. Vitamin K is necessary to activate several clotting factors such as II, VII, IX, and X. The infants, intestines are also sterile, which means that they are unable to synthesize vitamin K on their own. As a result, vitamin K injection in a dose of 0.5 to 1 mg is recommended by the American Academy of Pediatrics at birth to prevent complications related to hypovitaminosis K.

The American Academy of Pediatrics also recommends early administration of hepatitis B vaccine to medically stabilize the neonates over 2 kg and infants whose mothers are serology-negative to receive the initial dose before discharge from the hospital. If the mother is hepatitis B surface antigen positive, it is important to remember that the child also needs protection against acute hepatitis with the administration of hepatitis B immune globulin.

For both of these medications, administration is done by an IM route, usually in the thigh in the vastus lateralis muscle. It is important to remember to hold the thigh firmly and "pinch" the muscle, insert the needle into the body of the muscle at a 90° angle, aspirate the syringe plunger for blood, and administer the medication slowly, applying direct pressure after needle withdrawal.

The nurse should determine in which thigh the vitamin K was administered and administer the hepatitis vaccination in the opposite thigh to be able to differentiate adverse effects at the site.

SUGGESTED READINGS

AAP & ACOG. Transitional care and preventive care. In: *Guidelines for Perinatal Care*. 6th Ed. Washington, DC: ACOG; 2007, pp. 219–222.

Murray SS, McKinney ES. Normal Newborn: Process of adaptation and care of the normal newborn. In: *Foundations of Maternal-Newborn Nursing*. 4th Ed. St. Louis, MO: Saunders; 2006, pp. 450–467, pp. 508–535.

SUCTION THE MOUTH OF THE NEONATE BEFORE SUCTIONING THE NOSE

CATHERINE A. CHILDRESS, RN, MSN

WHAT TO DO: IMPLEMENT

The compression of the chest during a vaginal delivery forces some of the fetal lung fluid from the chest, although some moisture will remain in the lungs for several hours after birth. The neonates excrete some of this fluid through their airway. The neonate also experiences relaxation of the cardiac sphincter between the esophagus and the stomach, which can potentially lead to regurgitation of feedings into the airway. These excretions and other secretions produced by the neonate's airway can potentially block the neonate's airway.

One of the goals when caring for a neonate is to maintain an open airway. The neonate will occasionally require suctioning. The newborn's head should be positioned to the side to facilitate drainage. Typically, a bulb syringe is utilized for most situations. The mouth should be suctioned first to prevent the newborn from gasping and aspirating mucus or fluid. Once the mouth has been suctioned, then the nose can be suctioned as needed. It is important for the nurse to realize that suctioning can traumatize the tissues causing edema and respiratory difficulty.

The nurse should carefully monitor the neonate for signs and symptoms of airway compromise. The airway should be suctioned promptly and the parents should be taught the proper use of a bulb syringe.

SUGGESTED READINGS

Murray SS, McKinney ES. Normal newborn: Process of adaptation and care of the normal newborn. In: *Foundations of Maternal-Newborn Nursing*. 4th Ed. St. Louis, MO: Saunders; 2006, pp. 450–467.

Tell the Obstetrician That You Will Ready the Operating Room After Two "Pop Offs" with a Vacuum-Assisted Delivery

Catherine A. Childress, RN, MSN

WHAT TO DO: EVALUATE

One technique of operative vaginal birth is vacuum extraction to aid in the descent and rotation of the fetal head. Indications include shortening of stage two because of maternal exhaustion and ineffective pushing, a nonreassuring fetal heart rate pattern, failure of the presenting part to rotate and descend, or partial separation of the placenta.

In the last 15 years, the rate of vacuum-assisted deliveries has outnumbered forceps deliveries. McQuivey (2004) states that vacuum extraction is safe for both the fetus and the mother as long as the physician has correct placement and knows when to abandon the procedure. The technique used in vacuum extraction can reduce the risk of maternal or fetal injuries. Increased traction efforts cause cup detachments or "pop offs," a predisposing factor for many of the major complications of vacuum-assisted deliveries. To reduce injuries, the number of tractions should be limited to 4–5 and detachments to 2–3.

If the nurse applies the suction cup in a vacuum-assisted delivery, the suction should not go outside the green zone on the suction indicator. The nurse should not hesitate to tell the physician that she will get the obstetrical operating room ready for a cesarean section after 4 to 5 tractions or 2 to 3 pop offs.

SUGGESTED READINGS

McQuivey RW. Vacuum-assisted delivery: A review. *J Matern-Fetal Neonat Med*. 2004;16:171–179.

Murray SS, McKinney ES. Nursing care during obstetric procedures. In: *Foundations of Maternal-Newborn Nursing*. 4th Ed. St. Louis, MO: Saunders; 2006, pp. 364–388.

O'Grady JP, Pope CS, Patel SS. Vacuum extraction in modern obstetric practice: A review and critique. *Gen Obstet*. 2000;12:475–480.

Frozen breast milk should be thawed quickly under running water or overnight in the refrigerator

Catherine A. Childress, RN, MSN

WHAT TO DO: IMPLEMENT

The advantages of breast milk have been acknowledged for years. They include immunologic benefits, easier digestion, hypoallergenic, and potentially even more intelligence. While breast-feeding has some additional benefits including maternal bonding and improved jaw and motor control, some mothers experience difficulty with breast-feeding or their baby may be too ill to breast-feed. For these mothers, breast pumping and freezing becomes an option.

Breast milk can be frozen for 2 to 3 weeks if it will not be used within a few days of expression. Breast milk should be thawed quickly under running water, being careful not to subject it to extremely hot water or microwave ovens. Microwaving and high temperatures destroy the valuable components such as lysozymes, IgA, and lipase. Breast milk can also be thawed in the refrigerator overnight or in a bowl of warm water for 30 min.

The nurse should teach the breast-feeding mother to thaw breast milk quickly under warm running water. Advise her not to use hot water or the microwave. Explain to the mother that as an alternative, she can thaw the sealed bottle of milk in a bowl of warm water for over 30 min.

SUGGESTED READINGS

AAP & ACOG. Neonatal nutrition. In: *Guidelines for Perinatal Care*. 6th Ed. Washington, DC: ACOG; 2007, p. 245.

Neilson J. Return to work: Practical management of breastfeeding. *Clin Obstet Gynecol*. 2004;7(3):724–733.

NOTICE PERSISTENT AND INCREASING PERINEAL PAIN IN THE POSTPARTUM PATIENT

CATHERINE A. CHILDRESS, RN, MSN

WHAT TO DO: ASSESS

The patient with intractable postpartum pain must be appropriately assessed to determine its cause, particularly if it is increasing. Since pain is a normal postpartum phenomenon and inappropriate pain management may result in unrelieved pain, the first step in assessing the patient requires that the pain be effectively managed as a symptom. Then, an understanding of the possible causes can be addressed.

Women with severe postpartum lacerations of the birth canal can present with similar symptoms of severe pain in the perineal region that are often refractory to routine pain-control measures. The possibility of hematoma formation should also be considered by the nurse in the patient experiencing unrelenting pain. A hematoma forms when there is bleeding into the loose connective tissue while the overlying tissue remains intact. Postdeliveryhematomas may be found in the vulvar, vaginal, and retroperitoneal regions either as a course of routine delivery or when a forceps or vacuum delivery has occurred. The postpartum woman will complain of deep, severe, unrelieved pain and pressure in the perineal region.

Postpartum pain requires the administration of analgesics, usually narcotic analgesics to treat the symptoms. Small hematomas can be treated with ice packs and will generally reabsorb. Larger hematomas may require incision, evacuation, and ligation of the vessel. The postpartum nurse should screen patients upon admission for their level of pain and risk factors related to lacerations and postpartum hematomas.

SUGGESTED READINGS

Murray SS, McKinney ES. Postpartum maternal complications. In: *Foundations of Maternal-Newborn Nursing*. 4th Ed. St. Louis, MO: Saunders; 2006, p. 737.

Review the chart and patient history for risk factors of postpartum hemorrhage for early detection of uterine atony

Catherine A. Childress, RN, MSN

The uterine muscles contract in the postpartum period to return the uterus to its nonpregnant size and control bleeding. Should the uterus fail to contract and become "boggy," the patient can experience postpartum hemorrhage. Severe bleeding is the leading cause of maternal death. Uterine atony is the cause in 80% of primary postpartum hemorrhages.

Postpartum women with risk factors for uterine atony should be identified to facilitate early detection of this possible complication (see Table 414.1). An important risk factor to note is a history of postpartum hemorrhage and the precipitating factors.

Fundal assessment should be done frequently to identify early signs of uterine atony. Woman should be taught about the purpose of the uterine contractions, normal blood flow, and how to massage her uterus.

Suggested Readings

American College of Obstetrics and Gynecology. ACOG Practice bulletin: Clinical management guidelines for obstetricians-gynecologists number 76, October 2006: Postpartum hemorrhage. *Obstet Gynecol.* 2006;108(4):1039–1047.

MacMullen NJ, Dulski LA, Meagher B. Red alert perinatal hemorrhage. *Matern Child Nurs.* 2005;30(1):46–51.

Murray SS, McKinney ES. Complications of pregnancy. In: *Foundations of Maternal-Newborn Nursing.* 4th Ed. St. Louis, MO: Saunders; 2006, pp. 640–643.

Murray SS, McKinney ES. Physiologic adaptations to pregnancy. In: *Foundations of Maternal-Newborn Nursing.* 4th Ed. St. Louis, MO: Saunders; 2006, pp. 109–149.

THE NURSE SHOULD GIVE THE MEASLES, MUMPS, AND RUBELLA VACCINE TO THE POSTPARTUM WOMAN USING THE SUBCUTANEOUS METHOD

CATHERINE A. CHILDRESS, RN, MSN

WHAT TO DO: IMPLEMENT

The American Academy of Pediatrics (AAP) and the American College of Obstetricians and Gynecologists (ACOG) recommends offering the rubella vaccine to postpartum women who are susceptible to rubella. The Committee on Infectious Diseases recommends administering the rubella vaccination using the subcutaneous route of injection.

Preferred sites for the subcutaneous injection are the outer posterior aspect of the upper arm, the abdomen from below the costal margin to the iliac crests, and anterior thighs. When giving an injection with a 5/8 in. needle to the average patient, the needle should be inserted at a 45° angle or a ½ in. needle at a 90° angle. With obese patients, the nurse needs to pinch the skin and use a long enough needle (generally half the width of the skin fold to penetrate the fatty tissue). A 5/8 in.

needle at a 90° angle can inadvertently inject the muscle in an average patient or smaller.

AAP and ACOG recommend testing childbearing women for rubella immunity. The nurse should check the prenatal records of all postpartum women for their rubella immunity. If the woman is susceptible to rubella, she should receive the rubella vaccination. The nurse should identify an appropriate site, assess the woman's size, and determine the appropriate needle length and angle of injection.

SUGGESTED READINGS

AAP & ACOG. Perinatal infections. In: *Guidelines for Perinatal Care*. 6th Ed. Washington, DC: ACOG; 2007, p. 324.

Pickering LK, ed. *Red Book: 2006 Report of the Committee on Infectious Diseases*. 27th Ed. Elk Grove, IL: American Academy of Pediatrics; 2006.

Potter PA, Perry AG. Medication administration. In: *Fundamentals of Nursing*. 6th Ed. St. Louis, MO: Mosby; 2005, pp. 822–902.

Postpartum Units Are Not Intensive Care Areas

Lynda Cook Sawyer, RNC, BSN, MBA

Postpartum units are for mothers who have just given birth. In the hours and days following birth, the mother spends her time adjusting to her new role and taking care of herself while adapting to providing care for her newborn. Depending on the route of birth and the activities that occurred during birth, the mother may need assistance out of bed and back into bed, assistance to and from the bathroom, assistance with intravenous poles and fluid lines, and patient-controlled analgesia, and antibiotic pumps may need loading and alarm maintenance.

The staff members, on the other hand, spend their time obtaining her vital signs, rubbing the fundus, checking the episiotomy (if she has one) and/or abdominal incision (if she has one), managing her pain, answering her call light and questions, and providing safe assistance for mobility. In addition, there is a standard set of discharge teaching points that need to be reviewed with the new mother. If the postpartum unit combines the care of the well newborn with the care of the mother, then the postpartum nurse is providing nursing expertise to two patients—a pediatric patient and a maternity patient. Housekeeping activities for the new mother and her postpartum room are a must to complement "good nursing care"—her trash and linen need to be removed frequently and her mountains of gifts, balloons, plants, and flowers may need corralling just to declutter her space. She may also need assistance with her visitor traffic.

All of this is to say that the postpartum nurse and unit are very busy. The nurse-to-patient ratio recommendations from the Association of Women's Health, Obstetric and Neonatal Nurses (AWHONN), and the American College of Obstetricians & Gynecologists (ACOG) in agreement with the American Academy of Pediatrics (AAP) are usually interpreted to mean that each nurse can provide care to the maximum number of postpartum patients—six mothers or four couplets (mothers with their well babies). (Labor and delivery is 1:1–2 for an actively laboring patient and 1:1 for a high-risk patient, for Stage II of labor patient, or for the circulation of a cesarean section.)

What is traditionally overlooked is that these recommendations also come with qualifiers: "stable," "unstable," and "high risk." When the full intentions of the staffing recommendations are not implemented on a postpartum unit, the nurses become even busier caring for a wide spectrum of postpartum acuities. The patients, in the end, are professionally cared for, but the nursing staff members are ragged; they gather to assist each other with the management of a postpartum hemorrhage and a maternal postpartum seizure, and attend to a difficult-to-attain pain threshold or resuscitating an apneic newborn. These scenarios consume valuable nursing time during almost every shift—time that is not taken into account with the simple, but common, application of the low-risk postpartum nurse-to-patient ratio.

To add an incredibly high-risk postpartum patient to that mix is dangerous. Nursing care in a hospital setting is physically and purposefully compartmentalized around the levels of nursing care a patient needs: intensive care units have highly specialized monitoring equipment, technicians to monitor the equipment outputs, and a nurse-to-patient ratio of 1:1–2 patients; operating rooms are 1:1 while recovery areas are 1:1–2; and medical-surgical units and step-down areas will maintain a ratio anywhere from 1:3–6–8 depending on the individual hospital's leadership decisions. Labor and delivery units and their postpartum units, however, are governed by national standards and oftentimes by state regulations.

Learn to recognize the clinical story of a postpartum patient that dictates the need for a higher level of nursing care. Any mother needing cardiac or respiratory monitoring should be transferred to the nursing unit where that type of support is a primary skill with the correct staffing ratio to provide optimal care. If a mother needs vascular support and hemodynamic monitoring related to a severe hemorrhage during birth or interrelated disseminated intravascular coagulation, simply increasing her postpartum vital sign checks to once per hour on a postpartum unit where the staffing ratio is 1:4–6 is inadequate for rapid recognition of a change in patient status. Postpartum mothers with comorbidities needing medical treatment that are not primary specialties of perinatal nurses—diabetic crisis, neurologic disorders, infectious disease processes, trauma, etc.—should be reassigned to a department that can meet their medical needs.

"But, she's postpartum!" nurses will say. Yes, she is, but she is medically unstable first and postpartum second, and not the other way around. A perinatal nurse can be assigned to travel to her room once per shift and provide the postpartum care and assessments the new mother needs, but an intensive care unit (ICU) nurse cannot be assigned to the postpartum unit to provide the types of care this patient may need. Postpartum areas are not ICUs and being an expert perinatal nurse does not mean that the nurse is everything to every patient. Postpartum units are arranged for high volumes of ambulatory patients and high turnover rates of patient beds; their staffing plans are arranged for high patient-to-staff ratios and sharp fluctuations in census that can stress the already busy nursing staff...this is

not the nursing environment for a medically intensive patient, whether postpartum or not.

SUGGESTED READINGS

AAP & ACOG. Specialized counseling. In: *Guidelines for Perinatal Care*. 6th Ed. Washington, DC: ACOG; 2007, pp. 89–93.

Simpson KR, Creehan PR. *AWHONN's Perinatal Nursing*. 3rd Ed. Philadelphia, PA: Lippincott Williams & Wilkins; 2007.

MOTHERS OF INFANTS MORE THAN 23 WEEKS GESTATION HAVE A MILK SUPPLY READY-TO-FEED

LYNDA COOK SAWYER, RNC, BSN, MBA

WHAT TO DO: IMPLEMENT

Mothers do well to be reminded that they do have milk when their viable babies (>23 weeks gestation) are born. Colostrum, the first milk, is made during the end of the first and beginning of the second trimesters and is available in the lactiferous ducts as early as 20 weeks gestation. This is a normal, routine process for the mammary glands as the hormones of the embryo and placenta send messages to the body that pregnancy has occurred.

During the first 12 weeks of gestation, the vascular and lymph transport system of the mammary glands expands and branches in the presence of chorionic gonadotrophins. With the increased vascular circulation and the presence of estrogen and progesterone, the mammary gland begins the lengthening of milk ducts and the proliferation of milk producing cells within the alveoli of the mammary gland lobes. The mother will experience breast tenderness and increased nipple and areola sensation as well as darkening of the areolar pigmentation during this process.

When the placenta is fully formed and the embryo's human growth hormones begin to circulate through the maternal system, the mother's prolactin-inhibiting hormone is suppressed. This suppression allows her pituitary gland to release and freely circulate prolactin. In the presence of prolactin, the milk-producing cells in the mammary gland's alveoli are stimulated to begin the secretion process. The first milk, colostrum, is in production as early as 16 to 20 weeks gestation.

Why is milk not bursting forth, then, from the second trimester pregnant woman? A voluminous milk supply requires three steps: circulating and received prolactin—to stimulate the milk-producing cells to secrete copious amounts of milk; circulating and received oxytocin—to stimulate the muscle fibers that surround the clusters of milk producing cells to contract; and regular milk removals—to continue the cycle of "empty and produce" (supply and demand). Each of these steps is necessary to increase a milk supply, but they are effectively held in check by the functioning placenta attached to the uterine wall.

The placenta produces human placental lactogen that favors the mother's prolactin in its biochemical makeup. Human placental lactogen will occupy the prolactin receptor sites on the alveolar secretory cells, effectively shutting out the mother's own circulating prolactin. In the absence of the mother's prolactin, the milk-producing cells are restricted from the stimulation that is necessary to produce copious amounts of milk.

Full lactogenesis begins with the delivery of the placenta. The mother's circulating prolactin levels stay high, but the abrupt drop in progesterone levels and the disappearance of placental lactogen with the infant's birth and placental delivery automatically initiate the milk production in the mammary glands...regardless of gestational age. Encourage the mother to begin regular nursings or expressions for her viable newborn; her milk is there, and it is perfect for her baby.

SUGGESTED READINGS

Morhbacher N, Stock J. *The Breastfeeding Answer Book*. 3rd revised Ed. Chicago, IL: La Leche League International; 2003.

Riordan J. *Breastfeeding and Human Lactation*. Sudbury, MA: Jones & Bartlett; 2004.

KNOW NATURAL BIRTH AND ITS NUANCES BEFORE PRACTICING HIGH-RISK LABOR AND DELIVERY

LYNDA COOK SAWYER, RNC, BSN, MBA

WHAT TO DO: PLAN

Women's bodies are made to labor and give birth vaginally. The shape of an adult female pelvis, the hormones that circulate from puberty onward, the strength and power of their uterus, and the musculature and ligature in their lower abdomen and perineal areas combine to provide a perfect environment for the passage of a fetus. If you are unfamiliar with the actual workings of these factors as they join to birth a newborn or two into waiting hands, then you are missing quite a lot of your perinatal nursing education. You are destined to believe that babies can only be born with doctors, epidurals, intravenous fluids, sterile hospital environments, needles, scissors, episiotomies, fetal monitoring machines, stirrups, and nurse call bells. You will believe that babies

are "delivered," and never fully appreciate that babies can be "born."

But, even worse than all of that, you will project this belief on the families assigned to your care and the nurses assigned to your preceptorship. So, take the initiative to teach yourself natural childbirth. Find a mentor who practices natural childbirth and volunteer yourself to him or her as an assistant. Read textbooks, childbirth education books, and birth stories. Witness as many natural childbirths as you can—in person, on video tape, and on videostream via the internet or television.

SUGGESTED READINGS

Kelleher J. *Nurturing the Family: The Guide for Postpartum Doulas.* Philadelphia, PA: Xlibris Corporation; 2002.

Simkin P. *The Birth Partner: A Complete Guide to Childbirth for Dads, Doulas, and All Other Labor Companions.* 3rd Ed. Boston, MA: Harvard Common Press; 2007.

TAKE CHILDBIRTH CLASSES AND READ ALL THE BOOKS

LYNDA COOK SAWYER, RNC, BSN, MBA

WHAT TO DO: ASSESS

Mothers come to us from all walks of life and all educational backgrounds. A laboring woman and her support person(s) arrive at our facility for care in all states of emotional and physical preparedness. It is our job to meet them in their state of emotional and physical preparedness, not the other way around. For instance, a woman arrives, obviously very pregnant, clutching a pillow with one hand and a male support person's arm with the other. She stops at the entry door of the OB triage, turns to her companion, and begins to pant. He murmurs words of encouragement in her ear. After a moment, the woman stops the altered breathing, stands erect, and proceeds into the room. This being your first contact with the pair, your only determination can be that you have just witnessed a contraction.

But, what you don't know at this point could fill a small medical record all by itself—what is her name, what is the gestational age of the pregnancy, who is her obstetrical provider, what number pregnancy is this, what was the outcome of the other births (if any), what relationship is the basis for this male support, what is his name, are her membranes intact, has there been any vaginal bleeding, is the baby moving, is there more than one fetus, when did her contractions start, when did her contractions start to hurt, is she preregistered with your facility or any other one, what is her past medical history, allergies, and so on. There is a volume of detail that needs to be gathered directly from the woman, in conjunction with a whole other set of clinical data in order to provide a safe medical plan of care, including fetal heart rate, fetal lie, contraction frequency, duration, strength, maternal vital signs, and cervical dilatation.

The laboring woman brings a third aspect with her. She brings a preconceived perception of what her childbirth experience will be. This is vital for the healthcare team to know as this perception will underlie and motivate the woman's decision making and approach to labor and birth. For instance, if she lies on her side and breathes deeply and peacefully through contractions without any other verbalizations, and her support person physically moves in close and murmurs softly to her through every contraction, then it is possible they are practicing the Bradley Method of childbirth. If so,

neither partner will entertain or speak back to anyone attempting to elicit information during these moments. The support person could be her brother, her father, her lover, or a close male friend. She will have trained for an unmedicated birth and most likely will refuse a flowing intravenous line for mobility reasons. Upon cervical examination, it would not be abnormal to find her 8 cm, 9 cm, or completely dilated. On the other hand, the exact scenario may be observed for a couple that is completely in love with each other and she is extremely shy or scared. The labor is very early in the process, the contractions do not cause pain yet, and her cervical dilatation is fingertip. She was planning an early epidural and did not want to miss it by laboring one minute longer at home. She is presenting herself for hospital admission and expects the intravenous line and fluids as the first step in her pain management regimen.

Knowing the variations of childbirth preparation is your job. Early in your perinatal career, enroll as an observer in every single childbirth method you can locate. Sit through the entire series, from beginning to end. Read their parent handout materials and scrutinize their suggested reading lists for books you have not read yet. Develop a working relationship with the instructors. Contact independent childbirth educators that you find via an Internet or local Yellow Pages search for "childbirth." Introduce yourself and ask if you could sit through one of their childbirth series as a learning experience for your job. Most often, they will welcome you at no charge, but if an independent instructor requests a nominal fee, pay it—you will not be sorry. Read, read, and read. There is no need to purchase all of these books yourself—libraries and instructors will lend you books. If you prefer to own the really good ones, try eBay and other online discount sites.

In reality, your clients will expect and assume that you are at least as prepared as they are. You will be seen as the expert. Live up to that. This is their child's birth, not yours; the least you can do is meet them where they are and proceed professionally and lovingly from there.

SUGGESTED READINGS

Korte D, Scaer RM. *A Good Birth, A Safe Birth*. 3rd Ed. Boston, MA: Harvard Common Press; 1992.

Simpson KR, Creehan P. *AWHONN's Perinatal Nursing*. Philadelphia, PA: Lippincott Williams & Wilkins; 2007.

ABDOMINAL SUPPORT AFTER A CESAREAN SECTION IS A WELCOME GIFT

LYNDA COOK SAWYER, RNC, BSN, MBA

WHAT TO DO: IMPLEMENT

Cesarean sections, whether unplanned or scheduled, create a painful recovery that is often unexpected by the mother. Cesarean sections, like vaginal births, are considered by most of the lay public to simply be an alternate means by which a baby is produced to waiting arms. This is so entirely misleading that the new mother is often shocked and emotionally numb to discover that she cannot move about freely or care for her newborn as she had inevitably planned prior to the birth. You will not be able to fix this misconception for her, but you can provide her with strategies and physical support that will allow her to still care for her newborn as she recovers from major abdominal surgery.

The physical act of the surgical procedure itself must be placed into context. Whether it is a low transverse incision through the skin and uterus or, in case of an emergent cesarean, a horizontal incision through either or both the skin and uterus, the overlaying abdominal musculature has been similarly incised. The muscles of the abdomen are laid horizontally, vertically, and laterally. There is more than a single layer. These muscles work in harmony to provide the human being with skeletal movement that would not normally be associated with the abdominal area and therefore, their functional loss can be surprising. For instance, rolling from a supine position to a lateral position—who would think that this movement is almost entirely controlled by the muscles covering the intestines? Or rising from a laying position to a sitting position? Yes, it is the abdominal musculature that provides that ability. Sitting to standing? Bending at the waist and lifting with your arms? Granted, as in lifting, your biceps and triceps are exerting the power, but it is your abdominal and low back muscles that are providing the stability.

When the new mother is without this support, self-care becomes a chore; caring for her newborn becomes overwhelming. In the extreme, her new baby becomes the cause of the mother's inability to be a good mother and she may become depressed and withdraw altogether from the care of her infant.

When you are aware of the physical limitations, you can begin your nursing care of this mother with a gift: an abdominal binder. It is not a torture device, though it looks like one, and the relief that its proper placement brings is almost worth delaying its application by 8 to 12 h for the mother to experience the before and after effects, but that would be very cruel, indeed. The binder is slid under the patient's low back while she is lying on her back. The sides are brought up and overlapped across her abdomen. Velcro bands hold the sides in place. It does not need to be tight, just snug. While the mother is healing from the incised abdominal muscle wounds, the firmness of the binder provides the skeletal support she has lost. It allows her the autonomy to sit up in bed a little more naturally, to stand a little more erect, and to remain balanced as she lifts with her arms.

The cesarean section may be little more than a birthing method to a new mother, but the autonomy to care for her new baby is her goal. Knowing this, teach her the methods to do so and give her the physical support she needs to begin her journey of good motherhood... even if initially it resembles a torture device.

SUGGESTED READINGS

Connolly M, Sullivan D. *The Essential C-Section Guide: Pain Control, Healing at Home, Getting Your Body Back, and Everything Else You Need to Know about a Cesarean Birth.* New York, NY: Broadway; 2004.

Kelleher J. *Nurturing the Family: The Guide for Postpartum Doulas.* Philadelphia, PA: Xlibris Corporation; 2002.

TEACH NEW MOTHERS TO READ THEIR BABY'S CUES

LYNDA COOK SAWYER, RNC, BSN, MBA

WHAT TO DO: ASSESS

Babies are born with a set of reflexes that usually are necessary for their survival. Rooting, for example, is the natural reflex of a newborn to turn his face left or right in response to the stimulation of his left or right cheek. This reflex assists the infant in his quest to consume food through his mouth. Suckling is also a reflex. When an object is introduced into a baby's mouth, the reflex to create a seal with his lips and tongue is stimulated and the infant clamps down on the object and creates a negative pressure within his mouth (similar to using a straw). This effort, when used with a bottle, will initiate the flow of fluids from the bottle, through the nipple opening and into the baby's mouth. This effort when used with a pacifier will simply hold the pacifier in the infant's mouth.

There are also natural reflexes of a newborn that are not associated with feedings. Breathing for example, is an autonomic reflex associated with living, while the grasp reflex elicited by objects placed in the palms of the baby's hands or the balls of his feet is associated with bonding for the hopeful assurance of protection. The Babinski reflex—the fanning of the toes when an object is gently drawn along the sole of the newborn's foot—is a sign of a probably healthy central nervous system.

For instance, the snorting sound a newborn makes when otherwise sleeping peacefully should be interpreted as an early feeding cue. The newborn is beginning to rouse from a sleep state in response to an internal signal for glucose and is looking for his feeding source, mom, by smell. The next feeding cue offered on this continuum is the smacking of lips. Associated as an early attempt to latch on to a feeding source, the sound is usually loud enough to wake one or more adults. The newborn is not strong enough yet to coordinate many movements, but getting his hands to his mouth is a final feeding cue that is difficult to misinterpret.

Newborn expressions are also indicative of their needs. A sleeping baby with a furrowed brow is attempting very strongly to stay asleep. If identified by a parent, the activity surrounding the baby can be lessened or the newborn can be moved to a calmer place. Light and normal activities of daily living do not usually disturb the sleep cycles of a newborn, but unexpected sounds or activity might—chastising older siblings, a dropped dish crashing to the floor, or a sharp increase in the number of speaking voices.

Pain is expressed in its own groupings of cues—a piercing cry, arms and legs curled tightly toward the torso alternating with a longer than normal, but restless sleep cycle. This child needs pain relief—whether the pain is from a fresh circumcision or a food that is disagreeing with his digestive system, the source should be identified and resolved. Discomfort, on the other hand, is expressed through a mournful type of cry, an inability to sleep, and a driving desire to suckle, but not necessarily consume nutrition. Whether the cause of discomfort is a gas bubble, a tag from his clothing sticking to the back of his neck, or the soggy wetness of a diaper, the cue here is for the reason to be discovered and eliminated.

Newborns are gestated long enough (37 to 42 weeks) to breathe automatically upon birth, to bond for protection, and seek food for further growth, but not long enough (3 years) to be independent enough to walk, run, hide, communicate their needs through words and sign language, or to search for food when hungry. At birth, however, they can perform or display very specific and universal cues as to what they need at the moment. And, if received and interpreted correctly, the new parents and grandparents can begin participating in this baby's independence and care generously from the beginning.

SUGGESTED READINGS

La Leche League International. *The Womanly Art of Breastfeeding.* New York, NY: The Penguin Group; 2004.

Sears W. *The Baby Book: Everything You Need to Know about Your Baby from Birth to Age Two.* Boston, MA: Little, Brown and Company; 2003.

REMEMBER THAT PITOCIN CAN BE DANGEROUS

TERESA A. SLONIM, RN

WHAT TO DO: ASSESS AND EVALUATE

Oxytocin is a hormone secreted by the pituitary gland. It functions to stimulate milk ejection and may have a role in initiating labor during childbirth. Pitocin is the synthetic form of the hormone and is used commonly to induce labor, stimulate greater force during contractions, and is also used in the postpartum period to control hemorrhage. Pitocin is a very useful medication during the peripartum period, but as with all medications, there are contraindications and side effects do occur. The peripartum nurse needs to know how to appropriately assess and evaluate for these side effects.

Since the mother and baby are cared for as a "package" the side effects often relate to both of them. Remember that each contraction increases the pressure on the fetus as it attempts to make its descent. Hence, these contractions may be associated with hypoxia to the fetus and with asphyxia. As a result, mothers receiving pitocin are often placed on fetal heart monitoring for continuous recording of the fetal heart tones. This allows for early detection of fetal compromise or deterioration related to the administration of the drug.

Common side effects to the mother include increased pain related to the severity of the contractions.

The pain is an important symptom for the mother and may alter prior plans for a natural childbirth. The mother should be supported through this. The medication's side effects may also be manifest by "tetanic contractions," which are contractions that are longer and more intense than normal. The intensity of contractions also causes potential complications with placental insufficiency, abruption, and uterine rupture. Remember, the fetus is not immune to the effects of these contractions.

Finally, the administration of the drug may help to achieve its intended purpose—the delivery of the baby. However, the clinical effects of the drug may be unpredictable. The labor may progress more quickly than expected. Both the mother and the clinical team need to be prepared for this occurrence. Ensuring that the room and equipment are ready and monitoring for placental insufficiency, lacerations, tears, and the complications of a rapid descent are critical tasks for the nurse and the team.

SUGGESTED READINGS

http://www.childbirth.org/articles/pit.html. Accessed on April 15, 2009.
http://pregnancy.about.com/od/induction/a/risksinduction. htm. Accessed on April 15, 2009.
http://pregnancy.about.com/od/induction/a/pitocindiffers. htm. Accessed on April 15, 2009.

REMEMBER TO CONSIDER AND TEST FOR HELLP SYNDROME IN PATIENTS WITH SEVERE PREECLAMPSIA

TERESA A. SLONIM, RN

WHAT TO DO: ASSESS

Preeclampsia is an idiopathic condition of pregnancy characterized by hypertension and proteinuria which occurs after 20 weeks gestation. Preeclampsia can be classified as mild or severe depending upon the severity of the blood pressure, the degree of proteinuria, and end organ effects including visual changes, headache, reflex changes, and abnormalities in laboratory findings. Severe preeclampsia is important to diagnose and treat since it has implications for both the mother and the fetus.

The HELLP syndrome is a variant of severe preeclampsia that is characterized by Hemolysis, ELevated liver enzymes and Low Platelets and occurs in 2% to 10% of severely preeclamptic women. It increases the risk of a number of adverse outcomes including abruption of the placenta, renal and hepatic failure, maternal or fetal demise. Maternal mortality has been estimated as high as 25%.

The diagnosis of HELLP syndrome requires laboratory confirmation of a number of diagnostic tests including a platelet count <100,000, elevated liver transaminases, and hemolysis with the presence of fragmented red blood cells on the peripheral smear. The prothrombin time and partial thromboplastin time are usually normal.

Since the diagnosis depends upon laboratory testing and a high index of suspicion, it is important for the bedside nurse to be suspicious of the patient with severe preeclampsia and significantly elevated blood pressure so that appropriate testing can be performed including a complete blood count and liver function tests. Reassessment of the patient and encouragement of the physician to order appropriate testing may be important in assuring appropriate intervention.

SUGGESTED READINGS

Poole JH. Hypertensive disorders in pregnancy. In: Lowdermilk DL, Perry SE, eds. *Maternity and Women's Health Care*. 8th Ed. Philadelphia, PA: Mosby; 2004, pp. 229–237.

Stone J. HELLP syndrome: Hemolysis, elevated liver enzymes, and low platelets. *JAMA*. 1998;280:559–562.

REMEMBER TO ADMINISTER RH IMMUNE GLOBULIN AFTER MISCARRIAGE

TERESA A. SLONIM, RN

WHAT TO DO: IMPLEMENT

Rh immune globulin (IG) is administered intramuscularly to the postpartum mother and is important to prevent isoimmunization in mothers who are Rh negative and may experience transmission of Rh positive red blood cells from the fetus after delivery or during an invasive obstetrical procedure. The Rh IG helps to lyse the Rh positive cells and prevent an immune antibody response from occurring.

The Rh IG is administered intramuscularly within 72 h of birth, as prophylaxis at 28 weeks gestation or as prophylaxis for circumstances when there is the potential to have Rh positive fetal cells cross to the mother. These circumstances include amniocentesis, chorionic villous sampling, and miscarriage. A standard dosage is used. However, if there are concerns that dosage adjustment needs to be made, a Kleihauer-Betke test that identifies fetal blood in the mother can be performed.

When administering Rh IG, the nurse has several important safety checks that need to be performed. First, the lot number needs to be checked and recorded. Second, since Rh IG is usually considered a blood product, appropriate consent and cross-match needs to be performed. Finally, the expiration date on the product needs to be checked.

Rh IG is an important product to protect the mother from an immune reaction to the passage of fetal Rh positive red blood cells. While the approach is commonplace after delivery, the nurse needs to remember to administer it to the mother after miscarriage as well.

SUGGESTED READINGS

Cashion K. Nursing care of the post-partum woman. In: Lowdermilk DL, Perry SE, eds. *Maternity and Women's Health Care.* 8th Ed. Philadelphia, PA: Mosby; 2004, pp. 427–437.

KNOW WHEN TO SUSPECT AND HOW TO TREAT AMNIOTIC FLUID EMBOLISM

TERESA A. SLONIM, RN

WHAT TO DO: EVALUATE AND IMPLEMENT

Amniotic fluid embolism is a rare complication of labor or birth that results in an obstruction of the pulmonary artery by microscopic elements of the fetus and is associated with a high mortality rate. These elements may be cellular products of meconium, tissue, or hair that enter the mother's circulation and lead to respiratory distress, circulatory collapse, and coagulation problems.

The risk factors for amniotic fluid embolism include multiparity, abrupt labor, placental abruption, macrosomia, and intrauterine passage of meconium from fetal stress. The patient becomes agitated, restless, and acutely short of breath with tachycardia that progresses to respiratory failure and shock. The fetal elements activate the mother's coagulation system and lead to a bleeding diathesis.

The care is supportive and includes an assurance of the As, Bs, and Cs. The nurse needs to be sure that intravenous (IV) access is patent and that oxygen is administered. Isotonic IV fluids are administered for shock and the woman should be placed in a decubitus position to allow adequate venous return. Blood products need to be readily available and intensive care unit support is often needed. If the event occurs in the prepartum state, preparations for an emergent delivery need to be made.

Amniotic fluid embolism is an important complication that can occur in the prepartum, intrapartum, or postpartum patient. It is a devastating complication of childbirth associated with a high rate of maternal death. The nurse is instrumental in ensuring that this condition is identified, and treated, and that the mother and family are supported during this critical time.

SUGGESTED READINGS

Martin R, Leaton M. Amniotic fluid embolism. *Am J Nurs.* 2001;101:43–44.

Piotrowski KA. Labor and birth complications. In: Lowdermilk DL, Perry SE, eds. *Maternity and Women's Health Care.* 8th Ed. Philadelphia, PA: Mosby; 2004, pp. 227–289.

Preterm Labor Requires Dedicated and Supportive Care for the Mother and Fetus

Teresa A. Slonim, RN

WHAT TO DO: EVALUATE

The normal gestation for humans is 37 to 40 weeks. When the laboring process begins early, care needs to be taken of both mother and fetus, particularly if the fetus has not reached an appropriate gestational age for viability. Preterm labor is also an anxiety-provoking experience for the mother and family. Several important interventions can improve the outcomes for mothers experiencing preterm labor. The cause of the preterm labor should be investigated and a determination about stopping the contractions should be made.

The nurse caring for the preterm labor patient actually has two patients to care for, and appropriate attention needs to be directed to both mother and fetus. Many mothers are admitted to the hospital when they begin experiencing contractions and are put on activity restrictions. The fetus should be monitored to identify any distress. In addition, several interventions can be used to assist the mother. These include placing the mother on her side, supporting her emotionally through this stressful time, explaining to her the interventions that are being performed for the benefit of her baby. Direct and honest communication is important in allaying fears and answering questions. Ensuring that the mother is comfortable and vital signs are monitored to detect any changes are important. Often, tocolytic agents can be used to stop uterine contractions in the preterm patient.

Several medications are available to assist with stopping preterm labor. These include magnsesium sulfate, terbutaline, and ritodrine. The goal of terminating labor is to provide an opportunity for lung maturity or further fetal development. Magnesium is a commonly used medication to relax uterine muscles and stop premature contractions. It is administered by intravenous infusion and requires monitoring of urine output, reflexes, respiratory status, and serum levels to ensure its safe administration. If adverse reactions from magnesium occur, calcium can be administered to counteract the reactions. Terbutaline is a sympathetic agonist that is a smooth muscle relaxer and is administered subcutaneously or orally. The major adverse reactions include elevations in pulse, blood pressure, and respiratory rate. The indications for terminating preterm labor with tocolytics include a viable fetus, absence of signs of uterine infection or bleeding, and cervical dilation <6 cm.

The nurse caring for the patient with preterm labor is uniquely positioned to provide both clinical and emotional support at a very difficult time in the pregnancy. Continuous monitoring of the mother and fetus, particularly if tocolytics are being administered, needs to occur.

SUGGESTED READINGS

Piotrowski KA. Labor and birth complications. In: Lowdermilk DL, Perry SE, eds. *Maternity and Women's Health Care*. 8th Ed. Philadelphia, PA: Mosby; 2004, pp. 277–289.

Wichter P. Treatment of preterm labor. *J Perinatal Neonatal Nurs*. 2002;16:25–46.

KNOW THE RISKS ASSOCIATED WITH COMMON CONGENITAL MALFORMATIONS

TERESA A. SLONIM, RN

WHAT TO DO: PLAN

One of the most concerning aspects of pregnancy for the couple is the health and well-being of their unborn child. A congenital malformation draws on the couple's energy and emotion, placing them in a position of uncertainty about the health of their child. Some congenital malformations are associated with genetic alterations, and as maternal age increases, some of these genetic conditions also increase in frequency. However, others are not genetically transmitted and may be multifactorial in their origin, occurring as the fetus develops. It is important for the nurse to understand the risks associated with common congenital malformations to advise and counsel the pregnant or newly birthed couple. The most important thing to remember is that malformations often occur together, so the nurse should be careful about reassuring the parents since the complete constellation of findings may not be present at the outset and other malformations may present at a later date.

Obvious physical malformations may be present in the delivery room and affect many different organ systems of the body and the physical appearance of the newborn. These days, prenatal testing fortunately takes some of the uncertainty from the delivery room crisis phenomenon of needing to explain a malformation to the new parents. However, there are still occasions when a malformation may not have been known in the prenatal period. These malformations range from mild, such as web toes or extra digits, to major malformations including cleft lip and palate, neural tube defects, or abdominal wall defects. It becomes incumbent upon the nurse to provide a supportive role in the care of the parents by providing them with comfort, counsel, and guidance while making decisions. The parents experience a feeling of loss and grief because they fear that the dreams and expectations they held for their unborn child will be unrealized. The nurse has an important role in providing realistic expectations, encouragement, and support at this crucial time and engaging the parents in the important decisions that will need to be made on behalf of the baby.

While physically obvious malformations may be devastating, the presence of physical malformations that are internal may be equally devastating and just as severe even though they may not be visible. For example, congenital cardiac malformations are one of the more common congenital conditions of childhood and may present abruptly with cyanosis and shock shortly after delivery or in the period after birth with difficulty feeding, failure to thrive, respiratory distress, or a murmur identified in the nursery. While physically the baby may look "normal," there is no way for the nurse to predict the extent of the condition since further diagnostic testing will be needed. Comforting the parents through the uncertainty and potential loss of their child is important. Often, there is a long road ahead for these families consisting of multiple hospital stays, procedures, surgeries, and medications. Depending on the lesion, many children do very well and live normal life expectancies. However, the bedside nurse in the delivery room or nursery is not in a position to predict the outcome and needs to be supportive of the unknown.

The obstetrical nurse needs to know the common congenital malformations, their risks and supportive strategies, and how to counsel and educate the new parents when these conditions arise in their child during the peripartum period.

SUGGESTED READINGS

Chandler M, Smith A. Prenatal screening and women's perception of infant disability: A Sophie's choice for every mother. *Nurs Inq.* 1998;5:71–76.

Information and resources for the CHD community. Available at: http://www.congenitalheartdefects.com/. Accessed August 16, 2008.

Riper MV. Genetics. In: Lowdermilk DL, Perry SE, eds. *Maternity and Women's Health Care.* 8th Ed. Philadelphia, PA: Mosby; 2004, pp. 15–21.

TEACH EVERY WOMAN BREAST SELF-EXAMINATION...
YOU MAY SAVE A LIFE

TERESA A. SLONIM, RN

WHAT TO DO: IMPLEMENT

Breast cancer was diagnosed in nearly 187,000 women and was the fifth leading cause of death in 2004. The best time to provide effective care is when the diagnosis is made. Therefore, the identification of early breast cancer becomes an important strategy in improving mortality from this devastating disease. Breast self examination is an effective strategy for improving early detection.

Breast self examination should be taught to adolescent girls so that they can begin to practice the technique and create a lifelong habit of monthly examination. The familiarity of the woman with her breasts also improves her ability to detect subtle changes, often before their healthcare provider, and bring it to appropriate attention.

Breast self examination should be performed monthly, usually after the woman's period. Many women find it easier to perform the examination while showering; however, there are also components that can be performed in front of the mirror or in bed. The woman should begin with a visual inspection in front of the mirror for asymmetry, discharge, redness, swelling, or nipple irregularities. The examination can then include palpation of the breasts. Many women find it easier to use a soaped hand and a circular motion in all quadrants of the breast tissue including the "tail" that arises into the axilla. The pads of the finger tips should be used and a firm touch should be applied. The nipple should be squeezed between the fingers and thumb to express discharge. The approach is not as important as the need to assure that the woman uses a methodical approach that captures all areas of the breast. Identified areas of concern should be brought to the attention of a healthcare provider.

Not all identified masses are serious and the nurse can provide support for the woman who has identified an area of concern. After a physical examination by a healthcare provider, several diagnostic approaches can be used depending upon the age of the patient and the suspicion of the mass. An ultrasound can be used to asses a mass and determine if it is cystic in nature. Mammography is another technique that is helpful and should be performed as a routine screening modality every 1 to 3 years for women >40 years old.

While breast self examination by itself does not improve the mortality from breast cancer, in combination with clinical breast examination by a healthcare provider and appropriate diagnostic testing, it can improve the outcome. Nonetheless, there is value in having a woman understand her body and be able to identify changes and suspicious areas for further evaluation by her providers.

SUGGESTED READINGS

Breast cancer: Statistics. Available at: http://www.cdc.gov/cancer/breast/statistics/. Accessed August 16, 2008.

Mammography guidelines and recommendations and rationale for screening for breast cancer. Available at: http://yenoh93.medceu.com/index/courses/MammographyGuidelines.htm. Accessed August 16, 2008.

USE APPROPRIATE CARE IN A SPECULUM EXAMINATION

TERESA A. SLONIM, RN

A speculum is a useful piece of equipment for accomplishing an internal examination of the female reproductive organs and accomplishing the completion of the Papanicolaou (Pap) smear for the detection of cervical cancer. Unfortunately, many providers do not take appropriate care in the use of a speculum during a pelvic examination, which by its nature is already an uncomfortable procedure for many women.

There are a number of important preparatory steps that can be performed to ready the woman for examination. First, the woman should be made comfortable, asked to urinate prior to the procedure, placed in a room that has an appropriate temperature and provided with a gown and sheet to provide appropriate modesty and respect, and provided with techniques to assist with relaxation. Second, the tray needs to include all the equipment, supplies, and cultures that are needed so that there are no interruptions or unnecessary delays once the examination begins. Third, the speculum should be warmed and lubricated with water. Its insertion needs to be guided slowly through the introitus with care so that skin is not pinched. The woman should be encouraged to breathe slowly through her mouth. A valsalva may assist with the entry of the speculum.

Once the speculum is seated appropriately, the blades can be opened for the inspection of the cervix and the collection of specimens. Again, care during the opening and locking of the blades needs to taken since skin and tissues may be pinched or abraised during this procedure. After appropriate examination and specimen collection, the removal of the speculum also requires care. It should be unlocked, the blades allowed to collapse (ensure that the cervix is not entrapped in the ends of the blades), and withdrawn carefully, providing appropriate attention so that skin, hair, and tissue are not pulled or injured during the procedure.

A speculum examination is an important healthcare procedure. However, it is also uncomfortable for the patient. Nurses performing this examination require due diligence in the performance of the procedure to ensure that the woman is not injured or made unduly uncomfortable during the procedure.

SUGGESTED READINGS

Guide to a comfortable speculum exam. Project prepare: An innovative approach to breast and pelvic education. Available at: http://www.projectprepare.org/speculum.html. Accessed August 16, 2008.

Zdanuk JL. Assessment and health promotion. In: Lowdermilk DL, Perry SE, eds. *Maternity and Women's Health Care*. 8th Ed. Philadelphia, PA: Mosby; 2004, pp. 25–39.

KNOW THE SIGNS AND SYMPTOMS FOR AN ABUSIVE RELATIONSHIP

TERESA A. SLONIM, RN

WHAT TO DO: ASSESS AND EVALUATE

The nurse who focuses her career on women's health issues plays a pivotal role in assuring that women get the care they need and deserve. The traditional aspects of the health assessment for women include attention to medical and surgical conditions, medications and allergies, family and social history, and a menstrual and birth history. A physical assessment includes attention to the traditional aspects such as the examination of the skin, heart, and lungs, and abdominal examination, but also specific aspects such as the examination of the breasts and pelvis. With domestic violence estimated to occur in approximately 15% of women that present to healthcare providers for evaluation, the nurse who is concerned about domestic violence needs to be able to recognize the signs, assess its severity, and ensure the safety and follow-up of the victim. These occurrences have both short-and long-term consequences and represent an opportunity for the nurse to not only save a life, but also improve the quality of a life and support a family in crisis.

The assessment of the woman who presents for care should always include an assessment for potential abuse. Anxiety, returns for repeated evaluations, a changing story about injuries, bruises, hesitancy, and fear all characterize the range of findings in the victim of domestic violence. The nurse is required to have a high index of suspicion and recognize the constellation of signs and symptoms that characterize this syndrome. Once identified, the priority shifts to ensuring the victim's safety,

which may require the separation from the domestic partner, the involvement of police, and the finding of temporary housing. The nurse needs an appreciation for the duration of abuse, the kinds of abuse, and the pattern and severity of occurrences so that she can identify potential physical injuries by recommending appropriate diagnostic testing and identifying potential emotional injuries for counseling. Understanding the other members of the family unit, including children, is necessary so that appropriate measures for their protection are ensured. An assessment of the future safety of the victim and family needs to be made so that the woman is not discharged to the abusive relationship.

The care of the domestic violence victim includes a multidisciplinary approach including nurses, physicians, social workers, law enforcement, and counselors. The priority is ensuring the victim's present and future safety. Attention to the physical and emotional injuries and scars requires long-term counseling and empowerment of the victim.

SUGGESTED READINGS

Domestic violence assessment and intervention provided by the family violence prevention fund. National Association of Social Workers. Available at: http://www.socialworkers.org/pressroom/events/domestic_violence/assessment.asp. Accessed August 16, 2008.

Domestic violence homicide risk assessment. Women's Justice Center. 2004. Available at: http://www.justicewomen.com/dv_risk_assess.pdf. Accessed August 16, 2008.

Evaluating domestic violence programs. Available at: http://www.ahrq.gov/research/domesticviol/. Accessed August 16, 2008.

Endometriosis can Mimic a Number of Acute Intra-Abdominal Processes

Teresa A. Slonim, RN

WHAT TO DO: ASSESS

Endometriosis occurs when endometrial tissue is implanted in an extrauterine location, usually somewhere in the abdomen or pelvis. The patient may be asymptomatic or may experience abdominal or pelvic pain, symptoms of gastrointestinal illness including nausea, vomiting, and diarrhea. The pain is usually cyclical, occurring with the woman's menstrual cycle when the endometrium becomes hormonally active and may lead to changes in the pattern of bleeding. Depending on the location of the endometriosis, the pain may be exacerbated by sexual intercourse, exercise, and other routine activities.

Many women with endometriosis are asymptomatic, but others may experience disabling abdominal pain that mimics other acute intra-abdominal processes like acute appendicitis, ovarian torsion, diverticulitis, cholecystitis, and nephrolithiasis. This differential becomes important, particularly if the woman does not have a clear history of endometriosis or a pattern has not developed. The nurse must ensure that an appropriate assessment is performed including the location, quality, radiation, and temporizing and relieving factors. Importantly, cyclical symptoms in conjunction with the menstrual period can assist with the diagnosis. On occasion, laboratory and diagnostic testing may be performed, particularly if the symptoms are new in onset and the patient presents to the emergency department. For established endometriosis, the management is supportive, with many women achieving relief from non steroidal anti-inflammatory agents and rest. If severe, the patient may benefit from hormonal manipulation or perhaps even surgery. Endometriosis can lead to adhesions. So, it is important to rule out acute intra-abdominal processes, not only because of the similarities in pain, but also because the adhesions caused by endometriosis may cause intra-abdominal pathology that leads to an acute abdominal condition.

An assessment including a thorough history and physical examination is important for the woman with suspected or established endometriosis to ensure that there is no acute intra-abdominal process. Nurses can play an important role in assuring that this condition is not missed.

SUGGESTED READINGS

Fogel CI. Reproductive system concerns. In: Lowdermilk DL, Perry SE, eds. *Maternity and Women's Health Care*. 8th Ed. Philadelphia, PA: Mosby; 2004, pp. 47–57.
Nakad T, Isaacson K. Endometriosis. In: Carlson K, ed. *Primary Care of Women*. 2nd Ed. St. Louis, MO: Mosby; 2002.

LOOK AT THE PLACENTA...IT MAY PROVIDE INSIGHTS INTO WHAT IS WRONG WITH THE NEWBORN

TERESA A. SLONIM, RN

WHAT TO DO: ASSESS

The placenta functions as the baby's lifeline during pregnancy. An examination of the placenta after a seemingly uneventful pregnancy and birth can provide some additional insights into what the baby may have experienced (or is about to experience). There are several descriptions about the placenta that may be helpful.

There are a number of ways in which the umbilical cord inserts abnormally into the placenta; each one of these may jeopardize the easy flow of blood between the fetus and the mother. A velamentous insertion has the cord inserted into the amniotic membranes and not the substance of the placenta itself. These vessels are prone to rupture and the fetus may experience blood loss and hemorrhage. In a circumvallate placenta, there is an abnormal extension of the placental tissue beyond the margins. This can lead to peripartum bleeding.

The shape and characteristics of the placenta itself can provide important information. If twins or triplets are born, the placenta can provide information regarding monozygosity of the twins. Chorioamnionitis is an infection of the amniotic fluid. These infants may have peripartum difficulties and be born through amniotic fluid that is discolored or foul in odor. A placenta from a pregnancy affected by chorioamnionitis is likewise affected and may be discolored as well. An amnion nodosum is a specific finding of the placenta where it is covered with nodules. In this case, renal agenesis and Potters syndrome are the diseases that present themselves in infancy. Finally, placental infarction compromises the oxygenation and nutrition of the fetus and may jeopardize intrauterine growth, providing an explanation for the infant's size.

The placenta is an important part of the peripartum examination. The delivery room and nursery nurse should become familiar with the different appearances of the placenta and its implications for the baby.

SUGGESTED READINGS

Balsan MJ, Holzman IR. Neonataology. In: Zitelli BJ, Davis HW, eds. *Atlas of Pediatric Physical Diagnosis*. St. Louis, MO: Mosby; 1993, pp. 2.1–2.19.

FACILITATE MATERNAL–INFANT BONDING ESPECIALLY WHEN THERE ARE RISKS TO IT

TERESA A. SLONIM, RN

WHAT TO DO: IMPLEMENT

Often, healthcare providers become wrapped up in the needs to accomplish tasks and document findings. While these are important to the practice of nursing, one needs to remember that the nurse in the delivery room or newborn nursery has a role that transcends the years of motherhood that lie ahead of the patient and her baby. As a result, the nurse should be aware of problems with maternal–fetal bonding and be ready to intervene to protect and foster this relationship.

The stresses on maternal–infant bonding (MIB) begin long before its birth in the delivery room. The mother may be at risk because she is an adolescent, unmarried, or financially dependent. The pregnancy may have been unwanted and the mother may have made a decision regarding abortion, adoption, or delivery that she must now live with. Perhaps, she is questioning her decision or contemplating her ability to be a "good" parent. The mother's social support network may be unstable. The baby's father may not be present or engaged in the pregnancy. Even if present, the mother may perceive this to be because of guilt and not his interest in her or the baby.

After delivery, these issues are magnified, particularly if the mother or baby has problems during the delivery. If the mother and baby are unhealthy, additional barriers to bonding may occur. The mother may experience depression or mood disorders and struggle with their management. She may be unsuccessful at breast feeding. In these circumstances, isolation and loneliness are of concern, particularly if the mother does not have a support network. The infant may be vulnerable to abuse if this cycle continues.

The nurse has an obligation in the delivery room and nursery to encourage, complement, and facilitate the bonding of the mother with her baby. Encourage self care, breast feeding, and demonstrate how to perform these roles. Complement the mother for a job well done and coach her when difficulties arise. Assess her abilities, support network, and her relationship with the baby's father and her social network. Identify risks to bonding early and provide appropriate consultation, networking, and follow-up since the baby's life may depend upon it. Mothers who fail to bond effectively with their infants experience higher rates of abuse. Most importantly, let her know that she is not alone, and if at risk, provide her with meaningful community support. If you do not know the resources, provide guidance with the help of social services and the pediatrician. Ensure that you communicate your concerns with appropriate members of the team so that appropriate follow-up can occur after discharge.

MIB is a fundamental postpartum process, but a number of factors can jeopardize this important period. The nurse needs to recognize this important timeframe, identify risk factors to its success, foster the development of the new mother and her bonding with her infant, and foster appropriate postdischarge follow-up to ensure success.

SUGGESTED READING

Olsson J. The newborn. In: Kliegman RM, Jenseon HB, Behrman RE, et al., eds. *Nelson Textbook of Pediatrics*. 18th Ed. Philadelphia, PA: Saunders; 2007, pp. 41–43.

Know how to support the adolescent female (and her mother) during her first gynecologic examination

Teresa A. Slonim, RN

WHAT TO DO: IMPLEMENT

A gynecologic examination is often a memorable, yet, unpleasant event in a woman's life. Nurses can provide important support to the adolescent female who is presenting for her first examination by being honest, open, and direct in their approach.

Adolescent females often present for gynecologic care and the need for a rapport with these patients is important. A friendly face, a supportive environment, and an opportunity to ask questions and receive open and honest answers from a caring professional are some of the most rewarding aspects of providing gynecologic care to adolescents. Whether the reason for the visit is a complaint like vaginal bleeding or discharge or a routine evaluation, the adolescent needs a caring professional to deliver the care.

The skilled nurse can use this time to assess important aspects of gynecologic health. Is the patient sexually active, what does she know about sexually transmitted diseases, does she know if her mother or grandmother had any health problems or trouble with fertility? The questions need to be asked in an age-appropriate, yet, open manner. The adolescent's body is going through dramatic changes. She may have concerns about her breasts, vaginal discharge, or pubertal development. Inquire about her friends and relationships. If you demonstrate comfort with these conversations, she will be more likely to open up and ask questions that concern her.

The examination should be performed without the parents, making the role of the nurse much more important. The procedure should be explained, the equipment can be demonstrated, and the adolescent's modesty preserved. Clear communication from the physician and nurse to the patient during the examination is important.

A female chaperone should be present during the examination. Ask the patient to disrobe and provide appropriate gown and cover. She can be assisted to the dorsal lithotomy position and appropriately draped. Hold her hand and encourage her. Tell her how well she is doing and let her see your face. Explain the procedure to her. Encourage deep breaths, particularly during insertion of a speculum. When the examination is done, help her up and allow her to get dressed. After the results of the examination have been explained to her, ask her if she has any questions for you about the examination or other aspects of gynecologic health. This is often a good time to provide guidance about contraception, sexually transmitted diseases, and gynecologic health including human papillomavirus prevention.

SUGGESTED READINGS

Hewitt GD. The young woman's initial gynecological visit. The female patient. Available at: http://www.femalepatient.com/html/arc/sig/adoles/articles/031_09_025.asp. Accessed August 24, 2008.

Sanfilippo JS. Gynecologic problems of childhood: History and physical examination. In: Kliegman RM, Jenseon HB, Behrman RE, et al., eds. *Nelson Textbook of Pediatrics.* 18th Ed. Philadelphia, PA: Saunders; 2007, pp. 2273–2290.

KNOW HOW TO MANAGE THE ACUTELY TRAUMATIZED PREGNANT WOMAN

TERESA A. SLONIM, RN

WHAT TO DO: IMPLEMENT

Pregnancy is an important time in a woman's life. The pregnant woman prepares for motherhood and establishes an important role for herself during the pregnancy. When acute trauma intervenes, providers need an understanding of the physiologic changes, and also need to recognize how to manage the pregnant condition and for both the mother and fetus. The care of the acutely traumatized pregnant woman requires a multi-disciplinary team of providers including trauma surgeons, emergency department personnel, neonatologists, obstetrical personnel, and maternal–fetal medicine specialists. The mechanism of injury is important to consider in the pregnant woman. Blunt trauma to the abdomen may directly affect the fetus depending upon its severity. Penetrating trauma that violates the uterus often is poorly tolerated by the fetus. Pregnancy does not change the approach to the traumatized patient; a consideration of the As, Bs, Cs, and neurologic injury are the same, but an awareness of some important differences can be crucial in the acute setting.

Attention to airway, breathing, and circulation is critical for the traumatized woman. Particularly related to the assessment of "circulation," providers need to remember to position pregnant women on their side to allow adequate venous return from the lower extremities and enhance cardiac output. If there is concern for neurologic injury, appropriate techniques can be employed and the woman then log-rolled on the spine board to ensure adequate venous return. An assessment of heart tones of the fetus needs to be performed on every pregnant patient with trauma. This may require obstetrical personnel to come to the trauma bay. Of importance, consideration of both patients and the care of each needs to be considered when the pregnant trauma patient arrives.

Some important caveats regarding pregnancy and trauma need to be understood. First, pregnancy should be considered in any acutely traumatized young woman of child bearing age. In some situations, the patient may be as young as the 12–14-year-old child or the woman in her mid-to-late 40s. By asking about the last menstrual period, the nurse will have an understanding of a potentially pregnant patient and her needs. If the patient is unconscious, does not remember, or is nonspecific, a pregnancy test should be obtained. Second, the plasma, blood volume, and cardiac output are all increased in the pregnant woman. Therefore, typical signs of impending shock, including tachycardia and hypotension may present relatively late in the course of illness and may be unreliable indicators of the need for therapy. Third, the gravid uterus exits the pelvis at approximately the 12th week of pregnancy, beyond which point, the fetus becomes more susceptible to abdominal trauma. As the pregnancy progresses to the second and third trimesters, the infant grows inside the uterus, occupying more and more of its internal space and becoming more susceptible to maternal trauma. As the uterus grows, it also changes the relationships of intra-abdominal organs, influencing their function and susceptibility to injury as well.

Remember that the trauma patient requires an approach that is similar to other trauma patients, but that some specific changes related to pregnancy also need to be considered.

SUGGESTED READINGS

Trauma in women. In: *Advanced Trauma Life Support Student Course Manual*. 7th Ed. Chicago, IL: American College of Surgeons, Committee on Trauma Illinois; 2005, pp. 275–282.

THE NURSE IN THE DELIVERY ROOM NEEDS THE KNOWLEDGE, A PLAN, AND THE SKILLS TO CARE FOR A DEPRESSED NEWBORN

TERESA A. SLONIM, RN

WHAT TO DO: ASSESS, PLAN, AND IMPLEMENT

Delivery room (DR) care of the newborn is usually straightforward. Most babies are born to young healthy women, accompanied by caring partners at one of the most joyous times in life, the birth of a child. However, things may not always proceed as planned and the result may be a depressed newborn that needs resuscitation in addition to normal newborn care. The nurse in the DR needs to know what to do and how to do it to effectively resuscitate the newborn.

In the DR, the sound of a wailing infant is usually met with gratification by the staff, parent, and families, all of whom have been waiting for months for the moment to arrive. The dreams, ambitions, and fears all come together in a rush of emotion at that very moment. Some parents may not know the gender of their infant and may need to choose between a girl's name and a boy's name. Among the fears may be concerns for a congenital anomaly, the need to count ten fingers and ten toes for reassurance. Eager grandparents wait for the answers to their questions that both mom and grandbaby are alright. But when the cry doesn't start spontaneously, the mother, father, and DR staff all recognize that something may be wrong, and the nurse needs to be prepared to step in.

Prior to each delivery, the nurse should assure that the DR is appropriately prepared with the necessary equipment and personnel. The overbed warmer turned on to an appropriate temperature, dry towels, oxygen delivery and suction equipment, a bag valve system and appropriately sized masks, intubation equipment, resuscitation medications with appropriate delivery equipment, and most importantly, personnel skilled in the care of the newborn requiring resuscitation need to be present.

The approach to the infant in the DR begins with a rapid primary assessment and an approach to the As, Bs, and Cs. While the assessment takes place, the baby is warmed, dried, and stimulated, usually under an overbed warmer paying particular attention to the infant's inability to maintain normothermia. The baby is placed on its back with the head slightly lower than the trunk. A rolled towel may be placed under the shoulders to elevate the head. The airway is positioned and suctioned. Oxygen is provided to the spontaneously breathing infant during these initial phases of the resuscitation.

Relatively quickly, an assessment of the adequacy of breathing needs to be made. In most instances, this is done with attention to the breathing rate and whether it is in the normal range of 40 to 60, the presence of cyanosis or if the baby is "pinking up," and the depth and pattern of respirations appropriate for a newborn to accommodate to postuterine life. Alterations in these areas may imply difficulty with adapting to postuterine life, congenital heart disease, or transient respiratory problems of the newborn that need to be addressed. But, for now, the nurse needs to intervene and consider the possibilities later. Ineffective respirations require bag mask ventilation and may require tracheal intubation. In the newborn, the heart rate is heavily dependent on oxygenation, so the nurse can monitor the heart rate and improve ventilation based upon the heart rate responses. If the heart rate is <100, bag mask ventilation and oxygen should be provided.

After attention to breathing is accomplished, attention should turn to the circulatory system. The heart rate in the newborn is easily palpated at the umbilical stump. In the DR, heart rates <60 require an intervention with chest compressions and continued ventilation and oxygen delivery. If, despite these interventions, the heart rate remains <60, then medications, specifically epinephrine, should be administered. The APGAR scoring system needs to be used at 1 and 5 min to adequately assess the infant, but the nurse should not be distracted from the resuscitation to perform the APGAR.

Resuscitation in the DR is occasionally needed to assist the newborn in accommodating to extrauterine life. When this occurs, the nurse needs to be prepared and know when and how to intervene.

SUGGESTED READINGS

Neonatal resuscitation. In: *American Heart Association and American Academy: Pediatrics PALS Provider Manual*. Washington, DC: American Heart Association Press; 2002, pp. 337–358.

KNOW WHAT TO DO TO SUPPORT HIGH RISK MOTHERS WITH HEART DISEASE

TERESA A. SLONIM, RN

WHAT TO DO: IMPLEMENT

Pregnancy is a stressful time for a woman, not only emotionally, but also physically. While there is stress placed on all of the mother's body systems, the cardiovascular system goes through extensive changes with increases in blood volume, red cell mass, heart rate, and cardiac output, reductions in systemic vascular resistance, and the major changes that occur with the birth of a child. For a mother with a structurally normal and healthy heart, these changes are accommodated easily. For the mother with structural disease, including problems with valves, muscle, or sympathetics, pregnancy may represent an important and problematic time period.

Many women with cardiac disease during pregnancy can be classified according to the New York Heart Association (NYHA) functional classification system, which ranges from 1 to 4 depending on the severity of symptoms at various levels of activity. A "1" represents the normal or asymptomatic patient whereas a "4" represents severe functional impairment even at rest.

With newer and more modern approaches, pregnant women with heart disease can be supported throughout their pregnancy to deliver healthy infants.

There are conditions in which pregnancy is contraindicated because of the increased risk to the mother or fetus. These include pulmonary hypertension, complex cyanotic congenital heart disease, coarctation of the aorta, Marfan syndrome with aortic dissection, and poor ventricular function.

Pregnant women with heart disease may experience problems in their babies related to appropriate growth, development, and attainment of weight. In addition, mothers with congenital cardiac disease are more likely to have babies with congenital heart disease. The nurse plays a pivotal role in counseling women with heart disease who become pregnant before, during, and after their pregnancy. The nurse also has a role in ensuring that the mother receives appropriate physiologic support and understands her condition, medications, and ways to improve her overall health status. During the peripartum period, the nurses must ensure that they are prepared to take care of the mother's physiologic status and support her during the birth and afterwards.

SUGGESTED READINGS

Genovese SK. Antepartal hemorrhagic disorders. In: Lowdermilk DL, Perry SE, eds. *Maternity and Women's Health Care*. 8th Ed. Philadlephia, PA: Mosby; 2004, pp. 237–245.

KNOW HOW TO ADDRESS THIRD TRIMESTER BLEEDING

TERESA A. SLONIM, RN

WHAT TO DO: ASSESS AND IMPLEMENT

One of the more frightening experiences for a couple is vaginal bleeding that occurs late in pregnancy. In an instant, their hopes and dreams of the pregnancy and their unborn child become jeopardized. The delivery room nurse needs to have a working knowledge of the causes of late pregnancy bleeding and know when and how to intervene for the safety of the fetus, the mother, and the family.

A woman who presents for care in the third trimester with vaginal bleeding needs a quick assessment of the history to identify the potential causes. The mother should be assessed for stability, the hemodynamic status, and the condition of the fetus through fetal monitoring. An intravenous line can be started to ensure patency and a blood count, type, and crossmatch, and coagulation studies can be performed while the type of bleeding is identified.

Placenta previa is a condition that places the placenta near or over the internal os of the cervix. As a result, the heavily vascular structure of the placenta can cause abrupt onset of painless vaginal bleeding. Neither the mother nor infant may show signs of compromise and the uterus may be relaxed, but that does not lessen the urgency of this situation. An ultrasound examination should be performed to identify the location of the placenta. Once a normally implanted placenta is identified, a speculum examination looking for other causes of bleeding can be considered.

Placental abruption is another cause of bleeding in the third trimester that can have serious consequences. In these instances, the placenta begins to prematurely separate from the uterine wall. Placental abruption can be classified as mild, moderate, or severe depending upon the condition of the uterus, the degree of separation, and the condition of the mother and fetus. While bleeding may be obvious, there are also times when the bleeding may be covert. Other symptoms including pain, tenderness, and cardiovascular instability are common.

For either of these serious conditions of pregnancy, an action plan for delivery can be established once the diagnosis is made. The plan will depend upon the gestational age and condition of the fetus, maternal condition, ongoing blood loss, and presence of labor. If expectant management is decided, reevaluation of the mother and fetus need to be performed at regular intervals with a plan for urgent intervention as needed.

SUGGESTED READINGS

Genovese SK. Antepartal hemorrhagic disorders. In: Lowdermilk DL, Perry SE, eds. *Maternity and Women's Health Care*. 8th Ed. Philadelphia, PA: Mosby; 2004, pp. 237–245.

KNOW HOW TO OBTAIN LAB SPECIMENS FROM A NEWBORN

TERESA A. SLONIM, RN

There are occassionaly needs for important diagnostic testing to be performed on newborn infants. These include laboratory and radiology results. Not only are the specimens more difficult to obtain in this population, but they can also lead to diagnostic and procedural problems if done incorrectly.

The collection of blood specimens usually occurs by heelstick. It is relatively easy to perform, but may require the warming of the baby's heel to increase the circulation and ensure that there is ample blood for the specimen. It is important to have firm support on the infant, cleanse the area appropriately, and insert the lancet. The outer surfaces of the medial or lateral heel should be used. One of the most important complications from this procedure is necrotizing osteochondritis, which occurs when the lancet punctures the bone. Diagnostically, heelsticks are used to assess a hematocrit, glucose, capillary blood gas, and bilirubin levels, and may be, even electrolytes. Several problems may arise with the results of this testing. It is not uncommon for the sample from a heelstick to be hemolyzed, hence, the results of some laboratory tests like potassium may be falsely elevated.

When a venipuncture is performed for blood sampling, the arms, hands, and feet can be used. If an intravenous is running, the sample should not be drawn above the level of the IV. In addition, care should be exercised in "poking" around with the needle in the arm since this can lead to arterial puncture, nerve injury, and tissue damage.

A routine urine specimen can be obtained by placing a bag with adhesive in the perineal area for collection of the urine. It is important to remember that the technique depends upon the reason for the sample. If a specimen is needed for culture, a urinary catheterization may need to be performed. The collection of spinal fluid to rule out sepsis is an important and frequently performed procedure on babies. After cleansing of the area, a needle is placed in the lumbar interspaces to collect the specimen. Spinal fluid is usually clear and colorless in the normal baby, but may be colored and cloudy in the presence of infection. It is important to label the specimens and assure that the specific tests are appropriately ordered.

Some parents choose to have a circumcision performed for their sons. The surgical removal of the foreskin is a commonly applied nursery procedure with very low risk. The major complication is bleeding. In some patients, the presence of a bleeding diathesis may first become apparent during circumcision. Another important thing to remember is that previously, babies were not thought to experience pain. Now, there are reliable methods to address discomfort in babies undergoing painful procedures and the nurse should be fluent in their use and encourage the physician to use them for the sake of the baby.

The nurse will encounter procedures in the nursery and knowing the common approaches and pitfalls can help care for our most fragile patients.

SUGGESTED READINGS

Alden KR. Nursing care of the newborn. In: Lowdermilk DL, Perry SE, eds. *Maternity and Women's Health Care.* 8th Ed. Philadelphia, PA: Mosby; 2004.

KNOW HOW TO ASSESS THE NEWBORN INFANT

TERESA A. SLONIM, RN

WHAT TO DO: ASSESS AND EVALUATE

The assessment of the newborn infant is a fundamental job for the nurse in the delivery room and nursery, but because of the overwhelming number of "normal" newborns that are born in comparison to the number of ill newborns, the assessment gets skewed toward normal. Nurses in these settings need to be able to identify problems in three major areas, the normal newborn examination, attention to congenital conditions, and the premature newborn examination.

An assessment of the normal newborn begins with the As, Bs, and Cs of airway, breathing, and circulation. Newborns that are adapting well to postnatal life usually handle them without difficulty. Then, a head-to-toe assessment of the newborn's condition becomes important. An assessment of the gestational age, size, weight, anthropometric measurements, development, and reflexes needs to be performed. The nurse needs to recognize when there is a disparity between the report of a full term baby and the presentation of a much smaller infant with growth retardation. In addition, specifics like an understanding of birthmarks or physical findings related to the delivery itself such as cephalohematoma need to be assessed. There are important findings, particularly on the skin of the newborn, that may be normal. If the nurse has any doubts, she should consult other professionals since you can be sure that the parents will find out and want to know what it is.

The newborn assessment is also the time when the identification of congenital anomalies is most evident. After assessing hundreds of normal newborns, the identification of anomalies is important. It may start as simply as a question about the baby's facies, which may unravel a genetic syndrome. There may be obvious physical deformities like cleft lips or palates. The nurse has an obligation during the newborn assessment to remember the potential congenital anomalies and identify them if they exist. Evaluation of the head, eyes, ears, nose, and mouth followed by a cardiopulmonary examination with an assessment of murmurs and circulation is critical. The abdomen and pelvis can be evaluated next with attention to patency of the anus and evaluation of the genitalia. Finally, the extremities can be examined, identifying the number of digits on the limbs.

For the preterm newborn, the assessment becomes more complicated. These babies will often emerge with alterations in their vital signs, including their airway, breathing, and circulation. They stand the potential to be at higher risk for congenital anomalies. The cause for preterm birth is unknown and congenital anomalies are one etiology that needs to be ruled out. Finally, there are alterations in their physical examination due to preterm birth that need to be considered by the nurse. The presence of an odor on the baby, and the color of its skin and umbilical stump may provide clues to why preterm delivery occurred, and also provide insights into what may need to be done for the infant.

The newborn examination is a patient safety event waiting to happen. For the nurse that normally cares for well babies, there is a need to remain hypervigilant so that the subtle heart murmur is not missed. Nurses who are in crisis mode because of the frequency of dealing with ill preterm newborns need to be thorough in their assessment so that they do not get distracted by the As, Bs, and Cs and miss an obvious congenital malformation.

SUGGESTED READINGS

Alden KR. Nursing care of the newborn. In: Lowdermilk DL, Perry SE, eds. *Maternity and Women's Health Care*. 8th Ed. Philadelphia, PA: Mosby; 2004.

THE APGAR SCORE CAN PROVIDE AN OBJECTIVE MEANS OF COMMUNICATING A NEWBORN INFANT'S STATUS

TERESA A. SLONIM, RN

WHAT TO DO: ASSESS AND EVALUATE

Experienced nurses become really good at quickly identifying patients that are in trouble. This nursing intuition allows a quick appraisal of the situation and an almost automated response to the patient. The problem is that while often their intuition is correct, providers with whom they work have to deal with a range of nurses with different skills and expertise and as a result, a statement that a patient "doesn't look good" does not provide a lot of specificity for action to their colleagues. Nurses need a mechanism by which they can provide specific, objective, and direct information for their colleagues so that they can assist in caring for patients.

The APGAR score, created by Dr Apgar, is one such mechanism that has become so well entrenched in delivery room and nursery care that providers from all disciplines know its components and what a particular score means for a newborn infant. This is a mechanism to get everyone "on the same page" with a simple, yet reliable, means of communication.

The APGAR score rates a newborn's vital statistics across five dimensions, each with a score from 0 to 2. The maximum score is 10. Scores of 0–3 represent a severely distressed infant, 4–6 a moderately distressed infant, and 7–10 as one that is essentially without obvious distress. The infant is scored at 1 and 5 min after birth. Additional assessments can be made based on the need from the first two scores. The components of the APGAR score include heart rate, respiratory rate, muscle tone, reflex irritability, and appearance. Nurses who routinely work in the nursery or delivery room know when an infant is in trouble, and using the APGAR score gives them a reliable and objective means to communicate that to others at multiple stages in the care of the infant.

SUGGESTED READINGS

Alden KR. Nursing care of the newborn. In: Lowdermilk DL, Perry SE, eds. *Maternity and Women's Health Care*. 8th Ed. Philadelphia, PA: Mosby; 2004.

Casey B, McIntire D, Leveno K. The continuing value of the APGAR score for the assessment of newborn infants. *N Engl J Med*. 2001;344(7):467–471.

REMEMBER THAT PREGNANCY IS THE MOST COMMON CAUSE OF SECONDARY AMENORRHEA

TERESA A. SLONIM, RN

WHAT TO DO: ASSESS AND EVALUATE

Amenorrhea is the absence of menses and is classified as primary or secondary. Primary amenorrhea occurs when menarche has not occurred by 16 years of age. Secondary amenorrhea occurs when menses stop for three or more cycles or duration of 6 months. Of the two, primary amenorrhea is less common and may be associated with hormonal or anatomic problems that need to be investigated. Secondary amenorrhea may also occur for a variety of reasons, but the condition that needs to be ruled out first is pregnancy.

While many women keep track of their menstrual cycles, others have difficulty because of irregular cycles. Hence, it may not be unusual for them to go 30 or 60 days before becoming concerned. When one of these women presents for evaluation, a pregnancy test still needs to be performed to ensure that an unknown pregnancy is not the cause of the amenorrhea. Once this is done, a workup for other reasons can be undertaken.

Situational factors play a major role in the development of secondary amenorrhea. Stress, fatigue, excessive exercise, dietary deficiencies, and eating disorders may all lead to amenorrhea.

Hormonal reasons are another major reason for secondary amenorrhea and of them, problems with the thyroid are the most common. Hypothyroidism can present with a constellation of symptoms in addition to the amenorrhea, including fatigue, skin changes, weight gain, and temperature changes. Hypothyroidism can be tested for relatively easily with a blood test for a serum thyroid stimulating hormone. Other hormonal problems can lead to menstrual irregularities including the loss of menses. These include hyperprolactinemia syndromes and pituitary disorders.

Finally, medications can also cause menses to cease. Many medications administered to treat psychiatric illness can alter the hormonal response and lead to amenorrhea. Therefore, a drug history is very important in identifying the cause.

Amenorrhea is a condition that occurs with regularity in women. Differentiating the cause of this condition can often be done by history, but a pregnancy test should also be ordered as a first line of diagnostic testing.

SUGGESTED READINGS

Amenorrhea. Wrong diagnosis.com. Available at: http://www.wrongdiagnosis.com/p/pregnancy/book-diseases-2a.htm. Accessed August 20, 2008.

IS YOUR PATIENT JUST TIRED, OR IS THERE MORE TO THE STORY?

TERESA A. SLONIM, RN

WHAT TO DO: ASSESS AND EVALUATE

Women today are busy. They are busy with their careers, caring for a significant other and the kids, driving to and from activities, cleaning, shopping, and perhaps caring for aging parents. And, if you are a nurse, add shift work and weekend work to the list, and you have a setup for fatigue.

There are times though, when a woman raises concerns about fatigue that are outside of the ordinary. They have been handling the schedule, managing their house and job, but now they are complaining about something different. They are getting the usual amount of sleep, but are unrested. It is important for the nurse to identify when the symptom of fatigue becomes a concern and may represent an organic problem.

There are a number of emotional and physiologic factors that can cause fatigue and often accompany the busy lifestyles that many women have. From an emotional perspective, the nurse should inquire about the woman's relationships. Are they getting along with their spouse? How are their parents doing, and are finances a problem? Situational factors can certainly cause mood changes and lead to physical symptoms like fatigue. Most women will have developed coping mechanisms that allow them to adapt to these situations. However, on occasion, there are circumstances that may lead to major mood disorders like depression and require treatment. While fatigue is one symptom of depression, there are usually others including weight changes,

isolation, and loss of excitement that can help the nurse get clued into the illness. In addition, the woman may be experiencing grief over a recent death or illness of a friend or family member. Probing with specific questions can often be helpful.

From a physical perspective, there are a number of factors that can cause disease. Anemia or a reduction in the blood count either because of nutrition or menorrhagia can cause fatigue. Thyroid disorders including hypothyroidism can lead to fatigue, but may also be accompanied by changes in temperature tolerance, weight changes, and changes in skin and hair.

A variety of infections may lead to fatigue including the hepatitis viruses, Ebstein Barr Virus infection, and pneumonia. Rheumatologic conditions also may cause fatigue, but these are also often accompanied by other signs and symptoms. Finally, normal pregnancy alters the woman's body in a number of ways and can cause fatigue.

Fatigue is a nonspecific, yet, important sign for determining if a woman may be experiencing a clinical condition. While women in today's society are busier than ever, the search for an organic problem remains an important job for the nurse, who in the right situation can document, through a thorough history, the signs and symptoms that will lead to the diagnosis.

SUGGESTED READINGS

Fatigue. Wrong diagnosis.com. Available at: http://www. wrongdiagnosis.com/sym/fatigue.htm. Accessed August 20, 2008.

KNOW HOW TO HELP YOUR PATIENTS CONTROL THE SYMPTOMS OF MENOPAUSE

TERESA A. SLONIM, RN

WHAT TO DO: ASSESS AND EVALUATE

Menopause is described as amenorrhea or the cessation of menstruation for more than 1 year and results from the function of ovarian follicles. Women experiencing menopause demonstrate a number of symptoms including temperature changes, night sweats, mood swings, atrophy of the vaginal walls, and depression. There are a number of physiologic changes that also accompany menopause. The symptoms and some of these changes may be ameliorated by the administration of postmenopausal hormonal therapy with estrogen. Hormonal therapy is primarily targeted toward relief of symptoms. While many women may experience improvement of their symptoms, definitive evidence supporting this therapy from clinical trials is lacking.

Hormonal therapy can assist with the temperature, night sweats, and hot flashes of menopause. Estrogen therapy is felt to assist with the osteoporosis of aging, which is a normal effect of the aging process, although other therapies are as effective, including the administration of vitamin D and calcium. Estrogen therapy also has a number of risks that need to be considered before recommending its use in patients. Patients taking estrogen supplementation experience an increased risk of breast and endometrial cancer and cardiovascular disease including thromboembolic disease. Some studies suggest that the risk for colorectal cancer, gallbladder disease, and cognitive function are improved through the use of these agents.

Overall, there remains a lack of clarity for the use of estrogen therapy to assist with symptoms in the postmenopausal female. Its use in the short term, barring any contraindications, may assist those women with severe symptoms. Over the long term, the risks of major side effects increase, but other rationale for its administration may outweigh the risks of these complications. Finally, for the woman with contraindications to hormonal therapy, the administration of soy products, a serotonin reuptake inhibitor, or other agents may be helpful. A regimen of exercise, good nutrition, and appropriate rest can also be helpful.

SUGGESTED READINGS

Manson JE, Bassuk SS. The menopause transition and postmenopausal hormone therapy. In: Kasper DL, Braunwald E, Fauci AS, et al., eds. *Harrison's Textbook of Medicine*. 16th Ed. New York, NY: McGraw Hill; 2005.

452

ALWAYS PROVIDE HUMIDIFIED OXYGEN FOR PEDIATRIC PATIENTS

VANESSA L. FREVILLE, RN, BSN, CPN

WHAT TO DO: IMPLEMENT

Infants and children often present with alterations in their respiratory status that may require the use of oxygen to improve their oxygenation. There is a wide variety of noninvasive oxygen delivery devices available, including nasal cannulae, masks, and tents. The device used depends on the degree of hypoxemia and the patient's ability to tolerate the device.

For patients who require a low concentration of oxygen delivery, blow-by oxygen or a nasal cannula are usually appropriate. Infants and small children may be too uncooperative or agitated to maintain a cannula in place. In this case, a nasal cannula can be applied and secured to the face using tape or transparent occlusive dressing. As the patient's requirement for higher oxygen concentrations occurs, the need to advance to a mask or hood as an alternative delivery device allows for accommodation of the child's clinical needs. However, it is also important to ensure that the patient is not experiencing complications from the therapy.

One of the more common complications of prolonged oxygen therapy is the drying of the nasal passages and airway mucosa, which can lead to irritation and bleeding. Whenever possible, oxygen therapy should be humidified to prevent drying of the nasal membranes. Humidification can be provided in a number of ways including delivering the oxygen through a water bath, delivering it through a humidified tent, or ensuring that if the patient requires mechanical ventilation, the ventilator is equipped with a humidification device. Humidification is important as a means of ensuring good pulmonary toilet since dry and inspissated secretions are difficult for the patient to mobilize and the nurse to suction. While humidification is a benefit for patient comfort and improves respiratory status, there are also complications to the therapy that need to be considered. Infectious agents can occupy the reservoir and be inhaled through the oxygen tubing. Further, oxygen tubing, particularly ventilator tubing, often fills with condensate and may enter the patient's airway if the providers are not diligent about draining the tubing periodically.

Oxygen therapy has revolutionized the care of the sick child with respiratory conditions. Humidification is an important adjunct to providing this therapy.

SUGGESTED READINGS

Bailey P, Torrey SB, Wiley JF. Oxygen delivery systems for infants and children. 2008. Available at: http://www.uptodate.com/patients/content/topic.do?topicKey=ped_res/8392. Accessed August 2, 2008.

Dieckmann RA, Fiser DH, Selbst SM, eds. *Illustrated Textbook of Pediatric Emergency & Critical Care Procedures.* St. Louis, MO: Mosby; 1997.

USE ORAL SYRINGES TO ADMINISTER ORAL MEDICATIONS

VANESSA L. FREVILLE, RN, BSN, CPN

WHAT TO DO: IMPLEMENT

Medication errors are a major cause of preventable patient injury and have been found to occur at a rate of 5 per 100 medication orders. Such errors can occur in several ways including wrong dose, wrong person, and even wrong route. The practice of utilizing the "5 Rights" in medication administration is one standard approach in preventing medication errors. This practice involves ensuring that five items are correct prior to the administration of every medication, which are right patient, right medication, right dose, right time, and right route.

Up to 18% of medication errors involve the incorrect route of administration. The practice of drawing up oral medications for children into Luer-Lok syringes has led to serious medication errors with oral medications being given intravenously. To help alleviate this potential error, oral syringes have been designed and manufactured for use with oral medications. Oral syringes are now designed to be incompatible with IV tubing connectors and therefore should help reduce wrong route errors. This type of intervention is known as "forcing function" and uses the manufacturer's product design to eliminate errors in the environment.

However, it is important to note that using amber colored oral syringes may assist in avoiding the incorrect route type of error, but creates a potential for error that is related to the administration of clear, colorless medications, since the volume contained in the syringe is not clearly visible through the darkened syringe. This has led to several cases of empty syringes being labeled and dispensed from the pharmacy to patient care areas. Therefore, clear oral syringes may help to verify that the correct medication is contained in the syringe by allowing the provider to check the medication's color.

SUGGESTED READINGS

Boyce T. Oral syringe in acute care hospital: Audit and policy introduction. *Int J Pharm Pract*. 1999;11:R79.
ISMP Medication Safety Alert. *WHO Pharm Newslett*. 1999;4(11).
Kaushal R, Bates DW, Landrigan C, et al. Medication errors and adverse drug events in pediatric inpatients. *J Am Med Assoc*. 2001;285:2114–2120.

USE GLOVES WITH DIAPER CHANGES

VANESSA L. FREVILLE, RN, BSN, CPN

WHAT TO DO: IMPLEMENT

Infants are admitted to the hospital for a variety of reasons whether it is for respiratory infections, vomiting, diarrhea, or even surgical procedures. Despite the reason for admission, nursing care of infants and young children involves routine activities such as frequent diaper changes. Wearing gloves during routine diaper changes is often overlooked in nursing practice, especially when the infant or child presents with nongastrointestinal symptoms. According to the Centers for Disease Control (CDC) and Prevention, the routine use of gloves during diaper changes has not been considered mandatory practice. Standard precautions, however, include the use of gloves in addition to proper hand hygiene when touching blood, body fluids, secretions, excretions, and items contaminated with these fluids on all patients.

Infants and children admitted with diarrhea or suspected gastrointestinal infection should be routinely cared for using proper isolation precautions based on the suspected organism, which includes, at a minimum, wearing gloves. Still, a question remains though on whether to wear gloves routinely for every diaper change in the absence of gastrointestinal symptoms as a way to reduce cross-contamination to healthcare providers and other patients. To support the use of gloves with all diaper changes, the CDC states that the routine use of gloves for diaper changes in hospitalized children could minimize the potential transmission of colonizing microbes such as cytomegalovirus, *Clostridium difficile*, and *Citrobacter freundii* to another patient who might become infected. It is therefore very important for healthcare providers to utilize standard precautions of hand hygiene and use gloves in the routine changes of diapers in all hospitalized infants and children in an effort to reduce cross-contamination.

SUGGESTED READINGS

Committee on Infectious Diseases and Committee on Hospital Care. The revised CDC guidelines for isolation precautions in hospitals: Implications for pediatrics. *Pediatrics*. 1998;101:e13.

Recommendations for care of children in special circumstances. In: Pickering LK, ed. *Red Book: 2006 Report of the Committee on Infectious Diseases*. 27th Ed. Elk Grove, IL: American Academy of Pediatrics; 2006, p. 154.

USE PULSE OXIMETRY IN CHILDREN, BUT REMEMBER THAT IT ALSO HAS LIMITATIONS

VANESSA L. FREVILLE, RN, BSN, CPN

WHAT TO DO: ASSESS

Children admitted to the hospital or seen in the emergency department (ED) routinely have a set of vital signs taken including temperature, pulse, respirations, and blood pressure as an initial assessment in the course of their care. A trend in evaluating pulse oximetry in pediatrics as a fifth vital sign is developing rapidly. Pulse oximetry has been described as an accurate, simple, and noninvasive method of measuring arterial oxygen saturation (SaO_2) in patients. It accurately measures normal SaO_2 and reliably detects desaturation under a variety of conditions, and improves our ability to assess the cardiorespiratory status of infants and children. However, it is important for healthcare providers to realize that researchers have stated that routine pulse oximetry screening has not been carefully evaluated in the general pediatric population and that studies need to be performed to outline both benefits and problems of this technology before it is reliably used on a routine basis.

In the pediatric intensive care unit and the ED, infants and children often present with clinical complications that may reduce the accuracy of pulse oximetry. For example, dyshemaglobinemia, poor perfusion, pigmentation, and motion can all alter the accuracy of readings by either under- or over-estimating the results when compared with the gold standard of blood samples and co-oximetry. While pulse oximetry is a very valuable tool, it should not be the sole parameter for determining the patient's cardiorespiratory status. Other assessment findings and tools must be utilized along with pulse oximetry to ensure a more accurate picture of the patient's status. For example, the child's perfusion may be so poor that the oximeter is unable to detect a pulse or provide saturation. In these circumstances, respiratory status is not the problem; rather, the child has inadequate circulatory function and would be expected to have a resting tachycardia and signs of shock. It is therefore important for the healthcare provider to use a number of resources to determine the accuracy of the pulse oximetry readings and to optimize treatment and improve outcomes.

SUGGESTED READINGS

Mower WR, Sachs C, Nicklin EL, et al. Pulse oximetry as a fifth pediatric vital sign. *Pediatrics*. 1997;99(5):681–686.

Salyer JW. Neonatal and pediatric pulse oximetry. *Resp Care*. 2003;48(4):386–398.

LABEL ALL PATIENT TUBES, CATHETERS, AND DEVICES TO ENSURE THAT ROUTES ARE NOT CONFUSED

VANESSA L. FREVILLE, RN, BSN, CPN

WHAT TO DO: EVALUATE

Infants and children requiring medical care in the Intensive Care Unit (ICU) often have multiple tubes and devices to deliver medication and other needed therapies or to facilitate the delivery of care. To further complicate care, many of the lines and tubes look similar in size and color. Therefore, the identification of each line through the use of labeling at the distal end aids in preventing inadvertent administration of medications or treatment through improper lines. In addition, the use of multicolored labels adds further identification of the differences of the lines to aid in proper identification prior to use. These should be included in all handoffs from shift to shift and provider to provider. A key for the different tubes can be kept on the flow sheet or medication administration record that identifies which port to administer the medication through.

This is important. With the wrong route of administration being identified as a significant contributor to medication errors in hospitalized children, the confusion in tubes and routes becomes critical. As the number of medications increases, there are more opportunities for confusion and error. Medications that are to be administered by the enteral route can also be administered to the stomach or small bowel, depending upon which site is better for absorption, thus complicating the delivery of medications even via the enteral route. Two commonly confused medications are total parenteral nutrition (TPN) and intralipids, which are usually administered via the same central venous catheter, but at significantly different rates and for different durations. With inversion errors on two channel medication pumps, the patient may get the total daily dose of TPN in 6 h leading to significant electrolyte abnormalities and hyperglycemia.

When multiple tubes are protruding from a body cavity, one may be for drainage (eg. abscess), while the other may be for the infusion of nutrition or antibacterial agents. Using a tube for its intended purpose is essential to ensure that the patient gets the appropriate therapy and does not experience a complication. The labeling of tubes can go a long way in keeping providers organized.

SUGGESTED READINGS

Kaushal R, Bates DW, Landrigan C, et al. Medication errors and adverse drug events in pediatric inpatients. *J Am Med Assoc.* 2001;285:2114–2120.

Paparella S. Inadvertent attachment of a blood pressure device to a needleless IV "Y-site": Surprising, fatal connections. *J Emerg Nurs.* 2005;31(2):180–182.

The Institue of Healthcare Improvement. Reduce adverse drug events (ADEs) involving intravenous medications: Label all distal ports and tubing on all lines. Available at: www.ihi.org.

USE CAPNOGRAPHY DURING PEDIATRIC CONSCIOUS SEDATION

VANESSA L. FREVILLE, RN, BSN, CPN

WHAT TO DO: EVALUATE

Children with acute or chronic illnesses often have to undergo painful procedures which require the use of analgesia to obtain accurate results and treatment. In the clinical setting, both inpatient and outpatient children undergo procedures such as MRI and CT scanning which require the child to remain still for prolonged periods of time. The patient's young age, fear, and anxiety often create a challenge in obtaining accurate results due to the child's inability to remain still and follow commands throughout the procedure. For this reason, children may receive sedative and analgesic medications through conscious sedation in order to undergo such testing.

Several pharmacologic agents are used for conscious sedation in pediatrics, some of which can cause adverse effects such as respiratory depression and apnea. Traditionally, children undergoing conscious sedation are monitored via pulse oximetry and EKG according to facility policies. In addition, the use of capnography which involves measuring the amount of carbon dioxide that is exhaled during ventilation via a specialized nasal cannula can enhance the monitoring parameters of children during conscious sedation. End tidal CO_2 monitoring or capnography measurement is separate from oxygen saturation and thereby aids the clinician in identifying hypoventilation and apnea in the sedated patient at an earlier stage than conventional monitoring. Utilizing this added technology will enable the providers to more accurately titrate sedative medications to the desired effect, thereby reducing the risks associated with oversedation.

SUGGESTED READINGS

Levine DA, Platt SL. Novel monitoring techniques for use with procedural sedation. *Curr Opin Pediatr.* 2005;17(3):351–354.

McQuillen KK, Steele DW. Capnography during sedation/analgesia in the pediatric emergency department. *Pediatr Emerg Care.* 2000;16(6):401–404.

USE EMLA TO REDUCE PAINFUL VENIPUNCTURE AND VENOUS CANNULATION IN CHILDREN

VANESSA L. FREVILLE, RN, BSN, CPN

WHAT TO DO: IMPLEMENT

Children with acute or chronic illnesses often have to undergo painful procedures for appropriate diagnosis and treatment. Laboratory testing requires venipuncture to obtain a blood specimen and is a common procedure required to obtain necessary information for diagnosis and treatment. Venipuncture is often a painful and uncomfortable procedure for both children and adults. In addition, children are often afraid of hospitals and healthcare providers because of the experience of pain or discomfort. The reduction of pain and anxiety in treating pediatric patients is an important component of care for both the patients and parents. As a result, attending to and reducing pain in the care of patients has become an important focus for healthcare providers and regulating boards. Every effort to use available methods to reduce the anxiety and pain associated with procedures should be implemented.

Myths continue to exist that children do not experience pain the same way adults do and that pain has no untoward consequences in children. Nonpharmacologic methods of reducing anxiety and pain during procedures in pediatrics include, for example, distraction techniques, imagery, and allowing family presence.

Despite these efforts, the use of pharmacologic methods is often helpful in addition to the nonpharmacologic methods. Pharmacologic methods include the use of topical analgesics such as EMLA cream which contains 2% to 5% prilocaine and 2.5% lidocaine to numb the surface of the skin. There are a number of disadvantages including time, since the medication needs to be applied for at least 60 min prior to the painful procedure to reach its full effect. Therefore, the use of EMLA cream would not be beneficial in emergency situations where treatment and procedures need to be performed quickly.

Reducing anxiety and pain during procedures for pediatric patients is an important consideration when caring for them. EMLA cream, when topically applied 1 hour prior to procedure, provides effective dermal analgesia for venous cannulation and venipuncture.

SUGGESTED READINGS

Dieckmann RA, Fiser DH, Selbst SM, eds. *Illustrated Textbook of Pediatric Emergency & Critical Care Procedures*. St. Louis, MO: Mosby; 1997.

Santiago A, Abad P, Fernandez C, et al. Premedication with EMLA cream for ambulatory surgery in children. *Ambul Surg*. 2000;8(3):157.

Zempsky WT, Cravero JP. Relief of pain and anxiety in pediatric patients in emergency medical systems. *Pediatrics*. 2004;114(5): 1348–1356.

Avoid the use of bicarbonate and bolus insulin in pediatric DKA

Vanessa L. Freville, RN, BSN, CPN

Type I Diabetes Mellitus (IDDM) occurs most often in childhood and early adulthood and is the second most common chronic disease in children. The most serious complication associated with diabetes that contributes to increased morbidity and mortality of the disease is diabetic ketoacidosis (DKA). Approximately 30% of children who present with newly diagnosed IDDM present with DKA. Children and adolescents can also present with DKA after diagnosis when there is an intercurrent illness, vomiting, diarrhea, infection, emotional stress, or insufficient insulin administration.

DKA is a life-threatening catabolic condition which occurs as the result of insulin deficiency and is defined by the coexistence of hyperglycemia, ketosis, and metabolic acidosis. The treatment and management of DKA require an understanding of the pathophysiology which led to the acid–base, fluid, and electrolyte imbalances. One of the most serious complications of DKA is cerebral edema which accounts for 60% to 90% of all DKA-related deaths in children. Once cerebral edema develops, death occurs in 20% to 25% of patients. The key to management and treatment of DKA involves fluid resuscitation, electrolyte management, and insulin administration slowly and carefully to prevent increase in cerebral edema.

It is important to note that in severe DKA, acidosis with a pH of less than 7.0 and serum bicarbonate level <5 mEq/L can occur. This acid–base imbalance can be eventually corrected with insulin therapy and fluid resuscitation; however, bicarbonate treatment and insulin boluses are not used in children. It has been stipulated that bicarbonate administration in the treatment of acidosis secondary to DKA may worsen cerebral acidosis due to crossing the blood–brain barrier more slowly than carbon dioxide, thus leading to an increase in cerebral edema. In addition, it has been demonstrated that of all the therapeutic interventions in the treatment of DKA, only the administration of bicarbonate in DKA was associated with increased risk of cerebral edema. Bolus insulin therapy also causes dramatic swings in the glucose level and alters the osmolality of the serum; thereby also contributing to cerebral edema in pediatric patients.

The prevention of DKA in children and adolescents with diabetes is ultimately the primary goal of reducing complications associated with DKA. However, despite education and proper management of diabetes, DKA continues to occur and threaten the lives of children living with diabetes. With proper management, complications such as cerebral edema can be prevented in the treatment of DKA in children and adolescents, thus improving outcomes in morbidity and mortality.

SUGGESTED READINGS

Silverstein J, Klingensmith G, Copeland K, et al. Care of children and adolescents with type 1 diabetes: A statement of the American Diabetes Association. *Diabetes Care*. 2005;28(1):186–212.

Wolfsdorf J, Glaser N, Sperling MA. Diabetic ketoacidosis in infants, children, and adolescents: A consensus statement from the American Diabetes Association. *Diabetes Care*. 2006;29(5):1150–1159.

Yaffe S, Aranda JV. *Neonatal and Pediatric Pharmacology: Therapeutic Principles in Practice*. 3rd Ed. Philadelphia, PA: Lippincott Williams & Wilkins; 2005.

Isolation Precautions: Positive Until Proven Negative for RSV

Vanessa L. Freville, RN, BSN, CPN

WHAT TO DO: PLAN

Standard precautions are to be taken by healthcare providers during any patient contact; however, during certain circumstances, a higher level of protection is warranted. These "Transmission-based precautions" should be implemented when patients present with suspected symptoms for increased risk of nosocomial exposure, including diarrhea and certain respiratory infections in infants and young children. Transmission-based precautions include contact, droplet, and airborne precautions and vary in the time of utilization based on the suspected organisms.

Common infections in which infants require hospitalization include rotavirus and respiratory syncytial virus (RSV). Standard precautions are used throughout the diagnostic process and while awaiting test results for suspected organisms, it is important to remember that patients infected with these highly contagious organisms should be placed on transmission-based precautions in addition to standard precautions until a negative organism is ruled out. A study conducted by Alcasid et al. (2004) demonstrated that infants admitted to the hospital with suspected RSV were not appropriately isolated, thus leading to increased risk of nosocomial transmission and exposure. Healthcare providers may be increasing risk to both themselves and other patients throughout the first stages of treatment by using only standard precautions with organisms that require a higher level of protection.

The Centers for Disease Control and Prevention (CDC) supports the empiric use of contact, droplet and airborne precautions by stating that in many instances, the risk of transmitting a nosocomial infection may be highest before the definitive diagnosis is made and before precautions based on that diagnosis are implemented. While it is not possible to project or plan for all the patients needing these higher levels of precaution, certain clinical syndromes and conditions hold a higher risk to warrant the empirical use of transmission-based precautions until a definitive diagnosis can be made. Through the use of empiric transmission-based precautions with highly suspective organisms in pediatrics, the risk of cross-contamination and nosocomial infection can be greatly reduced.

SUGGESTED READINGS

Alcasid G, Garcia-Houchins S, Peev M, et al. Failure to institute appropriate isolation precautions for suspected respiratory syncytial virus (RSV) infection: Frequency and identification of risk factors. *Am J Infect Control*. 2004;32(3):e1.

MAINTAIN THERMOREGULATION DURING EXAMINATION OF THE NEWBORN

VANESSA L. FREVILLE, RN, BSN, CPN

WHAT TO DO: IMPLEMENT

Often newborns and infants are seen by healthcare providers in a variety of settings such as well check or emergency care. During these examinations, the infant or newborn is often undressed completely to perform a thorough physical examination of the skin and anatomical features. After prolonged exposure to the environment, especially in cold examination rooms, the newborn or infant can quickly become hypothermic, thus further complicating its condition. For healthcare providers, it is important to remember that infants, especially neonates, have difficulty controlling temperature since they have a large ratio of surface area to weight, poor insulation with less subcutaneous fat, and small mass. In addition, this population does not have the capacity to conserve heat by methods such as changing posture and adjusting clothing. They, therefore, rely on adults and healthcare providers caring for them to assist in ensuring that thermoregulation is maintained throughout the examination.

The ideal skin temperature for a 2-week-old full-term infant is 36 °C (96.8 °F) and 36.5 °C for a newborn. Loss of thermoregulation in the neonate leads to changes in oxygen consumption and metabolic rate. These changes can lead to further decompensation of the infant's condition. There are several ways of ensuring thermoregulation during the physical examination including maintaining a warm room temperature, bundling or clothing the infant as soon as possible, and using a radiant warmer when necessary. Using measures to ensure that thermoregulation is maintained during the physical examination and resuscitation of an infant or newborn is an important goal in the care of infants.

SUGGESTED READINGS

Bissinger, RL. Neonatal resuscitation. *Emedicine*. Available at: www.webmd. Accessed August 26, 2008.

Dieckmann RA, Fiser DH, Selbst SM, eds. *Illustrated Textbook of Pediatric Emergency & Critical Care Procedures*. St. Louis, MO: Mosby; 1997.

BE CAREFUL WHEN CATHETERIZING AN INFANT'S UNCIRCUMCISED PENIS

VANESSA L. FREVILLE, RN, BSN, CPN

WHAT TO DO: IMPLEMENT

Often, the placement of an indwelling urinary catheter in the care of ill children is necessary to document accurate urinary output. The procedure involves inserting an indwelling catheter by sterile technique into the urinary meatus and instilling a specified amount of saline into a balloon located at the tip of the catheter to help maintain it in place. Once in place, the catheter may cause some discomfort to the patient but generally poses no major complications. A number of risks for urinary catheterization include damage to the internal structures during placement, leakage around the catheter, and infection.

One specific complication of urinary catheterization related to uncircumcised pediatric male patients is the risk of paraphimosis. In most cases, paraphimosis occurs accidentally with the retraction of the foreskin during penile exam, cleaning, or urethral catheterization, and then remains retracted following the exam or procedure. Careful foreskin manipulation by healthcare professionals is the most important part in preventing paraphimosis. The development of paraphimosis after catheterization is not uncommon. Before the insertion of a urethral catheter in an uncircumcised male, the nurse or caregiver retracts the foreskin to prepare and drape the glans penis by sterile technique. Following the procedure, the retracted foreskin may be inadvertently left as such for several hours or even days before it is discovered. This failure to restore the foreskin to its original position sometimes leads to the development of paraphimosis.

In the majority of cases, the foreskin reduces on its own; however, if the foreskin remains in a retracted state, it then becomes predisposed to paraphimosis. Venous congestion and edema develop making it difficult to reduce the foreskin back to the normal position and the condition worsens. If untreated, ischemia and gangrene in the penis can result.

Since paraphimosis is often a condition that is almost always inadvertently induced, education and clarification of proper foreskin care to nurses and healthcare professionals may be all that is necessary to prevent this problem.

SUGGESTED READINGS

Dieckmann RA, Fiser DH, Selbst SM, eds. *Illustrated Textbook of Pediatric Emergency & Critical Care Procedures.* St. Louis, MO: Mosby; 1997.

Donohoe JM, Kim H, Brown JA. Paraphimosis. 2006. Available at: www.emedicine.com.

USE XYLOCAINE JELLY WITH URINARY CATHETERIZATION

VANESSA L. FREVILLE, RN, BSN, CPN

WHAT TO DO: IMPLEMENT

Often, the placement of a urinary catheter in the care of children is necessary to document accurate urinary output or for other medical purposes such as to obtain a sterile specimen for testing or to decompress a distended bladder in a patient with urinary retention. The procedure involves inserting a urinary catheter, either intermittent or indwelling, into the urinary meatus using sterile technique. The complications associated with urinary catheterization include pain, discomfort, infection, urethral trauma, emotional trauma, and dysuria following the procedure.

The procedure is only uncomfortable physically, but in the young child, it can be emotionally distressing and traumatic as well. With adequate preparation and skill, however, the procedure can be performed with limited discomfort and anxiety for both the child and the parent. Knowledge of child development and behavior is important in the approach to the child as well as the selection of appropriate equipment size and type of catheter. In addition, the use of a local anesthetic introduced into the urethra can assist in decreasing the pain and discomfort associated with catheter insertion. The use of 2% xylocaine jelly can help to alleviate the discomfort of catheter insertion in both males and females when used as a sterile lubricant prior to insertion. In addition, and most particularly, with male children, the use of 2% xylocaine jelly injected into the urinary meatus 3 to 5 min prior to catheter insertion can aid in not only anesthesia, but it also encourages urethral relaxation prior to catheter insertion.

While urinary catheterization can be distressing not only physically but also emotionally for children, adequate knowledge and skill in the use of appropriate equipment and 2% xylocaine jelly can significantly reduce the associated discomfort and anxiety.

SUGGESTED READINGS

Gray ML. Atraumatic urethral catheterization of children. *Pediatr Nurs*. 1996;22(4):306–310.
Robeson WLM, Leung AKC, Thomason MA. Catheterization of the bladder in infants and children. *Clin Pediatr*. 2006;45: 795–800.

CHECK NASOGASTRIC TUBE PLACEMENT PRIOR TO USE

VANESSA L. FREVILLE, RN, BSN, CPN

WHAT TO DO: ASSESS

Nasogastric tubes or NG tubes are used in pediatrics for a variety of diagnostic and therapeutic reasons including gastric lavage, stomach decompression, and enteral feeding. Most pediatric NG tubes are placed into the stomach through the nare with a confirmation of placement made prior to securing it with tape. Once in place, it can be used to aspirate stomach contents for diagnostic purposes, remove air placed into the stomach following bag-valve-mask ventilation, instill contrast for radiographic examinations, and provide nutrition or hydration via enteral feedings or oral replacement hydration fluids.

Complications can occur during the placement of an NG, including the displacement into the trachea or damage to the oropharyngeal mucosa. The placement of an NG tube is contraindicated in patients without a protective airway reflex, those with an esophageal stricture, recent alkali ingestion, penetrating cervical wounds, or cervical spinal injuries, and those with facial fractures or cribriform plate injuries.

Placement of an NG tube can be confirmed through the use of several methods. One of the most common techniques is hand aspiration of stomach contents. If the provider has doubts about whether the gastric secretions represent stomach contents, additional testing of the contents for pH level can be performed. The pH of gastric secretions is usually <5. Another common method involves injecting air through the NG using a syringe and listening with a stethoscope over the stomach for an air bolus or "whooshing" sound. If the provider doubts that the NG is in proper position,

an abdominal X-ray may be obtained to check for proper placement. Once placement is confirmed, the NG should be secured safely to the patients face and marked or measured from nare to tip for subsequent uses by other caregivers. Once secured, the frequent assessment of NG tube placement should be performed to ensure that migration or dislodgement has not occurred through coughing, vomiting, general activity, or accidental pulling from the pediatric patient.

When checking the placement of an NG tube, aspirated fluid, by itself, does not confirm placement since fluid can be aspirated from both the lungs and pleural space if improperly placed. In addition, a false-positive placement may involve the auscultation of injected air over the stomach area; however, these sounds may be transmitted sounds from the thorax to the upper abdomen. The only absolutely reliable method for determining placement of NG tubes is by radiographic examination. While radiographic testing is not always used in practice secondary to the attributable cost and risk of radiation exposure to the pediatric patient, bedside techniques such as aspiration of gastric contents and auscultation of air bolus over the abdomen prior to use should be routinely performed by nurses. Whenever the NG placement is in doubt, using bedside techniques, an abdominal radiograph should be obtained to confirm placement.

SUGGESTED READINGS

American Association of Critical-Care Nurses. Practice alert: Verification of feeding tube placement. 2005. Available at: www.aacn.org.

Dieckmann RA, Fiser DH, Selbst SM, eds. *Illustrated Textbook of Pediatric Emergency & Critical Care Procedures.* St. Louis, MO: Mosby; 1997.

Double-check all pediatric chemotherapy

Vanessa L. Freville, RN, BSN, CPN

WHAT TO DO: PLAN

Childhood cancer affects nearly 1 in 300 boys and 1 in 333 girls below 20 years of age. For some types of childhood cancer, the incidence has risen since the 1970s, but rates have been fairly stable in recent years. Chemotherapy is often used in the treatment of childhood cancer which involves three phases: induction, consolidation, and maintenance therapy. There are numerous types of chemotherapy drugs used in the treatment of childhood cancer, all of which have potential side effects and complications and require close patient monitoring to prevent drug toxicities and to ensure the early treatment of complications.

Despite stringent practices and protocols, it is important to ensure that dosages are calculated appropriately prior to administration. Rinke and colleagues have reported that as many as 85% of chemotherapy dosage errors have actually reached the patient, and of those, 15.6% required additional patient monitoring or therapeutic intervention. In addition, 48% of errors originated in the administration phase of the process and 30% originating in the dispensing phase, the most common errors related to improper dose.

One way to assist in reducing medication errors with pediatric chemotherapy is to implement a system and routine practice of double checking the dosage written between two medical professionals, either two chemotherapy certified nurses or a nurse with a physician. In addition, once the medication is received and prepared for administration, the dosage should again be double checked between two chemotherapy certified nurses or with a physician prior to administration. It is important to ensure that the volume of medication in the syringe or bag matches the order written if applicable and volume listed on the label. Through a systematic series of checks and balances from the point of order prescribing to the point of medication administration to the patient, pediatric chemotherapy administration errors can be greatly reduced.

SUGGESTED READINGS

Hay WW, Levin MJ, Sondheimer JM, et al., eds. *Current Diagnosis & Treatment in Pediatrics*. 18th Ed. New York, NY: McGraw-Hill; 2007.

National childhood cancer foundation and children's oncology group. Available at: www.curesearch.org.

Rinke ML, Shoe AD, Morlock L, et al. Characteristics of pediatric chemotherapy medication errors in a national error reporting database. *Cancer*. 2007;110(1):186–195.

USE APPROPRIATE PROTECTION FOR YOUR IMMUNOSUPPRESSED CANCER PATIENTS INCLUDING THE AVOIDANCE OF RECTAL TEMPERATURES

VANESSA L. FREVILLE, RN, BSN, CPN

WHAT TO DO: PLAN

Cancer affects nearly 11,900 children and adolescents in the United States. Nurses caring for pediatric oncology patients play an integral role in preventing further complications related to the child's condition. Complications related to the treatment of childhood cancer include neutropenia, anemia, and thrombocytopenia from the side effects of chemotherapy. Neutropenia is a reduction in the number of neutrophils that fight infection and is the most severe consequence of bone marrow suppression. Anemia is a reduction in RBCs and occurs secondary to myelosuppressive chemotherapy, radiation, or blood loss. Thrombocytopenia is defined as <100,000/mm^3 of circulating platelets and occurs as an adverse effect of chemotherapy.

Children presenting with fever and neutropenia secondary to chemotherapy treatment typically will usually have anemia and thrombocytopenia as well. In addition, children with immune deficiency from chemotherapy are at increased risk of developing many different infections. It is important to evaluate lab results carefully to appropriately treat the patient. Children with severe neutropenia, showing absolute neutrophil count (ANC) < 500, such as those undergoing chemotherapy are at risk for life-threatening infections secondary to a reduced ability to fight infection. A thorough assessment and prompt action are critical in the care of the febrile neutropenic child. As part of the management, it is important to avoid exacerbating the child's already compromised condition through treatment strategies. One way to avoid causing further complications is by avoiding all rectal temperatures, enemas, or suppositories in the neutropenic child to prevent causing perirectal injury secondary to impaired mucosal wall, thrombocytopenia, and neutropenia. Using safe practice in caring for the febrile neutropenic child along with providing prompt assessment and treatment improves the outcomes of treatment.

SUGGESTED READINGS

Baggott CR, Kelly KP, Fochtman D, et al. *Nursing Care of Children and Adolescents with Cancer*. 3rd Ed. Philadelphia, PA: WB Saunders; 2002.

Bryant R. Managing side effects of childhood cancer treatment. *J Ped Nurs*. 2003;18(2):113–125.

National Cancer Institute. 2005. Available at: www.cancer.gov.

Always place electrocardiogram (EKG) electrodes correctly

Lea E. Lineberry, RNIII, BSN, CCRN, CPN

WHAT TO DO: ASSESS

Many patients in acute care settings require standard bedside monitoring for the observation of their EKG. This monitoring provides a picture of the heart's electrical activity. A more comprehensive view of the heart can be provided by a standard 12-lead EKG. Each lead provides a different view of the heart's electrical activity based upon the placement of the electrode on the body. In bedside monitoring (usually 3 to 6 leads) and 12-lead EKGs, lead placement must be accurate to obtain high-quality EKG readings.

Research has demonstrated that the misplacement of electrodes for the standard 12-lead EKG produced differences in amplitude and waveform associated with different shifts in the QRS axis, particularly when the torso was used for limb lead placement. In a recent study, Jowett and colleagues (2005) noted these abnormal changes in 36% of patients with known normal EKGs.

Personnel responsible for the placement of electrodes (RN, LPN, EKG technologists) for bedside monitoring and 12-lead EKG recordings should receive competency validation in skin preparation and accurate electrode placement. Other competency validations should include the ability to define, recognize, and understand the basic pathophysiology of the EKG. The validity of the EKG used in bedside monitoring rests upon the competency and skill of the care provider to accurately place the electrodes on the patient. Skin preparation is also an important tool to obtain the most accurate reading possible. This preparation includes using electrodes that make good contact with the body. Prepasted electrodes are commonly used and effective. Daily changing of the electrodes will minimize artifact, thus decreasing the risk of erroneous interpretation of the EKG.

In the event of misplaced precordial leads, misinterpretation of the EKG can occur and may lead to an inaccurate diagnosis of ischemia. If there is a reversal of limb leads, this produces a variety of alterations in the EKG. In addition, if the patient has dextrocardia, proper documentation and communication to appropriate staff must occur so that leads are placed in correct position.

In conclusion, information contained in different perspectives from multiple leads can be used to improve recognition of EKG abnormalities. Correct placement of the electrodes reduces the chance of a misinterpretation in the EKG. It is important that all bedside monitoring and EKGs are obtained by utilizing a standard placement competency check off.

SUGGESTED READINGS

Jowett NI, Turner AM, Cole A, et al. Modified electrode placement must be recorded when performing 12-lead electrocardiograms. *Postgrad Med J*. 2005;81:122–125.

National Guideline Clearinghouse. Recommendations for the standardization and interpretation of the electrocardiogram. 2008. Available at: http://www.guideline.gov. Retrieved, June 28, 2008.

ENSURE THAT AN EMERGENCY MEDICATION SHEET IS AT THE BEDSIDE OF EVERY PATIENT

LEA E. LINEBERRY, RNIII, BSN, CCRN, CPN

WHAT TO DO: PLAN

Pediatric admissions to a children's hospital emergency room, medical floor, or intensive care unit occur regularly, as do adult admissions. The pediatric patient is different in size and stature and requires a different type of specialized care. Pediatric resuscitation is challenging to all caregivers that deal with children on a regular basis. Certain standards and principles of care must be applied to all pediatric emergency situations. One such standard of care is that there is a correct patient weight obtained and documented on admission and that emergency resuscitative care sheets are available for these patients at the bedside.

Pediatric resuscitation is challenging to even the most experienced pediatric caregiver. The ensuing panic that is sometimes generated when a "crashing" pediatric patient is admitted can snowball into a disorganized attempt at viable resuscitative efforts. Errors in decimal point placement, mathematical calculations, or expression of dosage have accounted for nearly two thirds of dosage errors in pediatric medication calculations. A higher risk for medication errors occurs in acute situations where there is no emergency system set in place for each individual patient. Some institutions use a color-coded system for patients of different sizes and weights. Others use a simple solution of placing an emergency medical sheet at the bedside for the individual patient according to size and weight.

Being prepared is the key to preventing errors in resuscitation management. The nurse plays an important role in this area. It is the responsibility of the nurse to ensure that properly sized and functioning equipment is available at the bedside when it is needed. One means of critical reference is the emergency medical sheet that can be placed at the bedside on admission and labeled with the patient's name.

Emergency reference guides are developed according to the size and weight of the patient. The weight is listed in kilograms and each medication is standardized and listed according to the weight. Dosing for standard resuscitation drugs, sedatives, anticonvulsants, muscle relaxants, anesthetics, and vasoactive drips are listed. This prepared list allows for ease of preparation, correct dosing in an emergency, and a controlled resuscitation environment that ultimately leads to fewer errors.

SUGGESTED READINGS

Curley MA, Moloney-Harmon PA. *Critical Care Nursing of Infants and Children*. Philadelphia, PA: Saunders; 2001.

Lesar TS. Errors in the use of medication dosage equations. *Arch Pediat Adolesc Med*. 1998;152(4):340–344.

REMEMBER YOUR UNITS AND DO NOT MISINTERPRET KILOGRAMS AND POUNDS

LEA E. LINEBERRY, RNIII, BSN, CCRN, CPN

WHAT TO DO: IMPLEMENT

Pediatrics refers to the care of infants, children, and adolescents. It differs from adult medicine in a variety of ways. Body size, weight, and the differences in family dynamics are just a few of the ways in which pediatric care is different. Children are not "little adults" and must be treated appropriate to their age and developmental status.

The competent nurse is the single most effective patient advocate. The continual growth in judgment, skills, attitude, and knowledge by the practicing registered nurse expands the expertise brought to the bedside for the benefits of patients. Clinical expertise can be defined as "the ability to integrate complex multisystem effects and understand the trajectory of illness and human response to critical illness" (Critical Care Nursing of Infants and Children). The competent pediatric nurse knows how to deliver the essentials of safe care and quality nursing practice. Understanding the age-specific competencies is critical for the competent pediatric nurse.

The growth parameters of acutely ill children should always be documented and followed while the child is a patient in the hospital. These values will serve as a baseline for the assessment of fluids and nutritional support. The weight also serves as a baseline for drug administration. The use of the metric system is referenced in most pediatric care practices. Upon admission, the actual weight of the child should be obtained. This is usually documented in kilograms. The conversion of kilograms to pounds is that 1 kg equals 2.2 lb. As a competent pediatric nurse, knowing this difference can mean avoiding medication and fluid management errors.

Since the appropriate dosing of medications depends on the weight of an infant or child, confusing kilogram weight and pound weight could be detrimental to the child. If a child is weighed on admission as 5 lb and the nurse transfers this to the chart as 5 kg, the potential for double dosing is apparent. The same could occur if the child is weighed on admission as 5 kg and the information is transferred as 5 lb, where inappropriate underdosing could occur.

Pediatric providers must implement strategies that adequately communicate patient information to all members of the healthcare team. Proper documentation of the patient's weight must be carefully placed on the chart in the correct measurement units.

SUGGESTED READINGS

Curley MA, Moloney-Harmon PA. *Critical Care Nursing of Infants and Children*. Philadelphia, PA: Saunders; 2001.

Money-Harmon PA, Czerwinski SJ. *Nursing care of the Pediatric Trauma Patient*. St. Louis, MO: Saunders; 2003.

REMEMBER YOUR UNITS AND DO NOT MISINTERPRET MICROGRAMS AND MILLIGRAMS

LEA E. LINEBERRY, RNIII, BSN, CCRN, CPN

WHAT TO DO: EVALUATE

Use of the metric system in the fields of medicine, nursing, and pharmacy is standard of practice. There are, however, errors that occur if the metric abbreviations are poorly written and misinterpretation occurs. The use of μg (micrograms) can be mistaken for mg (milligrams) and so, these have been removed from the Joint Commission on Accreditation of Healthcare Organizations (JCAHO) list of approved abbreviations. However, its use may appear in error and can cause transcription errors.

In 2003, JCAHO released its National Safety Goals with one of the goals being listed as "standardize the abbreviations, acronyms and symbols used throughout the organization, including a list of abbreviations, acronyms and symbols not to use" (The Joint Commission, 2003). Since that time, the list of unapproved abbreviations has been created and implemented. However, visual errors still occur as poor writing habits remain a part of the medical practice. For example, a prescription for a hydromorphone epidural could be written as 2μg/mL. The order is entered and mixed as 500mg in 250mL, with the dose labeling as "2mg/mL." The nurse interprets the medication incorrectly and administers the medication that is 1,000 times the originally ordered medication.

Even with JCAHO setting forth its initiative of unapproved abbreviations, errors still occur as these two units of measurement are used frequently in the medical field. Conversion inaccuracy occurs easily with micrograms and milligrams due to decimal point errors. The simplicity in which conversion of the two occurs by the moving of the decimal point three zeros either to the right or to the left is a common user error. The preparation that a nurse receives in school is necessary for avoiding mathematical errors at the bedside. Human factors such as poor staffing, fatigue, and hunger can affect the judgment of the overwhelmed and hurried nurse.

Errors involving the conversion of micrograms and milligrams still occur. The use of a system for verifying dosing is highly encouraged when it involves micrograms or milligrams. Many institutions employ such a system when pediatrics is involved; however, a system-wide policy of verification of certain medications that are in micrograms or milligrams could eliminate many more errors including some for the adult population.

SUGGESTED READINGS

JCAHO revises list of approved abbreviations. Retrieved, from US Pharmacist Web. 2003. Available at: http://www.uspharmacist.com/index.asp?show=article&page=8_1180.htm. Accessed June 28, 2008.

The Joint Commission. National Patient Safety Goals. The Joint Commission Web. 2003. Available at:http://www.jointcomission.org/PatientSafety/National PatientSafetyGoals/03. Accessed June 6, 2008.

PEDIATRIC LAB RESULTS: FALSE INTERPRETATION AND ITS CONSEQUENCES

LEA E. LINEBERRY, RNIII, BSN, CCRN, CPN

WHAT TO DO: EVALUATE

Patients who are admitted to the hospital are destined to have laboratory tests. The results will be processed and sent to the patient's unit, and then to the primary nurse who is caring for that particular patient. It is up to that nurse to properly interpret these findings and then report them to the physician in a timely manner. Some laboratory results are simple and easy to understand. Others require the involvement of the physician for interpretation and explanation of the laboratory findings. It is a significant part of the nurse's responsibility to avoid misinterpretation so that future treatment is not delayed.

Laboratory testing is often used, in combination with other diagnostic modalities, to assist the physician with defining a problem in a patient's care. The findings of each of these testing forms must be communicated appropriately to the physician and in a timely manner. The direct and immediate responsible party for interpretation is the physician; however, nurses must relay laboratory information to these physicians. The reporting of critical lab values is the responsibility of the laboratory; however, nurses must have insight into the meaning of those critical care results and know when to escalate and receive feedback on the next step of care.

There are several disease entities that are lab-specific. These diseases require a laboratory analysis that includes basic screening, selective monitoring, specific evaluations, and regularly scheduled follow-up screening. When patients with these diseases are admitted to the hospital, laboratory testing is a daily part of their hospital regimen. For example, a patient who has an oncologic problem will be followed for certain cell counts. If the nurse who is taking care of that patient fails to acknowledge what lab values are of significance to the patient, delays in treatment can occur or erroneous interventions could be implemented. An essential element of duty arises when a patient and his or her caregiver form a relationship. This duty requires the caregiver to act in a reasonable manner and within the standard of care (Logan, 1998). It is with this duty in mind that the nurses must be responsible for all aspects of care provided to their patients. This includes being knowledgeable in lab values and being able to interpret critical results and communicate them to the physician.

The misinterpretation of lab values can result in delayed or improper management necessary for the patient. There continues to be a need to define critical lab results for pediatrics, instead of using the adult standard lab value system for interpretation. Laboratory results remain one of the single most important means of assisting physicians in making diagnostic decisions. The responsible nurse has insight into and knowledge of laboratory values and can communicate any laboratory results that are critical to the physician.

SUGGESTED READINGS

Defining critical lab value to improve patient safety. Medical News Today website. 2007. Available at: http://www.medicalnewstoday.com. Accessed July 1, 2008.

Logan P. *Principles of Practice for the Acute Care Nurse Practitioner*. Stamford, CT: Appleton & Lange; 1998.

DECIMAL ERRORS AND MISCALCULATIONS IN PEDIATRIC DRUG DOSING

LEA E. LINEBERRY, RNIII, BSN, CCRN, CPN

Calculation errors are a well-recognized problem, especially in the field of pediatrics. The broad range of size and age contributes to the likelihood of calculation errors in children. Dosage equations account for a large number of errors in which adverse outcomes are presented. Whether there is a displacement of a decimal or a dosage is miscalculated, errors involving children continue to be very common. These errors may result in underdose or overdose of medications.

In the acute care setting, pediatric patients often require medications that are highly potent. These medications are calculated using body weight and usually administered by intravenous infusion. Drugs such as dopamine and epinephrine are only a couple of the highly potent drugs used in emergency situations that must be calculated properly and prepared appropriately for immediate infusion. One simple miscalculation or shifting of the decimal point could result in a significant overdose or underdose.

Complicated dosage regimens and confusion regarding the way dosage calculations are stated or expressed frequently appear to cause errors. Utilizing a system of verification could potentially eliminate pediatric medication errors. A double check on vasoactive drugs and other drugs used in the critical care setting is easy and cost-efficient.

Decimal point misinterpretation is often a common problem that causes medication dosage errors. As part of the 2003 JCAHO National Patient Safety Goals, any dosage that is less than 1 and documented using a decimal must have a zero preceding the decimal point. Any dosage that uses a whole number should never have a decimal point and zero following that number. The transcriber could easily miss the decimal point after the whole number and mistakenly interpret the dose as ten times higher than prescribed. Always remember, no trailing zeros and only leading zeros with decimal points.

Dosage miscalculations and decimal point errors are common and can be life threatening, especially to the pediatric patient. To avoid these types of errors, a system of verification with two nurses should be employed. The nurse must also take care to avoid any distraction when calculating doses and administering medications. A periodic review of mathematical calculation skills should be included in competency validations as well.

SUGGESTED READINGS

Curley MA, Moloney-Harmon PA. *Critical Care Nursing of Infants and Children*. Philadelphia, PA: Saunders; 2001.

Lesar TS. Errors in the use of medication dosage equations. *Arch Pediat Adolesc Med*. 1998;152(4):340–344.

Ensure the Correct Size and Placement of Blood Pressure Cuffs in Children

Lea E. Lineberry, RNIII, BSN, CCRN, CPN

WHAT TO DO: EVALUATE

Accurate blood pressure measurement in pediatrics is necessary as a reflection of the patient's cardiac status; the blood pressure can indicate certain disease entities and how well a patient is responding to treatment. Abnormalities, such as coarctation of the aorta and renal disease, can be recognized by first noting hypertension in the pediatric patient and the response to therapy can be ascertained by calculating the mean arterial pressure.

Blood pressure is best taken by auscultation or through use of noninvasive automatic equipment. Although nurses are taught blood pressure measurement techniques in school, the skill can deteriorate, and the blood pressure measurement obtained can be erroneous. As a result, diagnoses may be made incorrectly and inaccurate treatment may be started. Proper technique and skill in taking a blood pressure must be validated through competency evaluation on a periodic basis, particularly for the pediatric patient.

The bare right arm is typically the site of choice for blood pressure measurement. This site is preferred since standardized blood pressure tables reflect right arm readings, and left arm measurements can provide inaccurately low readings if the patient has coarctation of the aorta. Measurement in all four extremities should be obtained if there is a detection of hypertension. Systolic pressure in the thigh increases by >10 or more mm Hg than the arm after the first year of life. Always take the blood pressure in the arm that is not compromised by an arterial line, pulse oximeter, or intravenous line.

The selection of the appropriately sized blood pressure cuff is critical. The width of the cuff bladder should be at least 40% of the circumference of the arm, and the bladder length should cover at least 80% of the arm's circumference. If the size is questionable, always use the larger sized cuff for measurement. The inflatable part of the bladder should be centrally placed over the artery that is to be compressed. If the cuff is misplaced, erroneous readings may be obtained.

Blood pressure measurements can be accurately obtained if the cuff size is appropriate and placement is in correct position on the extremity. Pediatric nurses must be competent in the procedure for obtaining accurate blood pressure measurements. By periodic validation of bedside technical skills, practice can be current and up to date.

SUGGESTED READINGS

Curley MA, Moloney-Harmon PA. *Critical Care Nursing of Infants and Children*. Philadelphia, PA: Saunders; 2001.
Schell KA. Evidence-based practice: noninvasive blood pressure measurement in children. bNet: Business Network website. 2006. Available at: http://findarticles.com/p/articles/mi_m0FSZ/is_3_32/ai_n17213853/pg_8. Accessed July 1, 2008.

LANGUAGE BARRIERS CAN JEOPARDIZE YOUR PATIENT'S SAFETY

LEA E. LINEBERRY, RNIII, BSN, CCRN, CPN

WHAT TO DO: ASSESS

Hospital admissions are difficult for adults and even more difficult for children. However, the stress that is placed on the parents of a hospitalized child is even more significant. The ability to acknowledge in words and actions the parent's valuable and irreplaceable role during this critical time helps set the tone for the entire hospitalization. When a language barrier is added to the equation, the loss of control that affects these patients and their families is paramount. A language obstacle can affect the entire healing process and dramatically influence discharge planning.

Nurses are taught from the beginning of their careers that communication with the patient provides support and facilitates understanding of the treatment interventions necessary to appropriate care. Current practice includes serving an increasing number of diverse cultures that have their own health beliefs, values, and practices. Although cultural differences have been a part of the history of the United States, its healthcare system has been developed by its most dominant culture. Cultural and language barriers continue to exist; however, multicultural growth is taking precedent as more immigrants seek to maintain their culture.

The ability of the nurse to cross a language barrier during the hospitalization of a child, rests on being culturally competent and knowing how to address the problems that may be faced due to the language obstacle. The nurse does not have to be fluent in the language of the patient in order to provide quality care. Respect and an understanding of the available resources needed to enhance the child's hospitalization is all that is necessary.

In order to achieve cultural awareness, the nurse must come to a self understanding of her own beliefs and values. Ambivalence to language differences and how it can affect the child's hospitalization and discharge is no longer accepted practice. Nurses have to be committed to a goal of lifelong learning which includes acknowledging diversity and incorporating it into practice. Most institutions have methods of providing interpreters for use with language needs. It is the job of the patient's primary nurse to know how to provide this service. It is especially important when the child is ready for discharge. Discharge instructions must be communicated appropriately and accurately. The use of an interpreter will eliminate the possibility of erroneous instructions. Many children often have parents who can speak some English; however, they may misinterpret a vital piece of information necessary for discharge.

Children of different cultures are often admitted to the hospital and present with a language barrier. In order to facilitate proper communication, the nurse must be aware of all available resources that can be of use for assistance during hospitalization and at discharge.

SUGGESTED READINGS

Curley MA, Moloney-Harmon PA. *Critical Care Nursing of Infants and Children.* Philadelphia, PA: Saunders; 2001.

Leonard BJ. Quality nursing care celebrates diversity. The Online Journal of Issues in Nursing Website. Available at: http://www.nursingworld.org/MainMenuCategories/ANAMarketplace/ANAPeriodicals/OJIN/TableofContents/Volume62001/Number2May31/NursingCareDivers. Accessed July 2, 2008.

ENSURE THAT THE PERTINENT SEXUAL HISTORY IS OBTAINED ON ADOLESCENT PATIENTS AT ADMISSION

LEA E. LINEBERRY, RNIII, BSN, CCRN, CPN

WHAT TO DO: ASSESS

Pediatrics includes the transitional adolescent period that ranges from 12 to 18 (some say 21) years of age. More often than desired, the adolescent is required to become independent and move into adulthood. As society propels these children into early adulthood, hospitals are admitting children to the adult wards and young adults to the pediatric wards. When admitted, it is important that the past medical and sexual history be documented in the database.

Admission to the hospital is usually not planned and often accompanied by severe stresses. The adolescent, already in a transitional phase, must now deal with the threat of physical illness or injury. The hospital environment compounds this challenge with its structure, noises, equipment, and routines. The adolescent struggles to move into a realm of freedom outside of the hospital and with admission, often loses the ability to express needs, concerns, or desires. The ability to cope is challenged and the adolescent may rebel against all methods of care in an attempt to regain some form of control over this new environment.

The admission database usually consists of pertinent past medical history, a record of height, weight, current history, and vital signs. Often, the parent becomes the reliable source of information that the nurse addresses for history. Most adolescents, when ill, can release self control to others and will allow their parents to speak for them. This, however, does not give the child the opportunity to address sexual history in a way that is comfortable for him or her and leaves the caregiver without firsthand knowledge of issue of which the parent may be unaware.

Adolescent patients should be encouraged to verbalize questions and concerns. By providing the adolescent with positive support, respect, and some control over the environment, the nurse may be able to achieve acceptance in the patient's realm of understanding. They may be able to express themselves more openly to the nurse with the parent out of the room. A more detailed sexual history may then be obtained, but only after some form of trust is created.

Important parts of the adolescent patient's sexual history may be eliminated or obtained in error on admission if the parent is the only informant or is present during the history taking. Allowing the adolescent to speak openly without parents in the room may be the most adequate way to obtain accurate sexual history for the admission database.

SUGGESTED READINGS

Curley MA, Moloney-Harmon PA. *Critical Care Nursing of Infants and Children*. Philadelphia, PA: Saunders; 2001.
Kinney MR, Dunbar SB, Brooks-Brunn JA, et al. *AACN Clinical Reference for Critical Care Nursing*. St. Louis, MO: Mosby; 1996.

Pediatric critical care: Lack of knowledge and skill in bedside EKG interpretation

Lea E. Lineberry, RNIII, BSN, CCRN, CPN

WHAT TO DO: ASSESS

The pediatric critical care nurse is competent in areas of judgment, critical thinking, task management, and technical skills. Within the intensive care working environment, many technologic advances have developed that require the skill of use and interpretation. The use of continuous bedside electrocardiogram (EKG) monitoring is one type of technology that requires accuracy of interpretation to correctly inform the physician of changes.

Technologic advances, such as innovative treatment modalities, pacing algorithms, and radiofrequency catheter ablation, have significantly improved patient outcomes and improved management of cardiac rhythm disturbances in children and adults. The ability to accurately diagnose a rhythm disturbance is the ultimate responsibility of the physician; however, the bedside nurse must be able to recognize challenging and lethal arrhythmias. Being prepared through annual competency validation is essential in maintaining current knowledge of recognition and practices necessary to understand cardiac rhythms. The inability or lack of motivation of the critical care nurse to learn basic cardiac rhythms and lethal arrhythmias is unacceptable.

This knowledge can mean the difference in a child's life or possible death.

The American Heart Association provides classes in Pediatric Advanced Life Support. This course covers arrhythmias that typically occur in children and teaches the responder how to treat these disturbances in rhythms. However, it is not a substitute for adequate knowledge and skills necessary for the understanding and recognition needed in bedside EKG interpretation. If an abnormal rhythm occurs, the nurse must be able to acknowledge what the disturbance is.

Basic cardiac rhythms and lethal arrhythmias are a necessary part of the pediatric critical care nurse's knowledge and technical skill base. Many abnormal rhythms are caused by different underlying causes that may be identified by the nurse after interpreting the cardiac rhythm disturbance. Obtaining a detailed past medical history may also reveal symptoms or triggers of cardiac events that could later be associated with sudden cardiac death.

SUGGESTED READINGS

Curley MA, Moloney-Harmon PA. *Critical Care Nursing of Infants and Children*. Philadelphia, PA: Saunders; 2001.
Types of arrthymias in children. American Heart Association Website. 2008. Available at: http://www.americanheart.org/presenter.jhtml?identifier=7. Retrieved July 5, 2008.

MARFAN SYNDROME: PAY ATTENTION TO THE WARNING SIGNS

JEANNIE SCRUGGS GARBER, DNP, RN

WHAT TO DO: IMPLEMENTATION

Marfan syndrome is a connective tissue disorder and can result in minor to major complications with cardiovascular, eye, skin, and skeletal systems. "The most serious effects of Marfan syndrome involve the aorta, where the disease weakens the connective tissue in the walls of the aorta, making it more likely that the artery will enlarge, tear, or rupture, which can be life threatening" (Mayo Clinic, 2006). At times, the patient and family's first awareness of this syndrome is when symptoms progress to cardiovascular surgery.

Diagnosing Marfan syndrome can be challenging; however, the most common signs and symptoms are physical appearance of the patient. Individuals with Marfan syndrome are usually very tall with exceptionally long arms, legs, and torso. They also have very flexible joints and possibly visible chest wall abnormalities. According to the clinicians at the Mayo Clinic, the following can be used as diagnostic criteria for Marfan syndrome:

- Aortic dissection affecting the ascending aorta
- Dislocation of the lens of an eye
- Dural ectasia, expansion of the membrane that encloses the fluid around the spinal cord
- At least four skeletal problems such as chest deformities; long, thin arms and legs; flat footedness; and scoliosis
- Family history—having a parent, child, or sibling who meets the diagnostic criteria for Marfan syndrome
- Having an abnormal gene known to cause Marfan syndrome

Echocardiography can assist in identifying cardiovascular abnormalities related to this syndrome. Maron and colleagues report that the "clinical spectrum has gradually evolved, and it is now obvious that not all affected individuals demonstrate classic features of the disease, that a diverse and complex constellation of abnormalities that are variable in severity (but difficult to measure) is consistent with this vast clinical continuum, and that many of the physical findings attributable to this disease are subtle or commonly encountered in the general population."

There is no cure for Marfan syndrome. Patients are encouraged to maintain routine physical and eye examination schedules and to have a routine echocardiogram to monitor heart and blood vessel changes over time.

Marfan syndrome is a complex condition that warrants early diagnosis and careful management. Patients who are diagnosed early in life and maintain optimal health status may live productive lives.

SUGGESTED READINGS

Maron B, Moller J, Seidman C, et al. Impact of laboratory molecular diagnosis on contemporary diagnostic criteria for genetically transmitted cardiovascular diseases: Hypertrophic cardiomyopathy, long-QT syndrome, and marfan syndrome: A statement for healthcare professionals from the councils on clinical cardiology, cardiovascular disease in the young, and basic science. American Heart Association. *Circulation*. 1998;98:1460–1471.

Mayo Clinic. Marfan's syndrome. 2006. Available at: http://www.mayoclinic.com/print/marfan-syndrome/DS00540/DSECTION=all&METHOD=print. Accessed June 16, 2008.

Medicine.net (n.d.). Marfan Syndrome. Medicine.net. Available at: http://www.medicinenet.com/marfan_syndrome/page3.htm#8whattreatment. Accessed June 16, 2008.

BACK TO SLEEP: EXCEPT IN THE PICU

SHEILA LAMBERT, RN, MSN, CCRN

In 1992, the American Academy of Pediatrics (AAP) released its first policy statement on reducing the risk of Sudden Infant Death Syndrome (SIDS). The statement recommended that all healthy infants be placed supine to sleep in order to reduce the risks of SIDS. This paved the way for the "Back to Sleep" campaign, appropriately named for its recommendation to place healthy babies on their backs to sleep. Placing babies on their backs to sleep reduces the risk of SIDS, also known as "crib death." The term crib death is used because the infants are oftentimes found in their cribs. Since 1992, the percentage of infants placed on their backs to sleep has increased dramatically, and the rates of SIDS have declined by more than 50%. In fact, before the "Back to Sleep" campaign began to recommend back sleeping as the best way to reduce SIDS, more than 5,000 babies died annually from SIDS in the United States. But now, the number of babies who die of SIDS is less than 3,000 each year.

While the cause of SIDS is unknown, it is the leading cause of death in infants more than 1 month of age. Most SIDS deaths occur between the ages of 2 to 4 months. The majority of SIDS deaths occur in the colder months, with African–American babies being twice as likely to die of SIDS as white babies, and American–Indian babies being nearly three times more likely to die of SIDS than white babies. In addition, when infants sleep prone, the elevated risk of SIDS is increased by each of five factors: the use of natural-fiber mattresses, swaddling, recent illness, exposure to tobacco smoke, and the use of heating in bedrooms.

The infants admitted to the Pediatric Intensive Care Unit (PICU) are placed prone or side-lying for a variety of reasons such as postural drainage, comfort, or postoperative positioning for wound care. Parents view the PICU staff as the experts in care and will mimic this care when they arrive home. Prior studies have demonstrated that health care workers' professional advice is influential in determining infant care practices. It is essential that staff caring for infants be aware of the importance of a safe sleep environment and understand other modifiable risk factors for SIDS in order to adequately advise the infant's family.

It is imperative to incorporate education about placing infants on their backs for sleep into the discharge planning process. Families need to understand that their children were placed prone or side-lying in the ICU for medical reasons but should be placed on their back at home. When patients are admitted to the PICU or many Progressive Care Units, they are placed on monitors that are observed centrally as well as at the bedside—families will not have this capability at home. In addition, PICU nursing staff should make every attempt to support the back to sleep campaign and return infants to the supine position for sleep as soon as medically possible.

SUGGESTED READINGS

Back To Sleep. KeepKidsHealthy.com. Available at: http://www.keepkidshealthy.com/welcome/safety/back_to_sleep.html#What.

Ponsonby A, Dwyer T, Gibbons L, et al. Factors potentiating the risk of sudden infant death syndrome associate with the prone position. *N Engl J Med*. 1993;329(6):377–382.

SIDS: "Back to Sleep" Campaign. NIH. Available at: http://www.nichd.nih.gov/sids/sids.cfm.

STRIVE TO PROVIDE FAMILY-CENTERED CARE IN THE PEDIATRIC ENVIRONMENT

SHEILA LAMBERT, RN, MSN, CCRN

WHAT TO DO: PLAN

In pediatrics, it is difficult if not impossible to separate the child and family when developing a plan of care. Traditional approaches to delivering care at the bedside have positioned families as observers who remain outside the care processes. Family-centered practitioners recognize the vital role that families play in ensuring the health and well-being of children of all ages. This approach acknowledges that emotional, social, and developmental support are integral components of healthcare, promoting the health and well-being of individuals and families and restoring dignity and control to them.

Family-centered approaches lead to better health outcomes, wiser allocation of resources, and greater patient and family satisfaction. Family-centered care is based on the understanding that the family is the child's primary source of strength and support. Individuals who are most dependent on hospital care are also generally the most dependent on families, making family-centered care essential in pediatrics.

Family-centered care in pediatrics involves a complete change in the way care is delivered and the way that patients and families are addressed. In a family-centered care environment, the child is recognized as the "family's child" rather than "our patient". The definition of "family" may not be the same for each patient, but the family unit must be defined by the patient and family.

Families are increasingly demanding the opportunity to be more involved in the decision-making process during the hospitalization of a child. Family centered care requires an evolution from addressing or telling the patient or family what to do to fully embracing them as an important member of the team, to enhance care and reduce recovery times, Simply put, serving today's children means serving today's families.

There are several benefits to family-centered care. This approach greatly enhances patient and family satisfaction and staff satisfaction. It creates a supportive workplace, which encourages recruitment and retention of nurses, reduces healthcare costs by decreasing length of stay, and positions the institution more effectively in the marketplace. By providing information and involving families in a family-centered decision-making process, the risk of errors may also be reduced. Patient safety is a factor that has emerged as an area of importance among families, healthcare professionals, and regulatory agencies. The family is in a pivotal role to remind providers of things that they may be missing and to understand the care so that the child is treated appropriately.

There are numerous methods to support the environment of family-centered care. Bedside rounds by the healthcare team are instrumental in this approach. Families are able to contribute to rounds and hear information firsthand from the healthcare team. Mutual goals for the day and the length of stay can be set at this time. Bedside nursing rounds are another form of communication with the family to involve them in the care. During this time, the oncoming nurse can introduce himself or herself to the family, meet the patient, and further support the goals for the day or length of stay. Hourly rounding by the nursing staff is also an effective method to support this approach—nurses can use this time to teach and talk with families about the care of their child. In the family-centered care approach, it is important to avoid the use of the term visitor when referring to the family. The family is not a visitor to the child but rather a vital member of the team. Visiting hours should be removed if at all possible—24h visitation should be encouraged. Sleeping arrangements should be readily available to the family as well as showering and bathroom facilities. Meals should also be available to the families, since meal time is an important family time. The idea is to provide the basic necessities to further encourage the family to stay with the child if at all possible.

Another useful tool in the implementation of family-centered care is the use of a parent advisory board. Parent advisory boards consist of families and staff working together for the common goal of further enhancing the care in pediatrics. Families have firsthand knowledge of the care delivered and are wonderful resources in improving the care in pediatrics. The advisory boards generally meet monthly to review processes, provide insight, and offer suggestions.

Incorporating the principles of family-centered care into our practices in pediatrics improves the care of our patients and the satisfaction of the providers who partner with these patients and families during illness.

SUGGESTED READINGS

American Academy of Pediatrics Committee on Hospital Care. Family-centered care and the pediatrician's role. *Pediatrics.* 2003;112:691–696.

Johnson BH. Family-centered care: Four decades of progress. *Fam Syst Health: J Collab Fam Healthc.* 2000;18(2):137 157. Available at: www.familycenteredcare.org.

BE MINDFUL OF HAIR TOURNIQUETS

JEANNIE SCRUGGS GARBER, DNP, RN

WHAT TO DO: EVALUATE

Hair tourniquet syndrome is when hair or thread becomes wrapped around an infant or child's appendage, resulting in decreased circulation and discomfort. The presenting symptom is usually uncontrollable crying, but no other recognizable symptoms; therefore, the most common misdiagnosis is gastrointestinal upset. The diagnosis of hair tourniquet can be difficult since the hair or thread can be difficult to see, especially if it has cut into the skin. The most commonly affected appendages are the fingers, toes, and genitalia.

According to a case review by Strahlman, the majority of patients had toe involvement with hair being the constricting material. This usually occurred at approximately 4 months of age when the greatest postpartum hair loss for the mother was also experienced. The finger was the next most affected appendage with thread, more than hair, creating the problem. The third category involved genital strangulation and often led to questions of abuse. It is the role of the healthcare provider to educate parents to guide and prevent injuries that can occur as a result of a hair tourniquet.

Strahlman suggests that the following educational points be discussed with new parents:

- Expect hair loss in the first months after delivery
- Mothers with long hair should be cautious and aware of this concern
- Assess the child's appendages regularly to asses for hair tourniquets
- Inspect clothing for loose strings or hair
- Seek medical assistance immediately when hair tourniquets are found

To minimize risk of this syndrome going undiagnosed, physicians and healthcare providers must also gain awareness of the condition. Treatment options for hair tourniquet include removing the hair or thread with scissors, using a hair dissolver or surgical intervention. Antibiotics may also be used after removal to prevent infection.

Educating new parents and healthcare providers about prevention, diagnosis, and treatment of this syndrome will aid in minimizing emergent situations resulting from hair tourniquets. The healthcare provider must consider this diagnosis in infants when no other diagnosis is apparent and inconsolable crying continues.

SUGGESTED READINGS

Hair tourniquets. Available at: http://pedclerk.bsd.uchicago.edu/hairTourniquet.html. Accessed August 4, 2008.

Strahlman R. Toe tourniquet syndrome in association with maternal hair loss. *Pediatrics*. 2003;111(3):685–687.

Fentanyl Is a Very Effective Narcotic for Use in the ICU; However, It Can Cause Chest Wall Rigidity in Patients When Pushed Too Quickly

Sam Harvey and Sheila Lambert, RN, MSN, CCRN

WHAT TO DO: PLAN

Fentanyl is an analgesic and anesthetic agent with a potency of approximately 80 times that of morphine. fentanyl is a synthetic opioid and is administered both intravenously (IV) and transdermally. It is often referred to as Sublimaze, its trade name. Many analogues of fentanyl exist, such as sufentanil, a more potent derivative, and alfentanil, an extremely fast-acting analgesic. fentanyl has many uses in interoperative, postoperative, and chronic pain management. In fact, Fentanyl is often the drug of choice in achieving analgesia early in the patient's recovery period.

Despite its effectiveness, when fentanyl is quickly pushed IV, a patient's chest may become rigid and lead to severe respiratory failure. This side effect is most often encountered in neonates, although all age groups are susceptible. This is a side effect that must be immediately diagnosed and treated to ensure patient safety. Consequently, when fentanyl is administered, staff trained in airway ventilation and pharmaceutical counteraction through medication such as neuromuscular blocking agents must be present. Oftentimes, truncal rigidity may be so severe that traditional bag and mask ventilation may be ineffective. Additionally, truncal rigidity has been observed in the postoperative recovery room, heightening the importance of monitoring patients on a fentanyl drip early and throughout the period after administration. Although rare, some cases of respiratory depression have occurred through improper fentanyl distribution via a transdermal patch.

The administration of IV fentanyl is widely used in the ICU setting for its analgesic effect. Chest wall rigidity is a life-threatening event that requires immediate diagnosis and treatment in the ICU. Clinicians administering IV fentanyl should be adept at airway management and narcotic antagonists and neuromuscular blocking agents since this is the recommended treatment for this phenomenon.

Fentanyl has a long half-life of approximately 2 to 3 h and exhibits a biphasic decay curve in some individuals (approximately 25% to 50% of the population). This means that there is a secondary rise in the concentration of the drug about 45 to 60 min after injection. The exact mechanism of this is not known. It appears that much of the drug is taken up by the stomach and later released by

the small bowel where it is reabsorbed, thus the patient receives two divided doses instead of one.

If the patients were to experience chest wall rigidity following the administration of IV fentanyl, the first sign will be difficulty ventilating. This results from chest wall rigidity or rigidity of the glottis. Extreme difficulty will be encountered when attempting to ventilate with a bag-valve-mask. This phenomenon can mimic grand mal seizures as there may be a gross twitching of all extremities associated with the rigidity.

While there is a greater correlation between high dose fentanyl and chest wall rigidity, there are numerous reports of this occurring in low doses as well. Extreme caution and frequent assessment must be used regardless of the administered dose. The precise cause of truncal rigidity is unknown, although drug interaction could possibly be involved. Fentanyl is often used alongside benzyldiazepines and other drugs when truncal rigidity occurs, yet, cases of rigidity have been reported from fentanyl alone. Importantly, drugs used in combination with fentanyl often increase the potency of the duration and severity of the respiratory depression. In one study, 100 micrograms of fentanyl was administered before respiratory depression occurred. Experiments suggest that fentanyl may cause rigidity in the vocal chords as well, which represents a significant upper airway obstruction. Naxalone and other neuromuscular blocking agents have facilitated successful truncal relaxation, yet, these agents are not without their own side effects. Naxalone specifically increases dopamine concentrations in brain tissue and has a shorter elimination half-life than fentanyl. Therefore, even after successful muscular relaxation with Naxalone, the patient must be observed for several hours should the truncal rigidity manifest again. Nondepolarizing muscle relaxants may also be used with caution due to their relatively slow onset of action and significantly longer duration of action than fentanyl—this must be considered.

Although the side effects of pushing fentanyl too fast intravenously are severe, profound cases of truncal rigidity are rare compared to the number of successful fentanyl administrations. Therefore, it is of the utmost importance that fentanyl be dispensed not only in the appropriate amount but at the appropriate rate as well. As most cases of respiratory depression occur during fast administration of fentanyl, a slower means of administration is almost always preferred.

As the nurse at the bedside, it is important to understand that rigidity may occur with the use of fentanyl and the treatment methodologies that may be used. Frequent assessment of the patient receiving fentanyl is very important. If the patient is not ventilated, alert the respiratory practitioner that the patient is receiving fentanyl and that this may occur. In addition, ensure that you have the appropriate mask and ambu bag at the bedside, emergency drug sheet readily available for the patient's weight (in the PICU), and the code cart and/or emergent respiratory cart nearby.

SUGGESTED READINGS

Ackerman WE, Phero JC, Theodore GT. Ineffective ventilation during conscious sedation due to chest wall rigidity and intravenous midazolam and fentanyl. *Anesth Progr.* 1990;37:46–48.

Product Information: SUBLIMAZE(R) Injection, Fentanyl Citrate Injection. Decatur, IL: Taylor Pharmaceuticals; 2005.

BEWARE OF MUNCHAUSEN'S BY PROXY (MSP) IN CHILDREN WHO ARE THOUGHT TO PRESENT REPEATEDLY WITH VAGUE COMPLAINTS

JENNIFER BATH RN, BSN, FNE, SANE-A AND JEANNIE SCRUGGS GARBER, DNP, RN

WHAT TO DO: ASSESS

Munchausen's by Proxy (MSP) is another form of factitious disorder in which the caregiver inflicts or induces illness or injury on a dependent. It is similar to Munchausen syndrome in that the illness or injury is created or inflicted but instead of harming themselves, they harm someone in their care, usually a child. MSP is most often seen in infants with the mother being the one who most often perpetuates the disorder. These patients are willing to let their children undergo painful procedures, even surgery, to fulfill their need to be seen by healthcare providers as the heroic and tragic parental figure.

Certain characteristics are common in a person with MSP:

- Often it is a parent, usually a mother, but can be the adult child of an elderly patient
- Might be a healthcare professional
- Is very friendly and cooperative with the healthcare providers
- Appears quite concerned (some might seem overly concerned) about the child or designated patient
- Might also suffer from Munchausen syndrome (a related disorder in which the caregiver repeatedly acts as if he or she has a physical or mental illness when he or she has caused the symptoms).
- Sometimes displays gleeful excitement at the moment when life hands in the balance

Other possible warning signs of MSP in children include the following:

- The child has a history of many hospitalizations, often with a strange set of symptoms.
- Worsening of the child's symptoms generally is reported by the mother and is not witnessed by the hospital staff.

- The child's reported condition and symptoms do not agree with the results of diagnostic tests.
- There might be more than one unusual illness or death of children in the family.
- The child's condition improves in the hospital, but symptoms recur when the child returns home.
- Blood in lab samples might not match the blood of the child.
- There might be signs of chemicals in the child's blood, stool, or urine.

Some of the most common methods mothers use to cause signs and symptoms include suffocation, poisoning with ipecac or laxatives, and induced seizures.

The exact cause is unknown, as is the case with Munchausen syndrome. It is estimated that 1,000 of the 2.5 million child abuse cases reported per year are from MSP. MSP is more common in women than men. Diagnosing MSP is difficult since medical causes must be ruled out first. Once they are ruled out, a thorough investigation of the child, mother, and family medical history needs to take place.

MSP can be very difficult to treat. Treatment includes removing the victim from the caregiver. Other treatment modalities involve changing the inflictors, thinking and behavior along with psychotherapy. These patients are such accomplished liars that you cannot tell fact from fiction. A thorough history is very important with any patient, but especially with a child where you suspect that it may be MSP, because history is often the only way to diagnose the disease.

SUGGESTED READINGS

Cleveland clinic center for consumer health information. Available at: http://my.clevelandclinic.org/disorders/factitious_disorders/hic_munchausen_syndrome_by_proxy.aspx. Accessed August 8, 2008.

Hammer R, Moynihan B, Pagliaro E. *Forensic Nursing: A Handbook for Practice*. Boston, MA: Jones and Bartlett; 2006, p. 654.

Lynch V. *Forensic Nursing*. St. Louis, MO: Elsevier Mosby; 2006, pp. 82–84.

Ensure That Your Transport Team Is Prepared for Whatever Might Come in Its Way

Anthony D. Slonim, MD, DrPH

Pediatric patients are often referred from one healthcare institution to another for specialized services. When the need for transfer arises, an interfacility transport team is often used to provide the expertise that the child and family needs. The response is often consistent with the information that is being described by the referral facility. However, it must be remembered that the pediatric experience at the referral facility may vary and the child's condition may change between the time the call was received and the time the team arrives at the child's bedside. To be better prepared for these urgent or emergent transports, it is imperative that the transport team be ready to rescue the child from a deeper level of care than is being reported. For example, if the child is reported to be having respiratory distress, the team should be prepared to rescue the child from respiratory failure and intubate as needed.

In order to be better prepared, the team needs to have both the human and technologic resources readily available to safely transport the child. The transport team should have considerable pediatric and pediatric intensive care experience, know how to manage the As, Bs, and Cs of resuscitation and trauma, and have medical control that allows problems to be escalated and managed as they are needed. While some transport teams use a triage response and discharge a low or high acuity team based upon the child's severity, this can be difficult if all members of the team are not trained similarly and a low acuity team is dispatched but the child's needs exceed the capabilities of the team or its equipment. To avoid these challenges, the transport teams need to have the high acuity team on standby to intervene as needed if its services are needed. In addition, the teams should have regular drills to ensure that they function well as a team and have the requisite skills to effectively achieve stability of the patient.

As far as equipment is concerned, clearly, children vary in their size and weight and the equipment also needs to be available to handle the children regardless of their characteristics. A full range of equipment that extends from caring for the newborn in distress to the adult patient is necessary. A checklist should be available and the equipment on the transport vehicle validated against this checklist on a shift by shift basis to ensure that all the necessary equipment and medications are available.

The transportation of the critically ill or injured child is a serious matter that depends upon the appropriate personnel, equipment, and supplies. Ensuring that the team that is dispatched is appropriately equipped is essential to running a pediatric transportation program.

SUGGESTED READINGS

What is a Pediatric/Neonatal Critical Care Transport Team? American Academy of Pediatrics. Available at: http://www.aap.org/sections/pem/PediatricTransportTeam_final.pdf. Accessed August 3, 2008.

Woodward GA, Insoft RM, Pearson-Shaver AL, et al. The state of pediatric inter-facility transport: Consensus of the second national pediatric and neonatal interfacility transport medicine leadership conference. *Pediatric Emerg Care.* 2002;18:38–43.

INTRAVENOUS (IV) ACCESS: IT IS YOUR FRIEND, BUT CAN ALSO BE YOUR ENEMY

ANTHONY D. SLONIM, MD, DRPH

WHAT TO DO: EVALUATE AND IMPLEMENT

One of the most common hospital procedures is the establishment of intravenous (IV) access. In pediatrics, many a provider has spent hours at the bedside of a child attempting to get IV access throughout the day and night. Despite this common procedure, there are a number of important considerations in caring for the child with IV access problems.

The most important issue with IV access is being unable to obtain it. The acutely decompensated child needs IV access for fluid or medication administration and may worsen in front of your eyes if this is not accomplished in a timely manner. Providers always believe that they are one needle stick away from securing the IV, but the more time passes, the sicker the child gets, and the harder IV access gets to accomplish. Rapid and decisive approaches need to be taken to move quickly to larger and more central veins such as the external jugular vein or call consultation from colleagues in intensive care or emergency medicine. This is not a reflection on the providers, some babies are more difficult than others and we all have our "bad nights" when we are unable to gain access in the child with the largest veins. Try hard, escalate quickly to large veins or central access and if still unable to achieve, do not forget the intraosseous route for resuscitation.

Once IV access is achieved in children, the catheters usually remain in place until their indication is no longer present. In contrast to adult patients where routine catheter and central venous catheter changes are commonplace, in children, the risks and difficulty with gaining access prohibits routine line and catheter changes. Hence, these catheters usually stay in place for longer durations. The nurse needs to be aware of the difficulties with IV access including superficial and deep infections and thrombosis, mechanical problems like the shearing of the catheter tip and infiltrations, and the inadvertent introduction of air or substances particularly in the child with intracardiac defects. For patients with peripherally inserted central catheters (PICC), the limb may swell since the catheter occupies a major component of the vein inhibiting venous return. This by itself may not be an indication for removing the device, but if swelling is accompanied by local signs of erythema and systemic signs including fever and chills, consideration of removing the catheter and administering systemic antibiotics needs to occur.

The IV catheter is essential for providing care to hospitalized children. However, it has a number of important limitations that need to be considered by the bedside nurse.

SUGGESTED READINGS

Emergency vascular access in children. American College of Surgeons Committee on Trauma. Available at: http://www.facs.org/trauma/publications/vasaccess.pdf. Accessed August 3, 2008.

Schultz TR, Durning S, Niewinski M, et al. Multidisciplinary approach to vascular access in children. *J Spec Pediatr Nurs.* 2006;11(4):254–256.

KNOW HOW TO HANDLE THE DISLODGED TRACHEOSTOMY

ANTHONY D. SLONIM, MD, DRPH

WHAT TO DO: EVALUATE AND IMPLEMENT

For many pediatric patients, life saving and sustaining care in the newborn period has led to dependence upon a number of medical technologies. Tracheostomy is a very common intervention for children who require long-term mechanical ventilation, are unable to protect their airway due to poor neuromuscular control, or have laryngeal reconstruction due to congenital abnormalities. These children are often seen by pediatric nurses shortly after placement of the tracheostomy when many of them are admitted to the pediatric intensive care unit until their first tracheostomy change, but they can also be seen in the office setting or on the pediatric ward when they return for follow-up or acute deterioration.

The pediatric nurse needs to be familiar with the use of a tracheostomy to provide safe and effective care to these patients. There are a few important items that are required. These children often benefit from humidified oxygen or air to assist in moistening secretions, there should be a monitor to detect oxygen desaturations, and readily available suction. A replacement tracheostomy tube should be at the bedside, including one size larger and one size smaller. In the immediate postoperative setting, the nurses and intensive care specialist will want to discuss what was done in the operating suite and the location of any "stay sutures" in the event that the tracheostomy is dislodged. This will allow the visualization of the ostomy site itself if the tube needs to be reinserted and prevent the creation of a false tract in the early postoperative period.

For the more established tracheostomy, the nurse still needs the same supplies, but usually a tract is formed that allows the easy changing or passage of a new tracheostomy tube should the current one be dislodged or removed accidentally. Patients with cuffed tubes may be able to eat or speak and over the long term, the need for the tracheostomy may resolve. In the event of dislodgement, if the tube is unable to be replaced, the patients can have their airway managed and be intubated through the orotracheal route or nasotracheal route.

Tracheostomy is a life-saving intervention, but one that can also cause serious harm if managed incorrectly or if safety is not considered.

SUGGESTED READINGS

Abraham SS. Babies with tracheostomies: The challenge of providing specialized clinical care. American Speech-Language-Hearing Association. Available at: http://www.asha.org/about/publications/leader-online/archives/2003/q1/030318.htm. Accessed August 3, 2008. http://patienteducation.tv/trach_video.php. Accessed August 3, 2008.

Tran C. Considerations of pediatric tracheostomy. Baylor College of Medicine. Available at: http://www.bcm.edu/oto/grand/01202005.htm. Accessed August 3, 2008.

Ensure That Your Vital Signs Are Correct

Anthony D. Slonim, MD, DrPH

WHAT TO DO: ASSESS AND EVALUATE

Vital signs are the fundamental evaluative technique used for hospitalized patients. In many circumstances, this function is now relegated to the nurse's aide or technician. However, there is no more important routine and repetitive function for identifying emerging problems in the hospitalized patient than the vital signs. For hospitalized children, it is even more important.

Vital signs usually consist of an assessment of the temperature, pulse, respiratory rate, and blood pressure. While the scale upon which the temperature norms are based do not vary between children and adults, the scales for the other vital signs are dramatically different not only between children and adults, but also between children of different ages. Hence, the nurse needs to be aware of age-related normal vital signs when caring for children and evaluating their physiologic status based upon these parameters.

The pulse rate is rapid as a neonate (140 to 160 beats per min) and progressively slows as the child ages, reaching adult levels by 14 to16 years of age. Children respond to intravascular depletion through increasing their heart rate to maintain cardiac output. Hence, tachycardia in the resting state is a very sensitive measure of volume depletion and should be noted. In fact, the response to volume repletion in the hypovolemic or dehydrated child can often be assessed through the reduction in heart rate that accompanies the intervention.

Respiratory rate is another important vital sign. Children attempt to maintain their minute ventilation, which is the product of their respiratory rate times their tidal volume. As tidal volume decreases, because of atelectasis, pneumonia, or other pathologic state, the respiratory rate will increase to achieve minute ventilation. Tachypnea is important to detect and one of the most underappreciated vital signs. For children, the respiratory rate needs to be counted for a full minute rather than for 15 s and multiplied by 4. Children have periodic breathing and accuracy in determining the respiratory rate is critical to understanding their physiologic status.

Finally, blood pressure is important as well. However, in children, as mentioned above, the heart rate is a much more sensitive indicator to volume status than the blood pressure. When hypotension occurs in children, in contrast to adults, it is usually the end result of a long period of decompensation and one in which it is difficult to reverse. Further, the blood pressure in children is highly dependent upon the manner in which it was taken. Cuff size is very important and cuffs that are too snug will lead to false elevations in blood pressure as will assessments done while the child is crying from agitation or pain.

The vital signs are important to note and reassess on a routine basis in children. They can alert the astute clinician to the child in trouble, but need to be assessed in an appropriate manner and compared against age-appropriate normal values to determine if an intervention is needed.

SUGGESTED READINGS

King C, Henretig FM, eds. *Textbook of Pediatric Emergency Procedures.* 2nd Ed. Philadelphia, PA: Lippincott Williams & Wilkins; 2008, p. 26. Available at: http://books.google.com/books?id=qfcKjyZ6 xP4C&pg=PA23&lpg=PA23&dq=pediatric+vital+sign+measu rement&source=web&ots=yrWviRf7uy&sig=wpH8RWRfUhjr G7tm_pjYnJHeLCg&hl=en&sa=X&oi=book_result&resnum= 1&ct=result#PPA26,M1. Accessed August 3, 2008.

Confirmatory bias: Pay attention, bad things do happen to children...ignoring the warning and looking for alternative reasons will not make it get better

Anthony D. Slonim, MD, DrPH

WHAT TO DO: ASSESS, EVALUATE, AND IMPLEMENT

The care of sick children is one of the greatest privileges that a healthcare provider can have. However, it is not for everyone. So many times a provider that cares mostly for adults will say: "I could never care for a sick child—it would break my heart." While it is true that caring for sick children can occasionally be sad, there are also some very rewarding aspects to caring for sick children, not the least of which is that a child's body has a remarkable opportunity to compensate for physiologic dysfunction and sick children are resilient and can rebound from critical illness to a far greater extent than adults.

Nonetheless, when a sick child is being cared for, details need to be attended to and not ignored. The failure to respond to changing vital signs, alarms, or conditions may rob a child of his or her last chance at survival. Providers, however, find it so unconscionable that a child could be near death that they waste precious minutes validating their assessment, finding another provider to confirm their findings, or "overthinking" or rationalizing a finding that they wish not to be true because it could mean that the child might die.

As healthcare providers, we rely often on other members of the healthcare team for support and help in caring for patients. In fact, the whole system of consultation is built so that providers are empowered to ask for help if they require specialty advice in treatment. However, when a critical situation emerges, for example, finding a bradycardic or pulseless child, providers need to assess the situation quickly and act definitively. When a blood pressure cannot be obtained and the child is motionless and cold, finding another blood pressure machine or calling a colleague to assess the situation is unlikely to change the child's outcome. This is the time to trust your impulses, begin basic life support, and call for help.

Another example of this bias is when uncommon manifestations of common diseases occur in children. Most cardiac arrests in children result from respiratory insufficiency. However, there are times when a primary cardiac malfunction causes a cardiac arrest. Providers need to be aware of and ready to treat uncommon presentations of common conditions.

Finally, in critical situations, time moves quickly. Many can recall spending what seems like a few minutes in a code blue scenario but turns out to be over an hour of documented interventions on the code sheet. This is important, since for interventions like accessing the airway or vein or guessing about the "down time," our internal clocks are relatively unsophisticated when we are preoccupied with caring for the critically ill child. Hence, time is moving and the patient is still not intubated or does not have an IV. In these cases, a recognition of the time needs to be addressed head on and alternatives identified so that appropriate care can be delivered.

Heatlhcare providers are the last line of defense for a sick or dying child. It is critical that we rely on our assessment skills, integrate the facts and implement a plan that is decisive. An inability to have confidence in our assessment or make a decision may lead to a less than optimal outcome.

SUGGESTED READINGS

Confirmation bias. *The Skeptic's Dictionary*. Available at: http://www.skepdic.com/confirmbias.html. Accessed August 3, 2008.

Croskerry P. The importance of cognitive errors in diagnosis and strategies to minimize them. *Acad Med*. 2003;78:775–780.

Pines JM. Profiles in patient safety: Confirmation bias in emergency medicine. *Acad Emerg Med*. 2006;13:90–94.

Redelmeier DA. Improving patient care. The cognitive psychology of missed diagnoses. *Ann Intern Med*. 2005;142:115–120.

Remember How to Dose Medications for Extremely Overweight Children

Anthony D. Slonim, MD, DrPH

WHAT TO DO: EVALUATE

Obesity in the United States is on the rise and reaching epidemic proportions among a variety of demographics including children. There are a number of reasons for this, including inactivity and excess caloric intake. Both of these characteristics are particularly troublesome since they are also the risk factors for hypertension, diabetes, and coronary artery disease in the adult, all of which are major concerns for the health of the population.

Pediatric providers need to be cognizant of this trend in childhood obesity since there are opportunities to intervene with anticipatory guidance and improve the long-term healthcare of children. In addition, there are ramifications for drug dosing since all pediatric drugs are dosed based upon weight, and obesity affects the pharmacodynamics and kinetics of many medications.

The prescribing of medications to children is based upon weight and is one of the key clinical components that differentiates pediatric clinical care from adult clinical care. However, in the obese child, it is not unusual for the total daily dosage to exceed the adult dosage when based on a per kilogram weight. This is problematic. Calculations for children should be based upon the ideal body weight and not the actual body weight. When pediatric providers are faced with a total daily dose in excess of the adult dose, the adult dosage should be used. While it is true that the metabolism of medications is different between children of different ages and adults, the adult dose approach will prevent some of the unwanted toxicities that accompany large daily dosages. When clinical situations require appropriate serum levels for certain medications, these levels can be checked to ensure that the therapeutic targets are in range.

SUGGESTED READINGS

Calculations and Dosing Tools. Compendium of Pharmaceuticals and Specialties (CPS). 2008. Available at: http://www.pharmacists.ca/content/hcp/resource_centre/drug_therapeutic_info/pdf/CalcAndDosing_EN_26Feb08.pdf. Accessed August 8, 2008.

Dietz WH, Robinson TN. Clinical practice: Overweight children and adolescents. N Engl J Med. 2005;352:2100–2109.

REMEMBER THAT HYPOVOLEMIC SHOCK IS THE MOST COMMON TYPE OF SHOCK IN CHILDREN AND CAN OCCUR FROM CONDITIONS AS COMMON AS GASTROENTERITIS AND DIARRHEA

ANTHONY D. SLONIM, MD, DRPH

WHAT TO DO: ASSESS

Shock is the end result of problems with circulation that occurs either in the delivery of blood, oxygen, and nutritive substrate to the cells of the body or due to the inability of the cells to use the substrates delivered to them. Hypovolemic shock is the most common type of shock occurring in the pediatric age group and results from dehydration, hemorrhage, and plasma fluid losses that ultimately reduce the circulating vascular volume.

Dehydration is very common in children and can result from insufficient intake of fluids or excessive excretion of fluids that are out of proportion to intake, resulting in a net negative fluid balance. For most children, including those in third world countries, a regimen of oral rehydration works well and prevents hospitalization. For others, however, admission to the hospital and volume repletion with intravenous fluids become necessary.

Dehydration is usually characterized as mild, moderate, or severe depending on the extent of volume loss. Mild dehydration (<5%) is usually manifested by dry oral mucosa and skin, mild tachycardia, and a concentrated urine. Moderate dehydration (<10%) is characterized by lethargy, poor skin turgor, tachycardia, tachypnea, and a normal blood pressure. Severe dehydration manifests itself with overt signs of volume insufficiency and signs of inadequate perfusion of end organs including mental status changes, reduced urine output, and respiratory insufficiency.

Dehydration can be caused by a number of clinical conditions. The child who has been feeling ill and has poor oral intake or failure to thrive may not have taken in enough nourishment for sustenance. The kidney will do a remarkable job of holding onto water and concentrating the urine in these circumstances until the child begins to decompensate. Children also become dehydrated because of excess losses. Children with gastroenteritis and the symptoms of excessive vomiting and diarrhea may be unable to maintain their fluid balance. These children, particularly infants and small children, may decompensate clinically if rehydration is inadequate. For the acutely decompensated child with hypovolemia who is demonstrating signs of inadequate end organ perfusion, intravenous boluses of normal saline in 20 mL/kg are indicated to restore intravascular volume and organ perfusion. These can be repeated at regular intervals to improve the child's condition.

Children can decompensate to hypovolemic shock with common conditions like gastroenteritis. The administration of isotonic fluids is important to improve organ perfusion and dramatically improves the child's clinical condition as well. Nurses need to recognize just how quickly young children can become dehydrated and that early recognition and treatment can really help improve the child's condition.

SUGGESTED READINGS

Carcillo JA, Piva JP, Thomas NJ, et al. Shock and shock syndromes. In: Slonim AD, Pollack MM, eds. *Pediatric Critical Care Medicine*. Philadelphia, PA: Lippincott, Williams & Wilkins; 2006.

Hypovolemic shock. Available at: http://www.peppsite.com/docs/26540_CH04_83.pdf. Accessed August 4, 2008.

Remember to Obtain a Digoxin Level for Children with Dehydration or Renal Insufficiency, Who Take the Drug

Anthony D. Slonim, MD, DrPH

WHAT TO DO: EVALUATE, PLAN, AND IMPLEMENT

Digoxin is an important medication used in children with congenital and acquired heart disease, who experience cardiac insufficiency or failure. Digoxin is well tolerated in many children and has limited side effects. In contrast to adults, where digoxin levels are routinely followed to ensure that the therapeutic window is reached, children do not need routine digoxin levels performed. However, there are certain times when a digoxin level may be beneficial to the care of the child.

Since digoxin is excreted via a renal mechanism, children on digoxin, who become dehydrated or are suspected of having renal insufficiency, should have a digoxin level measured to ensure that there is no toxicity. However, digoxin levels need to be interpreted with caution. Even when high, the level itself does not imply that the child is toxic. Digoxin redistributes well to the tissues of the body and it is not unusual for children to have high levels, but they remain perfectly fine. The key decision is to understand if the high level is causing the child to be symptomatic. The most common side effect for digoxin toxicity is bradycardia. This can be identified by measuring the pulse. The child should be placed on a cardiac monitor and watched in the intensive care unit as the condition dictates.

Digoxin toxicity usually does not require treatment. If renal insufficiency or dehydration occurs, supportive care should be undertaken with correction of the dehydration. If the patient is symptomatic from the digoxin with hemodynamic compromise, an antidote, known as the Fab antibody fragment, can be used. The dosage calculation for this antidote is complicated and depends upon a number of assumptions. Nonetheless, for important and symptomatic toxicities, this is the treatment of choice.

Digoxin is a commonly used drug in children and nurses need to understand the value (or lack thereof) of serum digoxin levels.

SUGGESTED READINGS

Hougen TJ. Digitalis use in children: An uncertain future. *Progr Pediatr Cardiol.* 2000;12(1):37–43.

Husby P, Farstad M, Brock-Utne JG, et al. Immediate control of life-threatening digoxin intoxication in a child by use of digoxin-specific antibody fragments (Fab). *Paediatr Anaesth.* 2003;13(6):541–549.

Tuncok Y, Hazan E, Oto O, Guven H, et al. Relationship between high serum digoxin levels and toxicity. *Int J Clin Pharmacol Ther.* 1997;35(9):366–368.

REMEMBER THAT IRON DEFICIENCY ANEMIA IS NOT THE ONLY CAUSE OF ANEMIA IN CHILDREN

ANTHONY D. SLONIM, MD, DRPH

WHAT TO DO: ASSESS AND EVALUATE

Anemia is a reduction in the hemoglobin concentration in the red blood cells (RBCs). Hemoglobin is the major protein in RBCs and responsible for the transport of oxygen throughout the body. In fact, the majority of oxygen in the body is carried to tissues in this "bound" form where a very small proportion of oxygen is carried and dissolved in the blood. Anemia occurs because of blood loss from the body, insufficient production of RBCs, or the destruction of RBCs. Clinically, anemia is classified based upon the size of the RBCs, which is measured by the mean corpuscular volume (MCV). The normal MCV is 80 to 100 femtoliters (FL). Patients can be anemic and still have a normal MCV. This occurs through acute blood loss or the breakdown of RBCs (hemolysis). Microcytic anemia corresponds to an MCV of <80 FL and is usually caused by iron deficiency anemia, lead poisoning, excessive milk ingestion, thallasemia, or the anemia of chronic disease. Macrocytic anemia (MCV >100 FL) can occur from folate or B_{12} deficiency or hypothyroidism.

Many children with anemia may be asymptomatic. As the anemia progresses, so do the signs and symptoms, moving from slight pallor of the conjunctiva and oral mucosa to fatigue, breathlessness, and overt cardiac failure.

The treatment for anemia depends on the cause. Patients with acute blood loss may require a transfusion of RBCs to restore their oxygen carrying capacity. Those with deficiencies of iron, folate, or B_{12} may require dietary supplementation and a search for the underlying cause. There are some causes of anemia that require a specific search for the cause through diagnostic testing including thyroid function tests or a hemoglobin electrophoresis. However, in children, the most common cause is iron deficiency anemia, and in the healthy child, an empiric trial of supplemental iron may be all that is necessary. If this fails, then further evaluation for other causes may be indicated.

SUGGESTED READINGS

Iron Deficiency Anemia in Infants and Children: How to Prevent It. FamilyDoctor.org. Available at: http://familydoctor.org/online/famdocen/home/children/parents/kidshealthy/nutrition/751.html. Accessed August 8, 2008.

Irwin JJ, Kirchner JT. Anemia in children. American Family Physician. Available at: http://www.aafp.org/afp/20011015/1379.html. Accessed August 8, 2008

KNOW THAT THE CHILD ADMITTED WITH AN ACUTE INJURY WILL COME BACK UNLESS YOU EDUCATE THE PARENT AND THE FAMILY ON HOW TO PREVENT INJURY

ANTHONY D. SLONIM, MD, DRPH

WHAT TO DO: IMPLEMENT

Anticipatory guidance is one of the foundational elements of pediatric practice and can be performed both in the ambulatory setting during child visits and during hospitalization. The nurse has a major function in identifying the developmental stage of the child and helping the child and the parent to understand what trouble that child might get into and what injuries might result, based on the development. For example, infants who begin to crawl around the house need special attention paid to blockades at the top of stairs and side-rails on cribs to prevent accidental injury. As the preschool child begins to ride a tricycle, helmets and road safety should be taught in anticipation of increasing independence during school age.

Prevention strategies are classified as primary prevention, secondary prevention, and tertiary prevention strategies. Primary prevention strategies represent the anticipatory efforts that are made to prevent injury. These include public service announcements regarding bicycle safety, drug abuse prevention, and preventing firearms injuries with trigger locks. Secondary prevention is how the system is organized to respond to the injury once it has occurred. This includes emergency medical services that are kid-friendly and have appropriate staffing and equipment, the use of designated pediatric trauma centers, and healthcare personnel who are certified to care for the acutely traumatized or injured child. Tertiary prevention involves mitigating the effects of injury and reducing the disability that might accompany injury such as what occurs with rehabilitation.

Children will get hurt and there is no way to alleviate injuries during childhood. However, the pediatric provider has a role in ensuring that parents and children are knowledgeable about the things they can do to prevent accidental injury and ensuring that the skills for caring for these children once injured meet the highest standards available in our discipline.

SUGGESTED READINGS

Hsu A, Slonim AD. Preventing pediatric trauma: The role of the critical care professional. *Crit Conn*. 2006;1–3.

Keep watching for the missed injuries in hospitalized pediatric patients with trauma

Anthony D. Slonim, MD, DrPH

WHAT TO DO: PLAN

Trauma is the leading cause of death and disability in those less than 14 years of age. It also accounts for the largest proportion of years of productive life lost. In children, blunt trauma far exceeds penetrating trauma as a mechanism of injury and these are often to do with motor vehicle accidents and falls. The acutely traumatized child places the family in turmoil and is a leading cause of family discord, divorce, and financial ruin. Pediatric providers need to realize that the patient is not only the child in the bed but also the whole family.

Accompanying the demographic and social challenges with pediatric trauma are the very real clinical challenges. The child victim of multiple traumas often has injuries that affect multiple body regions including the head, thorax, abdomen or pelvis, and extremities. A systematic approach is imperative when assessing the critically ill child with trauma and begins with the primary survey of Airway, Breathing, and Circulation. Providers often get these issues immediately cared for. However, the multiple trauma patient requires a methodologic assessment that extends beyond the primary survey and assures a reassessment of injuries in different body regions with an attention to ongoing disability. Important adjuncts to this include plain radiography, bedside diagnostic testing, and CT scanning of the head and abdomen.

While the attention in the trauma bay is on the preservation of life, there are always injuries that are missed. Missed injuries in acute trauma patients have ranged from 3% to 25% and many of them can be serious. On the minor end of the continuum, missed fractures and extremity injuries are found, but missed injuries can also range to major organ dysfunction including aortic transaction or major organ trauma. The best way to improve upon missing injuries is to have a method for a head to toe assessment, regardless of injury site, that inspects and examines each body part in sequence and is not distracted by the injured area. The more the independent observers, the more likely a missed injury to be found.

Delays in diagnosis are important and common in the setting of pediatric trauma. All pediatric providers need to maintain a high index of suspicion during their assessments that aim to identify any injuries missed during the primary and secondary surveys, particularly those serious ones with long-term consequences.

SUGGESTED READINGS

Beaty JS, Chendrasekhar A, Hopkins J, et al. Missed injuries in pediatric trauma patients. *J Appl Res*. Available at: http://www.jarcet.com/articles/Vol3Iss1/CHENDRASEKHAR.htm. Accessed August 8, 2008.
Peery CL, Chendrasekhar A, Paradise NF, et al. Missed injuries in pediatric trauma. *Am Surg*. 1999;65(11):1067–1069.

REMEMBER THAT THE WHEEZING PATIENT MIGHT HAVE ASTHMA OR SOMETHING ELSE AS WELL

ANTHONY D. SLONIM, MD, DrPH

WHAT TO DO: ASSESS AND EVALUATE

Wheezing is an important clinical sign that presents as a whistling noise and represents an obstruction to airflow. In children, it is an important clinical sign that is common due to the relatively smaller diameter of the child's airways. There are a number of clinical situations that are highlighted when a wheezing child is brought to the hospital. However, the nurse needs to be cautious and ensure that the child is being treated for the correct condition. This is particularly important if the condition is not improving with treatment.

Bronchiolitis represents an important lower airway disease usually found in children less than 2 years of age. It is often caused by a viral respiratory infection in winter. One of the most common viruses causing this disorder is respiratory syncytial virus, which can be a very serious disease in premature infants and those with congenital heart disease. Patients with bronchiolitis have respiratory distress, wheezing, and oxygen desaturation. They are often hospitalized for supportive care and oxygenation during the acute phase. Often, the disease is self-limiting in healthy children, but occasionally, a serious or even deadly course may result.

Asthma is a chronic disease of airway obstruction caused by inflammation. It is characterized by acute exacerbations of disease interspersed in a chronic course. Asthma episodes can be triggered by a number of environmental causes including pet dander, cigarette smoke, and pollutants. The child with asthma will have respiratory distress, wheezing, and oxygen desaturation. Asthma is treated in the acute episode with beta agonists and steroids. On a more chronic basis, inhaled β-agonists and steroids can also be used depending on the severity of the condition.

Foreign bodies are an important clinical problem in children. It is not uncommon for a child to present with a foreign body in the airway, which is a small aspirated object and produces wheezing and an infiltrate on X-ray. In toddlers, this always needs to be considered since their ability to provide accurate history is questionable.

Gastroesophageal reflux disease (GERD) is an important problem for pediatric patients that usually do not present with acute wheezing, but may be mistaken in the subacute timeframe. GERD is often accompanied by "spitting up," vomiting and other symptoms including arching, but wheezing is a common enough accompaniment to warrant discussion.

Congestive heart failure (CHF) is a condition that has a number of causes depending upon the component of the heart that is most affected. Children can have conduction problems (arrhythmias), muscle problems (myocarditis), or valvular problems (mitral regurgitation) as the etiology for their CHF. Patients with CHF will look very similar to those with acute respiratory disease and have symptoms of respiratory distress, wheezing, and desaturation. CHF patients may also have elements of poor perfusion like cyanosis, poor capillary refill, and signs of shock if severe.

Wheezing is an important clinical sign for children and may be a manifestation of relatively minor or severe problems. Importantly, it is only a sign that requires that the healthcare professional interprets it and ensures that the interpretation is correct through repeated evaluations.

SUGGESTED READINGS

Wheezing. Available at: http://www.wrongdiagnosis.com/s/sleep_apnea/book-diseases-3b.htm. Accessed August 8, 2008.

REMEMBER THE SIDE RAILS ON THE CRIB

ANTHONY D. SLONIM, MD, DRPH

WHAT TO DO: IMPLEMENT

Patient falls are a major problem in acute care hospitals. There is an important emphasis on falls occurring during hospitalization and falls with injuries, which are classified as "never" events or events that should never occur to a patient during hospitalization. Patients fall during hospitalizations because of a number of reasons including weakness, the effects of medications, instability related to their illness, and slipping on the floor. While falls occur far less frequently in pediatrics, there are still a number of things that need to be kept in mind to keep children safe during hospitalization, including the use of protective equipment and side rails.

Maintaining a safe environment for patients is important. In pediatrics, the equipment used in caring for patients is different than those for adults, but the safety features need to be remembered and consistently used. For younger infants, cribs are often used during hospitalization to provide a safe and comfortable environment for

the child to sleep. These cribs are often significantly raised off the floor to provide an ergonomically improved environment for providers, but this also increases the distance to the floor if the child should accidentally fall. Providers need to make sure that they elevate the side rails on the cribs when they are finished providing care at the bedside or if they need to turn their back and remove their eyes from the child. Ensuring that the appropriately sized patients are placed in cribs is also important. Older and larger children may be able to climb over the top of the side rails. In these cases, ensuring that the child is assessed or a canopy is placed over the top is important for ensuring protection of the child.

Equipment used to care for children have safety features that need to be ensured. Incorporating these safety processes into our care of hospitalized children is essential for ensuring their safety.

SUGGESTED READINGS

Razmus I, Wilson D, Smith R, et al. Falls in hospitalized children. *Pediatr Nurs.* 2006;32(6):568–572.

KNOW THAT THERE ARE MULTIPLE CAUSES FOR CONJUNCTIVITIS

SAM HARVEY AND ANTHONY D. SLONIM, MD, DrPH

WHAT TO DO: ASSESS

Conjunctivitis, commonly known as "pink eye," is the most common disease affecting the eye across the world and is very common in children. The symptoms of the condition include itching, foreign body and burning sensations, and redness of the eye. The four classes of conjunctivitis are bacterial, viral, allergic, and toxic agent, all defined by their respective etiologies (Fig. 496.1).

Determining the causative agent involved in a patient's conjunctivitis is important in establishing the proper treatment for the condition. Bacterial conjunctivitis can be chronic or acute. The most common causative agents are *Streptococcus pneumoniae, Haemophilus influenzae*, and *Staphylococcus aureus*. Bacterial conjunctivitis usually appears with acute redness, burning, and discharge. Exudate is usually apparent in the morning, but is often variable. It may be difficult to open the eye due to exudate adhesion. One of the worst bacterial conjunctivitis agents is *Chlamydia*, and a condition known as trachoma can occur alongside chlamydial conjunctivitis. Trachoma is the leading cause of treatable blindness and is characterized by many of the same symptoms as conjunctivitis in addition to photophobia.

Viral conjunctivitis is very common at schools and other public places because it is highly contagious.

Adenovirus and herpes simplex virus most often cause viral conjunctivitis. Adenovirus is the virus responsible for the highly contagious form. Many of the symptoms are similar to bacterial conjunctivitis, yet some distinct symptoms include lid edema and dilation of the conjunctival blood vessels (hyperemia). Viral conjunctivitis usually persists longer than bacterial conjunctivitis—for a duration of two weeks. Epidemic keratoconjunctivitis is a seasonal disorder that rapidly spreads among people in close contact such as household members, students, and healthcare workers. Many outbreaks of this disorder are connected to improper swimming pool chlorination.

Allergic conjunctivitis is most often characterized by a hypersensitivity to allergic rhinitis, although the reaction may be completely independent. Unique symptoms include extreme itching, secretion of tears, and severe photophobia. Discharges are usually stringlike and mucosal in nature due to intense rubbing of the eyes. The condition is more common among children and young adults than adults.

Lastly, toxic conjunctivitis is the least severe of the classes and is characterized by similar symptoms to allergic conjunctivitis, which are less severe. The condition can stem from a reaction to medication, exposure to chlorine in swimming pools, toxic gases in industrial plants, and many other minor irritants such as smoke, aerosols, acids, and alkalis.

SUGGESTED READINGS

Smeltzer S, Bare B, Hinkle J, et al. *Textbook of Medical-Surgical Nursing*. Philadelphia, PA: Lippincott Williams & Wilkins; 2008.

Viola RS. Conjunctivitis. In: Rakel R, Bope ET, eds. *Conn's Current Therapy*. 56th Ed. Philadelphia, PA: W. B. Saunders; 2004.

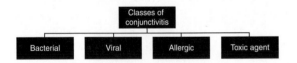

FIGURE 496.1. Four classes of conjunctivitis.

UNDERSTAND THE DANGER OF AN ACUTE ASTHMA EXACERBATION

SAM HARVEY AND ANTHONY D. SLONIM, MD, DRPH

WHAT TO DO: ASSESS

Asthma is an obstructive lung disease caused by chronic inflammation of the airways. The pathophysiology involves mucosal hyperresponsiveness, mucosal edema, and excessive mucus production. Asthma is widespread; approximately 1.9 million visits to emergency departments were reported in 2002. Fortunately, asthma is one of the few easily prevented and treated obstructive lung disorders. Although the disease may occur at any age, children are the most susceptible age group. The disease is characterized by acute episodes that are generally short lived; therefore, most asthmatics regard their condition as a disruption in pursuing daily activities and schedules (Fig. 497.1). All of these symptoms serve to narrow the airway diameter available for respiration.

A predisposition to asthma is most often exposure to allergens. These allergens can range from dust to pollen, though chronic overexposure leads more easily to asthma. Most patients have a specific allergen that precipitates an acute asthmatic response characterized by

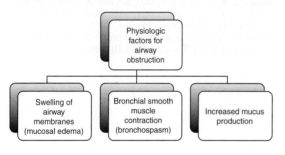

FIGURE 497.1. The physiology of asthma.

symptoms such as cough, dyspnea, and wheezing. Asthma "attacks" occur most often in the morning or evening, and sometimes may be caused by excessive exercise. Due to the allergic nature of asthma, prevention is an important tool in reducing the number of acute exacerbations. If the specific etiologic agent can be identified, its removal from the patient's environment may alleviate the most severe symptoms.

Treatment for asthma generally involves a step-by-step process at the onset of an attack. Quick-relief medications such as β-adrenergic agonists and anticholinergics are available for immediate topical administration via inhalers. For extraordinary asthma cases, long-acting asthma control medications are available. Corticosteroids are the most effective anti-inflammatory medication available, but newer drugs such as leukotriene modifiers are other options. These medications are administered via an inhaler but are much more long lasting than other alternatives. Therefore, the medication has the ability to prevent attacks in short succession.

Self-care is appropriate and manageable for most asthmatics. A device known as a peak flow meter, which measures the highest volume of airflow during a forced expiration can inform patients when their respiration is in danger and there is a need for intervention. Carefully designed asthma management symptoms, when properly implemented, allows asthmatics to live lives interrupted only occasionally by an outstanding attack.

SUGGESTED READINGS

Centers for Disease Control and Prevention. *Fast Stats Sheet: Asthma.* Atlanta, GA: National Center for Health Statistics; 2004.
Smeltzer S, Bare B, Hinkle J, et al. *Textbook of Medical-Surgical Nursing.* Philadelphia, PA: Lippincott Williams & Wilkins; 2008.

BE MINDFUL OF THE OPPORTUNITIES FOR A CHILD TO BE POISONED DURING HOSPITALIZATION

ANTHONY D. SLONIM, MD, DRPH

WHAT TO DO: ASSESS

With over 1 million children being poisoned in the United States annually, pediatric poisoning has become an important issue for pediatric providers. Children often present emergently to care after ingesting a chemical agent or a loved one's medications. Older children may purposefully attempt ingestion as a gesture of suicide. The approach to managing treatment depends upon both the timing for recognition and the substance ingested. The approach begins with attention to airway, breathing, and circulation, and is followed by decontamination, monitoring for organ decompensation and failure, and assuring that physiologic support is provided in the postingestion period. These approaches often include cardiac monitoring and serial laboratory testing. There is always the opportunity for providing guidance to parents and families after an ingestion on preventive actions they can take to ensure that chemicals are locked up and secured.

The problem is that the hospital is also a place where medications and chemicals can be sought out and ingested by children. In the hospital environment, providers need to be aware that the medications, equipment, and chemicals they use every day to care for and protect patients can also be a problem for a hospitalized child. Nurses need to have an appreciation for the developmental level of the hospitalized child and the mischief they can get into, particularly as they start to feel better and approach discharge. Ensuring that medication rooms, cabinets, and drawers are locked is important from a medication safety perspective. The nurse also needs to recognize that there are other environmental dangers that are potential sources of injury for the hospitalized child. These include ensuring that housekeeping carts remain locked, mop buckets are emptied when they are unattended, electrical sockets are covered, and dangerous equipment is stored away from where children might be able to access them.

The hospital can be a dangerous place for the inquisitive child who is hospitalized. It is important for the nurse to identify and remedy potential hazards so that children do not get injured or poisoned during their hospitalization.

SUGGESTED READINGS

Broderick M. Pediatric poisoning! RNWeb. Available at: http://rn.modernmedicine.com/rnweb/article/articleDetail.jsp?id=119738. Accessed August 8, 2008.

Bryant S, Singer J. Management of toxic exposure in children. *Emerg Med Clin North Am.* 2003;21(1):101.

CHECK THE SETTINGS ON THE OVERBED WARMERS ON HOSPITALIZED INFANTS AND MONITOR THE PATIENT'S TEMPERATURE

ANTHONY D. SLONIM, MD, DRPH

WHAT TO DO: EVALUATE

Maintaining normothermia is an important part of caring for infants and small children. Hypothermia has a number of adverse physiologic consequences, which are exaggerated for infants. A number of strategies are used clinically to ensure that infants remain warm in the nursery, including bundling and overbed warmers. When these devices are used in pediatrics, it is important to ensure that they are used safely and that babies do not become overheated or burned.

Overbed warmers are equipped with a temperature sensor that is usually placed on the baby to monitor the radiant heat from the warmer. Ensuring that the sensor is working appropriately is important, but it is also important to continue to monitor and evaluate the baby. Signs of overheating include fever, tachycardia, restlessness, and even dehydration. The nurse needs to ensure that the equipment and the patient are continually monitored for adverse effects that can cause harm. Children may also become hypothermic if the sensor is not working appropriately and the warmer shuts down automatically. This can be monitored through the baby's temperature, but can also be identified through slower heart and respiratory rates.

In addition to under- or over-heating, the infant can be burned by these overbed warmers. This is particularly important since the baby's skin is exposed to ensure that temperature is maintained. Unfortunately, the application of medicinal creams, salves, and ointments to improve the healing of common skin rashes becomes a medium for binding the heat and accelerating tissue destruction. It is not unusual for babies to receive serious skin burns from the application of excessive heat to their skin, particularly in the setting of a topical medication.

The use of equipment to improve the care of patients requires attention to the equipment and the patient. Ensuring that infants do not become burned from overbed warmers is important during their hospitalization.

SUGGESTED READINGS

Batistich SP, Clark MX. Burn following use of the Suntouch warmer. *Anaesthesia*. 2006;61(11):1124–1125.

Hammer SG. Second degree burn from a toe warmer. *Wisconsin Med J*. 1999;98(7):4.

ENSURE THAT YOU HAVE THE RIGHT PATIENT

ANTHONY D. SLONIM, MD, DRPH

WHAT TO DO: ASSESS

Patient identification is an imperative for delivering the correct care. Children cannot self-identify with certainty like adults can. Therefore, the objective validation and use of two patient identifiers are important for delivering care to children, particularly if the parent is not present. Even when the parent is present, two objective identifiers become important when there is more than one child in the room for treatment as often occurs when children present for well child checks and immunizations.

Much of the care delivered to patients is individualized to needs, which makes assurances of identification for procedures like medication administration, blood administration, and surgical procedures specific for patients. Ensuring that the patient is correctly identified and the therapy is matched to the appropriate patient is a fundamental, yet often overlooked, part of the procedure for patients.

Even when the procedure is part of the routine care of patients, identification is important. For example, the delivery of nutrition is a fundamental component of care for hospitalized children. In the nursery or pediatric ward, the administration of breast milk from a refrigerator to the incorrect infant is an important and concerning adverse event for providers and families alike. There are other important dietary problems that can manifest themselves. Patient allergies are also important, particularly in children, and the delivery of foods with allergens to childern may result in adverse reactions. The childern may not be able to identify that they are allergic to the food and even if they know, may eat it anyway since they cannot understand or link the consumption to an illness.

Patient identification underlies everything we do for patients as healthcare professionals to ensure that we deliver the individualized care for patients. Failure to appropriately identify patients is a problem with potentially serious consequences.

SUGGESTED READINGS

Drenckpohl D, Bowers L, Cooper H. Use of the six sigma methodology to reduce incidence of breast milk administration errors in the NICU. *Neonat Netw*. 2007;26(3):161–166.

The Institute for Safe Medication Practices. Preventing accidental IV infusion of breast milk in neonates. Available at: http://www.ismp.org/newsletters/acutecare/articles/20060615.asp. Accessed August 8, 2008.

Vanitha V, Narasimhan KL. Intravenous breast milk administration—a rare accident. *Ind Pediatr*. 2006;43(9):827.

Note: Page numbers in *italics* denote figures; those followed by a t denote tables.

blood component therapy, 207
blood transfusion reaction, 206
bone marrow transplantation (BMT), 233
cancer patient education, 218
cancer prevention, 229
cancer treatment, 218
central venous access devices (CVADs), 213, 221
cervical cancer screening, 230
chemotherapy
  administration medication error, 209
  body surface area
    height role, 215
    weight role, 215
  dosage, 215
  infusions, peripheral IV site placement, 224
  orders, 216
  personal protective equipment, 211
eosinophils, 232
hazardous drug administration, 210
high dose methotrexate (HDM), 216
hypercoagulable syndromes, 231
isotonic solutions, 207
leukemia, 219
lymph node swelling, 234
methotrexate, 212
packed red blood cells (PRBCs) administration, 205
pressure ulcers, 217
sickle cell crisis, 226
tumor lysis syndrome, 225
vincristine administration, 223
Hemolysis, elevated liver enzymes and low platelets (HELLP)
  syndrome, 467
Heparin, 44, 62
High dose methotrexate, 216
Hormonal therapy, menopause, 488
β Human chorionic gonadotrophic (HCG), 435
Hyperbaric oxygen therapy (HBO), 359
Hypercoagulable syndromes, 231
Hypertension, 281
Hypoglycemia, 38
Hypomagnesemia, 274
Hyponatremia, 275
Hypothyroidism, 177
Hypovolemic shock, 527

I

Institute for Safe Medication Practices (ISMP),
  31–32, 35
Insulin
  dose, 181–182
  physiology, 179–180
Insulin dependent diabetes mellitus (IDDM), 175
Intensive care unit (ICU), 45
International normalized ratio (INR), 21
Interprofessional education (IPE), 8
Intra-aortic balloon pump (IABP), 165
Intracranial pressure (ICP), 162
Intravenous (IV) access
  drug administration, 29
  electrolyte replacement therapy, 39
  pediatric nursing, 522

J

Joint Commission on Accreditation of Healthcare Organization's
  (JCAHO), 37
  labeling medications, 41
  look alike sound alike medications 27
  standards, 254–255
  wrong-site surgeries, 333

L

β-Lactam antibiotics, 25
Latex allergies, 89
Leukemia, 219
Look-alike sound-alike drug names, 27
Low cardiac output syndrome, 367
Lymph nodes (LN), 234

M

Malignant hyperthermia (MH), 350
Marfan syndrome, 514
Maternal–infant bonding, 477
Measles, mumps, and rubella (MMR) vaccine, 458
Medical nursing
  behavioral and psychiatric, 137
    alcohol abuse, 135
    alcoholism assessment, 138
    bipolar disorder, 128
    borderline personality disorder, 127
    CIWA protocol, 129
    confused patients, 132
    dementia, 139
    depressed patients, 133
    electroconvulsant therapy (ECT), 126
    fear and anxiety, 134
    postpartum depression, 131
    psychiatric problems, 130
    schizophrenia, 125
    violent behavior, 136
  conscious sedation
    fentanyl, 292
    midazolam, 292
  critical care
    acute respiratory distress syndrome (ARDS), 158
    arterial lines, 155
    cardiovascular and pulmonary systems, 169
    chronic obstructive lung disease, 168
    critically ill patients, intrahospital transfers, 157
    dampened waveforms, 163
    disseminated intravascular coagulation (DIC), 159
    dynamic hyperinflation, 169
    intra-aortic balloon pump (IABP), 165
    intracranial pressure monitoring (ICP), 162
    mechanical ventilation, 168
    temporary invasive pacing, 166
  cytarabine
    acute myelogenous leukemia (AML), 220
    dosing, 220
  diabetes
    adolescent patients, 175
    blood glucose management, 171 172
    foot ulcer, 176